W

D0875353

PEDIATRIC CLINICAL CHEMISTRY

PEDIATRIC CLINICAL CHEMISTRY

A Survey of Reference (Normal) Values, Methods,
and Instrumentation, with Commentary

Second Edition

Samuel Meites, *Editor in Chief*
Professor, Department of Pediatrics, Ohio State University
Clinical Chemist, Children's Hospital, Columbus, OH

Contributing Editors:
Thomas A. Blumenfeld
Larry W. Clark
Leonard K. Dunikoski, Jr.
Keith B. Hammond
Jocelyn M. Hicks
J. Gilbert Hill
John E. Sherwin
Elizabeth K. Smith

Virginia S. Marcum, *AACC Book Editor*

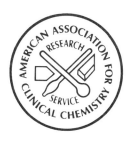

The American Association for Clinical Chemistry
1725 K Street, N.W.
Washington, DC 20006

Related books from the American Association for Clinical Chemistry:

The Neonate: Clinical Biochemistry, Physiology, and Pathology, Donald S. Young and Jocelyn M. Hicks, Eds. (Vol. 2, Current Topics in Clinical Chemistry)

Aging—Its Chemistry, Albert A. Dietz, Ed. (Proceedings of the Third Arnold O. Beckman Conference in Clinical Chemistry)

Selected Methods for the Small Clinical Chemistry Laboratory, Willard R. Faulkner and Samuel Meites, Eds. (Vol. 9, Selected Methods; available late 1981)

Library of Congress Cataloging in Publication Data:

Pediatric clinical chemistry.

Includes indexes.
1. Children—Diseases—Diagnosis. 2. Diagnosis, Laboratory. 3. Chemistry, Clinical. I. Meites, Samuel. [DNLM: 1. Chemistry, Clinical—In infancy and childhood. QY 90 P371]
RJ51.L3P43   1981   618.92'00756   80–66259
ISBN 0-915274-12-4

Printed in the United States of America.

Contributors

ADAMS-MAYNE, MABELLE E., Clinical Chemist, Department of Pathology, Texas Children's Hospital, Houston, TX.

APPLEGARTH, DEREK A., Director, Biochemical Diseases Laboratory, Children's Hospital, Vancouver, B.C., Canada.

BARNES, G. L., Director, Department of Gastroenterology, Royal Children's Hospital, Melbourne, Parkville, Victoria, Australia.

BEAUDET, ARTHUR L., Pediatric Genetics Laboratory, Baylor College of Medicine, Houston, TX.

BLUMENFELD, THOMAS A., Assistant Professor of Clinical Pathology, Columbia University College of Physicians & Surgeons, and Director, Microchemistry Laboratory, Columbia-Presbyterian Medical Center, New York, NY.

BOECKX, ROGER, Children's Hospital National Medical Center, Washington, DC.

BOWERS, GEORGE N., Jr., Director, Clinical Chemistry Laboratories, Hartford Hospital, Hartford, CT.

BUFFONE, GREGORY J., Director, Clinical Chemistry, Texas Children's Hospital, and Assistant Professor of Pathology, Baylor College of Medicine, Houston, TX.

CAFFO, ALBERT L., Technical Service, E. I. DuPont, Wilmington, DE; formerly, Nutrition/Trace Metals Laboratory, Children's Hospital, Columbus, OH.

CEJKA, JAN, Immunochemistry Laboratory, Children's Hospital of Michigan, Detroit, MI.

CHENG, MARY H., Clinical Laboratory, Children's Hospital of Los Angeles, Los Angeles, CA.

CHESKIN, H. S., Graduate Research Assistant, Department of Pathology, Columbia University College of Physicians & Surgeons, Columbia-Presbyterian Medical Center, New York, NY.

CLARK, LARRY W., Laboratory, Norton Children's Hospital, Louisville, KY.

COLLE, ELEANOR, Department of Endocrinology, Montreal Children's Hospital, Montreal, Quebec, Canada.

CONNELLY, JOHN F., Director of Clinical Biochemistry, Department of Clinical Biochemistry, Royal Children's Hospital, Melbourne, Parkville, Victoria, Australia.

DAVIES, H. E., Senior Scientific Officer, Department of Clinical Biochemistry, Royal Children's Hospital, Melbourne, Parkville, Victoria, Australia.

DELVIN, EDGARD E., Assistant Head, Genetics Unit, Shriner's Hospital for Crippled Children (Quebec) Inc., Montreal, Quebec, Canada.

DUNIKOSKI, LEONARD K., Jr., Director, Clinical Chemistry, Perth Amboy General Hospital, Perth Amboy, NJ.

DUPONT, CLARE, Montreal Children's Hospital, Montreal, Quebec, Canada.

EHLERS, PEARL WEHRMAN, Chemistry Supervisor, Children's Mercy Hospital, Kansas City, MO.

FISHER, DELBERT A., Professor, Department of Pediatrics, U.C.L.A. School of Medicine, Harbor General Hospital, Torrance, CA.

FREER, DENNIS E., Department of Pathology, University of California–Davis Medical Center, Sacramento, CA.

FRIEDMAN, SHLOMO, Associate Professor, Pediatrics, Division of Hematology/Oncology, Department of Pediatrics, State University of New York at Buffalo, and the Children's Hospital of Buffalo, Buffalo, NY.

GLASSMAN, ARMAND B., Professor and Chairman, Department of Laboratory Medicine, Medical University of South Carolina, Charleston, SC.

GOODMAN, JUDY, Cleveland Clinic, Cleveland, OH.

GUTHRIE, RICHARD A., Chairman, Department of Pediatrics, The University of Kansas School of Medicine–Wichita, Wichita, KN.

HAMMOND, KEITH B., Director, Pediatric Microchemistry Laboratory, University of Colorado Medical Center, Denver, CO.

HARRIS, DAVID I., Pediatric Geneticist, Genetic Counseling Center, The Children's Mercy Hospital, Kansas City, MO.

HICKS, JOCELYN M., Director of Clinical Laboratories, Children's Hospital National Medical Center, and Associate Professor, Department of Child Health and Development, and Department of Pathology, George Washington University School of Medicine, Washington, DC.

HILL, J. GILBERT, Head, Service Division, Department of Biochemistry, The Hospital for Sick Children, and Associate Professor, Department of Clinical Biochemistry, University of Toronto, Toronto, Ontario, Canada.

HOFFMAN, WILLIAM H., Director, Endocrinology, Children's Hospital of Michigan, Detroit, MI.

HOWANITZ, JOAN H., Department of Pathology, Division of Clinical Pathology, State University of New York, Upstate Medical Center, Syracuse, NY.

HOWANITZ, PETER J., Department of Pathology, Division of Clinical Pathology, State University of New York, Upstate Medical Center, Syracuse, NY.

JOHANSON, ANN J., Professor, Department of Pediatrics, University of Virginia Medical Center, Charlottesville, VA.

JOHNSON, THOMAS R., Associate Director, Medical Services, Ross Laboratories, Division of Abbott Laboratories (USA), Columbus, OH.

KALLNER, ANDERS, Department of Clinical Chemistry, Karolinska Institute, Huddinge University Hospital, Huddinge, Sweden.

KNIGHT, JOSEPH A., Associate Professor of Pathology, Director of Clinical Pathology, Department of Pathology, College of Medicine Medical Center, University of Utah, Salt Lake City, UT; formerly Director, Clinical Laboratories, Primary Children's Medical Center, Salt Lake City, UT.

LEBENTHAL, EMANUEL, Chief, Gastroenterology, Children's Hospital, and Associate Professor of Pediatrics and Chief, Division of Gastroenterology and Nutrition, State University of New York at Buffalo, Buffalo, NY.

LEE, PING-CHEUNG, Director, Gastroenterology Laboratory, Children's Hospital, and Associate Research Professor, State University of New York at Buffalo, Buffalo, NY.

LEVITT, MONTE J., Biodecision Laboratories, Inc., Pittsburgh, PA.

LI, PHILIP K., Director of Clinical Laboratories, The Children's Hospital of Buffalo, Buffalo, NY.

LONSDALE, DERRICK, Cleveland Clinic, Cleveland, OH.

LUM, GARY M., Assistant Professor, Pediatrics and Medicine (Nephrology), and Head, Pediatric Renal and Dialysis Services, University of Colorado Health Sciences Center, Denver, CO.

LUSHER, JEANNE, Director, Division of Hematology and Coagulation, Children's Hospital of Michigan, Detroit Medical Center, Detroit, MI.

MARTIN, RICHARD F., Fort Hamilton Hughes Memorial Hospital Center, Hamilton, OH.

MEITES, SAMUEL, Professor, Department of Pediatrics, Ohio State University College of Medicine, and Clinical Chemist, Children's Hospital, Columbus, OH.

MURRAY, ROBERT L., Associate Director, Biochemistry, Lutheran General Hospital, Park Ridge, IL.

NG, WON G., Enzyme Laboratory, Children's Hospital of Los Angeles, Los Angeles, CA.

NYHAN, WILLIAM L., Professor and Chairman, Department of Pediatrics, University of California Medical Center, San Diego, CA.

O'BRIEN, WILLIAM E., Pediatric Genetics Laboratory, Baylor College of Medicine, Houston, TX.

OSBERG, IRIS M., Assistant Director, Pediatric Microchemistry Laboratory, University of Colorado Medical Center, Denver, CO.

PESCE, MICHAEL A., Director, Special Chemistry Laboratory, Columbia-Presbyterian Medical Center, Babies Hospital, New York, NY.

PETERSON, ROBERT G., Assistant Professor, Department of Pediatrics, School of Medicine, University of Colorado Health Sciences Center, Denver, CO.

PINTER, JOYCE K., Fort Hamilton Hughes Memorial Hospital Center, Hamilton, OH.

ROY, CLAUDE C., Professor of Pediatrics, Pediatric Gastroenterology Unit, Pediatric Research Center, Hopital Sainte-Justine, Montreal, Quebec, Canada.

SCHMITT, KARL W., Associate Pathologist—Pathologist in Charge of Microbiology, Serology and Radioisotopes, Department of Laboratory Medicine, St. Luke's Hospital, Milwaukee, WI.

SHERWIN, JOHN E., Director of Chemistry, Valley Children's Hospital, Fresno, CA.

SMITH, ELIZABETH K., Director of Chemistry, Department of Laboratories, Children's Orthopedic Hospital and Medical Center, Seattle, WA.

SPENCER, W. W., Chemistry Laboratory, St. Elizabeth Medical Center, Dayton, OH.

STARK, R. I., Assistant Professor of Pediatrics, Columbia University College of Physicians & Surgeons, Columbia-Presbyterian Medical Center, New York, NY.

STATLAND, BERNARD E., Director of Clinical Chemistry, Department of Pathology, University of California–Davis Medical Center, Sacramento, CA.

STEINER, PAULA, Clinical Chemistry Laboratory, Cincinnati General Hospital, Cincinnati, OH.

TOONE, JENNIFER, Biochemical Diseases Laboratory, Children's Hospital, Vancouver, B.C., Canada.

TRAVERS, HARRY, Children's Hospital of the Kings Daughters, Norfolk, VA.

UNDERWOOD, LOUIS E., Associate Professor of Pediatrics, University of North Carolina at Chapel Hill, Chapel Hill, NC.

VAN WYCK, JUDSON J., Professor of Pediatrics, University of North Carolina at Chapel Hill, Chapel Hill, NC.

WALFISH, PAUL G., Associate Professor, Department of Medicine, University of Toronto, and Director, Thyroid Research Laboratory and Endocrine Service, Mount Sinai Hospital, Toronto, Ontario, Canada.

WHITTAKER, CARL, Fort Hamilton Hughes Memorial Hospital Center, Hamilton, OH.

WOLF, PAUL L., Professor of Pathology, University of California Medical Center, San Diego, University Hospital, San Diego, CA.

Preface

The first edition of this book was published in 1977. Judging from its "best-seller" reception, the book at least partly filled a need. This response, of course, has brought joy and gratitude to us—the publishers and editors. We were aware that we had made only a beginning on the ingathering and collation of reference values for pediatric clinical chemistry; however, we felt sufficiently encouraged to refine and enlarge our efforts in a second edition.

Accordingly, in autumn of 1978, we appealed through an announcement to members of the American Association for Clinical Chemistry, to the large and worldwide readership of *Clinical Chemistry*, and in particular to laboratory directors in children's hospitals in the United States and Canada, for volunteers to contribute reports on analytes measured in pediatric chemistry laboratories, and for writers to supply critical commentaries. Participants were asked to provide data on a standardized report form, spelling out details concerning reference values, sources of data, analytical methods, sampling, instrumentation, and other pertinent information. Included in the announcement was a lengthy list of analytes on which information was sought. The goal of this work was, and remains, to show the reader how to meet the unique needs of the pediatric laboratory (and patient), as well as to provide "reference" values.

The outcome is this second edition, which now awaits your judgment. The number of analytes reported (200) and the reports on each analyte have expanded considerably beyond the first edition. Contributors increased from 14 to 68, a healthy sign for the future. Commentary, we hope, is more sophisticated. As with other purely voluntary enterprises of this size, not every subject is covered adequately. For this and other unintentional shortcomings of this text, the Editors are solely responsible.

Each of our contributors deserves a hearty toast from their colleagues in the pediatric world, and in clinical chemistry, but certain of them merit special commendation for providing an extraordinary number of reports on analytes, or for writing commentary on subjects they had not personally selected. We salute Roger Boeckx, Gregory J. Buffone, John F. Connelly, Joan H. Howanitz, Peter J. Howanitz, Joseph A. Knight, Philip K. Li, Iris M. Osberg, Michael A. Pesce, and Paul L. Wolf.

We have introduced a departure from our first edition that we hope our readers will find especially useful: four chapters are included from material that was submitted originally as commentary but was too comprehensive to be so used. These, together with two solicited chapters, add much to the presentation of the practice and interpretation of pediatric diagnostic testing. This additional information is presented in Chapters 4 and 6–10.

We have not yet discarded several tests that are either outmoded (including sulfobromophthalein and leucine aminopeptidase) or rarely performed; time must pass before it becomes clear that the old ones will not be resurrected. Among the less frequently performed tests are tests for blood volume, tubular reabsorption of phosphorus, several leukocytic enzymes, trace minerals, and vitamins. Our goal includes the printing of pediatric reference values for clinical chemistry, regardless of the current popularity of the tests involved, so that this text may truly be a resource for those needing data for purposes of research and development.

This text would not have been possible without support from several key people and hospitals. Although this is a "stock" expression of appreciation, it is nonetheless true. The Contributing Editors thank their individual pediatric institutions for generously providing them the time and, above all, the environment in which to make their contributions. The term "hospital," however, should be taken to include people in administration, on the medical staff, at the library, and above all, in the clinical chemistry laboratory. Although many individuals have provided material for this text, only a few have served as editors, among whom may be counted only one fulltime professional, A.A.C.C. Book Editor Virginia S. Marcum; if this book has gained in polish, clarity, and consistency over the first edition, much of the credit must go to her for close scrutiny and constructive criticism of its contents. Finally, we owe thanks to Lois P. Meites for typing the initial manuscript while eyeing its contents for the inevitable errors of omission and commission, an experience she gained from typing the first edition.

The Editor-in-Chief expresses a special note of thanks to the staff of the Children's Hospital of Columbus, Ohio, for their devotion to the care of children by translating compassion and medical and technical skills into the reality of relieving human suffering.

The Editors
August, 1980

The Editor-in-Chief dedicates this edition to his five-year-old grandson, John, and his generation. May they, in their moment of history, try—as we have tried—to pass on something worthy, however short-lived, for the children to come.

Contents

Chapter 1. Introduction

Samuel Meites

This book records reference (normal) ranges for children on a wide variety of more than 200 analytes, collated as much as possible from reports submitted by many clinical laboratories, primarily situated in pediatric centers. The ranges indicated are usually based on a mean ± 2 standard deviation (2 SD), unless otherwise indicated.

But a larger purpose is intended. The current "state of the art" of a pediatric clinical chemistry laboratory is also presented, to provide the reader useful information on analytical methods and instrumentation, and essential details concerning sample volume, collection, and preservation. Through the introductory material, the commentaries, and the appendices, the reader may also learn about the choice and variety of tests available, as well as some of the rationale in using and interpreting these tests. The book expresses the unique and demanding features of the laboratories serving children; above all, however, the material is intended to be practical and contemporary.

How Information Is Presented in This Text

Each analyte is reported in this text in the following format:

Name of Test:

The names of the tests are presented alphabetically. When appropriate, a name is followed by the common abbreviation of trivial name. If an enzyme is the topic, the systematic Enzyme Commission (EC) name and number are given.

Specimen Tested:

The body fluid or material to be analyzed is stated.

Laboratories Reporting:

The number indicates the number of laboratories that submitted reports on the analyte.

Reference (Normal) Values:

These are presented according to age (and sex, if appropriate). Many analytes do not display an age-related gaussian distribution of reference values; or when they do, that distribution may be the case only for some ages. Percentiles, therefore, may be reported, or simply the ranges found useful by experience or in the literature.

1

Note: When no specific age is listed with the report, the values indicated are for adults, but are used in interpreting data for children.

The units reported are either traditional or SI units *(1);* when traditional units are used, SI units are reported, if appropriate, in parentheses. Values per milliliter or per deciliter can easily be converted by the reader to values per liter.

When similar analytical methods are used, the values reported have been combined. In some instances, despite methodological differences, reports are combined because they are essentially similar, e.g., glucose by glucose oxidase and by hexokinase.

Sources of Reference (Normal) Values:

Three sources for these data are: *(a)* institutional, i.e., those data acquired by a reporting institution for its own use; *(b)* from the literature, including publications by the reporting laboratory; and *(c)* experimentally derived, but not formally reported. Frequently cited references are listed in Appendix 6, and are referred to by number (e.g., "text ref. *4*") to avoid constantly repeating the full citation. This practice is also followed when citing sources of information for the analytical methods.

Specimen Volume, Collection, and Preservation; Patient Preparation:

The volume refers to the volume of specimen used in the test, not to the volume of blood or body fluid collected. Specific information for blood collection is provided when indicated; the reader should refer to Chapter 3 on blood-collection and skin-puncture techniques. The anticoagulant, if not stated, should be assumed to be heparin in all cases. Instructions or precautions in collection are presented.

Attention is given to the stability, preservation, and storage of the materials to be tested, as given by those submitting these reports, and as reported in the literature *(2–5).*

Patient preparation is presented for those instances when special instructions are important, e.g., special feeding, fasting, dosage for injection, or timed specimen collection.

Analytical Method:

References are cited in detail and, when necessary, according to the laboratory reporting; instrumental and kit methods are included (manufacturers' addresses are listed in Appendix 5).

Enzyme Data:

This information generally includes:
1. Enzyme unit definition.
2. Buffer, pH.
3. Substrate, pH.

4. Reaction temperature, i.e., the temperature actually used for the determination.

5. Temperature reported, i.e., the temperature to which the results are factored and reported.

Instrumentation:

Instruments and special devices used are named. The manufacturers' addresses are listed in Appendix 5.

Note: Supplementary information may be given in added notes. When warranted, instrumentation may be combined with the analytical method. Some topics, e.g., patient preparation, may be omitted when there is no special report to make.

Commentary:

The contributing editors and invited commentators for this book have briefly discussed factors critically affecting results, whether dealing with reference values, methods, or instrumentation, from the specific viewpoint of pediatric clinical chemistry. The commentators may choose to include data of their own, which may differ somewhat from the reported data; this is a reflection of the current state of knowledge, or the lack thereof.

Nonstandard (or IFCC-Recommended) Abbreviations Used

whole blood	B
cerebrospinal fluid	CSF
competitive protein binding	CPB
day	d
ethylenediaminetetraacetate	EDTA
female	F
freezer (-20 °C)	FR
gas–liquid chromatography	GLC
hemoglobin	Hb
"high-performance" liquid chromatography	HPLC
male	M
month	mo
plasma	P
radial immunodiffusion	RID
radioimmunoassay	RIA
refrigerator (4 °C)	RR
room temperature (23–27 °C)	RT
serum	S
standard deviation	SD
Système International d'Unités	SI units
tris(hydroxymethyl)aminomethane	Tris
urine	U
week	wk
year	yr

1. Lippert, H., and Lehmann, H. P., *SI Units in Medicine.* Urban and Schwarzenberg, Baltimore, MD, 1978.
2. Young, D. S., Pestaner, L. C., and Gibberman, V., Effects of drugs on clinical laboratory tests. *Clin. Chem.* **21,** 1D–432D (1975). Special issue.
3. Henry, R. J., Cannon, D. C., and Winkelman, J. W., *Clinical Chemistry Principles and Technics,* 2nd ed. Harper and Row, Hagerstown, MD, 1974.
4. Schwartz, M. K., Interferences in diagnostic biochemical procedures. *Adv. Clin. Chem.* **16,** 1–45 (1973).
5. Tietz, N. W., *Fundamentals of Clinical Chemistry,* 2nd ed. W. B. Saunders, Philadelphia, PA, 1976.

Chapter 2. Reference Values: An Overview

Samuel Meites

The Unique Laboratory for Pediatric Clinical Chemistry

A recent study of children's hospitals in the United States concluded that several major factors contribute to the greater costs of caring for pediatric patients, compared with costs for adults (1). Children's hospitals must offer more specialized services and facilities, arising from the specific needs of children, particularly infants, and the greater variety and acuteness of diseases encountered. Children's hospitals also serve wider geographical areas than do general hospitals of similar size. Because of the complex mix of specialties required to treat the child adequately, organized research and educational programs must be maintained. It is no wonder, then, that costs are greater: the children's hospitals are unique, which, in turn, arises from the fact that the child is unique.

The uniqueness of children's hospitals in providing specialized services is well illustrated in their clinical chemistry laboratories. It has been repeatedly advocated (2–4) that, to give these same services when children occupy a small portion of the general hospital (perhaps representing only 15% of the patient load), the laboratory *must* allocate a separate, segregated area for pediatric services, with distinct, dedicated staffing. Laboratories of children's hospitals employ almost twice as many technologists as do general hospitals of comparable size. In part, this happens because relatively small institutions must furnish 24-h services, owing to the greater intensity and variety of disease, mentioned previously; but also there is the need to spend more time with the patient, to use analytical micromethods that are often more time-consuming and less mechanized than their "macro" counterparts used for adults, to offer screening procedures for metabolic disorders, and to provide costly analytical services for drugs, nutrition, trace metals, and endocrinology, to name a few. The list is long.

Moreover, there is a constant need for adapting for pediatric use those technological advances designed, however unintentionally, for the adult. This means that research and development are a constant and often obligatory requirement, if improvement in pediatric patient care is to be encouraged.

Consider a modest example of the unique character of the pediatric clinical laboratory. Cystic fibrosis of the pancreas is the most common lethal genetic disorder of Caucasians (5); its incidence is about 1 : 2500. Diagnosis is based on family history, chronic pulmonary disease, malabsorption, and the results of sweat analysis. Where does our community get the laboratory support required by the physician to establish the diagnosis, i.e., the collection and analysis of sweat sodium chloride as recommended by the Cystic Fibrosis Foundation? What we can offer is clearly stated under **Sweat Electrolytes** in this text. If the infant with diagnosed cystic fibrosis is then hospitalized, perhaps dehydrated and in metabolic acidosis, what special microtechniques will we offer to monitor the fluid therapy instituted? The answers are presented here under **Acid–Base, Blood Gases** and elsewhere.

Uniqueness of Pediatric Reference Values

This book deals with another facet of the child's distinct character, the changing pattern of "normative" laboratory data as a consequence of birth, development, nutrition, maturation, pubescence— all lumped together as "age-related" or "sex-related" changes. In short, these changes, when they occur, are neither abnormal nor indicative of disease, yet they may be far removed from the norms of the adult. Nowhere is this more dramatically illustrated than in the enzyme panorama shown in Figure 1. If one uses the upper limit of the adult reference value as a basis for comparison, these enzymes display gross increases at various ages. Strangely, the lower limits of the child's reference values are also usually several multiples above the lower limits of adults (Figure 2). That certain isoenzymes are more prevalent within each enzyme class, e.g., the bone isoenzyme in alkaline phosphatase, does not explain why the pronounced increase occurs. In transient infant hyperphosphatasemia, the increases of alkaline phosphatase are literally scores of multiples above the adult upper limit (6, 7); moreover, in addition to the bone-derived isoenzyme, there is an enzyme present that resembles the liver isoenzyme. What we need to learn, therefore, is the mechanism by which the isoenzymes enter into plasma, particularly in the newborn, as well as their origin.

Nor should one think only in terms of a scale of highly increased values. There are significant deficiencies of enzymes in the newborn. As discussed in Chapter 8, on gastrointestinal function, the infant's duodenal fluid has a much lower concentration of digestive enzymes than the adult's. It is no wonder, then, that the values for (e.g.) amylase and lipase in plasma reflect this deficiency. Here we must think about the mechanisms for enzyme induction and production, and individuals' variability in maturation.

Our knowledge of pediatric reference values in clinical chemistry has a relatively short history, in part because the science of clinical chemistry has had only a brief life span (8). Certainly a major impetus

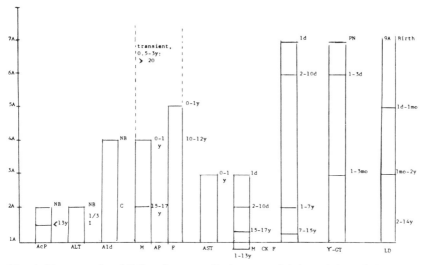

Fig. 1. Enzymes in childhood: upper limits as multiples of the adult upper limit (1A)

AcP, acid phosphatase; ALT, alanine aminotransferase; Ald, aldolase; AP, alkaline phosphatase; AST, aspartate aminotransferase; CK, creatine kinase; γ-GT, gamma-glutamyltransferase; LD, lactate dehydrogenase; PN, premature newborn; NB, newborn; C, child; I, infant. See Chapter 5 for Enzyme Commission (EC) identification of each enzyme

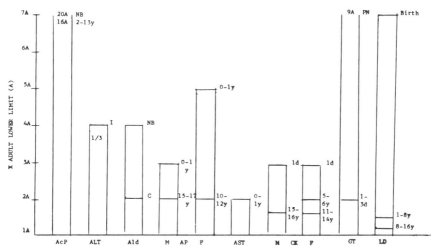

Fig. 2. Enzymes in childhood: lower limits as multiples of the adult lower limit (1A)

Abbreviations as in Fig. 1

towards assessing health and disease from the biochemical standpoint was the development of suitable analytical techniques and instrumentation for testing body fluids and tissues; qualitative testing preceded quantitative.

The substances or analytes we now measure are primarily of recent discovery. Fölling demonstrated a biochemical basis for phenylketonuria in 1934 *(9)*. The genetic and biochemical basis for this disorder, established by Jervis *(10,11)* not long afterwards, served as the forerunner of a truly remarkable search into and discovery of hundreds of hereditary defects initiated and predicted at the opening of this century by Garrod *(12)*. Folin published his monumental work on blood analysis in the first quarter of this century.

Instrumental analysis was a powerful force broadening the horizons of clinical chemistry. The spectrophotometer, pH meter, electrophoretic apparatus, and flame photometer—and even the oldest obsolete instruments such as the hand spectroscope and manual colorimeter—were only comparatively recently applied to clinical chemistry. The introduction of the syringe for use with venipuncture was a major advance in making blood available for analysis by a simple technique.

Our purpose here is not to explore the factors that form the foundation of clinical chemistry but to show that our knowledge of reference values, in general, is preliminary, even infantile. In pediatrics, we have only belatedly come to grips with the problem, but the situation for adults is hardly more advanced.

Some Origins of Pediatric Reference Values

The application to pediatrics of newer advances in blood analysis was often delayed because the volume of blood required was excessive. Qualitative testing on readily available urine promoted considerable progress in metabolic screening, endocrinology, and toxicology, but development of practicable microchemical techniques for blood analysis lagged. Consequently, studies on age-related reference values in children were often sparse, superficial, and isolated.

Even when valid studies on children were reported, there was delay, sometimes for many years, in their acceptance. The tendency in diagnosis was to use adult reference values that were themselves inadequately established because of insufficient sampling, variation in quality of analytical techniques, and inadequate concern about variables affecting the data other than age and sex (e.g., diet, exercise, drugs, sample quality, and preservation). To confirm this tendency, the reader has only to inspect the texts in pediatrics and clinical pathology used by medical schools in the first half of this century.

Good studies of pediatric reference values appeared, however, when analytical micromethods became available. This is well illustrated in the truly remarkable paper by Bullock *(13)*, published in 1930, on age-related variation of serum inorganic phosphorus. In sampling his population, Bullock considered the following variables: (a) persons with conditions that could influence serum inorganic phosphorus were eliminated from the study; (b) children one year or younger were given cod liver oil and sunbaths; (c) both breast-fed and bottle-fed babies were included, with the bottle-fed babies receiving well-balanced formulas of fresh cow's milk or dried milk; (d) older children followed routine dietary instructions; (e) adults not receiving a fair amount of green vegetables were excluded; (f) any of the subjects examined who displayed clinical signs (described in the paper) of rickets was eliminated from the study; (g) blood samples were taken over a seven-month period, out of consideration for possible seasonal variability; (h) blood from the longitudinal sinus or venipuncture was collected into a dry syringe; (i) blood was kept cold until determinations were made; (j) determinations were made within 2.5 h of blood collection; (k) samples were obtained at about the same time of day—at noon before eating, while the subject was at rest; (l) about an equal number of males and females, blacks and whites, were sampled; (m) the population sampled was chosen over the entire life span, from birth to old age; and (n) the analytical technique for inorganic phosphorus was that of Fiske and Subbarow (14), still used today. What is more, in publishing his paper, Bullock critically and thoroughly reviewed the existing literature.

Figure 3 shows the average changes in inorganic phosphorus Bullock observed on the 307 subjects he tested. The principal findings of this Figure have been well confirmed, and include: the higher-than-adult values that occur in childhood; the initial increase in serum inorganic phosphorus over the first few months of life; and the gradual decrease in concentration throughout childhood. Although Bullock could not reach a firm conclusion, he noted that girls show phosphorus values somewhat lower than boys in the 10- to 13-year-old group, and that their values level off at the time of cessation of bone growth, at 16–17 years; that is in contrast to young men, whose phosphorus and bone growth plateau at 19–20 years. The bar lines in the figure (see legend), taken from the recent work of Cherian and Hill (15), show that the more extensive recent studies generally affirm Bullock's work.

Alkaline phosphatase. Another major work on age- (and sex-) related reference values is the study by Clark and Beck on plasma alkaline phosphatase activity in the growing child, reported in 1950 (16), and extending the pioneering efforts of Bessey and Lowry (17) and Harrison et al. (18). Clark and Beck sampled 623 children and adults ranging in age from birth to 28 years, and observed well-defined trends. After a decrease (albeit still at three- to fourfold the adult value) in the first year of life, the values remain on a plateau to age 10. At this time, the values in boys show an increase to age 13 before decreasing, whereas girls' values decrease "precipitously,"

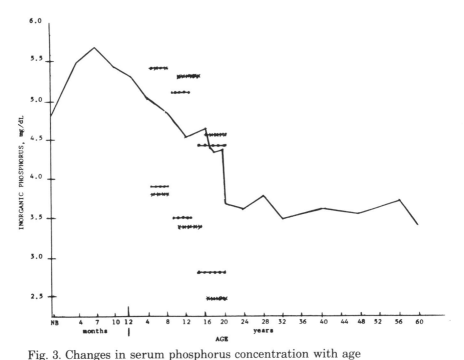

Fig. 3. Changes in serum phosphorus concentration with age

Solid line, values reported by Bullock *(13);* x—x, 5th and 95th percentiles for males, ●—●, 5th and 95th percentiles for females, from Cherian and Hill *(19)*

remaining below the values for males at least to age 27 years. Harrison et al., however, had shown that girls also reach peak alkaline phosphatase activity in pubescence, which has been confirmed most recently (1978) by Cherian and Hill *(19).* In general, the enzyme activity paralleled the rate of bone growth; this relationship was substantiated by inhibition studies with taurocholate, before isoenzyme measurements were known. For further discussion of alkaline phosphatase, see Bowers' commentary in this text (pp 73–77).

Two important factors making possible the study by Clark and Beck were the availability of an ultramicro technique for the analysis of alkaline phosphatase activity, and sophisticated instrumentation. They used the method of Bessey et al. *(20)* and the Beckman DU spectrophotometer. Plasma samples from the 623 subjects, in 16 age groupings, were obtained by skin puncture and analyzed in duplicate.

Calcium. Our knowledge of reference values for total plasma calcium in the newborn is illustrative of several aspects of the historical development of clinical chemistry, and its belated application to the pediatric patient, particularly to the neonate *(21).* To establish reference values for the newborn, three facts must be considered: *(a)* the need to distinguish values obtained for the premature or low-birth-weight infant from those obtained on the full-term or normal-weight infant, *(b)* the overlap between the lower limits of normocalcemia in a healthy neonate with the upper limits of a neonate who has true hypocalcemia, and *(c)* the time required for neonatal calcium concentrations to reach "stable" (adult) values.

In contrast with inorganic phosphorus and alkaline phosphatase, where changes occur over many years and are related strongly to bone growth, plasma calcium displays its principal change within the first month of life, and mostly in the first week. To obtain reference values, therefore, it is necessary that "healthy" premature and full-term newborns be studied over a short period of time, and consequently, that ultramicro analytical techniques be available for analysis of calcium in samples obtained by skin puncture. The latter objective has been met, but comparatively few studies have been made with newer techniques, and much more analyses must be done. The data available, however, point to the lower limit of plasma calcium in the newborn as being well below the limits for the adult; the lower limit for the premature infant is, in turn, below that of the full-term newborn *(22–24)*. All of this takes place, as mentioned, within the first week of life; adult values are reached at about one month *(25)*.

1. *Study to Quantify the Uniqueness of Children's Hospitals. Summary of Major Findings.* The National Association of Children's Hospitals and Related Institutions, Inc., Wilmington, DE, 1978, 16 pp.
2. Natelson, S., The analytical laboratory of neonatology. In *Clinical Chemistry,* D. T. Forman and R. W. Mattoon, Eds. American Chemical Society, Washington, DC, 1976, pp 95–152.
3. Avery, G. B., Neonatal physiology: Basis for the laboratory needs of the nursery. In *The Neonate,* D. S. Young and J. M. Hicks, Eds. John Wiley and Sons, New York, NY, 1976, pp 89–94.
4. Hicks, J. M., and Young, D. S., Obligations of the pediatric clinical laboratory. In *The Neonate* (see ref. *3*), pp 325–336.
5. Nadler, H., Rao, G. J., and Taussig, L. M., Cystic fibrosis. In *The Metabolic Basis of Inherited Disease,* 4th ed., J. B. Stanbury, J. B. Wyngaarden, and D. S. Frederickson, Eds. McGraw-Hill, New York, NY, 1978, pp 1683–1710.
6. Posen, S., Lee, C., Vines, R., Kilham, H., Latham, S., and Keefe, J. F., Transient hyperphosphatasemia of infancy—an insufficiency recognized syndrome. Case report. *Clin. Chem.* **23**, 292–294 (1977).
7. Wieme, R. J., More on transient hyperphosphatasemia in infancy—an insufficiently recognized syndrome. *Clin. Chem.* **24**, 520–522 (1978). Letter.
8. Caraway, W. T., The scientific development of clinical chemistry to 1948. *Clin. Chem.* **19**, 373–383 (1973).
9. Fölling, A., Uber Ausscheidung von Phenylbenztraubensaure in den Harn als Stoffwechselanomalie in Verbindung mit Imbezzillität. *Hoppe-Seyler's Physiol. Chem.* **227**, 169 (1934).
10. Jervis, G. A., Phenylpyruvic oligophrenia: Introductory study of 50 cases of mental deficiency associated with excretion of phenylpyruvic acid. *Arch. Neurol. Psychiatry* **38**, 944–963 (1937).

11. Jervis, G. A., The genetics of phenylpyruvic oligophrenia. *J. Ment. Sci.* **85**, 719–762 (1939).
12. Garrod, A. E., *Inborn Errors of Metabolism.* Oxford University Press, London, 1909.
13. Bullock, J. K., The physiological variation in the inorganic blood phosphorus content at the different age periods. *Am. J. Dis. Child.* **40**, 725–740 (1930).
14. Fiske, C. H., and Subbarow, Y., Colorimetric determination of phosphorus. *J. Biol. Chem.* **66**, 375–400 (1925).
15. Cherian, A. G., and Hill, J. G., Percentile estimates of reference values for fourteen chemical constituents in sera of children and adolescents. *Am. J. Clin. Pathol.* **69**, 24–31 (1978).
16. Clark, L. C., Jr., and Beck, E., Plasma "alkaline" phosphatase activity. I. Normative data for growing children. *J. Pediatr.* **36**, 335–341 (1950).
17. Bessey, O. A., and Lowry, O. H., Nutritional assay of 1200 New York State School children. Division of Nutrition and Physiology, the Public Health Research Institute of the City of New York, 1978.
18. Harrison, A. P., Roderuck, C., Lesher, M., Kaucher, M., Moyer, E. Z., Lameck, W., and Beach, E. F., Nutritional status of children: VIII. Blood serum alkaline phosphatase. *J. Am. Diet. Assoc.* **24**, 503–509 (1948).
19. Cherian, A. G., and Hill, J. G., Age dependence of serum enzymatic activities (alkaline phosphatase, aspartate aminotransferase, and creatine kinase) in healthy children and adolescents. *Am. J. Clin. Pathol.* **70**, 783–789 (1978).
20. Bessey, O. A., Lowry, O. A., and Brock, M. J., A method for the rapid determination of alkaline phosphatase with five cubic millimeters of serum. *J. Biol. Chem.* **164**, 321–329 (1946).
21. Meites, S., Normal total plasma calcium in the newborn. *CRC Crit. Rev. Clin. Lab. Sci.* **6**, 1–18 (1975).
22. Cockburn, F., Brown, J. K., Belton, N. R., and Forfar, J. O., Neonatal convulsions associated with primary disturbance of calcium, phosphorus, and magnesium metabolism. *Arch. Dis. Child.* **48**, 99–108 (1973).
23. Jukarainen, E., Plasma magnesium levels during the first five days of life. *Acta Paediatr. Scand. Suppl.*, 222 (1971).
24. Rosenkranz, A., Der Serumkalziumspiegel beim Frühgeborenen in den ersten Lebenstagen. *Paediatr. Paedol.* **2**, 367–381 (1966).
25. Dormandy, T. L., and Begum, R., The plasma calcium and magnesium response to standard metabolic loads in infants. In *Mineral Metabolism in Paediatrics*, D. Barltrop and W. L. Burland, Eds. F. A. Davis, Philadelphia, PA, 1969, pp 31–50.

Chapter 3. Skin-Puncture and Blood-Collecting Techniques for Infants[1]

Samuel Meites and Monte J. Levitt

The Committee on Pediatric Clinical Chemistry (CPCC) of the American Association for Clinical Chemistry describes here selected techniques for performing skin puncture[2] and collecting blood from newborns and older infants. This description is based on a consensus of eight individuals at major pediatric centers, and variations in approach are duly noted. Unfortunately, the "state of the art" sometimes does not permit distinct choices in recommendations. Nevertheless, this paper should serve as a guide to preferred current practice and as a reference for future development and selection.

Skin-puncture and blood-collecting techniques, and the quality of the blood obtained, have been described in much detail in several texts and many books and articles. Although a few of these will be cited at the outset (1–13), we will not present a historical review of the subject.

The National Committee for Clinical Laboratory Standards (NCCLS) has published a proposed "standard" for collecting blood by skin puncture for patients of all ages (14). While there is, and should be, some overlap of interests and details, this chapter is concerned exclusively with the infant, and with blood-collecting techniques intended for pediatric clinical chemistry. The information presented here is intended to supplement and strengthen the NCCLS in its efforts to establish standards for materials and practice in this routine but critical manipulation.

Skin-puncture blood-collecting technique should be used on infants primarily to avoid venipuncture,[3] because (a) microvolumes of blood

---

[1] This chapter was originally published in slightly modified form in *Clin. Chem.* **25**, 183–189 (1979), as a Proposed Selected Method. The Evaluators were Thomas A. Blumenfeld, Keith B. Hammond, Jocelyn M. Hicks, J. Gilbert Hill, John E. Sherwin, and Elizabeth K. Smith. Mention of a specific manufacturer does not constitute endorsement.

[2] The term skin puncture ("dermipuncture") is deliberately selected to avoid the more specific but less accurate term, "capillary" puncture. Although capillary blood (from arterioles, venules, and capillaries) predominates, at least traces of contaminating interstitial and intracellular fluid are likely to be present and cannot be ignored.

[3] Physicians alone perform venipuncture for blood-chemistry determinations in all but one of the institutions of the CPCC, and exclusively perform arterial punctures in all of them. Nurses may sample indwelling arterial catheters for blood-gas determinations.

are desirable to obviate anemia *(10)*, *(b)* veins must be reserved for parenteral therapy *(11,12,15)*, *(c)* frequent sampling is essential to monitor acid–base status and respiratory distress *(11,12,15)*, and *(d)* venipuncture is excessively hazardous in such patients *(10,13,16–18)*. For adults, skin puncture is often preferable for similar reasons, as when veins are difficult to tap owing to their small size or location, or because of obesity or burns, or when the patient cannot be properly restrained.

The CPCC finds among its members that the mean number of chemistry tests ordered per requisition varies between four and six, and that the number of skin punctures required to complete each order averages 1.0 to 1.5. If it is assumed that a uniform skin-puncture technique is being used, the volume of blood available from a single puncture depends on the size and health of the infant. The volume of plasma or serum that generally can be obtained from a premature newborn is about 100 to 150 μL, and about twice this volume from a full-term newborn. Because of the relatively high hematocrit of the neonate, these volumes correspond to about 0.4 to 0.7 mL of whole blood. Larger volumes are obtained from adults and older children *(14)*.

About 75 to 95% of all requests for chemical tests on blood (excluding p_{O_2}) in a pediatric institution are performed on samples obtained by skin puncture.[4] The rest involve venous or arterial puncture, or specimens collected from indwelling arterial catheters—procedures not generally performed by laboratory personnel.[3] Despite the greater risk, these procedures are used when the volume of blood required exceeds the volume available from skin puncture—e.g., when there are combined orders from hematology, microbiology, and (or) immunology, as well as from the chemistry laboratory—or when blood from skin puncture may be invalid to use, as in the case of certain enzymes or p_{O_2} measurement.

For the neonate, the skin-puncture technique provides sufficient blood for performing routine as well as urgent ("stat") procedures, on a 24-h per day basis *(15,19,20)*. These procedures include Na, K, Cl, CO_2, pH, p_{CO_2}, p_{O_2} (but see below), glucose, bilirubin, and Ca, and may also include measurements of urea, total protein, and osmolality. In addition, neonatal screening for metabolic disorders, particularly phenylketonuria and hypothyroidism, may be legally required. The validity of blood obtained by this technique has been well documented for chemistry tests. There is as yet no agreement, however, on the suitability of this blood vs arterial blood for p_{O_2} determinations, particularly for the "sick" newborn. At best, the CPCC can state that, in view of their experience and the fairly voluminous literature

---

[4] The institution of J.G.H. is an exception. Only 10% of blood samples for clinical chemical use are obtained via skin puncture. Arterial puncture for blood gases (primarily p_{O_2}), however, is not excluded from this figure, as it is from the others.

(11,21–38), p_{O_2} determinations via skin-puncture blood must be judiciously ordered, obtained by highly skilled personnel, and interpreted cautiously. It is hoped that the use of the transcutaneous electrode will resolve this vexing problem *(39–42)*.

Methods for Skin Puncture and Blood Collection

Warming the Site

For collecting samples for measurement of blood gases (pH, p_{CO_2}, p_{O_2}), the CPCC unanimously recommends warming the site before the puncture. Warming increases the rate of arterial blood flow (reddening) in the area, thus helping to assure that the test data will be validly comparable with those for arterial blood, and increasing the volume of blood available for collection.[5] For tests other than blood gases, such warming apparently does not affect the analytical data, but does make collection easier *(43)*. There are several choices of warming materials, but the most convenient is a cloth towel or washcloth, soaked in hot, running tap water at 39 to 44 °C. Temperatures exceeding 44 °C may cause burns *(44)*. The patient's foot or hand is wrapped in the cloth for 3–10 min. Once the cloth is applied, the wrapped extremity may be encased in a plastic bag to assure greater heat retention, and to keep the patient's bed dry.

Note: Evaluator J.G.H. uses "Infra-Rub Analgesic Cream" (Whitehall Labs. Ltd.), as well as "Col Pac Hydrocollator" (Chattanooga Pharmacal Co.). Evaluator K.B.H. uses "T-Pac" (Kay Laboratories Inc.).

Nursing personnel in neonatal units may perform the procedure. If so, the unit and laboratory personnel must coordinate their efforts, so that blood is collected just at the end of the warming period.

Site of Puncture

The least-hazardous site (Figure 1) of heel puncture for the neonate is medial to a line drawn posteriorly from the middle of the great toe to the heel, or lateral to a line drawn posteriorly from between toes 4 and 5 to the heel *(2,3,14,45)*. In older infants, the palmar (fleshy) surface of the distal phalanx of the second, third, or fourth fingers may be punctured, the middle finger being the first choice. The thumb, great toe, or ear lobe are seldom if ever used. To avoid contaminating the blood sample, edema must not be present at the puncture site.

Skin Puncture

Antiseptic. Isopropanol/water (70/30 by vol, "70%") is currently

---

[5] Submitter S.M. has observed this in a study of prewarming technique. Prewarming had little effect on the volume obtained from adults, in contrast to the increased volume from infants.

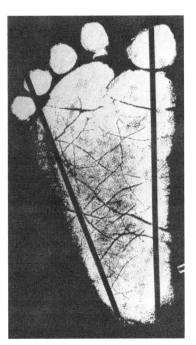

Fig. 1. Optimal sites for heel puncture of the newborn *(59)*.

The newborn's calcaneus (heel bone) does not extend medial to a line drawn posteriorly from the middle of the great toe or lateral to a line drawn posteriorly between the 4th and 5th toes. To avoid puncturing the calcaneus, the skin puncture should be performed outside of these two lines. (Footprint reproduced with permission from Grune & Stratton, Inc., New York, NY, from the cover of ref. 6)

the antiseptic favored for cleansing the puncture site.[6] Several manufacturers sell sterile, disposable absorbent pads soaked with 70% isopropanol.[7]

Note: Submitter S.M. reports that in a brief study of bacterial growth from adult fingers placed directly on blood-agar plates, after various pretreatments, the following data were obtained. *No treatment* (control): 40 of 40 (100%) cultures showed growth in 48 h at 37 °C; *sterile isopropanol (70%) swab, wiped dry with nonsterile gauze pad:* six of 20 (30%) cultures showed growth in 48 h; *sterile isopropanol (70%) swab, air-dried:* three of 20 (15%) cultures showed growth in 48 h; *sterile isopropanol (70%) swab, wiped dry with sterile gauze pad:* six of 60 (10%) showed growth in 48 h. From these data one would conclude that the last technique is preferable.

Drying the puncture site. After the puncture site is washed with isopropanol, the area must then be wiped dry with a sterile sponge.[8] Dryness is essential, to avoid hemolysis by alcohol or water. Ethyl

---

[6] Evaluator K.B.H. uses Wescodyne (West Chemical Products Inc.), 9 mL diluted with 2 L of water. Povidone-iodine ("Betadine") is not recommended for skin disinfection when skin-puncture blood is drawn for analysis *(46)*.

[7] Absorbent Alcohol Dab TPCO (Hospital Supply Corp.); Alcohol Prep-Pad (MED PAC Corp. or Dynamed Corp.); Preptic Swab (Johnson & Johnson); Kendall (Webcol) no. 5818, Boston, MA; STERI-WIPE Alcohol Swab No. 951 (Holland-Rantos Co., Inc.).

[8] Johnson's Gauze Sponges, folded, 2 × 2, 8 ply (Johnson & Johnson).

Table 1. Tip Dimensions of Several Currently Used Lancets for Skin Puncture[a]

Lancet[b]	Maximum length, mm	Maximum width, mm
Becton-Dickinson Long Point Microlance	4.85	2.25
Esta Steri Phoenix Blood Lancet	3.65	1.50
Medipoint Blood Lancet	3.50	1.50
Feather Blood Lancet	3.50	1.40
Sherwood Monolet Lancet	2.75	0.50
Becton-Dickinson Microlance	2.50	1.55
Propper Sera Sharp	2.50	1.20

[a] Data obtained by Thomas A. Blumenfeld.
[b] Lancets are available via usual suppliers of clinical laboratory equipment.

ether is not used for two reasons: its rapid evaporation cools the skin surface and it is a fire hazard.

Depth of puncture. For the neonate, the depth of puncture must not exceed 2.5 mm, to avoid penetrating bone (calcaneus) *(13,45,59)*. Osteomyelitis is a potential complication of skin puncture *(47)*.

Devices for skin puncture. The skin-puncturing device favored by the Committee is a disposable, sterile lancet. Only certain lancets, however, have tips 2.4 mm long or less as required for the newborn (Table 1).[9] Longer tips (to 5 mm) are suitable for older children, but should *not* be used on neonates younger than six months. Use of surgical blades, without appropriate control of the cutting edge and depth of puncture, is strongly discouraged for the infant.[10]

Follow-up of skin puncture. Once the blood collection is completed, and while the patient's foot is held above heart level, either a sterile gauze pad or cotton swab is pressed to the puncture site until bleeding stops. This critical step may prolong the collection to as much as 10 to 15 min, even longer in some instances. Most of the CPCC do not favor the use of adhesive bandages for infants who are six months old or younger, because the neonate's skin is sensitive to the adhesive, and because of the potential, though undocumented, hazard of the infant's placing it in his mouth and aspirating it.

Note: Submitter S.M. reports that cases of ingestion of adhesive bandages placed on *fingers* of older infants are not uncommon, and recommends that bandages not be used at all on children who are under two years of age.

---

[9] The CPCC generally favors the BD MICROLANCE (Becton-Dickinson), and the Monolet lancet by Monoject (Sherwood Medical Industries, Inc.).

[10] A suitable device incorporating a surgical blade has recently been developed *(48)*.

Blood Collection

Grasp the infant's heel with a moderately firm grip, with your forefinger at the arch of the foot, and your thumb placed well below the puncture site, at the ankle. Make the puncture in one continuous, deliberate motion, in a direction almost perpendicular to the puncture site. The pressure with the thumb is eased and re-applied as drops of blood form and are allowed to flow into the appropriate containers. Avoid "milking" (massaging) because this causes hemolysis and mixes interstitial and intracellular fluid with the blood sample.

For finger puncture, place your thumb either below or above, and well away from, the puncture site. As with the heel, make the puncture in one continuous, deliberate motion, in a direction almost perpendicular to the puncture site. Again, moderately firm pressure is applied without massage.

The first drop of blood must be assumed to contain an excess of intracellular and interstitial fluid, with surface debris. It is discarded by wiping it off with a sterile pad.

When filling capillary collection tubes for pH–blood gas determinations, maintain the patient's heel at approximately body (horizontal) level throughout the collection to avoid venous stasis (a good practice for clinical chemical samples in general); hold the collecting tube in a nearly horizontal position and allow it to be filled as long as there is sufficient blood present to cover the tip. If blood is being drawn into the capillary faster than it is replaced, withdraw the tube slightly, moving it back into position when there is sufficient blood present. If air is inadvertently drawn into the tube, discard it and replace it with a new one.

Sealing capillary tubes for blood gases, and mixing with anticoagulant. Once the capillary tube is filled with bubble-free blood, seal one end with "wax" (see Table 2) to a depth of about 4 mm *(9).*

Note: To mix the sample before sealing, gently invert the capillary tube several times. When the blood is ready for analysis, one end of the tube (with about 2 mm of the blood) is scored, broken, and discarded.

A small piece of iron wire, about 5 mm long, is then inserted into the tube. The second end is then sealed to a depth of about 2 mm. This should force out some of the wax on the other end. Mixing is then done by moving the iron wire back and forth inside the tube with the help of a magnet.

Labeling. At present there is no completely satisfactory technique for labeling containers in a manner that not only is convenient and applicable to the various containers used but also assures foolproof identification of the sample. Two procedures are in vogue: *(a)* direct inscription on the container and *(b)* affixing adhesive labels. Capillary tubes may be labeled directly with fine-tipped pens,[11] or by wrapping

---

[11] Fine Tip Marker, S/P P1226 (Scientific Products).

Table 2. Containers for Blood Collection

Container[a]	Remarks
Blood gases (pH, p_{CO_2}, p_{O_2}):	
Natelson glass collecting pipets, 75- and 250-μL volumes, ammonium heparin.	To mix, insert metal "fleas" or mixing bars, after filling.[b] Seal with caps, or sealing wax. Mix by use of a magnet. *Source:* many laboratory suppliers.
Blood-collecting pipet kits and component parts, supplied by manufacturers of blood-gas apparatus.	Kits containing glass capillaries, sealing wax, metal mixing bars, and magnets. *Source:* laboratory suppliers of Corning, IL, and Radiometer equipment.
Caraway glass tubes, 370-μL volume, ammonium heparin.	Mix and seal as above, or by inversion. *Source:* many laboratory suppliers.
Electrolytes (CO_2, Cl, K, Na) and general chemistry:	
Microhematocrit glass capillary tubes 1.1–1.2 mm i.d., 75 mm long, ammonium heparin.	Plasma obtained. Mix and seal as above.
Micro sample tubes, polyethylene, 250 μL, lithium heparin; larger sizes (400-, 500-μL) for general chemistry, with and without heparin.	Plasma obtained. Seal with attached cap. Mix by inversion.[c] *Source:* Kew Scientific and Beckman Instruments, Inc.
B-D Microtainer, polypropylene, 600 μL, silicone separator *(58).*	Serum obtained. Seal with accompanying cap. Centrifuge at 6000 $\times$ g. *Source:* Becton-Dickinson and Co.

[a] Containers listed here are all commercially available.
[b] Mixing without a flea is also possible by gently inverting the capillary before sealing.
[c] For collecting electrolytes, fill two 250-μL tubes, one for CO_2/Cl, another for Na/K. Shake the first drop entering the tube to its bottom. All further drops should then flow along the path of the first drop, if the tube is held in a nearly vertical position.

a small adhesive label (flag) around them, or by attaching the label to a test tube into which the capillaries are placed for transport. Adhesive labels on which accession numbers are printed, coinciding with and detachable from the request form, are popularly used. Larger containers are more readily labeled by either of the two procedures. Evaluator J.M.H. uses computer-generated labels.

Containers. Table 2 details the various containers used by the CPCC for blood collection. For blood gases the favored container is a heparinized glass Natelson tube, but capillary tubes of other dimensions are also used, as well as the larger-bore Caraway tube.

Several different containers are used in collecting blood for electrolyte assay. The advantage of using small-bore glass capillary tubes is that if blood is hemolyzed in one tube (affecting the potassium concentration), it may be discarded without compromising the quality of the specimen in the other capillary tube, whereas if a specimen collected into a single tube is hemolyzed, the entire specimen cannot be used and a second blood sample must be collected from the patient. Alternatively, multiple plastic microtubes may also be used. For measuring CO_2 content, there is no convincing evidence that specimens collected into capillaries are more valid than those collected into single, larger-bore plastic or glass tubes. Indeed, plasma from several glass capillaries is often pooled into a plastic tube before electrolytes are determined.

All of the glass capillary tubes listed in Table 2 are heparinized. The Natelson tube and the plastic microtubes may be obtained with or without heparin. There are different views within the CPCC, as well as in the literature (49–51), concerning the utility of plasma vs serum for determining electrolytes in particular, and for chemical tests generally. Those who favor plasma claim that more plasma may be obtained from an unclotted blood specimen than serum from a clotted one, and that contamination is less likely, because clotting may disrupt platelets and mechanically promote hemolysis. This hemolysis may partly relate to the relatively greater mechanical fragility of erythrocytes in the newborn's blood (52,53). Obviously, for quantitating serum proteins and for electrophoresis, serum is essential; hence, containers with no anticoagulant are used.

Almost without exception, heparin is the anticoagulant of choice for containers used in collecting skin-puncture blood for chemical tests; the lithium and ammonium salts of heparin are most suitable. They have not been reported to be a source of interference in determining blood gases, electrolytes, or in most other chemical procedures, with some exceptions (54).

Note: Submitter S.M. finds that lithium-heparinized vs unheparinized microcentrifuge tubes show only about 0.2% differences between the respective means for Na, K, and Ca. For Na and K, a standard containing 140 and 5 mmol/L, respectively, was placed into 20 heparinized and 20 unheparinized tubes and measurements were compared. For Ca, 1.25 and 2.5 mmol/L standards were each placed into 10 heparinized and 10 unheparinized tubes and measurements compared.

Specimen Transport

In general, sealed specimens for blood gases should be immersed in ice-water during transport. Plastic containers, with dimensions suitable for holding the tubes containing the specimen, as well as small enough to be carried on the blood collecting tray (Figure 2), are readily fashioned from discarded shipping containers. These are half-filled with water and then stored in the freezer between collections. Water is added before collection. Many variations are possible.

Blood pH is stable for about 2 h at 0 °C (11,55). Glycolysis in the erythrocytes and leukocytes of whole blood causes a decline in pH,

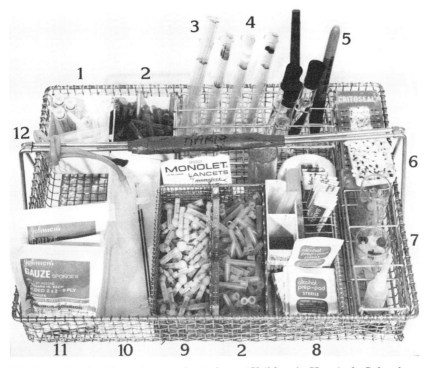

Fig. 2. A blood-collector's tray for infants (Children's Hospital, Columbus, OH)

Items in numerical order, clockwise: *(1)* unheparinized plastic microcentrifuge tubes; *(2)* heparinized (blue-colored) plastic microcentrifuge tubes, 250, 400, and 500 µL; *(3)* heparinized Natelson tubes, 75 µL; *(4)* capillary micropipets used in measuring blood for glucose determinations; *(5)* marking pen for labels; *(6)* sealing "wax" for Natelson and capillary (hematocrit) tubes; *(7)* Microtainer tubes, 600 µL, *(8)* alcohol pads, *(9)* lancets for skin puncture, *(10)* ice-water container, with submerged Natelson tubes for pH determination, *(11)* sterile gauze sponges, *(12)* mouth-tubing for use with capillary micropipets. Unnumbered items are used in blood collection for hematological tests. Manufacturers of the above items are indicated in the text

which is measurable after about 20 min of standing at room temperature *(11,55)*. It is best not to store samples for p_{CO_2} determination for longer than 30 min in ice-water *(55)*, and storage of samples for p_{O_2} for longer than 1 h is not recommended *(56)*.

Centrifugation of Microsamples

Table-top, high-speed centrifuges,[12] specifically designed for centrifuging microtubes, are currently used. Attaining forces up to about 10 000 to 13 000 × g, they separate plasma or serum within 1 to 2

---

[12] Beckman Microfuge B or 152 Microfuge; Eppendorf Micro Centrifuge 5412 or Micro Centrifuge 3200 (via major U.S. distributors); Fisher Centrifuge 59. Evaluator J.G.H. uses a Janetzki TH 12 micro centrifuge, distributed by Jena Instruments Ltd.

min. In this respect, they are much more efficient than the slower and bulkier floor centrifuges. The microcentrifuges have become routine instruments for the clinical microchemistry laboratory. Smallbore glass capillary tubes are readily spun in special centrifuges for hematocrit determinations or in the usual centrifuges.

Discussion

A "free" flow of blood is not obtained from skin puncture of infants, particularly those who are dehydrated or in shock. With the techniques described here, moderate pressure near the puncture site *must* be maintained to assure the flow. Drops of blood usually form on the skin surface, one by one. Necessarily, blood is exposed to air by this technique, but this is unrelated to the question of which container to use (capillary vs larger-bore tube) and how the container may affect the quality of the sample for blood-gas determination.[13]

Hemolysis is an undesirable complication of skin puncture that cannot be ignored (57). Even on carefully following the techniques recommended here, one may expect that about 3% of specimens from patients 0–13 days old may still show visible hemolysis. Such specimens must not be used in assays where hemolysis or contaminating cellular material affects the results (43). If blood is collected into multiple containers, any tube showing hemolysis may be discarded, or only used appropriately.

There is some tendency to assume that analytical data obtained with blood from skin puncture are the same for adults and infants. Comparison of analytes determined in venous vs skin-puncture blood in adults shows small but significant differences in glucose, calcium, total protein, and potassium, and little difference in lactate dehydrogenase (EC 1.1.1.27) (13,43,49). The issue is far from resolved, because previous studies and observations have not generally indicated such differences. The question as to whether lactate dehydrogenase and aldolase (EC 4.1.2.13) activities are the same in samples from either source remains to be proved for infants.

The volume of blood required for tests has been diminishing gradually, sometimes dramatically, within the past few years, thanks to efforts by clinical chemists and manufacturers. A long-standing goal of the clinical microchemist has been to remove sample volume as a limitation to clinical laboratory analysis. Recent progress moves that goal within reach.

---

[13] Readers may discover for themselves how little loss in p_{CO_2} and CO_2 content there is in the collecting process. Using reference sera (e.g., Versatol Acid-Base; General Diagnostics) with p_{CO_2} values of approximately 20, 40, and 60 mmHg, one may simulate the collecting technique by allowing serum to drip off a fingertip from a dropper into the appropriate container, then centrifuging the specimen before analysis. Results show little loss at 20 and 40 mmHg, and a small but significant loss at 60 mmHg. For observations in the literature see references 2,9,11,21–24,26, and 31.

1. Langner, P. H., Jr., and Fies, H. L., Blood sugar values of blood obtained simultaneously from the radial artery, antecubital vein, and the finger. *Am. J. Clin. Pathol.* **12,** 559–562 (1942).

2. Pincus, J. B., Gittleman, I. F., Saito, M., and Sobel, A. E., A study of plasma values of sodium, potassium, chloride, carbon dioxide, carbon dioxide tension, sugar, urea, and the protein base-binding power, pH and hematocrit in prematures on the first day of life. *Pediatrics* **18,** 39–48 (1956).

3. Kaplan, S. A., Yuceoglu, A. M., and Strauss, J., Chemical microanalysis: Analysis of capillary and venous blood. *Pediatrics* **24,** 270–274 (1959).

4. Wilkinson, R. H., *Chemical Micromethods in Clinical Medicine,* Charles C Thomas, Springfield, IL, 1960, pp 19–25.

5. Meites, S., and Faulkner, W. R., *Manual of Practical Micro and General Procedures in Clinical Chemistry.* Charles C Thomas, Springfield, IL, 1962, pp 5–9.

6. Mabry, C. C., Roeckel, I. E., Gevedon, R. E., and Koepke, J. A., *Recent Advances in Pediatric Clinical Chemistry.* Grune and Stratton, New York, NY, 1968, pp 4–9.

7. O'Brien, D., Ibbott, F. A., and Rodgerson, D. O., *Laboratory Manual of Pediatric Micro-Biochemical Techniques,* 4th ed. Hoeber, New York, NY, 1968.

8. Natelson, S., *Techniques of Clinical Chemistry,* 3rd ed. Charles C Thomas, Springfield, IL, 1971, pp 92–95.

9. Siggaard-Andersen, O., *The Acid-Base Status of the Blood,* 4th ed. Williams & Wilkins, Baltimore, MD, 1974, pp 149–151.

10. Blumenfeld, T. A., Clinical applications of microchemistry. In *Microtechniques for the Clinical Laboratory,* M. Werner, Ed. John Wiley, New York, NY, 1976, pp 1–15.

11. Dell, R. B., and Winters, R. W., Microanalysis of blood acid-base status. In *Microtechniques for the Clinical Laboratory* (see ref. *10*), pp 179–203.

12. *Pediatric Clinical Chemistry,* 1st ed., S. Meites, Ed. American Association for Clinical Chemistry, Washington, DC, 1977.

13. Blumenfeld, T. A., Infant blood-collection and chemical analysis. *Diagn. Med.* **1,** 58–66 (1978).

14. *Standard Procedures for the Collection of Diagnostic Blood Specimens by Skin Puncture, Proposed Standard: PSH-4,* NCCLS, 771 E. Lancaster Ave., Villanova, PA 19085, 1977.

15. Natelson, S., The analytical laboratory of neonatology. In *Clinical Chemistry,* D. T. Forman and R. W. Mattoon, Eds. (ASC Symposium Series, **36**), American Chemical Society, Washington, DC, 1976, pp 95, 152.

16. Garrow, E., and Kushnick, J., Management of femoral artery obstruction. Complication of femoral venipuncture. *Am. J. Dis. Child.* **110,** 570–571 (1965).

17. Asnes, R. S., and Arendar, G. M., Septic arthritis of the hip: A complication of venipuncture. *Pediatrics* **38,** 837–841 (1966).

18. McKay, R. J., Jr., Diagnosis and treatment: Risks of obtaining samples of venous blood in infants. *Pediatrics* **38,** 906–908 (1966).

19. Ryan, G. M., Toward improving the outcome of pregnancy. Recommendations for the regional development of perinatal health services. *Obstet. Gynecol.* **46,** 375–384 (1975).

20. Avery, G. B., Neonatal physiology: Basis for the laboratory needs of the nursery. In *The Neonate,* D. S. Young and J. M. Hicks, Eds. John Wiley & Sons, New York, NY, 1976, pp 89–94.

21. Gambino, S. R., Collection of capillary blood for simultaneous determinations of arterial pH, CO_2 content, p_{CO_2}, and oxygen saturation. *Am. J. Clin. Pathol.* **35**, 178–183 (1961).
22. Gandy, G., Grann, L., Cunningham, N., Adamsons, K., Jr., and James, L. S., The validity of pH and p_{CO_2} measurements in capillary samples in sick and healthy newborn infants. *Pediatrics* **34**, 192–197 (1964).
23. Koch, G., Comparison of carbon dioxide tension, pH and standard bicarbonate in capillary blood and in arterial blood. *Scand. J. Clin. Invest.* **17**, 223–229 (1965).
24. Langlands, J. H. M., and Wallace, W. F. M., Small blood-samples from ear-lobe puncture; a substitute for arterial puncture. *Lancet* **ii**, 315–317 (1965).
25. Desai, S. D., Holloway, R., Thambiran, A. K., and Wesley, A. G., A comparison between arterial and arterialized capillary blood in infants. *S. Afr. Med. J.* **41**, 13–15 (1967).
26. Koch, G., and Wendel, H., Comparison of pH, carbon dioxide tension, standard bicarbonate and oxygen tension in capillary blood and in arterial blood during the neonatal period. *Acta Paediatr. Scand.* **56**, 10–16 (1967).
27. MacIntyre, J., Norman, J. N., and Smith, G., Use of capillary blood in measurement of arterial p_{O_2}. *Br. Med. J.* **iii**, 640–643 (1968).
28. Siggaard-Andersen, O., Acid-base and blood gas parameters—arterial or capillary blood? *Scand. J. Clin. Lab. Invest.* **21**, 289–292 (1968).
29. Bannister, A., Comparison of arterial and arterialized capillary blood in infants with respiratory distress. *Arch. Dis. Child.* **44**, 726–728 (1969).
30. Mountain, K. R., and Campbell, D. G., Reliability of oxygen tension measurements on arterialized capillary blood in the newborn. *Arch. Dis. Child.* **45**, 134–138 (1970).
31. Winquist, R. A., and Stamm, S. J., Arterialized capillary sampling using histamine iontophoresis. *J. Pediatr.* **76**, 455–458 (1970).
32. Garg, A. K., "Arterialized" capillary blood. *Can. Med. Assoc. J.* **107**, 16 (1972).
33. Glasgow, J. F. T., Flynn, D. M., and Swyer, P. R., A comparison of descending aortic and "arterialized" capillary blood in the sick newborn. *Can. Med. Assoc. J.* **106**, 660–662 (1972).
34. Hofford, J. M., Dowling, A. S., and Pell, S., More about arterialized capillary blood measurements. *J. Am. Med. Assoc.* **224**, 1297 (1973).
35. Hunt, C. E., Capillary blood sampling in the infant: Usefulness and limitations of two methods of sampling, compared with arterial blood. *Pediatrics* **51**, 501–506 (1973).
36. Olivia, J. V., Spellman, S., Podgainy, M., and Gittleman, B., Earlobe capillary blood for estimating arterial oxygen tension. *J. Am. Med. Assoc.* **223**, 1388 (1973).
37. Oxygen therapy in the newborn infant. Statement by the Fetus and Newborn Committee of the Canadian Paediatric Society. *Can. Med. Assoc. J.* **113**, 750 (1975).
38. Karna, P., and Poland, R. L., Monitoring critically ill newborn infants with digital capillary blood samples: An alternative. *J. Pediatr.* **92**, 270–273 (1978).
39. Evans, N. T. S., and Naylor, P. F. D., The systematic oxygen supply to the surface of human skin. *Respir. Physiol.* **3**, 21–37 (1967).
40. Huch, R., Lübbers, D. W., and Huch, A., Reliability of transcutaneous monitoring of arterial p_{O_2} in new born infants. *Arch. Dis. Child.* **49**, 213–218 (1974).

41. Huch, R., Huch, A., Albani, M., Gabriel, M., Schulte, F. J., Wolf, H., Rupprath, G., Emmrich, P., Stechele, U., Duc, G., and Bucher, H., Transcutaneous p_{O_2} monitoring in routine measurement of infants and children with cardiorespiratory problems. *Pediatrics* **57**, 681–690 (1976).

42. Huch, A., and Huch, R., Transcutaneous, noninvasive monitoring of p_{O_2}. *Hosp. Prac.* **11**, 43–52 (1976).

43. Blumenfeld, T. A., Hertelendy, W. G., and Ford, S. H., Simultaneously obtained skin-puncture serum, skin-puncture plasma, and venous serum compared, and effects of warming the skin before puncture. *Clin. Chem.* **23**, 1705–1710 (1977).

44. Moritz, A. R., and Henriques, F. C., Jr., Studies of thermal injury, II. The relative importance of time and surface temperature in the causation of cutaneous burns. *Am. J. Clin. Pathol.* **23**, 695–720 (1947).

45. Blumenfeld, T. A., Turi, G. K., and Blanc, W. A., Optimum site and depth for newborn heel punctures. *Pediatr. Res.* **12**, 444 (1978).

46. Van Steirteghem, A. C., and Young, D. S., Povidone-iodine ("Betadine") disinfectant as a source of error. *Clin. Chem.* **23**, 1512 (1977).

47. Lilien, L. D., Harris, V. J., Ramamurthy, R. S., and Pildes, R. S., Neonatal osteomyelitis of the calcaneus: Complication of heel puncture. *J. Pediatr.* **88**, 478–480 (1976).

48. Fenton, L. J., Bertie, B., Gaines, J., and Cipriani, J., A superior method for obtaining blood from the heel of the newborn infant. *Clin. Pediatr.* **16**, 815–816 (1977).

49. Haymond, R. E., and Knight, J. A., Venous serum, capillary serum, and capillary plasma compared for use in determinations of lactate dehydrogenase and aspartate aminotransferase activities. *Clin. Chem.* **21**, 896–897 (1975).

50. Lum, G., and Gambino, S. R., A comparison of serum versus heparinized plasma for routine chemistry tests. *Am. J. Clin. Pathol.* **61**, 108–113 (1974).

51. Ladenson, J. H., Tsai, L.-M. B., Michael, J. M., Kessler, G., and Joist, J. H., Serum versus heparinized plasma for eighteen common chemistry tests. *Am. J. Clin. Pathol.* **62**, 545–552 (1974).

52. Goldbloom, R. B., Fischer, E., Reinhold, J., and Hsia, D. Y.-Y., Studies on the mechanical fragility of erythrocytes. I. Normal values for infants and children. *Blood* **8**, 165–169 (1953).

53. Sjöln, S., The resistance of red cells in vitro. *Acta Paediatr. Scand.* **43**, Suppl. 98, 1–92 (1954).

54. Young, D. S., Pestaner, L. C., and Gibberman, V., Effects of drugs on clinical laboratory tests. *Clin. Chem.* **21**, 1D-432D (1975). Special issue.

55. Gambino, S. R., pH and p_{CO_2}. *Stand. Methods Clin. Chem.* **5**, 169–194 (1965).

56. Gambino, S. R., Oxygen, partial pressure (p_{O_2}) electrode method. *Stand. Methods Clin. Chem.* **6**, 171–182 (1970).

57. Michaëlsson, M., and Sjöln, S., Haemolysis in blood samples from newborn infants. *Acta Paediatr. Scand.* **54**, 325–330 (1965).

58. Hicks, J. M., Rowland, G. L., and Buffone, G. J., Evaluation of a new blood-collecting device ("Microtainer") that is suited for pediatric use. *Clin. Chem.* **22**, 2034–2036 (1976).

59. Blumenfeld, T. A., Turi, G. K., and Blanc, W. A., Recommended site and depth of newborn heel skin punctures based on anatomical measurements and histopathology. *Lancet* **i**, 230–233 (1979).

Chapter 4. Some Effects of Growth and Development on Pediatric Clinical Chemistry

Thomas R. Johnson

Physical growth is usually considered a progressive increase in length or height and weight of the individual. Indeed, the body's growth is the net result of an increase in cell number and size of various tissues. However, there are other growth patterns distinctive of parts and organs of the body, as shown in Figure 1. The growth patterns of organ systems are characterized as general, neural, genital, and lymphoid types. Physical development often may be considered as the changes in function, form, or size of various organs and of the organism as a whole. The following discussion illustrates some effects of growth and development on pediatric clinical chemistry.

The liver, for example, tends to follow the general growth pattern. Laboratory tests of liver function show several different patterns of change at the molecular or enzyme levels (1), as seen in Table 1.

Brain weight, the most easily measured index of brain growth, essentially defines the neural growth pattern. Weight of the brain in the newborn is about 300 to 350 g. By one year of age, its weight has more than doubled and is about two-thirds that of the adult. Brain function, possibly at the molecular level, increases tremendously throughout childhood and well into adult life, yet brain weight gain during this time (350 to 400 g) is relatively small (2).

The genital growth pattern is typically that of the testes and ovaries. The uterus of the female fetus and newborn is relatively large. During the early weeks of life the uterus undergoes involution; its later growth tends to parallel that of the ovaries (Figure 2).

The lymphoid system includes the spleen and thymus, lymph nodes, circulating and tissue-bound lymphocytes, and some other characteristic aggregates of lymphoid cells such as the tonsils. The pattern of development followed by lymphoid tissue is somewhat unusual in comparison with other organs and systems. Lymphoid tissue is well-developed at birth but proportionately small; it increases rapidly in relative size until the child is 10 or 11 years old. The child's lymphoid tissue is adult size by about six years of age; the adult size is actually exceeded before puberty, after which the tissues slowly atrophy.

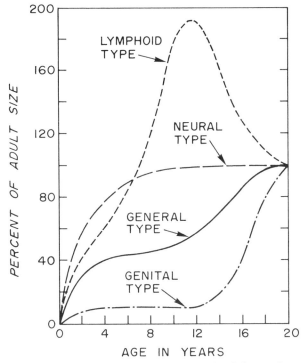

Fig. 1. Main types of postnatal growth of the various parts and organs of the body

After Scammon, The measurement of the body in childhood. In *The Measurement of Man*, Harris et al., University of Minnesota Press, Minneapolis, MN, 1930

Immunologic and Hematologic Tests

Functionally, the infant has the capacity to respond to a large number of antigens at birth. However, there are both quantitative and qualitative differences from the adult, which can be illustrated by a variety of differences between adult and child responses and differences in reference (normal) values for laboratory test results. Prolonged or "excessive" IgM antibody synthesis, the hallmark of the immature immunologic response, is seen after congenital intrauterine infections or after immunization of the young infant. The normal infant, born without significant antigenic stimulation, has little circulating IgM and IgA; IgG is almost completely derived from the mother by selective transport across the placenta. This exogenous (maternal) source of immunoglobulin suppresses the ability of the infant to synthesize his or her own IgG. As the maternal IgG (half-life about 21 days) is catabolized, its concentration in the infant de-

Table 1. Age-Related Changes in Size and Function of the Liver (1)

Age	Mean wt, g		Distance below costal margin, cm	BSP clearance, %[a]	Enzyme acty, U/L		Total cholesterol	Total bilirubin	Direct bilirubin
	M	F			Aspartate aminotransferase	Alanine aminotransferase		mg/dL	
Neonate									
Birth	124	125		10–20	16–74	1–25	50–120	<12	0–1
1–5 d	300	240	1.8	4	9–67	16–36	70–190	<1	0–1
Infant (1–12 mo)			1.5	5			135–250	<1	0–1
Preschool									
2 yr	400	390	1.1						
3 yr	460	450	1.0		6–30	7–23			
4 yr	510	500	0.6						
5 yr	555	550	1.0		5–25				
School child									
8 yr	665	685	0.9	5	26–28	2–15	135–250	<1	0–1
10 yr	770	810	1.0		24–27				
Adolescence									
12 yr	950	960	1.2	5	22–23	2–15	135–250	<1	0–1
14 yr	1150	1180	0.9		20–22				
Adult	1630	1415		5	4–40	4–35	130–270	<1	0–1

[a] Clearance of 5 mg of sulfobromophthalein per kilogram of body wt. in 45 min.

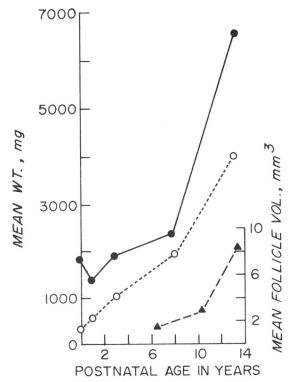

Fig. 2. Increments in ovarian (○) and uterine (●) weights and volumes of largest atretic follicles (▲) in human ovaries from birth to 14 years of age

Adapted from Ross, G. T., and Vande Wiele, R. L., The ovaries. In *Textbook of Endocrinology*, 5th ed., R. H. Williams, Ed. W. B. Saunders Co., Philadelphia, PA, 1974, p 372. Used with permission

creases to about 200 to 300 mg/dL by about six months of age. The adult concentration of IgM is reached at about one year of age, IgG at about five years, and IgA at about 10 years *(3)*.

Diagnosis of a suspected immunoglobulin deficiency in early childhood depends on accurate interpretation of several screening tests:

1. *Total and fractional protein determination.* Both low total protein and a high albumin/globulin ratio are anticipated because of the lower total globulin concentration (Tables 2 and 3).

2. *Isohemagglutinin determination.* Naturally occurring antibodies to the blood-group substances, mostly of the IgM class, are consistently present after about two years of age in all normal individuals of blood groups A, B, or O (Table 3). Their absence is presumptive evidence of IgM deficiency.

Table 2. Relation of Serum Protein Concentrations (g/dL) to Age: Mean ± 1 SD, and Range

	Total proteins	Albumin	Alpha-1	Alpha-2	Beta	Gamma
Cord blood:	6.22 ± 1.21 (4.78–8.04)	3.23 ± 0.82 (2.17–4.04)	0.41 ± 0.10 (0.25–0.66)	0.68 ± 0.14 (0.44–0.94)	0.74 ± 0.30 (0.42–1.56)	1.28 ± 0.23 (0.81–1.61)
1–3 mo:	5.64 ± 1.04 (3.64–7.38)	3.41 ± 0.72 (2.05–4.46)	0.24 ± 0.09 (0.08–0.43)	0.74 ± 0.24 (0.40–1.13)	0.59 ± 0.20 (0.39–1.14)	0.66 ± 0.24 (0.25–1.05)
4–6 mo:	5.43 ± 0.84 (4.29–6.10)	3.46 ± 0.36 (3.17–3.88)	0.17 ± 0.04 (0.12–0.25)	0.67 ± 0.11 (0.52–0.84)	0.61 ± 0.14 (0.44–0.76)	0.61 ± 0.26 (0.24–0.90)
7–12 mo:	6.54 ± 0.76 (5.10–7.31)	3.62 ± 0.60 (3.22–4.31)	0.35 ± 0.15 (0.15–0.55)	0.99 ± 0.30 (0.78–1.46)	0.79 ± 0.16 (0.63–0.91)	0.84 ± 0.36 (0.32–1.18)
13–24 mo:	6.66 ± 0.93 (3.69–7.50)	3.63 ± 0.80 (1.89–5.03)	0.31 ± 0.15 (0.09–0.58)	0.88 ± 0.42 (0.41–1.36)	0.77 ± 0.31 (0.36–1.41)	1.09 ± 0.32 (0.36–1.62)
25–36 mo:	6.98 ± 0.48 (6.38–8.06)	4.11 ± 0.78 (3.57–5.50)	0.23 ± 0.09 (0.19–0.26)	0.89 ± 0.14 (0.68–1.09)	0.67 ± 0.14 (0.47–0.91)	1.08 ± 0.28 (0.73–1.46)
3–5 yr:	6.65 ± 0.85 (4.88–8.06)	3.95 ± 0.57 (2.93–5.21)	0.21 ± 0.08 (0.08–0.40)	0.70 ± 0.15 (0.43–0.99)	0.67 ± 0.11 (0.47–1.01)	1.13 ± 0.31 (0.54–1.66)
6–8 yr:	6.95 ± 0.55 (5.97–7.94)	4.03 ± 0.45 (3.26–4.95)	0.22 ± 0.09 (0.09–0.45)	0.67 ± 0.10 (0.50–0.83)	0.72 ± 0.11 (0.45–0.93)	1.31 ± 0.32 (0.70–1.95)
9–11 yr:	7.43 ± 0.84 (6.32–9.00)	4.24 ± 0.79 (3.16–4.97)	0.30 ± 0.07 (0.12–0.38)	0.75 ± 0.27 (0.67–0.87)	0.84 ± 0.16 (0.63–1.02)	1.46 ± 0.41 (0.79–2.03)
12–16 yr:	7.25 ± 0.85 (6.25–8.75)	4.26 ± 0.64 (3.19–5.13)	0.19 ± 0.07 (0.09–0.32)	0.71 ± 0.15 (0.50–0.97)	0.68 ± 0.15 (0.48–0.88)	1.40 ± 0.31 (1.08–1.96)
Adult:	7.41 ± 0.96 (6.44–8.32)	4.31 ± 0.59 (3.46–4.78)	0.23 ± 0.06 (0.16–0.30)	0.61 ± 0.14 (0.51–0.86)	0.81 ± 0.22 (0.59–1.06)	1.45 ± 0.46 (0.68–2.11)

Protein fractions determined by cellulose acetate electrophoresis *(4).*

3. *Examination of bone marrow for plasma cells.* This is of diagnostic significance only for children more than five years old; before this, marrow examination of normal infants and children shows very few plasma cells.

4. *Schick test.* Normal individuals who have been adequately immunized with diphtheria toxoid should have a negative reaction to Schick toxin. A positive Schick test in a well-immunized individual is presumptive evidence of IgG deficiency.

5. *Serum electrophoresis on media such as paper or cellulose acetate.* This test indicates the approximate total gamma-globulin content and is generally reliable when gamma-globulin exceeds 500 mg/dL.

6. *Immunoelectrophoresis.* This procedure delineates the three major gamma-globulin classes—IgG, IgM, and IgA.

Confirmation of normal IgG, IgA, and IgM concentration is by a quantitative technique. Table 3 shows the variation in immunoglobulin concentrations with age and the broad range of reference (normal) values. Each laboratory that measures immunoglobulins should establish its own set of age-related reference values. Results of immuni-

*Table 3. Relation of Immunoglobulin and Isohemagglutinin (IHA)
Concentrations to Age* (4)

Age	Mean ± 1 SD (and range), mg/dL			Mean IHA titer (and range)
	IgG	IgA	IgM	
Cord blood:	1086 ± 290 (740–1374)	2 ± 2 (0–15)	14 ± 6 (0–22)	0 [a]
1–3 mo:	512 ± 152 (280–950)	16 ± 10 (4–36)	28 ± 14 (15–86)	1:5 [b] (0–1:10)
4–6 mo:	520 ± 180 (240–884)	22 ± 14 (11–52)	36 ± 18 (21–74)	1:10 [b] (0–1:160)
7–12 mo:	742 ± 226 (281–1280)	54 ± 17 (22–112)	76 ± 27 (36–150)	1:80 [c] (0–1:640)
13–24 mo:	945 ± 270 (290–1300)	67 ± 19 (9–143)	88 ± 36 (18–210)	1:80 [c] (0–1:640)
25–36 mo:	1030 ± 152 (546–1562)	89 ± 34 (21–196)	94 ± 23 (43–115)	1:160 [d] (1:10–1:640)
3–5 yr:	1150 ± 244 (546–1760)	126 ± 31 (56–284)	87 ± 24 (26–121)	1:80 (1:5–1:640)
6–8 yr:	1187 ± 289 (596–1744)	147 ± 35 (56–330)	108 ± 37 (54–260)	1:80 (1:5–1:640)
9–11 yr:	1217 ± 261 (744–1719)	146 ± 38 (44–208)	104 ± 46 (27–215)	1:160 (1:20–1:640)
12–16 yr:	1248 ± 221 (796–1647)	168 ± 54 (64–290)	96 ± 31 (60–140)	1:160 (1:10–1:320)
Adult:	1274 ± 280 (664–1825)	227 ± 53 (59–311)	127 ± 46 (45–205)	1:160 (1:10–1:640)

[a] Isohemagglutinin activity is rarely detectable in cord blood.
[b] 50% of normal infants will not have isohemagglutinins at this age.
[c] 10% of normal infants will not have isohemagglutinins at this age.
[d] Beyond this age all normal individuals (except blood type AB) have isohemagglutinins.
Immunoglobulins determined by immunochemical techniques.

zation with well-characterized antigens (e.g., diphtheria toxoid, teta-
nus toxoid, salmonella vaccine), in terms of specific antibody produced
and plasma cell development, also may be used to establish immuno-
competence *(4)*.

The thymus appears to confer specific immune properties to certain
leukocytes, termed T cells or T lymphocytes. Whether the lability
of the thymus weight during infancy and childhood has any relationship to counts of circulating leukocyte is unknown. The extreme
variability of leukocyte counts in the newborn, for example, has led
to skepticism concerning their diagnostic value. Christensen and
Rathstein *(5)* compared counts of leukocytes obtained from capillary
blood from heel punctures with those from arterial and venous blood
samples obtained simultaneously from indwelling umbilical arterial

and venous catheters. They found that arterial samples had a lower leukocyte count (77% of the capillary count), and venous samples were also consistently lower. Perhaps more importantly, in counts made before and after procedures that caused vigorous crying (circumcision, physical therapy of the chest, or heel puncture), the total leukocyte count increased an average of 146%. Sixty minutes appeared to be sufficient for the counts to return to baseline values after a stressful procedure. The data from this study indicate that in any single neonate the total leukocyte count varies according to the site of sampling and the muscular activity or stress of the infant. It would be interesting to study older infants and children to determine whether similar responses occur and, if so, to elucidate the mechanisms involved. These effects are important because high leukocyte counts may lead the clinician mistakenly to suspect an infection.

The range of reference values at a given age or stage of development, as well as other variables that may affect tests, enables the clinician to interpret the blood picture of a specific infant or child. For example, reports of "normal childhood values" have exhibited considerable variation. Defining reliable normal standards has been complicated by differences in methods, insufficient numbers of observations at different ages, mixing data of premature and full-term newborns, and incomplete data. The hematologic status of infants and children has been investigated extensively, and many of these complicating factors have been eliminated. Although Tables 4 and 5 were prepared from data obtained several years ago, more recent hematologic indices obtained with an electronic cell counter for infants up to 12 weeks old are similar. Table 6 defines the "lower limits of normal" for hemoglobin concentration and packed cell volume (hematocrit) for individuals of a given age. Until better standards are devised, values less than these represent anemia. Recent observations indicate that the average hemoglobin concentration of American blacks is approximately 1 g/dL less than that of whites. Whether this difference is due to a genetic mechanism or to environmental conditions is still unknown.

From birth until approximately one week of age, hemoglobin concentration and packed cell volume measurements are higher for capillary (skin-puncture) blood samples than for venous blood samples; in the first few hours after birth these results may differ by as much as 22%. This difference gradually diminishes during the first week of life.

Within one or two days after birth, the bone marrow becomes relatively hypoactive, resulting in a gradual decline in hemoglobin concentration during the first few weeks of neonatal life. This "physiologic anemia" is more marked in the premature infant than in the full-term one, but does not cause impaired oxygenation because the decreasing concentration of hemoglobin F (fetal hemoglobin) and

Table 4. Hematologic Values (Mean ± 1 SD) for Full-Term Infants, Children, and Adults (6)

Age	Hemoglobin (Hb), g/dL	Hematocrit (packed RBC vol), mL/dL	Erythrocytes (red cell count), $10^6/\mu L$	Mean corpuscular vol (MCV), μm^3/erythrocyte	Mean corpuscular hemoglobin (MCH), pg/erythrocyte	Mean corpuscular hemoglobin concn (MCHC), g/dL of erythrocytes
Cord blood	17.1 ± 1.8	52 ± 5	4.64 ± 0.5	113 ± 6	37 ± 2	33 ± 1
1 d	19.4 ± 2.1	58 ± 7	5.3 ± 0.5	110 ± 6	37 ± 2	33 ± 1
2–6 d	19.8 ± 2.4	66 ± 8	5.4 ± 0.7	122 ± 14	37 ± 4	30 ± 3
14–23 d	15.7 ± 1.5	52 ± 5	4.92 ± 0.6	106 ± 11	32 ± 3	30 ± 2
24–37 d	14.1 ± 1.9	45 ± 7	4.35 ± 0.6	104 ± 11	32 ± 3	31 ± 3
30–50 d	12.8 ± 1.9	42 ± 6	4.1 ± 0.5	103 ± 11	31 ± 3	30 ± 2
2–2.5 mo	11.4 ± 1.1	38 ± 4	3.75 ± 0.5	101 ± 10	30 ± 3	30 ± 2
3–3.5 mo	11.2 ± 0.8	37 ± 3	3.88 ± 0.4	95 ± 9	29 ± 3	30 ± 2
5–7 mo	11.5 ± 0.7	38 ± 3	4.21 ± 0.5	91 ± 9	27 ± 3	30 ± 2
8–10 mo	11.7 ± 0.6	39 ± 2	4.35 ± 0.4	90 ± 8	27 ± 3	30 ± 1
11–13.5 mo	11.9 ± 0.6[a]	39 ± 2	4.44 ± 0.4[a]	88 ± 7[a,b]	27 ± 2	30 ± 1
1.5–3 yr	11.8 ± 0.5	39 ± 2	4.45 ± 0.4	87 ± 7[b]	27 ± 2	30 ± 2
5 yr	12.7 ± 1.0	37 ± 3	4.65 ± 0.5	80 ± 4[b]	27 ± 2	34 ± 1
10 yr	13.2 ± 1.2	39 ± 3	4.80 ± 0.5	81 ± 6	28 ± 3	34 ± 1
Adults						
M	15.5 ± 1.1	46 ± 3.1	5.11 ± 0.38	90.1 ± 4.8[c]	30.2 ± 1.8[c]	33.7 ± 1.1[c]
F	13.7 ± 1.0	40.9 ± 3	4.51 ± 0.36			

[a] Three months after administration of 250 mg of elemental iron to normal infants (to exclude iron depletion): Hb, 12.3 (11.1–13.7) g/dL; erythrocytes, 4.98 (4.2–5.5) × $10^6/\mu L$; MCV, 78.9 (70–84) μm^3/erythrocyte; MCHC, 31 (30–33) g/dL of erythrocytes.
[b] Recent data establish the lower limits of normal for MCV (μm^3/erythrocyte) at 10 to 17 mo of age as 70, at 1.5 to 4 yr as 74, at 4 to 7 yr as 76. These values are helpful when the MCV is used as a screening test for iron-deficiency anemia and thalassemia trait.
[c] Average of M & F values.

Table 5. Hematologic Values (Mean ± 1 SD) for Low-Birth-Weight Infants (6)

Wt and gestational age at birth	Age at testing	Hemoglobin, g/dL	Hematocrit, mg/dL	Reticulocytes, %
<1500 g, 28–32 wk	3 d	17.5 ± 1.5	54 ± 5	8.0 ± 3.5
	1 wk	15.5 ± 1.5	48 ± 5	3.0 ± 1.0
	2 wk	13.5 ± 1.1	42 ± 4	3.0 ± 1.0
	3 wk	11.5 ± 1.0	35 ± 4	—
	4 wk	10.0 ± 0.9	30 ± 3	6.0 ± 2.0
	6 wk	8.5 ± 0.5	25 ± 2	11.0 ± 3.5
	8 wk	8.5 ± 0.5	25 ± 2	8.5 ± 3.5
	10 wk	9.0 ± 0.5	28 ± 3	7.0 ± 3.0
1500–2000 g, 32–36 wk	3 d	19.0 ± 2.0	59 ± 6	6.0 ± 2.0
	1 wk	16.5 ± 1.5	51 ± 5	3.0 ± 1.0
	2 wk	14.5 ± 1.1	44 ± 5	2.5 ± 1.0
	3 wk	13.0 ± 1.1	39 ± 4	—
	4 wk	12.0 ± 1.0	36 ± 4	3.0 ± 1.0
	6 wk	9.5 ± 0.8	28 ± 3	6.0 ± 2.0
	8 wk	9.5 ± 0.5	28 ± 3	5.0 ± 1.5
	10 wk	9.5 ± 0.5	29 ± 3	4.5 ± 1.5
2000–2500 g, 36–40 wk	3 d	19.0 ± 2.0	59 ± 6	4.0 ± 1.0
	1 wk	16.5 ± 1.5	51 ± 5	3.0 ± 1.0
	2 wk	15.0 ± 1.5	45 ± 5	2.5 ± 1.0
	3 wk	14.0 ± 1.1	43 ± 4	—
	4 wk	12.5 ± 1.0	37 ± 4	2.0 ± 1.0
	6 wk	10.5 ± 0.9	31 ± 3	3.0 ± 1.0
	8 wk	10.5 ± 0.9	31 ± 3	3.0 ± 1.0
	10 wk	11.0 ± 1.0	33 ± 3	3.0 ± 1.0

increasing concentration of erythrocyte 2,3-diphosphoglycerate shifts the hemoglobin–oxygen dissociation curve to the right. These changes allow the hemoglobin to "unload" relatively more oxygen at the tissue partial pressure of oxygen ($p_{O_2} = 40$ mmHg).

At approximately two months of age, erythropoiesis increases, thereby increasing the proportion of reticulocytes in the blood and, gradually, the hemoglobin concentration. If adequate amounts of iron and other essential nutrients are provided, the infant maintains a total erythrocyte volume commensurate with overall rate of growth (6).

Thyroid-Function Tests

The thyroid gland also profoundly affects growth and development. A normally functioning thyroid gland promotes body growth, skeletal

Table 6. *Lower Limits of Normal Hemoglobin and Hematocrit at Sea Level, by Age* (6)

Age	Hemoglobin, g/dL	Hematocrit, %
7 mo–4 yr	11.0	33
5–9 yr	11.5	34.5
10–14 yr	12.0	36
Adult, M	14.0	42
Adult, F	12.0	36
Pregnant women	11.0	33

maturation, brain differentiation, normal mental development, increased metabolic rate, and normal cutaneous texture, including growth and luster of hair. These are undoubtedly not separate functions but rather part of a total pattern regulated by thyroid hormones.

The diagnosis of thyroid disorders has particular significance in pediatric patients. Diseases of the thyroid gland usually present with recognizable clinical manifestations. At times, however, clinical diagnosis is difficult (e.g., in hypothyroidism), and biochemical confirmation becomes necessary.

Numerous laboratory tests have been devised for diagnosis of thyroid disorders. This diversity is largely attributable to the complex mechanisms of biosynthesis, distribution, metabolism, and regulatory systems of thyroid hormones. An added requisite in pediatrics is the awareness of age-related alterations in the concentration of thyroid hormones, because the values observed differ between pre-term and full-term infants, between neonates and older children, and between older children and adolescents (Tables 7–9).

Recently, mass screening for infantile thyroid dysfunction has been undertaken because hypothyroidism ranks high among the metabolic disorders that lead to mental deficiency. Replacement therapy based on early diagnosis restores physiologic function and prevents mental retardation. A filter-paper technique for the measurement of tetraiodothyronine (thyroxine, T_4) and thyroid-stimulating hormone (TSH; thyrotropin) is now used in neonatal nationwide screening programs.

Thyroid-function tests are based on examining:

1. Biosynthetic pathway metabolites (blood concentration of thyroid hormones or incorporation of precursors). Tests based on hormonal biosynthetic pathways include radioactive iodine uptake (RAIU), thyroid scintigram, and the perchlorate discharge test; those based on blood concentrations include protein-bound iodine (PBI), total and free T_4 and triiodothyronine (T_3), free T_4 index and resin T_3 uptake (RT_3U), and thyroid-binding globulin (TBG) capacity and (or) concentration.

2. Hormones that regulate thyroid gland function, including tests

Table 7. Thyroxine Concentration at Various Ages, as Measured by RIA (7)

Age	No.	Thyroxine, μg/dL		
		Mean	SE	Range
Premature, cord blood gestation age:	2683[a]			
30 wk		9.4		5.7–15.6
35 wk		10.1		6.1–16.8
40 wk		10.9		6.6–18.1
45 wk		11.7		7.1–19.4
Full-term neonates (h after birth):				
1	12	12.5		
18	13	13.5		
24	21	16		
68	18	14.5		
96	6	13		
120	6	12.5		
Infants, 6 wk:	15	10.3	0.4	7.8–12.7
Children:				
1 yr		11.0		
1–5 yr		10.5		7.3–15.0
5–10 yr		9.3		6.4–13.3
10–15 yr		8.1		5.6–11.7
15 yr		7.6		
Adolescents, M:				
Tanner Stage I	25	10.7	0.2	
II	25	9.4	0.3	
III	16	8.9	0.5	
IV	11	8.5	0.4	
V	11	8.4	0.6	
Adolescents, F:				
Tanner Stage I	14	10.1	0.4	
II	14	10.3	0.4	
III	10	10.2	0.6	
IV	11	8.9	0.4	
V	13	10.8	0.4	
Adults, 21–45 yr:	33	8.3	1.7	

[a] Total no. of premature infants.

for thyroid-releasing factor (TRF; thyroliberin) and TSH concentrations, TRF stimulation, and T_3 suppression.

3. Metabolism of thyroid hormones (these tests are of little clinical use, however).

4. Metabolic effects of thyroid hormones, including tests for basal metabolic rate, bone age from roentgenograms, serum cholesterol, alkaline phosphatase, carotene, blood urea nitrogen (BUN), and hemoglobin concentrations.

5. Immune mechanisms, including tests for thyroglobulin and mi-

Table 8. Triiodothyronine Concentration at Various Ages as Measured by RIA (7)

Age	T_3, ng/dL			
	No.	Mean	SE	Range
Full-term neonates,	114	97.5	1.0	80–120
cord blood:	29	48	3.0	11–90
	26	50.5	3.6	
Full-term neonates, time after birth:				
15 min	6	79	13	44–136
1 h	12	293		
1.5 h	6	191	16	136–231
24 h	4	262	41	182–353
24 h	15	419		
48 h	4	191	37	127–287
69 h	19	220		
72 h	26	125	8	63–256
Children:	195[a]			
1 yr		176		
1–5 yr		168		105–269
5–10 yr		150		94–241
10–15 yr		133		83–213
15 yr		125		
Adolescents, M:				
Tanner Stage I	25	139	4	
II	25	121	5	
III	16	134	7	
IV	11	146	7	
V	11	131	8	
Adolescents, F:				
Tanner Stage I	14	140	5	
II	14	143	5	
III	10	139	10	
IV	11	137	6	
V	13	128	6	
Adults, 21–45 yr:	33	126	23	

[a] Total no. of children.

crosomal antibodies, long-acting thyroid stimulator (LATS), and lymphocyte function.

6. Morphology and histochemical characteristics of thyroid tissue, to aid in the diagnosis of chronic lymphocytic thyroiditis, certain enzyme deficiencies, and thyroid gland malignancy.

Many data have been published on new tests of thyroid-hormone concentration in the normal young population, but often only on a small number of subjects and involving use of different laboratory methods. The values from cord blood, newborns, toddlers, school children, and young adults presented in Tables 7 through 9 are de-

Table 9. Thyroid-Stimulating Hormone (Thyrotropin) Concentration at Various Ages, as Measured by RIA (7)

Age	No.	TSH, micro-int. units/mL		
		Mean	**SE**	**Range**
Neonates (cord blood), gestation age:				
22–24 wk	22	9.6	0.93	2.4–20
38–40 wk	16	9.6	0.93	
Full-term	98	9.6		u–33 [a]
Full-term	20	5.5		2.1–10.7
Full-term neonates, time after birth:				
10 min	11	61	7.9	11–99
30 min	20	86	6.8	13–149
1 h	16	68	4.8	43–92
1.5 h	22	49	3.9	12–80
2 h	7	48	9.4	14–80
3 h	15	37	4.2	16–72
24 h	7	17.1	3.0	8.6–33
48 h	12	12.8	1.9	5.0–23.0
Children, 1–15 yr:	195	1.9		0.6–6.3
Adolescents, M:				
Tanner Stage I	25	8.5	0.6	
II	23	8.7	0.5	
III	16	10.8	1.0	
IV	11	12.5	1.2	
V	11	15.7	2.7	
Adolescents, F:				
Tanner Stage I	13	10.5	0.9	
II	14	9.8	1.6	
III	10	7.4	1.4	
IV	11	8.3	2.5	
V	13	8.9	1.1	
Adults, 21–45 yr:	33	3.1	0.6	

[a] u, undetectable.

rived from papers in which a large number of specimens have been analyzed and the same radioimmunoassay (RIA) has been used.

Serum T_4 by RIA is lower in the cord blood of prematures than in full-term infants. The serum T_4 increases in full-term infants to a peak 24 h after birth, then decreases during the next five days. From age one to 15 years, the concentration of serum T_4 gradually drops. Although boys experience a gradual decrease in T_4 values by RIA as they mature sexually, girls do not.

Serum T_3 by RIA peaks at about 24 h of age. Over the next 15 years the T_3 concentration decreases to a nadir, where it remains during early adult life. In neither sex does T_3 change with sexual development.

The concentration of TSH in cord blood is greater in prematures than in full-term infants. During the first minutes after birth, TSH increases rapidly and peaks about 30 min after birth, then decreases steadily over the next 48 h. During childhood, TSH concentrations are relatively stable: In boys there is a significant increase as sexual maturation progresses; in girls no significant change occurs with sexual maturation.

For assessing thyroid function, determination of serum T_4 concentration by RIA is satisfactory. Generally, no other determination is necessary. Rarely, T_3 by RIA will also be helpful. A few patients with clinical hyperthyroidism have normal serum T_4 but high T_3, or "T_3 toxicosis" (7).

Tests of Carbohydrate Metabolism

The oral glucose-tolerance test (OGTT), while useful in the diagnosis of diabetes mellitus, is often of little value and is difficult to interpret in the child with idiopathic hypoglycemia. The addition of concurrent hormone assays, especially insulin, has stimulated renewed interest in this test.

Concentrations of plasma insulin measured by RIA in the basal, postabsorptive, or fasting states are low in young term or pre-term infants, comparable with values found only after prolonged fasting in the adult. Depending on the sensitivity of the assay, activities have varied from 2 to 30 micro-USP units/mL. The plasma-sampling site is important in the newborn because the prehepatic portal system sampled via an umbilical catheter can give results quite different from those obtained at a peripheral venous or arterial sampling site. Portal venous blood contains the highest insulin concentration, because hepatic extraction is very high (at least 50% in the adult). There is no definitive information on hepatic extraction of insulin in the very young, but simultaneous sampling of portal and peripheral venous blood during an OGTT indicates significant differences. Some investigators have commented on the wide variations of basal plasma insulin values in pre-term infants less than 24 h after birth, and have also observed no relationship between plasma insulin and glucose. Urinary excretion of insulin in the healthy newborn increases sixfold between the first and fifth day of life. Excretion is independent of renal function.

The OGTT, properly performed, is valuable, especially in absorptive defects, e.g., monosaccharide malabsorption and celiac disease. Normal fasting blood glucose values vary between 50 and 90 mg/dL. The insulin peak occurs by 30 min after glucose ingestion, with a median of 60 micro-USP units/mL. Insulin concentrations in children tend to be less than in adults. A flat OGTT curve may indicate failure of absorption, from various causes. A diphasic curve has been observed in glycogen storage disease.

The *intravenous* glucose tolerance test circumvents the variability of gastrointestinal motility and absorption, but is of limited diagnostic value. Various doses and techniques have been used, and several techniques for analyzing the data have been used in children and adults. The absolute values from 5 to 60 min after infusion may be plotted semilogarithmically, with log glucose concentration on the ordinate and time (in minutes) on the abscissa. Alternatively, the difference between each value and the fasting blood sugar value may be similarly plotted. At least four points must be plotted; a straight line is usually obtained between 10 and 45 min. The slope of this line is the glucose disappearance rate, expressed as percent per minute. Results during the initial hour of the tolerance test are used to determine a single rate constant. In diabetes mellitus the disappearance rate is slow; in hyperinsulinism the rate is rapid.

The later portion of the prolonged intravenous GTT (60 to 360 min) indicates glucose homeostasis and rebound. Usually, a slight hypoglycemic dip below the control fasting concentration is observed at 75 to 90 min, with stabilization by 120 min. In some hypoglycemic states with a rapid initial rate, failure of maintenance of normal blood sugar is indicated by a hypoglycemic phase that persists between 60 and 360 min. This is why the prolonged period of observation is recommended *(8)*.

Carbohydrate Digestion and Absorption Tests

Carbohydrate digestion begins in the mouth with the action of salivary amylase on starch. Gastric acidity in the adult rapidly inactivates salivary amylase, but the low production of gastric acid by the infant may not be as effective in inactivating salivary amylase in the infant; salivary amylase approaches adult values, but pancreatic amylase does not reach adult values for several months after birth (Tables 10 and 11). Thus, salivary amylase may play a more important role in starch digestion for the infant than for the adult. Human milk and cow-milk-based formulas, the primary food sources of infants, provide carbohydrate in the form of lactose. Some infants receive commercially prepared formulas containing various amounts of sucrose and (or) partly hydrolyzed starch (dextrins). As indicated in Figure 3, sucrase and maltase attain maximum activity by the eighth month of gestation, whereas the increase in lactase activity occurs closer to term. Infants born during the seventh and eighth months of gestation may be able to hydrolyze only about one-third the quantity of lactose hydrolyzed by full-term infants after the first day of life. The fact that otherwise healthy premature infants are relatively deficient in intestinal lactase activity provides the basis for providing low-lactose feedings in the dietary management of premature infants *(9)*.

Table 10. Development of Digestive Enzymes (9)

Age	Gastric analysis					Mean glucose absorption, mg/h per cm of bowel
	Mean HCl production[a]	Mean vol of gastric juice, mL/h	Pepsin, mean pg/h per kg of body wt	Intrinsic factor, mean[b]	Serum gastrin, pg/mL (mean ± SEM)	
Birth	8.1/0.01	3.3	40	8	64 ± 125	70[c]
3–8 d	14.4/0.02	3.7	60	17.8	151 ± 15.8	
10–17 d	34.4/0.12	4.0	150	29.2	—	
25–32 d	26.4/0.02	6.4	240	27.9	193 ± 28	
60–90 d	34.8/0.01	13.4	280	34.4	—	
4–9 yr	114.2/0.1	42.5	—	79.5	215 ± 37	
Adult	91.2/0.19	143.2	600	78.7	<90	200[d]

[a] Titratable acid obtained during 1 h of intermittent suction after administration of Histalog, 1.0 mg/kg of body wt; values expressed as ratio of (mEq/L) to (mEq/h per kilogram of body wt).
[b] Ratio of hourly output of intrinsic-factor-bound B_{12} to totally bound B_{12} in gastric juice.
[c] In three infants.
[d] In two adults.

Table 11. Development of Digestive Enzymes: Duodenal Fluid Analysis (9)

Age	Mean (and range), per kilogram of body wt[a]				Bile salts	
	Vol, mL	α-Amylase, units[b]	Trypsin, mg[b]	Lipase, U	Total, mmol/L	Glycine/taurine[c]
Premature[d]						
Birth, before feeding	44 (4.3–152)	0.88 (0–3.6)	60 (0–482)	77 (3–343)		
24 h after first feeding	55 (16–98)	0.62 (0.2–1.4)	43 (1.6–148)	66 (2–209)	<2	<2/1
1 wk	82 (17–168)	2.07 (0.2–8.2)	233 (5–660)	329 (7–1249)		
4 wk	90 (34–187)	1.67 (0–4.6)	196 (0.9–660)	284 (11–730)		
Children, 9 mo–13 yr	390 (180–810)	665 (160–2150)	765 (215–2000)	1465 (350–5000)	>2	>2/1

[a] 50 min after injections of pancreozymin (2 units/kg) and secretin (2 units/kg).
[b] Full-term infants had slightly lower enzyme activities 1 wk after birth.
[c] Ratio of glycine conjugates to taurine conjugates.
[d] n = 36, wt = 2.0 to 2.4 kg.

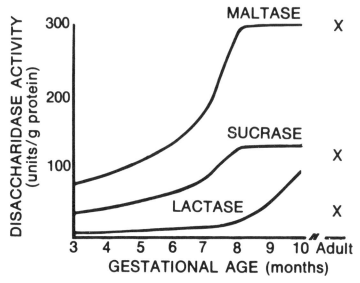

Fig. 3. Disaccharidase activity in jejunal mucosa of human fetus in relation to lunar months of gestational age

Modified from Auricchio, S., et al., *Pediatrics* **35,** 944 (1965), and reproduced from ref. *9*

These are but a few examples of how age, stage of development, and other variables are important to proper interpretation of pediatric clinical chemistry values. At a time of increasing precision in laboratory methods, knowledge of techniques and variables affecting results is essential to the physician who must interpret and act on the results of these tests.

1. Johnson, T. R., Development of the liver. In *Children Are Different: Developmental Physiology,* 2nd ed., T. R. Johnson, W. M. Moore, and J. E. Jeffries, Eds. Ross Laboratories, Columbus, OH, 1978, pp 155–160.
2. Johnson, T. R., Morphologic development of the brain and the appearance of reflexes. *Ibid.,* pp 31–37.
3. Frenkel, L. D., and Bellanti, J. A., Development and function of the lymphoid system. *Ibid.,* pp 177–183.
4. Park, B. H., and Ellis, E. F., Changes in serum protein and immunoglobulins with age. *Ibid.,* pp 185–189.
5. Christensen, R. D., and Rathstein, G., Pitfalls in the interpretation of leukocyte counts of newborn infants. *Am. J. Clin. Pathol.* **72,** 608–611 (1979).
6. Shumway, C. N., Development of the red blood cell and hemoglobin. In *Children Are Different (op. cit.),* pp 197–201.
7. Abbassi, V., Aceto, F., Jr., and Hung, W., Thyroid function in relation to age. *Ibid.,* pp 79–89.
8. Cornblath, M., Pancreatic function in relation to age. *Ibid.,* pp 161–175.
9. Greene, H. L., Gastrointestinal development. *Ibid.,* pp 149–154.

Chapter 5. Analytes

This chapter lists reference (normal) ranges for children for a wide variety of analytes, as reported by many clinical laboratories, primarily those in pediatric centers. The ranges presented are based on the mean value ± 2 SD, unless otherwise indicated. For a further discussion of the details of analyte presentations and what they include, see Chapter 1.

Acetaminophen

Specimen Tested:

P.

Laboratory Reporting:

1.

Reference (Normal) Values:

Therapeutic range: 10–20 mg/L
Toxic concentration: related to interval between drug ingestion and measurement in plasma; see nomogram (Figure 1).

Sources of Reference (Normal) Values:

Rumack, B. H., and Matthew, H., Acetaminophen poisoning and toxicity. *Pediatrics* **55,** 871–876 (1975).

Specimen Volume, and Collection:

1 mL. Avoid heparin as anticoagulant.

Analytical Method and Instrumentation:

Glynn, J. P., and Kendal, S. E., Paracetamol measurement. *Lancet* **i,** 1147–1148 (1975); Mace, P. F. K., and Walker, G., Salicylate interference with plasma-paracetamol method. *Lancet* **ii,** 1362 (1976); Wiener, K., and Hooper, J., Plasma-paracetamol estimation. *Lancet* **i,** 701 (1976). Spectrophotometer.

Commentary—J. Gilbert Hill

Acetaminophen is widely used as an alternative to acetylsalicylic acid in the treatment of mild pain and fever, and normally is well tolerated by patients of all ages. However, accidental or deliberate

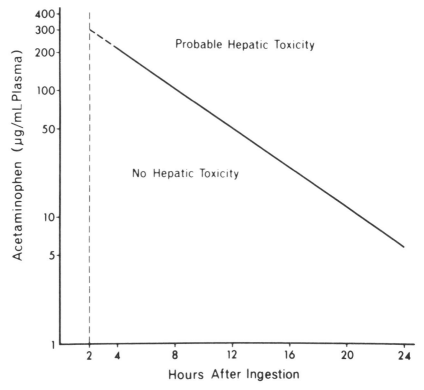

Fig. 1. Nomogram of plasma or serum acetaminophen concentration vs. time since acetaminophen ingestion

From *1*, used with permission

overdose can lead to serious hepatic toxicity, and a significant number of deaths have been attributed to the drug.

Acetaminophen is normally quickly absorbed from the upper gastrointestinal tract, with peak concentrations in plasma occurring 1 h after therapeutic doses and by 4 h after an overdose.

When given in therapeutic amounts, most of the drug is metabolized in the liver to form nontoxic sulfate and glucuronide conjugates, which are excreted in urine. In addition, a small portion of the drug is metabolized by the cytochrome P-450 mixed-function oxidase enzyme system to form a potentially toxic intermediate, which is rendered harmless by reaction with hepatic glutathione. With an overdose of acetaminophen, the sulfate and glucuronide pathways become saturated, forcing a larger amount of the drug to be metabolized via the P-450 pathway. In turn, the capacity of the hepatic glutathione to inactivate the potentially toxic intermediate is exceeded, resulting in hepatic cellular necrosis.

N-Acetylcysteine has been shown to be a very effective antidote to acetaminophen overdose, probably by restoring hepatic glutathione amounts to normal, or by acting as an alternative substrate for detoxification of the toxic intermediate. The decision to treat with N-acetylcysteine requires knowledge of plasma acetaminophen concentrations in relation to the time since drug ingestion, and a valuable nomogram (Figure 1) has been provided by Rumack and Matthew *(1).*

Relatively simple spectrophotometric techniques have been very valuable for measuring acetaminophen in plasma *(2–4),* but the need for a correction factor to compensate for coexisting salicylate *(5)* or the use of an extraction step *(6)* implies a potentially hazardous lack of specificity. The measurement technique of choice is currently HPLC *(7).*

1. Rumack, B. H., and Matthew, H., Acetaminophen poisoning and toxicity. *Pediatrics* **55,** 871–876 (1975).
2. Glynn, J. P., and Kendal, S. E., Paracetamol measurement. *Lancet* i, 1147–1148 (1975).
3. Mace, P. F. K., and Walker, G., Salicylate interference with plasma-paracetamol method. *Lancet* ii, 1362 (1976).
4. Wiener, K., and Hooper, J., Plasma-paracetamol estimation. *Lancet* i, 701 (1976).
5. Rosenbaum, J. M., Broer, H. H., and Shields, J., Misleading results in cases of coexisting acetaminophen and salicylate overdose. *Clin. Chem.* **26,** 673–674 (1980).
6. Meola, J. M., Emergency determination of acetaminophen. *Clin. Chem.* **24,** 1642–1643 (1978).
7. Miceli, J. N., Aravind, M. K., Cohen, S. N., and Done, A. K., Simultaneous measurements of acetaminophen and salicylate in plasma by liquid chromatography. *Clin. Chem.* **25,** 1002–1004 (1979).

Acetone (Ketone) Screening Test

Specimen Tested:
S, U.

Laboratories Reporting:
2.

Reference (Normal) Values:
Negative (< 50 mg/L, as acetoacetate) for both body fluids

Sources of Reference (Normal) Values:
Institutional, and package insert for Ames Keto-Diastix.

Specimen Volume, Collection, and Preservation:
10 μL to 0.3 mL. Deliver to lab immediately; 30% loss in 1 d at RT; stable for 2 d in RR or FR.

Analytical Method:

Keto-Diastix and Acetest tablets (Ames): acetoacetic acid and acetone (but not β-hydroxybutyric acid) react with nitroprusside to produce a purple-colored compound; report is semiquantitative. Free, A. H., and Free, H. M., Urinalysis, critical discipline of clinical science. *CRC Crit. Rev. Clin. Lab. Sci.* **3**, 481–531 (1972); Free, H. M., Smeby, R. R., Cook, M. H., and Free, A. H., A comparative study of qualitative tests for ketones in urine and serum. *Clin. Chem.* **4**, 323–330 (1958). Kova Trol Human Urine (dried) with diluent (ICL Scientific) used for quality control.

Beta-*N*-Acetyl-D-Hexosaminidase
(EC 3.2.1.52; 2-acetamido-2-deoxy-β-D-hexoside)

Specimen Tested:

P.

Laboratories Reporting:

1.

Reference (Normal) Values:

< 3 yr: 1151 ± 788 arbitrary units; range: 404–1760 (40–60.3% of adult values)
> 4 yr: 570 ± 536 arbitrary units; range: 320–963 (53–76% of adult values)

Sources of Reference (Normal) Values:

Institutional.

Specimen Volume, Collection, and Preservation:

2 mL of heparinized blood. Place on ice and separate plasma as soon as possible.

Analytical Method:

Refer to D. A. Applegarth (see list of **Contributors**); assay for the specific activity of *N*-acetyl-hexosaminidase by measuring the release of 4-methylumbelliferone (4-MU) from 4-MU-*N*-acetyl-β-D-glucosaminide. Isoenzyme B is heat stable and is measured by heating at 60 °C for 5 min to destroy isoenzyme A.

Enzyme data:

1. Enzyme unit definition: 1 arbitrary unit = the amount of enzyme that cleaves 1 nmol of 4-MU-*N*-acetyl-β-D-glucosaminide per hour per milliliter of plasma at 37 °C.
2. Buffer, pH: 10 mmol/L citric acid–20 mmol/L sodium phosphate, 4.4.

3. Substrate, final buffer–substrate pH: 1 mmol/L 4-MU-*N*-acetyl-*β*-D-glucosaminide, approx. 4.4.
4. Reaction temperature: 37 °C.
5. Temperature reported: 37 °C.

Commentary—Derek A. Applegarth

Hexosaminidase A activity in plasma or serum is markedly deficient in Tay–Sachs disease. Differing thermal stabilities of isoenzymes A and B allow total hexosaminidase and isoenzyme B activities to be measured and isoenzyme A activity to be calculated. The percentage of the A isoenzyme is used to assess heterozygosity for Tay–Sachs disease. No laboratory should embark on heterozygosity testing for Tay–Sachs disease without substantial analytical experience in this area of metabolism.

Total hexosaminidase activities are higher at birth and decrease to adult values by about three years of age. Conversely, the percentage of isoenzyme A is lower at birth and increases to adult values by about three years of age. Therefore, carrier detection in young children is difficult and best avoided.

Acid–Base, Blood Gases

pH

Specimen Tested:

B.

Laboratories Reporting:

8.

Reference (Normal) Values:

Age	Source of blood	pH range[a]
Newborn	Skin puncture; arterial	7.33–7.49
2 d–1 mo	Skin puncture; arterial	7.32–7.43
1 mo	Skin puncture; arterial	7.34–7.43
2 mo–1 yr	Skin puncture; arterial	7.34–7.46
Child and adult	Skin puncture; arterial	
M		7.35–7.45
F		7.36–7.44
	Venous	7.32–7.42

[a] Blood obtained by skin puncture follows "arterialization" by preheating the puncture site for 3 to 10 min at 40–42 °C. No distinction is made between premature and full-term newborns in the pH range listed.

Source of Reference (Normal) Values:

Institutional; Gambino, S. R., pH and p_{CO_2}. *Stand. Methods Clin. Chem.* **5,** 192–193 (1965)

Specimen Volume, Collection, and Preservation; Patient Preparation:

75 to 200 µL. Arterialized blood is collected into heparinized Natelson tubes; for further details see Chapter 3 of this text. Transport the pH tubes in an ice-water bath; pH decreases, however, because of continuing glycolysis, particularly in the newborn.

Analytical Method:

All laboratories measure pH with pH meters that are part of blood-gas equipment listed in next section.

p_{CO2}, p_{O2}

Specimen Tested:

B.

Laboratories Reporting:

8.

Reference (Normal) Values:

		mm Hg[a]	
Age	**Source of blood**	p_{CO_2}	p_{O_2}
Newborn	Skin puncture; arterial	26.8–40.4	60–76
2 mo–2 yr	Skin puncture; arterial	26.4–41.2	
Child and adult	Skin puncture; arterial		80–105
M		36.2–46.2	
F		33.1–43.1	
	Venous	40–50	25–47

[a]See note under pH reference values. p_{CO_2} may be indirectly obtained from pH by the Astrup method (below), or by calculating from the Henderson–Hasselbalch equation from pH and CO_2 content, by using the Siggaard-Andersen nomogram. All three, pH, p_{CO_2}, and p_{O_2}, may be obtained directly from blood-gas analyzers. The collection of valid skin-puncture specimens for p_{O_2} determination requires extra skill. The reference values cited above make no distinction between premature and full-term newborns. *Note:* 1 mm Hg = 133 Pa.

Sources of Reference (Normal) Values:

See sources under **pH.**

Specimen Volume, Collection, and Preservation; Patient Preparation:

See footnote above, footnote to pH values, and Chapter 3 of this text.

Analytical Method and Instrumentation:

The analytical methods are related to the instrumentation used.

1. **Astrup technique** (p_{CO_2}): Astrup, P., and Siggaard-Andersen, O., Micro methods for measuring acid–base values of blood. *Adv. Clin. Chem.* **6**, 1–28 (1963). Radiometer Acid–Base Analyzer PHM 72 Mk 2, and Radiometer BMS 3 Mk 2 Blood Micro System.

2. **Calculation of p_{CO_2} from CO_2 content and pH:** Use nomogram or tables for the Henderson–Hasselbalch equation. Siggaard-Andersen, O., Blood acid–base alignment nomogram. Scales for pH, p_{CO_2}, base excess of whole blood of different concentrations, plasma bicarbonate, and plasma total-CO_2. *Scand. J. Clin. Lab. Invest.* **15**, 211–217 (1963); Siggaard-Andersen, O., *The Acid–Base Status of the Blood*, 4th ed. Williams & Wilkins Co., Baltimore, MD, 1974, pp 51–71. **Calculated p_{CO_2}:** Beckman CO_2/Cl Analyzer (also Beckman Astra 8) with pH from Radiometer Acid–Base Analyzer PHM 72. **Direct pH, p_{CO_2}, p_{O_2}:** Corning Model 165, 168, and 175 pH/Blood Gas Analyzers; IL 513, 813 Blood Gas Analyzers (Instrumentation Laboratory Inc.); Radiometer ABL-2 Blood Gas Analyzer (The London Co.).

Note: Quality control for all techniques: General Diagnostics Blood G.A.S. Control; Versatol Acid–Base; Accept; Dade Quantra.

Commentary—Robert G. Petersen

Analytical methods for the determination of pH, p_{O_2}, and p_{CO_2} have become quite uniform, at least with regard to their theoretical basis. Measurements of pH are performed with electrochemical cells of small volume and constant temperature control at 37 °C. The determination of p_{O_2} has usually involved a cell based on the Clark electrode, which allows efficient equilibration of the cell with the oxygen tension of the blood sample. Carbon dioxide tension has been determined most widely by one of two principles. In the first, described by Severinghaus and Bradley *(1)*, CO_2 diffuses out of the sample to equilibrate across a CO_2-permeable membrane into a standard solution of potassium chloride and sodium bicarbonate. The influence of the CO_2 in solution upon the pH of the reference solution is measured, and the hydrogen-ion concentration in the cell is related to the carbon dioxide tension in the sample. The second method, described by Siggaard-Andersen et al. *(2)*, involves equilibrating two reference CO_2 gases [usually 4% and 8% CO_2 (40 and 80 mL/L)] against two portions of the sample. Determination of the pH in the two equilibrated portions of the cell allows for the measurement of p_{CO_2} as well as a calculation of the bicarbonate concentration in the blood sample.

The large ranges indicated for normal values do not reflect differences in instrumentation, but rather differences related to collection of the samples. The most striking difference is the difference between p_{O_2} measured in skin-puncture blood and in arterial blood. Variations may occur because of various techniques of heel warming, or because the baby is crying (see Chapter 3), but one study *(3)* has reported a lack of any correlation with arterial p_{O_2} when skin-puncture p_{O_2} values exceed 40 to 50 mmHg. In that report, skin-puncture values were always less than in the corresponding arterial samples. This may be due to the diminished perfusion in extremities in sick neonates *(4)*.

Newer methods for the determination of p_{O_2} and p_{CO_2} by transcutaneous monitoring *(5)* have shown quite dramatic changes in these values, in p_{O_2} in particular *(6)*, given routine handling of the neonate, including blood sampling. For these reasons, best results of neonatal blood-gas determination will come from the nurseries where samples are obtained "non-invasively" through indwelling arterial catheters.

1. Severinghaus, J. W., and Bradley, A. F., Electrodes for blood p_{O_2} and p_{CO_2} determination. *J. Appl. Physiol.* **13,** 515 (1958).
2. Siggaard-Andersen, O., Engel, K., Jorgensen, K., and Astrup, P., A micromethod for determination of pH, carbon dioxide tension, base excess, and standard bicarbonate in capillary blood. *Scand. J. Clin. Lab. Invest.* **12,** 172 (1960).
3. Mountain, K. R., and Campbell, D. G., Reliability of oxygen tension measurements on arterialized capillary blood in the newborn. *Arch. Dis. Child.* **45,** 134 (1970).
4. Kidd, L., Levison, H., Gemmel, P., Aharon, A., and Swyer, P. R., Limb flow in the normal and sick newborn. *Am. J. Dis. Child.* **112,** 462 (1966).
5. Huch, A., Huch, R., Arner, B., and Rooth, R., Continuous transcutaneous oxygen tension measured with a heated electrode. *Scand. J. Clin. Lab. Invest.* **31,** 269 (1973).
6. Versmold, H. T., Onken, D., Hopner, F., and Riegel, K. P., Transcutaneous monitoring of p_{O_2} in the sick newborn. In *Intensive Care in the Newborn,* L. Stern, B. Friis-Hansen, and P. Kildeberg, Eds. Masson, New York, NY, 1976.

CO₂ Content

Specimen Tested:

P, S.

Laboratories Reporting:

5.

Reference (Normal) Values:

	mmol/L
Cord blood:	15.0–20.2
Child:	18–27
Adult:	24–35

Sources of Reference (Normal) Values:

Institutional; Overman, R. R., Ettledorf, J. N., Bass, A. C., and Horn, G. B., Plasma and erythrocyte chemistry of the normal infant from birth to two years of age. *Pediatrics* **7**, 565–576 (1951).

Specimen Volume, Collection, and Preservation:

10 to 30 μL. Collect into dry, heparinized or non-heparinized capillary or polyethylene centrifuge tubes with caps (see Chapter 3, on blood collection). Transport in an ice-water bath.

Analytical Method and Instrumentation:

Beckman CO_2/Cl Analyzer, Astra 8; standby: Natelson microgasometer (Scientific Industries); Natelson, S., Routine use of ultramicro methods in the clinical laboratory. *Am. J. Clin. Pathol.* **21**, 1153–1172 (1951); Sternberg, J. C., Buzza, E., and Lillig, J., Simultaneous electrochemical determination of total CO_2 and chloride. 9th International Congress on Clinical Chemistry Procedures, 1975.

Actual Bicarbonate (calculated from pH and p_{CO_2})

Laboratories Reporting:

4.

Reference (Normal) Values:

	mmol/L
Newborn:	17.2–23.6
Infant:	19–24
2 mo–2 yr:	16.3–23.9
Child:	21–27; 18–25
Adult, M:	20.1–28.9
F:	18.4–28.8

Sources of References (Normal) Values:

Institutional.

Commentary—Garry M. Lum

The major anions in serum are chloride and bicarbonate. Changes in the normal concentrations of these anions certainly may accompany alterations in the major cations such as sodium. However, bicarbonate can also be affected in its role as primary buffer in defense of acid–base balance.

In severe volume depletion, for example, decreases in serum chloride will usually accompany decreases in sodium. Because the kidneys will increase their reabsorption of urinary sodium to expand intravascular volume in this situation, there will be an accompanying renal reabsorption of bicarbonate, thus satisfying ionic balance, and possibly producing an alkalemic state if losses of chloride are severe and not replenished.

Acidemic states usually produce low concentrations of bicarbonate in serum. In many cases the decrease in buffer is the result of accumulation of acid products, which will result in the production of unmeasured anions that satisfy the ionic balance while appearing to produce a discrepancy in total ions (the "anion-gap" = cations Na^+ and K^+ minus anions Cl^- and HCO_3^-). Alternatively, the acidemic state may be the result of a decrease in renal reabsorptive capacity of bicarbonate, with concomitant chloride absorption increasing to satisfy ionic balance, and there is no apparent "anion-gap."

Thus, the determination of chloride and bicarbonate are very helpful in assessing several clinical conditions and suggesting likely etiologies, depending on variable combinations of the major contributing serum ions and the acid–base status.

Standard Bicarbonate

Laboratory Reporting:

1.

Reference (Normal) Values:

	mmol/L
Premature:	18–26
Full-term:	20–26
1–2 yr:	20–25
2 yr–adult:	22–26

Sources of Reference (Normal) Values:

Institutional, based on pH measurement after equilibration of whole blood to a p_{CO_2} of 44 mmHG at 37 °C; Jorgensen, K., and Astrup, P., A simple electrometric technique for the determination of carbon dioxide tension in blood plasma, total content of carbon dioxide in plasma, and bicarbonate content in separated plasma at a fixed carbon dioxide tension (40 mmHg). *Scand. J. Clin. Lab. Invest.* **8,** 130 (1956).

Base Excess

Laboratories Reporting:

2.

Reference (Normal) Values:

mmol/L

Newborn: −10.0 to −2.0
2 mo–2 yr: −6.6 to 0.2
Child–adult: −2.3 to 2.3; −4 to −3

Sources of Reference (Normal) Values:

Institutional.

Acid Phosphatase (EC 3.1.3.2; orthophosphoric-monoester phosphohydrolase, acid optimum)

Specimen Tested:

P, S.

Laboratories Reporting:

1.

Reference (Normal) Values:

U/L

Newborn: 7.4–19.4
2–13 yr: 6.4–15.2
Adult, M: 0.5–11.0
    F: 0.2–9.5

Sources of Reference (Normal) Values:

Institutional.

Specimen Volume, Collection, and Preservation:

100 μL. Separate sample immediately and store in FR. Do not use fluoride-, heparin-, or oxalate-treated plasma; EDTA is recommended. Unless acidified, sample loses 10 to 50% of activity in 5 h at RT. Do not use hemolyzed or lipemic serum. Add 1.8 mg of disodium citrate monohydrate per milliliter of serum, or 1 μL of dilute (200 mL/L) acetic acid per 100 μL of serum. Acidified serum is stable for 7 to 8 d at RT.

Analytical Method:

Berger, L., and Rudolph, G. C., Alkaline and acid phosphatase. *Stand. Methods Clin. Chem.* **5,** 211–221 (1965).

Enzyme Data:

1. Enzyme unit definition: 1 IUB unit (U) is the activity by which 1 μmol of p-nitrophenol is produced per minute at 37 °C and pH 4.7.
2. Buffer, pH: citrate, 4.8.
3. Substrate: p-nitrophenylphosphate (disodium salt), 15.2 mmol/L.
4. Reaction temperature: 37 °C.
5. Temperature reported: 37 °C.

Instrumentation:

Beckman Model 25 spectrophotometer.

Commentary—Paul L. Wolf

Acid phosphatase (AcP) is a ubiquitous enzyme. Its serum activity is greater in growing children and is derived primarily from osteoclasts associated with bone growth. The major adult disease in which AcP plays a major role is as a tumor marker for carcinoma of the prostate; the enzyme is utilized to establish diagnosis and to follow the efficacy of therapy. The usual substrate has been α-naphthyl phosphate; more recently, thymolphthalein monophosphate is being used, to increase specificity for the prostatic isoenzyme. However, to identify the prostatic acid phosphatase (PAP) and to increase the sensitivity for identifying stage-A disease, a radioimmunoassay for PAP has recently been developed. [Colorimetric procedures are well known to fail to detect stage-A disease (1).] Various other diseases are associated with increased serum concentrations of AcP, including bone lesions (both benign and malignant), such as Paget's disease and osteogenic sarcoma; liver disease, such as viral hepatitis and metastic cancer; hematologic conditions, such as hemolysis and thrombocytopenia; and storage diseases, such as Gaucher's disease and Niemann–Pick disease (2).

The primary reason to assay serum AcP in pediatrics is in the diagnosis of Gaucher's disease or other storage diseases. Increased serum AcP has also been associated with osteogenic sarcoma and giant cell tumors of bone. The higher enzyme activity in the serum of children is physiologic, resulting from increased osteoclastic activity in growing bone.

Chen et al. (3) studied the AcP activity in 78 individuals younger than 18 years of age (49 children 12 years old and 29 adolescents) by using Babson's procedure with α-naphthyl phosphate in citrate buffer (70 mmol/L, pH 5.2) as the substrate. They found that serum AcP activity in normal children exceeded that of adults and that the fraction contributing to the higher value in children was the tartrate-resistant isoenzyme. The activity of this isoenzyme in children's sera is age-dependent, being highest in infants and decreasing slowly to age 14 years, then decreases sharply afterwards to normal adult values. It is derived from bone and is non-prostatic in origin.

Thus, the interpretation of AcP activity in children must contain an awareness that, physiologically, AcP is increased from a bone source. If the AcP activity is greater than the physiologic increase, a pathologic cause should be considered, most likely a bone lesion, such as a giant cell tumor or osteogenic sarcoma. Next, one should consider a storage disease, especially Gaucher's disease. Finally, thrombocytopenia may be associated with an increased serum AcP, especially in idiopathic thrombocytopenic purpura, in which AcP is liberated from the platelets.

1. Foti, A. G., Cooper, J. F., Herschman, H., and Malvaez, R., Detection of prostatic cancer by solid-phase radioimmunoassay of serum prostatic acid phosphatase. *N. Engl. J. Med.* **297,** 1357–1361 (1977).
2. Wolf, P. L., and Williams, D., *Practical Clinical Enzymology.* John Wiley & Sons, Inc., New York, NY, 1973, pp 110–111.
3. Chen, J., Yam, L. T., Janckila, A. J., Li, C. Y., and Lam, W. K. W., Significance of "high" acid phosphatase activity in the serum of normal children. *Clin. Chem.* **25,** 565–569 (1979).

Commentary—Roger L. Boeckx

Acid Phosphatase as a Marker for Semen in Cases of Sexual Assault

Even in pediatric practice, we are occasionally faced with the problem of sexual assault. Although most victims of sexual assault seen in pediatric centers are adolescent girls, we do occasionally see young children, even infants, who have been abused sexually.

It is common practice to collect samples of vaginal fluid from the victim, usually by using a swab. One such sample should be collected specifically for the assay of acid phosphatase.

Acid phosphatase is secreted into the seminal fluid by the prostate gland. The enzyme from the prostate can be measured by the use of specific substrates *(1)*. By using the method of Roy et al. *(2)*, which is specific for prostatic acid phosphatase, it has been shown that normal seminal plasma contains 68 to 360 kU of acid phosphatase per liter. Assuming a normal ejaculate volume of 2 to 6.5 mL, we can assume that from 130 to 2000 U of prostatic acid phosphatase will be deposited in the vagina during intercourse. In my laboratory, the method of Lantz and Eisenberg *(3)* is used for sampling, preservation, and measurement of acid phosphatase. Swabs are placed in 2.5 mL of a solution of buffered (pH 7.4) bovine serum albumin (5 g/dL) in saline. An aliquot of this solution is then analyzed by the method of Roy et al. *(2)*. A value of 50 U per sample or higher is considered "semen positive."

Normal acid phosphatase activity in non-coital women is less than 10 U/L *(3)*. Various studies of the survival of seminal acid phosphatase in the vagina have been published. Schumann et al. *(4)* summarized the literature and, adding their own data, concluded that vaginal acid phosphatase returns to normal pre-coital values in approximately 48 h. In a large study of volunteers and alleged sexual assault cases, Findley *(5)* found that 100% of women had increased acid phosphatase values immediately after intercourse; 8 h later 83% were positive; 40% were positive after 24 h; and 11% were positive after 72 h.

1. Pragay, D. A., Casey, S. J., and Grotthelf, J., Use of different chemical methods for acid phosphatase in cases of rape. *Clin. Biochem.* **10**, 183–187 (1977).
2. Roy, A. V., Brower, M. E., and Hayden, J. E., Sodium thymolphthalein monophosphate: A new acid phosphatase substrate with greater specificity for the prostatic enzyme in semen. *Clin. Chem.* **17**, 1093–1102 (1971).
3. Lantz, R. K., and Eisenberg, R. B., Preservation of acid phosphatase activity in medico-legal specimens. *Clin. Chem.* **24**, 486–488 (1978).
4. Schumann, G. B., Badawy, S., Peglow, A., and Henry, J. B., Prostatic acid phosphatase. Current assessment in vaginal fluid of alleged rape victims. *Am. J. Clin. Pathol.* **66**, 944–952 (1976).
5. Findley, T. P., Quantitation of vaginal acid phosphatase and its relationship to time of coitus. *Am. J. Clin. Pathol.* **68**, 238–242 (1977).

Adenine Phosphoribosyltransferase (EC 2.4.2.7; AMP:pyrophosphate phosphoribosyltransferase)

Specimen Tested:

B.

Laboratory Reporting:

1.

Reference (Normal) Values:

Newborn: 870–1430 arbitrary units
Child–adult: 426–838

Source of Reference (Normal) Values:

Institutional (experimental): Borden, M., Nyhan, W. L., and Bakay, B., Increased activity of adenine phosphoribosyltransferase in erythrocytes of normal newborn infants. *Pediatr. Res.* **8**, 31–36 (1974); Sweetman, L., Hoch, M. A., Bakay, B., Borden, M., Lesh, P., and

Nyhan, W. L., A distinct human variant of hypoxanthine–guanine phosphoribosyltransferase. *J. Pediatr.* **92,** 385–389 (1978).

Specimen Volume, Collection, and Preparation:

10 μL of heparinized whole blood. The enzyme is usually stable for about two weeks. Blood should be shipped at RT as soon as possible after collection. A "control" blood should also be sent for comparison.

Analytical method:

Bakay, B., Telfer, M. A., and Nyhan, W. L., Assay of hypoxanthine–guanine and adenine phosphoribosyl transferases. A simple screening test for the Lesch–Nyhan syndrome and related disorders of purine metabolism. *Biochem. Med.* **3,** 230–243 (1969).

Enzyme Data:

1. Enzyme unit definition: 1 arbitrary unit = 1 nmol of AMP transformed per minute per milliliter of packed erythrocytes
2. Buffer, pH: Tris/HCl/phosphate, 7.4
3. Substrate, pH: [8-^{14}C]adenine-5-phosphoribosyl-1-pyrophosphate, 7.4.
4. Reaction temperature: 60 °C.
5. Temperature reported: 60 °C.

Instrumentation:

Beckman LS-250 liquid scintillation system.

Commentary—David J. Harris

The best-known disorder of purine metabolism in childhood is the Lesch–Nyhan syndrome. The hyperuricemia in this disorder is due to deficient activity of hypoxanthine phosphoribosyltransferase (EC 2.4.2.8; HPRT). The method described is well validated, and involves only small quantities of blood. Because the disorder is rare, and the enzyme sufficiently stable to permit forwarding of samples to a central laboratory, hospitals generally do not perform this assay "in-house."

Partial deficiencies of HPRT are associated with some cases of gout. Detection of the partial defects may allow the development of preventive strategies. Screening programs may detect new variants. To date, there is no clinical disorder associated with low adenine phosphoribosyltransferase activity. Study of the activity of this enzyme is useful in understanding the regulation of the purine pathways in hyperuricemic syndromes.

See also **Hypoxanthine phosphoribosyltransferase.**

Adrenocorticotropin, ACTH (Corticotropin)

Specimen Tested:

P.

Laboratory Reporting:

1.

Reference (Normal) Values:

At 0800 to 1000 hours: 20–100 pg/mL

Sources of Reference (Normal) Values:

Radioimmunoassay Manual, 4th ed., Nichols Institute, San Pedro, CA, 1977.

Specimen Volume, Collection, and Preservation:

4 mL. Collect venous blood with a chilled *plastic* syringe containing heparin (1000 int. units/mL). Transfer to chilled test tubes (polystyrene or siliconized glass). Centrifuge immediately in a refrigerated centrifuge. Freeze the separated plasma immediately.

Analytical method:

Berson, S. A., and Yalow, R. S., Radioimmunoassay of ACTH in plasma. *J. Clin. Invest.* **47,** 2725–2751 (1968).

Commentary—Elizabeth K. Smith

Corticotropin (ACTH) is a polypeptide hormone secreted by the anterior pituitary. Regulation of ACTH release is controlled by corticotropin-releasing factor (CRF; corticoliberin) from the hypothalamus, and by negative feedback by cortisol from the adrenal cortex. Secretion is episodic and follows a diurnal rhythm, with increased concentrations in the morning and low ones at night. The principal action of ACTH is to stimulate steroidogenesis by the adrenal cortex. The episodic release and diurnal rhythm in ACTH secretion are responsible for the episodic release and diurnal rhythm in cortisol secretion.

ACTH secretion is stimulated by a variety of stressful stimuli: surgery, anesthesia, vasopressin, hypoglycemia, etc. ACTH increases markedly in primary adrenocortical insufficiency (Addison's disease) and in patients with Cushing's syndrome, in which pituitary ACTH hypersecretion is the cause of adrenocortical hyperplasia. ACTH is suppressed in patients with primary hypopituitarism and in patients receiving exogenous glucocorticoid therapy.

The peripheral, circulating concentration of ACTH shows little variation with age or sex. Blood should be drawn from a fasting patient between 0800 and 1000 hours. Observe special precautions in handling and processing. Because of potential losses from improper handling and because of difficulties in assay, specific measurement of ACTH is less valuable than results from indirect function tests. Such tests include the determination of cortisol after ACTH suppression by dexamethasone or the stimulation of ACTH by blockage of cortisol biosynthesis with metyrapone, leading to increased plasma concentration of 11-deoxycortisol in patients with an intact pituitary–adrenal axis.

Alanine Aminotransferase, ALT (EC 2.6.1.2; L-alanine:2-oxoglutarate aminotransferase)

Specimen Tested:

P, S.

Laboratories Reporting:

6.

Reference (Normal) Values:

Age	U/L
"Infant"	up to 54; a range of 27–54 includes about one-third, and 0–27 about two-thirds, of healthy infants
< 2 yr	3–37
2–8 yr	3–30
8–16 yr	3–28
"Adult"	3–35; M: 7–46, F: 4–35

Sources of Reference (Normal) Values:

Institutional: text ref. 2; Sitzmann, F. C., Die Enzymdiagnostik bei Erkrankungen in Kindesalter. *Arch. Kinderheilkd. Beih.* **57**, 1–59 (1968); Cheng, M. H., Lipsey, A. I., Blanco, V., Wong, H. T., and Spiro, S. H., Microchemical analysis for 13 constituents of plasma from healthy children. *Clin. Chem.* **25**, 692–698 (1979).

Specimen Volume, Collection, and Preservation:

5 to 100 μL of plasma from heparinized collection tubes. The enzyme is stable for 3 d at RT, 1 wk in RR.

Analytical Method:

Wroblewski, F., and LaDue, J. S., Serum glutamic pyruvic transaminase in cardiac and hepatic disease. *Proc. Soc. Biol. Med.* **91**, 569–

571 (1956); Henry, R. J., Chiamori, N., Golub, O. J., and Berkman, S., Revised spectrophotometric methods for the determination of glutamic-oxalacetic transaminase, glutamic-pyruvic transaminase, and lactic acid dehydrogenase. *Am. J. Clin. Pathol.* **34,** 381–398 (1960); Rodgerson, D. O., and Osberg, I. M., Sources of error in spectrophotometric measurement of aspartate aminotransferase and alanine aminotransferase activities in serum. *Clin. Chem.* **20,** 43–50 (1973); Abbott A-Gent reagents; Union Carbide CentrifiChem; BMC optimized kit No. 15925. Kinetic methods measure rate of disappearance of NADH and of L-alanine converted to pyruvate. Reagents include lactate dehydrogenase, DL-alanine, $NADH(Na_2)$, α-ketoglutarate, and phosphate buffer.

Enzyme Data:

1. Enzyme unit definition: 1 IUB unit (U) = that activity transforming 1 μmol of alanine to pyruvate per minute.
2. Buffer, pH: KH_2PO_4/Na_2HPO_4, 7.30 $\pm$ 0.15 at 25 °C.
3. Substrate, pH: L-alanine (337 mmol/L of reaction mixture), and α-ketoglutarate (8 mmol/L of reaction mixture), 7.30 at 25 °C.
4. Reaction temperature: 30 °C (6 labs.); 37 °C (2 labs.).
5. Temperature reported: 30 °C (7 labs.); 37 °C (1 lab.).

Instrumentation:

ABA-100, VP (Abbott); Union Carbide CentrifiChem; Beckman TR Enzyme Analyzer; Gilford Stasar II spectrophotometer.

$$* \qquad * \qquad *$$

Specimen Tested:
S.

Laboratory Reporting
1.

Reference (Normal) Values:

Age	No.	U/L
Newborn	23	0–34
6 wk–18 mo	24	0–53
18 mo–16 yr	255	0–35
Adult	150	0–50

Sources of Reference (Normal) Values:

Pediatric patients' charts were reviewed to exclude active infections, inflammatory disease, malignancy, and anemia by the criteria of Guest, G. M., and Brown, E. W., Erythrocyte and hemoglobin of the blood in infancy and childhood. *Am. J. Dis. Child.* **95,** 486–509 (1957). These 452 patients were selected from a total of 1209. Sera were analyzed with a Technicon smac to obtain the "reference" or "expected" values reported.

Specimen Volume, Collection, and Preservation; Patient Preparation:

0.47 mL of serum. Venous blood obtained. Patients, except infants, were fasted overnight.

Analytical Method:

Method essentially the same as that cited in preceding report: Henry et al., *op. cit.;* Kessler, G., Rush, R., Leon, L., Delea, A., and Cupiola, R., Automated 340 nm measurement of SGOT, SGPT, and LDH. In *Advances in Automated Analysis,* **1,** Technicon International Congress, 1970, Miami, FL. Thurman Associates, 1971, pp 67–74 (Technicon Instrument Corp.); the Technicon method involves a three-point rate reaction, with zero-order kinetics.

Enzyme Data:

Essentially similar to the method cited in preceding report. Temperatures used for analysis and report: 37 °C.

Instrumentation:

Technicon smac (high speed, computer-controlled biochemical analyzer); Technicon method no. SG4-0022 PC6.

Commentary

See Commentary for **Aspartate Aminotransferase.**

Albumin

Specimen Tested:

P, S.

Laboratories Reporting:

9.

Reference (Normal) Values:

Age	g/L	mmol/L	No. of patients [a]
Newborn, cord blood (S)	36–44		
Newborn	24–48; 29–48		25
Newborn to infant	20–55		
1 wk, premature	33–40		
1 wk, full-term	30–51		
2 mo	30–45	0.46–0.69	
Infant	23–38		
6 wk–3 yr	35–47		71
1 yr, premature	37–44		
1 yr, full-term	45–48		
2 mo–5 yr	37–53	0.57–0.82	
Child	38–54		
3–5 yr	38–50		48
4 yr and older	45–53		
5–8 yr	40–56; 37–48	0.62–0.86	75
8–13 yr	30–55		111
8–14 yr	38–58	0.59–0.89	
13–16 yr	35–49		119
14–16 yr	40–60	0.62–0.92	
16 yr–adult	35–55	0.58–0.80	
Adult	38–52; 38–54; 30–55		150
M:	42–55		
F:	37–53		

[a] Study made with the Technicon SMAC analytical system on 450 pediatric patients screened for disease.

Sources of Reference (Normal) Values:

Institutional; Cheng, M. H., Lipsey, A. I., Blanco, V., Wong, H. T., and Spiro, S. H., Microchemical analysis for 13 constituents of plasma from healthy children. *Clin. Chem.* **25,** 692–698 (1979); Electro-Nucleonics Gemeni Albumin Package Insert R1-1, P/N: 902091-1, Nov. 1977.

Specimen Volume, Collection, and Preservation:

2.5 to 30 μL. Stable 4 to 7 d at RT, 2 wk to 1 mo in RR, and up to 6 mo in FR. Reject samples showing hemolysis (and lipemia). Ultracentrifuge lipemic specimens with Beckman Airfuge for 5 min at 85 000 rpm, or blank lipemic specimens appropriately.

Analytical Method:

All laboratories reporting use a version of the dye-binding method with bromcresol green: Doumas, B. T., Watson, W. A., and Biggs, H. G., Albumin standards and the measurement of serum albumin with bromcresol green. *Clin. Chim. Acta* **31,** 87–96 (1971); Pierce Spectru BCG Albumin Reagent; Gindler, E. M., and Westgard, J.

O., Automated and manual determination of albumin with bromcresol green and a new ionic surfactant. *Clin. Chem.* **19**, 647 (1973), abstract; Electro-Nucleonics GEMSAEC and Gemeni Albumin kit; Gustafsson, J.E.C., Improved specificity of serum albumin determination and estimation of "acute phase reactants" by use of the bromcresol green reaction. *Clin. Chem.* **22**, 616–622 (1976); General Diagnostics Albu-Strate kit; Worthington Albumin Reagent (Bromcresol Green); Rodkey, F. L., Direct spectrophotometric determination of albumin in human serum. *Clin. Chem.* **11**, 478–487 (1965); American Monitor Albumin kit.

Instrumentation:
Abbott ABA-100 Bichromatic Analyzer; Technicon SMA and SMAC/ SDM System; Gilford Stasar II and III spectrophotometers; Electro-Nucleonics GEMSAEC and Gemeni; Hitachi 102 spectrophotometer; Coleman Jr. II spectrophotometer; Aminco Rotochem II.

Commentary—Gregory J. Buffone

All of the contributors use a bromcresol green (BCG) dye-binding method for albumin determinations, with some requiring as little as 3 μL of specimen. The BCG method has been recommended as a standard method, so reagent formulation has become fairly uniform between laboratories.

Variation in the time of the absorbance reading for the BCG procedure can cause significant differences in the results for patients' samples in which the α_1 and α_2 fractions are increased in concentration and the albumin is decreased (e.g., nephrotic syndrome and acute inflammation) *(1)*. Specificity of BCG dye-binding can be improved by making the absorbance measurement before the α_1 and α_2 fractions begin to react with the dye (< 20 s) *(1,2)*.

1. Webster, D. A., Study of the interaction of bromocresol green with isolated serum globulin fractions. *Clin. Chim. Acta* **53**, 109–115 (1974).
2. Webster, D., The immediate reaction between bromocresol green and serum as a measure of albumin content. *Clin. Chem.* **32**, 663–665 (1977).

Aldolase (EC 4.1.2.13; D-fructose-1,6-bisphosphate D-glyceraldehyde-3-phosphate-lyase)

Specimen Tested:
P, S.

Laboratories Reporting:
4.

Reference (Normal) Values:

	3 labs.	1 lab.[a]
Newborn	Up to 4 × adult	17.5–47.8 U/L
Child	Up to 2 × adult	8.8–23.9
Adult	Up to 8 U/L	4.4–12.0

[a] Uses Bio-Dynamics/*bmc* kit (collidine buffer, pH 7.4); see below.

Sources of Reference (Normal) Values:

Institutional.

Specimen Volume, Collection, and Preservation:

25 to 200 μ/L. Specimen *must* be free of hemolysis. Separate P or S immediately to avoid contact with clot. Stable for 5 h at RT, 5 d in RR, 2 wk in FR.

Analytical Method:

Pinto, P. V. C., Kaplan, A., and Van Dreal, P. A., Aldolase, II. Spectrophotometric determination using an ultraviolet procedure. *Clin. Chem.* **15**, 349–360 (1969); Wolf, P. L., Williams, D., Tsudaka, T., and Acosta, L., *Methods and Techniques in Clinical Chemistry*, Wiley-Interscience, New York, NY, 1972; Leuthardt, F., and Wolf, H. P., Fructose-1-phosphate from liver. In *Methods in Enzymology*, **1**, S. P. Colowick and N. O. Kaplan, Eds. Academic Press Inc., New York, NY, 1955, p 320; Bio-Dynamics/*bmc* "Reagent Set" Reagents Aldolase, enzymatic; Calbiochem-Behring Aldolase UV.

Enzyme Data:

1. Enzyme unit definition: 1 IUB unit (U) is that activity catalyzing the transformation of 1 μmol of substrate per minute, determined as micromoles of DPNH produced per minute.
2. Buffer, pH: Tris, 7.0.
3. Substrate, pH: fructose-1,6-diphosphate/triose phosphate isomerase, 7.0.
4. Reaction temperature: 37 °C.
5. Temperature reported: 37 °C.

Instrumentation:

Abbott ABA-100 Bichromatic Analyzer; Aminco Rotochem II; Beckman 25K spectrophotometer.

Commentary—Paul L. Wolf

Serum aldolase in the neonate is fourfold the adult activity, and in children is twice that of the adult. Adult values are attained by the time the child reaches puberty *(1)*.

Aldolase is a ubiquitous enzyme, its greatest activity being in skeletal muscle. Other tissues that contain the enzyme are heart, liver, brain, lung, kidney, small intestine, erythrocytes, and platelets.

Serum aldolase and the skeletal muscle isoenzyme cleave the substrate fructose-1,6-diphosphate but not fructose-1-phosphate. The liver isoenzyme cleaves both substrates. Because aldolase is present as a stable enzyme in erythrocytes, the serum used for analysis should not be hemolyzed.

The greatest usefulness of determining the enzyme is in the diagnosis of Duchenne's muscular dystrophy. Aldolase activity is increased before clinical symptoms are apparent and tends to decrease as the dystrophic process progresses. Because creatine kinase (CK) tends to remain increased longer, however, there is greater clinical interest in CK in the diagnosis and follow-up of muscular dystrophy. Aldolase may also be increased in polymyositis, dermatomyositis, limb-girdle muscular dystrophy, myotonic dystrophy, and rhabdomyolysis. It is usually not increased in neurogenic muscular atrophy.

The only other clinical indication for assessing the enzyme is in hepatic disease, especially acute viral hepatitis, where it follows the same course as aspartate aminotransferase, and viral pancreatitis in children.

It is unknown why the neonate has so much more activity than the adult. Perhaps it is related partly to the physiologic hemolysis in the neonate, or to the release of enzyme from traumatized fetal skeletal muscle during birth, or to the presence of mother's aldolase in the fetus from labor. Other possibilities include increased activity from the hyperplastic adrenal in the neonate. Experimentally, corticotropin (ACTH) stimulates aldolase activity (2); the enzyme may also be needed for carbohydrate metabolism.

1. Emanuel, B., West, M., and Zimmerman, H. J., Serum enzymes in disease. XII. Transaminases, glycolytic and oxidative enzymes in normal infants and children. *Am. J. Dis. Child.* **105**, 261–264 (1963).
2. Schapira, F., Hyperaldolasémie plasmatique provoquée par la cortisone et l'ACTH. *C. R. Seances Soc. Biol. Paris* **148**, 1997–2000 (1954).

Aldosterone

Specimen Tested:

S.

Laboratory Reporting:

1.

Reference (Normal) Values:

Patient on high-salt diet; in supine position: 2–9 ng/dL

Source of Reference (Normal) Values:

Radioimmunoassay Manual, Nichols Institute, San Pedro, CA, 1977, pp 182–183.

Specimen Volume, Collection, and Preservation; Patient Preparation:

1 mL. Patient on diet with regular salt intake.

Analytical Method:

RIA after Sephradex LH-20 chromatography with [³H]aldosterone indicator; Ito, T., Woo, J., Honing, R., and Horton, R. A., A rapid radioimmunoassay for aldosterone in human peripheral plasma. *J. Clin. Endocrinol. Metab.* **34**, 106–112 (1972).

Commentary—Peter J. and Joan H. Howanitz

Aldosterone, secreted by the zona glomerulosa of the adrenal cortex, enhances sodium reabsorption and potassium secretion in the distal tubule of the kidney. Its secretion is regulated by multiple complex feedback mechanisms. The most important regulator of aldosterone secretion is the renin/angiotensin system, which responds to changes in plasma volume. Other important factors influencing aldosterone secretion include corticotropin (ACTH) and potassium.

Aldosterone concentrations in serum may be measured by RIA. Because of inadequate antibody specificity, most procedures require initial solvent extraction of the sample, followed by chromatographic separation of aldosterone from interfering steroids. Thus, these methods not only are tedious, but require a large amount of specimen. Recently, RIA of serum aldosterone without use of extraction or chromatography has been described *(1)*. A summary of RIA methods for aldosterone has recently been published *(2)*.

During normal pregnancy, aldosterone concentrations in the mother increase significantly from the first to the third trimester, decreasing precipitously in the postpartum period *(3)*. Aldosterone in amniotic fluid ranges from 100 to 1000 ng/dL, but shows no correlation with gestational age *(4)*. Umbilical vein aldosterone concentrations are about twice that of the mother *(5)*. During the first week of life, aldosterone concentrations vary widely (<1 to 445 ng/dL) but tend to be high *(6)*. Decreased aldosterone clearance, as well as decreased sensitivity of the renal tubule to the hormone, may be responsible for these high concentrations. Studies indicate that these concentrations vary inversely with age: infants have higher concentrations than children *(5);* in adults, the concentration tends to decline with advancing age *(1)*.

The main use of aldosterone measurements is in the diagnosis of primary aldosteronism. This diagnosis can be suspected in individuals with hypertension, hypokalemia, and inappropriate kaliuresis. The increased production of aldosterone associated with this syndrome may be difficult to document; thus, multiple laboratory determinations usually are performed. An isolated aldosterone measurement made with no attention to patient preparation is of little clinical value. Even when time of sampling, posture, dietary sodium, and potassium are controlled, it is difficult to discriminate between primary aldosteronism and other forms of hypertension by using only aldosterone measurements (7). However, patients with primary aldosteronism have aldosterone in the range of 30 ng/dL, which is not suppressed with saline infusion (500 mL of 9 g/L saline from 0800 to 1200 hours), whereas aldosterone concentrations in patients who have other forms of hypertension are less than 10 ng/dL after saline infusion (7). Other suppression tests also have been used to separate individuals with primary aldosteronism from patients with other forms of hypertension. For example, use of the synthetic mineralocorticoid Florinef (fludrocortisone), 0.6 mg/d for three days, has met with fair success.

Aldosterone has also been measured after stimulation of the renin/angiotensin system by volume depletion. In patients with low or hyporesponsive renin activity, aldosterone measurements are made after administration of a diuretic. A typical protocol involves ingestion of 80 mg of furosemide at 0900 hours with specimens for aldosterone obtained 3 h later. Before testing, patients are maintained on a normal intake of sodium, and remain upright during the test. Under these conditions, aldosterone concentrations in patients with primary aldosteronism exceed 15 ng/dL, while values for normal individuals are less than 15 ng/dL (8).

Adrenal venography, with measurements of aldosterone in adrenal and vena cava blood, is helpful in localizing adenomas and identifying bilateral adrenal hyperplasia. In a large series of patients, the concentration of aldosterone in venous plasma draining unilateral adrenal adenomas averaged about 7000 ng/dL, while in venous plasma from the opposite adrenal and from the inferior vena cava, concentrations were about 100 ng/dL (9). Infusion of synthetic ACTH during simultaneous sampling of both adrenal veins improves the efficiency of the localization technique (10).

Aldosterone values have also been studied in patients with disorders of the adrenal gland. Markedly increased aldosterone concentrations are seen in some patients with 21-hydroxylase deficiency without salt loss (11), but are decreased in salt-losing 21-hydroxylase deficiencies (12). Values are also decreased in 17-hydroxylase, 18-hydroxylase, and 18-hydroxydehydrogenase deficiencies, as well as in adrenal insufficiency (13,14). Isolated deficiency of aldosterone has been described in hyporeninemic hypoaldosteronism, which is usually associated with diabetes mellitus or renal disease *(15)*.

1. Tan, S. Y., Noth, R., and Mulrow, P. J., Direct non-chromatographic radioimmunoassay of aldosterone: Validation of a commercially available kit and observations on age-related changes in concentrations in plasma. *Clin. Chem.* **24,** 1531–1533 (1978).
2. Vecsei, P., Hackenthal, E., and Ganten, D., The renin–angiotensin–aldosterone system. *Klin. Wochenschr.* **56,** 5–21 (1978).
3. Weir, R. J., Brown, J. J., Fraser, R., Lever, A. F., Logan, R. W., McIlwaine, G. M., Morton, J. J., Robertson, J. I. S., and Tree, M., Relationship between plasma renin, renin-substrate, angiotensin II, aldosterone and electrolytes in normal pregnancy. *J. Clin. Endocrinol. Metab.* **40,** 108–115 (1975).
4. Aderjan, R., Rauh, W., Vecsei, P., Lorenz, U., and Ruttgers, H., Determination of cortisol, tetrahydrocortisol, tetrahydrocortisone, corticosterone, and aldosterone in human amniotic fluid. *J. Steroid Biochem.* **8,** 525–528 (1977).
5. Sippel, W. G., Becker, H., Versmold, H. T., Bidlingmaier, F., and Knorr, D., Longitudinal studies of plasma aldosterone, corticosterone, deoxycorticosterone, progesterone, 17-hydroxy-progesterone, cortisol, and cortisone determined simultaneously in mother and child at birth and during the early neonatal period. I. Spontaneous delivery. *J. Clin. Endocrinol. Metab.* **46,** 971–985 (1978).
6. Raux-Eurin, M. C., Pham-Huu-Trung, M. T., Marrec, D., and Girard, F., Plasma aldosterone concentrations during the neonatal period. *Pediatr. Res.* **11,** 182–185 (1977).
7. Grim, C. E., Weinberger, M. H., Higgins, J. T., and Kramer, N. J., Diagnosis of secondary forms of hypertension. *J. Am. Med. Assoc.* **237,** 1331–1335 (1977).
8. Melby, J. C., Diagnosis and treatment of hyperaldosteronism and hypoaldosteronism. In *Endocrinology*, L. J. DeGroot et al., Eds. Grune and Stratton, New York, NY, 1979, pp 1225–1234.
9. Nicolis, G. L., Mitty, H. A., Modlinger, R. S., and Gabrilove, J. L., Percutaneous adrenal venography. *Ann. Intern. Med.* **76,** 899–909 (1972).
10. Weinberger, M. H., Grim, C. E., Hollifield, J. W., Kem, D. C., Ganguly, A., Kramer, N. J., Yune, H. Y., Wellman, H., and Donohue, J. P., Primary aldosteronism. *Ann. Intern. Med.* **90,** 386–395 (1979).
11. Parth, K., Zimprich, H., Swoboda, W., Brunel, R., and Bohrn, E., Congenital adrenal hyperplasia: Simultaneous determination of plasma aldosterone and 17-hydroxy-progesterone. *Acta Endocrinol. (Copenhagen)* **87,** 148–157 (1978).
12. Bartter, F. C., Adrenogenital syndromes. In *Congenital Adrenal Hyperplasia*, P. A. Lee et al., Eds. University Park Press, Baltimore, MD, 1977, pp 9–18.
13. Rovner, D. R., Conn, J. W., Cohen, E. L., Berlinger, F. G., Kem, D. C., and Gordon, D. L., 17 α-Hydroxylase deficiency. A combination of hydroxylation defect and reversible blockade in aldosterone biosynthesis. *Acta Endocrinol. (Copenhagen)* **90,** 490–504 (1979).
14. Ulick, S., Diagnosis and nomenclature of the disorders of the terminal portion of the aldosterone biosynthetic pathway. *J. Clin. Endocrinol. Metab.* **43,** 92–96 (1976).
15. Schambelan, M., and Sebastian, A., Hyporeninemic hypoaldosteronism. *Adv. Intern. Med.* **24,** 385–405 (1979).

Alkaline Phosphatase, ALP (EC 3.1.3.1; orthophosphoric-monoester phosphohydrolase, alkaline optimum)

Specimen Tested:

P, S. (See *Specimen volume, etc.*, note on use of plasma.)

Laboratories Reporting:

1. [*Ed. note:* Among the serum enzymes tested on children, none has received more study than alkaline phosphatase (ALP). For this reason, we are especially fortunate to present below the scholarly report and, further on, the commentary of Dr. Bowers. Because of its particular merit, this material on ALP is given separate emphasis, so that it may readily serve as a model for future reference. The valid data from the other laboratories follow.]

Reference (Normal) Values:

See Figure 1.

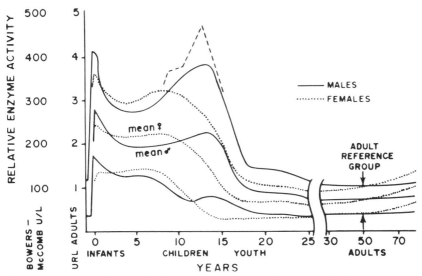

Fig. 1. Variation of upper limits, mean, and lower limits of alkaline phosphatase activity with age and sex.

Upper lines represent upper limits of reference intervals; *middle lines*, the mean; and *lower lines*, the lower limits. *Dashed line* indicates extreme increased values found in healthy boys by Clark and Beck (see reference *3* in Bowers' Commentary). *y*-axis: U/L according to method of Bowers and McComb, and upper reference limits (URL) for values found in adults

Sources of Reference (Normal) Values:

McComb, R. B., Bowers, G. N., Jr., and Posen, S., *Alkaline Phosphatase*. Plenum Press, New York, NY, 1979, Ch. 9, Sec. 9.2.

Specimen Volume, Collection, and Preservation;
Patient Preparation:

10 μL. See Bowers' Commentary for further details of collection and preservation. Heparinized plasma may be used, but not plasma from other anticoagulants. Analyze within 2 to 4 h of collection; otherwise, store in RR, but do not freeze.

Analytical Method:

See Chapter 13 in McComb et al., *op. cit.*, and Bowers' Commentary.

Enzyme Data:

See Bowers' Commentary and Table 1 there.
1. Enzyme unit definition: 1 IUB unit (U) = that enzyme activity catalyzing the transformation of 1 μmol of substrate per minute.
2. Buffer, pH: 2-amino-2-methyl-1-propanol, 10.5.
3. Substrate, pH: *p*-nitrophenyl phosphate, 10.5.
4. Reaction temperature: 29.77 °C.
5. Temperature reported: 29.77 °C.

*   *   *

Laboratories Reporting:

8.

Reference (Normal) Values:

See facing page.

Sources of Reference (Normal) Values:

Institutional; Cheng, M. H., Lipsey, A. I., Blanco, V., Wong, H. T., and Spiro, S. H., Microchemical analysis of 13 constituents of plasma from healthy children. *Clin. Chem.* **25**, 692–698 (1979); special institutional study of 450 patients selected to exclude disease, with the Technicon SMAC analytical system; Penttilä, I. M., Jokela, H. A., Vitala, A. J., Heikkinen, E., Nummi, S., Pystynen, P., and Saastamoinen, J., Activities of aspartate and alanine aminotransferases and alkaline phosphatase in sera of healthy subjects. *Scand. J. Clin. Lab. Invest.* **35**, 275–284 (1975).

Analytical Method and Enzyme Data:

In addition to those in the previous report: Morgenstern, S., Kessler, G., Auerbach, J., Flor, R. V., and Klein, B., An automated *p*-nitrophenyl-phosphate serum alkaline phosphatase procedure for the AutoAnalyzer. *Clin. Chem.* **11**, 876–888 (1965); Bessey, O. A., Lowry,

| Age[a] | U/L (Bowers–McComb method) | | | |
| | Reported at 30 °C | | Reported at 37 °C | |
	Lower	Upper	Lower	Upper
Cord blood, S			83	183
Newborn	20–72	210–225	62–95	95–368
1 mo–1 yr	50–85	232–260		
0–2 yr			80	270
6 wk–18 mo			118	354
2 mo–24 mo			115	460
1 yr–10 yr	65	265		
18 mo–3 yr			81	339
2–5 yr			80–115	220–391
2–8 yr	65	210		
3–10 yr			108	295
5–8 yr			60	230
6–7 yr			115	460
8–9 yr			115	345
8–12 yr			60	280
9–15 yr	60	290		
10–11 yr				
M			75–115	336–347
F			96–115	414–437
10–13 yr, F	10	250		
10–15 yr, M	55	295		
12 yr			159	387
12–13 yr				
M			127	403
F			92	336
12–14 yr			60	320
13–14 yr				
M			100	420
F			12	284
13–21 yr, F	30	130		
14–15 yr				
M			78	446
F			78	212
14–16 yr			30	250
15–16 yr				
M			43	267
F			35	117
15–21 yr, M	20	180		
16–18 yr				
M			58	331
F			35	124
16–adult	30	190		
M			20	110
F			20	90
Adult	20	75–80	30	115
M			41	137
F			39	118

[a] Both sexes unless otherwise indicated.

O. H., and Brock, M. J., A method for the rapid determination of alkaline phosphatase with five cubic millimeters of serum. *J. Biol. Chem.* **164,** 321–329 (1946); McMichael, J., Serum alkaline phosphatase. *Br. Med. J.* **i,** 786 (1968); Massod, M. F., Werner, K. R., and McGuire, S. L., Kinetic determination of serum alkaline phosphatase activity. *Am. J. Clin. Pathol.* **54,** 110–117 (1970); Fishman, W. H., and Ghosh, N. K., Isoenzymes of human alkaline phosphatase. *Adv. Clin. Chem.* **10,** 255–370 (1967); Amador, E., and Urban, J., Transphosphorylation by human alkaline phosphatases. *Am. J. Clin. Pathol.* **57,** 167–172 (1972); Yong, J. M., Origins of serum alkaline phosphatase. *J. Clin. Pathol.* **20,** 647–653 (1967); Standard method for the determination of alkaline phosphatase activity (Recommendation of the German Society for Clinical Chemistry). *J. Clin. Chem. Clin. Biochem.* **10,** 281–291 (1972).

Instrumentation:

Note: Specimen volume required for analysis varies markedly with the instrumentation used. In general, pediatric microanalysis is in the range of 5 to 50 μL for this enzyme.

Beckman TR Enzyme Analyzer with Beckman alkaline phosphatase kit; Electro-Nucleonics GEMSAEC; Abbott ABA-100 Bichromatic Analyzer with A-Gent reagent; Union Carbide CentrifiChem; Technicon SMA II and SMAC systems; Harleco UltraZyme PLUS ALP reagent; Worthington Diagnostics Alkaline Phosphatase (PNP) Reagent Set.

*   *   *

Laboratory Reporting:

1.

Reference (Normal) Values:

Age, yr	U/L (Bowers–McComb Method, 30 °C)			
	M		F	
	5th percentiles	95th percentiles	5th percentiles	95th percentiles
Up to 0.99	146	477	154	442
1.00–1.99	146	333	154	415
2.00–4.99	146	291	154	341
5.00–6.99	146	291	154	341
7.00–9.99	153	316	162	354
10.00–12.99	149	362	135	393
13.00–14.99			78	322
15.00–16.99	92	365		
15.00–17.99			47	122
17.00–18.99	70	176		
18.00–over			31	86
19.00–over	54	126		

Sources of Reference (Normal) Values:

Up to age 4.99 yr: Clark, L. C., Jr., and Beck, E., Plasma alkaline phosphatase activity. 1. Normative data for growing children. *J. Pediatr.* **36,** 335–341 (1950). **Age 5 yr and older:** Cherian, A. G., and Hill, J. G., Age dependence of serum enzymatic activities (alkaline phosphatase, aspartate aminotransferase, and creatine kinase) in healthy children and adolescents. *Am. J. Clin. Pathol.* **70,** 783–789 (1978); institutional.

Note: All other data as in preceding report.

*   *   *

Laboratory Reporting:

1.

Reference (Normal) Values:

Newborn: 1–4 × adult
Through childhood: 1–3 × adult
Adult: 26–57 U/L

Sources of Reference (Normal) Values:

Institutional.

Analytical Method:

Babson, A. L., Greely, S. J., Coleman, C. M., and Phillips, G. E., Phenolphthalein monophosphate as a substrate for serum alkaline phosphatase. *Clin. Chem.* **12,** 482–490 (1966); General Diagnostics Phosphastrate alkaline substrate.

Enzyme Data:

1. Enzyme unit definition: 1 IUB unit (U) of ALP = that amount of enzyme activity liberating 1 μmol of end product per minute under the conditions specified in the test.
2. Buffer: 2-amino-2-methyl-1-propanol.
3. Substrate, pH: phenolphthalein monophosphate dicyclohexylamine, 10.15 (9.9 at 37 °C).
4. Reaction temperature: 37 °C.
5. Temperature reported: 37 °C.

Instrumentation:

Abbott ABA-100 Bichromatic Analyzer.

Commentary—George N. Bowers, Jr.

Reference (Normal) Values

As shown in Figure 1 (p 69), the total ALP activity in human

serum varies considerably with age and to a lesser extent with sex
(1). Kay first reported such differences in 1930 *(2)*, and numerous
workers using many methods have confirmed, extended, and refined
these observations (e.g., *3–6*). The reference intervals given in the
reports—particularly those submitted by Hill, which were based on
measurements of 1033 individuals five to 20 years old *(6)*—very adequately differentiate the significantly higher reference limits in pediatric populations from those in adults. (For greater details and
other influences, see Chapter 9, Section 9.2, of ref. *1*.)

These age-dependent differences in total ALP activity can largely
be explained by the presence of increased "bone" isoenzyme in the
young *(1)*. During periods of accelerated bone growth, particularly
in adolescent boys at about 13 to 15 years of age, the increase of
bone isoenzyme in serum can occasionally result in *transient* activity
of total ALP that is five- to sevenfold the upper reference limits of
adults, as shown in Figure 1 *(3,4)*. When physicians and laboratory
scientists are knowledgeable as to an individual's peer group reference values and to these marked transient physiological increases
associated with rapid growth spurts, many "problems" related to
hyperphosphatemia in infants, children, and particularly in adolescents are resolved.

Blood Collection and Preservation

The site of blood collection (venous, capillary, arterial, or cord)
makes little difference, provided that concentration of blood from
prolonged tourniquet stress or dilution from extravasation of tissue
juices is avoided. Serum is the preferred specimen *(1)*. Heparinized
plasma can also be used, but *do not* use EDTA-treated, citrated, or
oxalated plasma. Freshly separated serum held at RT (23 °C) should
be analyzed within 4 h or refrigerated at 4 °C and assayed as soon
thereafter as possible *(7)*. Freezing and lyophilization can markedly
decrease activity by causing conformational changes in ALP(s). Special precautions to regain full activity may be required with some
commercial control materials *(1,7,8)*.

Methods

Most of the reference values submitted here are from methods
involving *p*-nitrophenyl phosphate as substrate and 2-amino-2-
methyl-1-propanol as buffer. Sample volumes range from 10 to 200
μL, and the sensitivity for pediatric microchemical needs seems more
than adequate. Although these methods look similar, there are many
significant differences in substrate concentrations, buffer strength,
pH, reaction temperature, and the procedural steps by which magnesium and sample are introduced. These methodologic differences
cause activity to vary considerably, so that reference values established for one set of methodologic conditions should not be transferred
from one method to another. For example, Table 1 shows the metho-

Table 1. Changes in the Bowers and McComb Method, and in Reference Values, as the Method Has Been Further Developed

	Year (ref.)			
	1966 *(9)*	1972 *(10)*	1975 *(11)*	1979 *(1)*[a]
Substrate, mmol/L	4	14	15	16
Buffer, mmol/L	750	750	800	1000
Magnesium, mmol/L				
Final	0.1	0.1	0.1	1
Preincubation	0	0	0	4
pH (30 °C)	10.15	10.30	10.30	10.50
Sample volume, μL	100	100	100	50
Total volume, μL	3000	3000	3000	3050
Volume ratio (sample : total)	1 : 30	1 : 30	1 : 30	1 : 61
Temperature, °C	30	30	30	29.77[b]
Molar absorptivity of *p*-nitrophenol in buffer (L × mol^{-1} × cm^{-1})	18 750	18 750	18 800	19 050
Reference values, U/L				
Adults, 20–60 yr	20–80	20–90	20–90	25–100
Children, 2–10 yr	80–300	80–330	80–330	100–350
Girls, 10–13 yr	90–360	90–400	90–400	110–400
Boys, 13–15 yr	100–400	100–450	100–450	125–500

[a] Similar preincubation and final reaction conditions are currently being used with the Perkin-Elmer KA-150 instrument; the serum sample is 10 μL and the total volume is 200 μL, giving a ratio of 1 : 20. The assay time is only 10 s.
[b] Gallium melting-point standard as provided by NBS/SRM 1968 *(12)*.

dologic changes in the "Bowers and McComb" procedure(s) over the years and demonstrates how these changes affect the upper reference limit *(1,9–11)* at or near 30 °C *(12)*. What is not readily apparent in the latest (1979) modification *(1)* is that the enzyme sample (serum or control) is now being preincubated only with magnesium, and exposure between serum and buffer is minimized by addition of buffer/substrate mixture to initiate the final reaction. This procedural change *(a)* saturates the enzyme(s) with magnesium, and *(b)* minimizes contact of the enzyme(s) with chelating-type impurities in some lots of buffer that may cause a time-dependent inactivation by binding or removing zinc from the active center of the ALP molecule.

Instrumentation

Because of the high molar absorptivity of the product, *p*-nitrophenol, in alkaline solution near 400 nm, almost any photometer can be adapted to make these *p*-nitrophenyl phosphate colorimetric determinations of ALP, either by simple sampling techniques or by more sophisticated continuous-monitoring procedures. These methods have been adapted to numerous automated systems with little difficulty; however, the constraints of reagent addition sequences in some systems will not permit the recent procedural changes for preincubation in magnesium and limiting exposure to the 2-amino-2-methyl-1-propanol buffer. As noted in Table 1, modern kinetic analyzers can follow the initial progress curve for very short periods (e.g., 10 s) because of their extremely stable photometers and electronic processing of the signals. Analytical precision for measuring serum ALP in clinical laboratories has been reported to be as good as 2 to 3% (CV) for within-day runs (1), but typically increases to 5% for long-term studies of day-to-day intralaboratory performance (13); CVs reportedly range from 17 to 28% for interlaboratory proficiency surveys (1,-14,15). It is difficult to determine just how much imprecision is due to the chemical variables (reagents and procedure) and how much to instrument variability.

Interpretation

With the possible exception of familial hypophosphatasia (16), few if any diseases or critical diagnostic decisions are made on the basis of ALP measurements alone. Nonetheless, more of these measurements are requested by physicians today than any other enzyme test, except possibly asparate aminotransferase (1). Therefore, both the physician and the laboratory scientist are repeatedly faced with the problem of the clinical significance of hyperphosphatasemia in healthy persons as well as in sick patients. Let me stress once again that all interpretations must be made with the proper reference values, especially in the pediatric age group, and that extreme physiological increases can be associated with the growth spurts of puberty.

Medications may increase alkaline phosphatase values in children; for example, the chronic therapeutic use of anticonvulsant drugs such as dilantin and phenobarbital is regularly associated with higher values. Transient hyperphosphatasemia of infancy has been described and is said to be under-recognized (17,18). Persistent hyperphosphatasemia presents problems in differential diagnosis because it occasionally, although only rarely, alerts one to an otherwise occult disease (e.g., malignancy); more often, however, hyperphosphatasemia unassociated with other signs and systems can lead to costly diagnostic workups that often fail to resolve the problem and leave both the physician and patient wondering. In such situations, isoenzyme fractionation is frequently requested. Physicians need to realize that it is usually the skill, experience, and consultative advice of the laboratory scientist that help resolve problems requiring the quantitation of isoenzymes, rather than the inherent separating power of the fractionating techniques.

1. McComb, R. B., Bowers, G. N., Jr., and Posen, S., *Alkaline Phosphatase*. Plenum Press, New York, NY, 1979, pp 531–538.
2. Kay, H. D., Plasma phosphatase. I. Method of determining some properties of the enzyme. *J. Biol. Chem.* **89**, 235–247 (1930).

3. Clark, L. C., Jr., and Beck, E., Plasma "alkaline" phosphatase activity. I. Normative data for growing children. *J. Pediatr.* **36,** 335–341 (1950).
4. Sereny, G., and McLaughlin, L., Serum alkaline phosphatase values in normal adolescents. *Can. Med. Assoc. J.* **102,** 1400–1401 (1970).
5. Fleisher, G. A., Eickelberg, E. S., and Elveback, L. R., Alkaline phosphatase activity in the plasma of children and adolescents. *Clin. Chem.* **23,** 469–472 (1977).
6. Cherian, A. G., and Hill, J. G., Age dependence of serum enzymatic activities (alkaline phosphatase, aspartate aminotransferase, and creatine kinase) in healthy children and adolescents. *Am. J. Clin. Pathol.* **70,** 783–789 (1978).
7. Massion, C. G., and Frankenfeld, J. K., Alkaline phosphatase: Lability in fresh and frozen human serum and lyophilized control material. *Clin. Chem.* **18,** 366–373 (1972).
8. Smith, A. F., and Fogg, B. A., Possible mechanisms for the increase in alkaline phosphatase activity of lyophilized control material. *Clin. Chem.* **18,** 1518–1523 (1972).
9. Bowers, G. N., Jr., and McComb, R. B., A continuous spectrophotometric method for measuring the activity of serum alkaline phosphatase. *Clin. Chem.* **12,** 70–89 (1966).
10. McComb, R. B., and Bowers, G. N., Jr., Study of optimum buffer conditions for measuring alkaline phosphatase activity in human serum. *Clin. Chem.* **18,** 97–104 (1972).
11. Bowers, G. N., Jr., and McComb, R. B., Measurement of total alkaline phosphatase activity in human serum. *Clin. Chem.* **21,** 1988–1995 (1975).
12. Mangum, B. W., and Thorton, D. D., Eds., *The Gallium Melting-Point Standard.* National Bureau of Standards Special Publication 481, Washington, DC, 1977.
13. Burnett, R. W., Accurate estimation of standard deviations for quantitative methods used in clinical chemistry. *Clin. Chem.* **21,** 1935–1938 (1975).
14. Whitehead, T. P., Browning, D. M., and Gregory, A., A comparative survey of the results of analyses of blood serum in clinical chemistry laboratories in the United Kingdom. *J. Clin. Pathol.* **26,** 435–445 (1973).
15. Strömme, J. H., Björnstad, P., and Eldjarn, L., Improvement in the quality of enzyme determinations by Scandinavian laboratories upon introduction of Scandinavian recommended methods. *Scand. J. Clin. Lab. Invest.* **36,** 505–511 (1976).
16. Bartter, F. C., Hypophosphatasia. Chapter 51 in *The Metabolic Basis of Inherited Disease*, 3rd ed., J. B. Stanbury, J. B. Wyngaarden, and D. S. Fredrickson, Eds. McGraw-Hill, New York, NY, 1972, pp 1295–1304.
17. Posen, S., Lee, C., Vines, R., Kilham, H., Latham, S., and Keefe, J. F., Transient hyperphosphatasemia of infancy—an insufficiently recognized syndrome. *Clin. Chem.* **23,** 292–294 (1977).
18. Wieme, R. J., More on transient hyperphosphatasemia in infancy—an insufficiently recognized syndrome. *Clin. Chem.* **24,** 520–522 (1978). Letter.

Commentary—Paul L. Wolf

Identifying the major source of ALP in the serum of children is important because its function is related to the tissue in which it is present. As is well known, the highest physiologic activity of the enzyme is found in growing children and is secreted into serum by osteoblasts, which produce the enzyme as an important function in the calcification of growing bone. The child's serum also normally contains a liver isoenzyme and may contain an intestinal isoenzyme if the child has blood type B or O and is a secretor.

Clark and Beck studied ALP in children and showed that the high activity in infants decreases during the second year, but remains somewhat increased at a constant value until puberty (1). A rapid decline to normal adult values occurs at age 9 in girls and age 11 in boys. The enzyme activity was still at adult values at age 17. Fleisher et al. (2), studying serum ALP in 854 healthy students, found that prepubertal girls had somewhat greater upper limits than did boys; the enzyme values peaked at ages 11–12 years in girls and 13–14 years in boys, with highest values of 1100 U/L in boys and 900 U/L in girls. Woodward and Kenny (3) found that growing bone contains at least 10-fold as much ALP as adult bone. Low serum ALP activity has occurred in myxedema, hereditary hypophosphatasia, deficiencies of vitamin C and B_{12}, and achondroplasia (4). The bone and liver isoenzymes are markedly diminished or absent in hereditary hypophosphatasia, but the intestinal isoenzyme persists (5). Phosphoethanolamine, present in increased quantities in the urine of these patients, is considered to be the natural substrate for ALP. With vitamin B_{12} deficiency ALP activity is decreased, possibly because vitamin B_{12} may act as a cofactor for the enzyme.

ALP also functions in the synthesis of collagen. Therefore, the increase of ALP in serum in children also reflects the growth of connective tissue. An important source of ALP is vascular endothelium.

When the activity of serum ALP in children is found to be increased, but is not related to physiologic bone growth, a pathologic lesion may be present in any of several various organs.

An increased total serum ALP activity may represent a combination of various isoenzymes from (e.g.) liver and bone, related to metastasis of a malignant lesion to both sites.

In children various liver lesions such as viral or toxic hepatitis and giant cell hepatitis will cause a two- to fivefold increase in ALP; biliary atresia may cause a 10- to 15-fold increase. This increase during liver disease results from decreased secretion of liver ALP into bile and regurgitation of ALP into the circulation through the sinusoids. In addition, with cholestasis, bile ductule cells increase their synthesis of this enzyme. Thus, an increase in liver ALP is a sensitive indicator of cholestasis.

Other important causes of an increased serum ALP in children are cardiac failure from passive congestion of the liver; organization of pulmonary, splenic, and kidney infarcts; celiac disease; cystic fibrosis associated with malabsorption states and ulcerative colitis; and ectopic production of ALP by a malignant neoplasm, the Regan isoenzyme (6–8).

Thus, the major pathologic causes for increased serum ALP in children are liver diseases (such as viral hepatitis, giant cell hepatitis, or toxic hepatitis) and various bone diseases, including infiltrates associated with leukemia, lymphoma, storage diseases such as Gaucher's disease, metastatic neoplasma (such as neuroblastoma), and primary lesions (such as osteogenic sarcoma). In addition, osteomalacia caused by rickets, vitamin-D-resistant rickets, and the osteomalacia associated with secondary hyperparathyroidism of renal insufficiency must be considered.

1. Clark, L. C., Jr., and Beck, E., Plasma alkaline phosphatase activity. I. Normative data for growing children. *J. Pediatr.* **36,** 335–341 (1950).
2. Fleisher, G. A., Eickelberg, E. S., and Elveback, L. R., Alkaline phosphatase activity in the plasma of children and adolescents. *Clin. Chem.* **23,** 469–472 (1977).
3. Woodward, H. Q., and Kenney, J. M., The relation of phophatase activity in bone tumors to the deposition of radioactive phosphorus. *Am. J. Roentgenol.* **47,** 227 (1942).
4. Wolf, P. L., Clinical significance of an increased or decreased serum alkaline phosphatase level. *Arch. Pathol. Lab. Med.* **102,** 497–501 (1978).
5. Danovitch, S. H., Baer, P. N., and Laster, L., Intestinal alkaline phosphatase activity in familial hypophosphatasia. *N. Engl. J. Med.* **278,** 1253–1260 (1968).
6. Kattwinkel, J., Taussig, L. M., Statland, B. E., and Verter, J. I., The effects of age on alkaline phosphatase and other serologic liver function tests in normal subjects and patients with cystic fibrosis. *J. Pediatr.* **82,** 234–242 (1973).
7. Dijkman, J. H., and Kloppenborg, P. W. C., Increased serum alkaline phosphatase activity in pulmonary infarction. *Acta Med. Scand.* **180,** 273–281 (1966).
8. Nathanson, L., and Fishman, W. H., New observations on the Regan isoenzyme of alkaline phosphatase in cancer patients. *Cancer* **27,** 1388–1397 (1971).

Alkaline Phosphatase, Heat-Labile

Specimen Tested:

P, S.

Laboratory Reporting:

1.

Reference (Normal) Values:

Up to 35% of the total activity in adults is heat-labile (bone-derived phosphatase).

Sources of Reference (Normal) Values:

Institutional; Fishman, W. H., and Ghosh, N. K., Isoenzymes of human alkaline phosphatase. *Adv. Clin. Chem.* **10,** 255–370 (1967).

Specimen Volume, Collection, and Preservation; Patient Preparation:

50 μL. Plasma from heparin anticoagulant only. See **Alkaline Phosphatase** for further information.

Analytical Method:

Method of McComb–Bowers, described under **Alkaline Phosphatase.**

Instrumentation:

Beckman TR Enzyme Analyzer, with Beckman Enztrate Alkaline Phosphatase kit.

Alkaline Phosphatase Isoenzymes

Specimen Tested:

P, S (cord blood).

Laboratory Reporting:

1.

Reference (Normal) Values:

Total isoenzyme acty: 26–208 U/L

Bone isoenzyme acty: 13–169 U/L

Sources of Reference (Normal) Values:

Institutional, based on analysis of 79 specimens.

Specimen Volume, Collection, and Preservation; Patient Preparation:

20 μL. Cord blood (umbilical venous and arterial), collected into heparinized containers, then centrifuged at 2500 $\times$ g for 5 min, and serum (or plasma) stored frozen at -20 °C. No differences observed between P and S.

Analytical method:

Statland, B. E., Nishi, H. H., and Young, D. S., Serum alkaline phosphatase: Total activity and isoenzyme determinations made by use of the centrifugal fast analyzer. *Clin. Chem.* **18,** 1468–1474 (1972).

Enzyme data:

As described by Bowers (first report given, p 70) under **Alkaline Phosphatase.**

Instrumentation:

Aminco Rotochem with Rotofill automatic dispensing pipettor–dilutor.

Alpha-Amino Acid Nitrogen

Specimen Tested:

U.

Laboratory Reporting:

1.

Reference (Normal) Values:

| | | α-Amino acid nitrogen | | |
Age	No.	mg/d	mg/kg body wt. per day	mg/mg of creatinine
1 mo–1 yr	50	10–70	0.5–10.5	0.05–0.87
1–5 yr	42	15–125	0.5–8.4	0.03–0.67
5–10 yr	34	30–175	0.5–7.6	0.04–0.44

Sources of Reference (Normal) Values:

Applegarth, D. A., Hardwick, D. F., and Ross, P. M., Creatinine excretion in children and the usefulness of creatinine equivalents in amino acid chromatography. *Clin. Chim. Acta* **22,** 131–134 (1968); Khachadurian, A., Knox, W. E., and Cullen, A. M., Colorimetric ninhydrin method for total alpha-amino acids of urine. *J. Lab. Clin. Med.* **56,** 321–332 (1960).

Analytical Method:

Quantitate α-amino acid nitrogen by using a reaction with ninhydrin after the removal of ammonia: Moore, S., and Stein, W. H., Photometric ninhydrin method for use in the chromatography of amino acids. *J. Biol. Chem.* **176,** 367–388 (1948); Rosenblum, R., Wolfman, M., and Leiter, L., A correction for the interference of total alpha-amino acid nitrogen in plasma by the ninhydrin photometric method. *J. Lab. Clin. Med.* **54,** 132–135 (1959); Hotchkiss, R. D., The assimilation of amino acids by respiring washed *Staphylococci. Arch. Biochem.* **65,** 302–318 (1956).

Specimen Volume, Collection, and Preservation:

5-mL aliquot of 24-h collection. Store U in FR during collection, and until analysis.

Commentary—David J. Harris

For detecting inborn errors of amino acid metabolism, this procedure is relatively nonspecific and may miss a significant increase in the excretion of a single amino acid *(1)*. For the day-to-day management of patients, specimens for screening tests should be easily obtained; on the other hand, collection of 24-h urine samples from young infants is often difficult. More specific qualitative tests with sufficient sensitivity can be done on spot urine samples and require less equipment and time.

1. Scriver, C. R., and Rosenberg, L. E., *Amino Acid Metabolism and Its Disorders.* W. B. Saunders, Philadelphia, PA, 1973.

Amino Acids

In Cerebrospinal Fluid

Laboratories Reporting:

3.

Reference (Normal) Values:

	Concn, μmol/L[a]			
Amino acid	1–24 mo (1)	3 mo–10 yr (1)[b]	Child (2)[c]	Adult (2)[c]
Alanine	<51.8	13.1–45.0	<38.8	5.6–67.3
α-Amino-*n*-butyric acid			<2.6	0–19.4
γ-Aminobutyryllysine				0–0.5
Arginine	<35.3	8.05–24.6	<29.3	2.3–39.7
Asparagine		3.0–18.9*		tr–30.3
Aspartic acid	<12.3	0.3–2.3*	<9.3	0–27.1
Citrulline	<41.0		<27.8	0.5–3.7
Cystine			trace	0–22.9
Ethanolamine			<6.7	5.8–25.0
Glutamic acid		0.2–59.1*	<14.7	0–163
Glutamine	<916.7		<753.4	71.0–890
Glycine	<51.8	1.90–9.08	<38.8	3.0–67.3
Histidine	<32.9	0–14.0	<23.9	4.5–35.5
Homocarnosine			<2.7	0–5.4
Isoleucine	<11.7	1.3–7.7	<10.1	1.8–11.4
Leucine	<23.4	3.3–21.2	<21.8	3.8–26.7
Lysine		5.96–26.1	<18.6	17.3–37.7
Methionine		0.7–5.0	<3.2	1.2–14.1
N-ϵ-Methyllysine				0–4.5
Ornithine		1.91–6.89	<8.5	1.7–9.3
Phenylalanine		4.24–36.4	<7.5	1.1–15.7
Phosphoethanolamine				1.7–8.1
Proline				tr–23.5
Serine[d]	<61.2	25.1–52.7	<45.7	14.3–69.5
Taurine	<20.0	3.11–11.2	<22.4	3.2–12.0
Threonine	<46.7	11.4–36.3	<36.5	10.1–48.0
Tryptophan	<4.4		<4.1	0–12.7
Tyrosine	<26.4	5.35–17.3	<15.8	3.8–16.0
Valine	<43.8	7.6–20.3	<39.7	6.0–27.5

[a] Numbers in parentheses indicate no. of labs. reporting.
[b] Values are reported for 5th and 95th percentiles, or, if indicated by *, for ranges observed.
[c] Combined ranges of two reports (lower to higher). Values are generally at 3 SD.
[d] Significant trend with age.

Sources of Reference (Normal) Values:

Applegarth, D. A., Edelsten, A. D., Wong, L. T. K., and Morrison, B. J., Observed range of assay values for plasma and cerebrospinal fluid amino acid levels in infants and children aged 3 months to 10 years. *Clin. Biochem.* **12**, 173–178 (1979); Liappis, F. N., Jäkel, A., and Bantzer, P., Verhalten der freien Aminosäuren im Liquor cerebrospinalis von Kindern. *Klin. Paediatr.* **189**, 155–160 (1977); Plum, C. M., Free amino acid levels in the cerebrospinal fluid of normal humans and their variation in cases of epilepsy and Spielmeyer–Vogt–Batten disease. *J. Neurochem.* **23**, 595–600 (1974); institutional.

Specimen Volume, Collection, and Preservation; Patient Preparation:

0.2 to 1.0 mL. Fasting sample preferred. Deproteinize without delay. Store in FR.

Analytical Method and Instrumentation:

Ion-exchange chromatography; Durrum (Dionex) 500 Amino Acid Analyzer; Technicon Amino Acid Analyzer, Type AAA-1.

In Blood

Specimen Tested:

P, S.

Laboratories Reporting:

5.

Reference (Normal) Values:

See page 84.

Sources of Reference (Normal) Values:

Institutional; Scriver, C. R., and Rosenberg, L. E., *Amino Acid Metabolism and Its Disorders*, W. B. Saunders Co., Philadelphia, PA, 1973, p 42; Applegarth et al., *op. cit.;* Dickinson, J. C., Rosenblum, H., and Hamilton, P. B., Ion-exchange chromatography of the free amino acids in the plasma of the newborn infant. *Pediatrics* **36**, 2–13 (1965); Scriver, C. R., and Davies, E., Endogenous renal clearance rates of free amino acids in prepubertal children. *Pediatrics* **36**, 592–598 (1965); Scriver, C. R., Amino acid metabolism in the newborn. In *The Neonate*, D. S. Young and J. M. Hicks, Eds. Wiley, New York, NY, 1976, pp 148–149; Stein, W. H., and Moore, S., The free amino acids of human blood plasma. *J. Biol. Chem.* **211**, 915–926 (1954); Scriver, C. R., Clow, C. L., and Lamm, P., Plasma amino acids: Screening, quantitation and interpretation. *Am. J. Clin. Nutr.* **24**, 886 (1971); Dickinson, J. C., Rosenblum, H., and Hamilton, P. B., Ion-exchange

Upper section — values in μmol/L:

Age	Alanine	α-Amino-n-butyric acid	Arginine	Asparagine	Aspartic acid	Citrulline	Cystine ½	Glutamic acid	Glutamine	Glycine	Histidine	Hydroxyproline	Isoleucine
16 d–4 mo[a]	239–345		53–71		17–21		33–51			178–248	64–92		31–47
1–3 mo	134–416	1–34	21–74	6–33	0–8	6–36	11–38			105–222	42–83		32–87
Newborn	236–410	6–29	22–88		tr–17	9–28	39–92	18–95		224–514	44–102		26–53
0–5 yr[b]	167–295				0–14			72–172		178–248	47–97		40–55
3 mo–6 yr[c]	158–393	12–36	33–122	72–144	3–12	9–47	23–49	15–77	475–746[d]	127–295	25–101		16–74
6 mo–3 yr	109–607	2–40	33–111	9–99		8–34	11–63	19–100	343–696	80–296	58–131		33–123
9 mo–10 yr	99–313	9–38	11–86	18–99	0–20	12–30	18–77			56–308	24–112		26–94
Child	137–665	4–38	28–150		4–20	8–42	45–77	7–250	486–806	110–319	24–127	25	25–120
6–18 yr, M	203–507	12–36	54–130	34–62	0–14	20–52	36–55	7–63	360–740	166–302	66–106	0–50	43–95
F	193–545	8–36	44–124	32–60	0–14	19–47	39–58	9–65	459–723	158–302	64–104	0–44	38–90
Adult, 18–77 yr, M	241–597	10–42	37–141	36–63		19–55	51–68	28–92	517–773	152–320	67–111	0–42	48–120
F	199–547	6–38	27–123	29–65		15–55	43–67	20–72	408–748	72–528	55–111	0–34	38–90
Adult, M + F	188–522	tr–65	23–118	30–69	tr–29	18–92	33–117	3–107	396–711	81–362	55–128		38–121

Lower section — values in μmol/L:

Age	Leucine	Lysine[e]	Methionine	1-Methylhistidine	3-Methylhistidine	Ornithine	Phenylalanine	Proline	Serine	Taurine	Threonine[e]	Tryptophan	Tyrosine	Valine[e]
16 d–4 mo[a]	56–98	107–163	15–21			39–61	45–65	141–245	104–158		141–213		33–75	123–199
1–3 mo	43–165	37–168	4–39			26–117	24–80	77–324	76–152	0–53	64–225		29–135	96–291
Newborn	46–109	114–268	9–41			49–151	42–110	107–277	94–243	74–216	114–335		42–99	80–246
0–5 yr[b]	86–128	106–175	10–20			38–71	44–52	62–180	75–149		59–105		44–67	143–194
3 mo–6 yr[c]	42–143	88–205	6–27			28–93	35–92	40–332	93–161	12–84	41–125		26–83	86–317
6 mo–3 yr	63–224	89–302	10–49	5–33		30–114	36–108	52–528	83–206	29–78		12–66	41–154	155–366
9 mo–10 yr	45–178	45–151	3–29				23–69	51–185		19–115	33–128	21–91	11–122	57–283
Child	56–222	71–181	11–43	0–33		36–107	26–91	68–454	79–206	32–115	42–95	21–82	41–141	116–373
6–18 yr, M	94–174	117–233	17–37			21–81	44–76	72–324	71–171	0–228	84–196		48–88	176–288
F	79–159	108–220	16–36			19–75	39–71	58–286	73–181	0–240	74–202		43–87	156–272
Adult, 18–77 yr, M	76–168	136–260	20–44			29–101	40–72	99–379	68–160	40–282	102–190		42–102	178–326
F	106–214	115–251	17–37			18–90	47–83	70–266	69–185	27–235	74–234		35–87	147–271
Adult, M + F	78–201	97–235		0–25	0–12	38–91	41–70	1–497	83–206	35–191	108–331	20–61	31–96	159–315

[a] 12 infants after 6–8 h fast. [b] 16 infants and children up to 5 yr. [c] 5th and 95th percentiles. [d] Range of values found. [e] Shows significant trends with age. tr, trace amount.

chromatography of the free amino acids in the plasma of infants under 2500 gm at birth. *Pediatrics* **45,** 606–613 (1970); Snyderman, S. E., Holt, L. E., Jr., Norton, P. M., Rottman, E., and Phansalkar, S. V., The plasma aminogram. I. Influence of the level of protein intake and a comparison of whole protein and amino acid diets. *Pediatr. Res.* **2,** 131–144 (1968); Armstrong, M. D., and Stave, U., A study of plasma free amino acid levels. II. Normal values for children and adults. III. Variations during growth and aging. *Metabolism* **22,** 561–569, 571–578 (1973).

Specimen Volume, Collection, and Preservation; Patient Preparation:

As reported for CSF. Minimum fasting, 2 h.

Instrumentation:

As reported for CSF; also, Liquimat III (Labotron-Kontron), with Spectra-Physics SP-4000 Integrator.

In Urine

Laboratories Reporting:

4.

Reference (Normal) Values:

See page 86.

Sources of Reference (Normal) Values:

Institutional; Gitlitz, P. H., Sunderman, F. W., Jr., and Hohnadel, D. C., Ion-exchange chromatography of amino acids in sweat collected from healthy subjects during sauna bathing. *Clin. Chem.* **20,** 1305–1312 (1974).

Specimen Data, Analytical Method, Instrumentation:

As for CSF and P; also, Technicon Multiple Amino Acid Analyzer.

Commentary—Jocelyn M. Hicks

Plasma

The primary reason for quantitating amino acids in plasma is to confirm a clinically suspected inborn error of amino acid metabolism in a child. In such disorders the abnormal amino acid concentration is usually three- to 10-fold greater than normal values. Although variation in the concentration of plasma amino acids is dependent upon age, time of day, and relation to feeding, these variations are not great enough to interfere with the recognition and identification of a child with a primary disorder of amino acid metabolism.

Amino acid	Amount excreted, μmol/L				
	0–5 yr	1 mo–3 yr	Child	3–15 yr	Adult
Alanine	29–370	0–183	43–367	0–292	200–1040
α-Aminoadipic acid		0–41		0–50	
α-Amino-*n*-butyric acid	5–39	0–18		0–20	3–29
Arginine		0–10	tr–37	0–29	0–60
Asparagine		0–80		0–106	88–300
Aspartic acid	5–278	0–45	0–75	1–65	155–390
β-Alanine		0–28		0–67	
β-Aminoisobutyric acid	95–540	0–91		0–104	12–1040
Carnosine		0–145		7–163	
Citrulline		0–4		2–6	
Cystathionine		0–17		0–26	
Cystine, ½	7–50	0–33	22–86	0–40	40–308
Ethanolamine			120–416		297–802
Glutamic acid	7–121	0–19	tr–55	0–20	0–84
Glutamine					290–1030
Glycine	111–1372	0–335	134–1250	0–893	458–4240
Histidine	21–844	0–338	215–905	0–751	430–2310
Isoleucine	5–38	0–20	0–17	0–21	0–36
Leucine	2–53	0–25	tr–59	0–55	16–123
Lysine	20–384	0–95	40–714	0–100	25–1950
Methionine		0–34	0–tr	0–40	0–152
1-Methylhistidine		0–95		0–262	48–2560
3-Methylhistidine		0–60		0–197	180–390
Ornithine	4–113	0–11	tr–22	0–14	0–44
Phenylalanine	8–61	0–46		0–89	44–220
Phosphoethanolamine		3–39	19–127	3–63	
Proline		0–22		0–38	
Serine	29–552	0–164	66–383	0–318	240–650
Taurine	133–2165	0–228	75–1000	0–545	90–1710
Threonine	9–579	0–73	43–282	0–145	110–840
Tryptophan	6–49				
Tyrosine	4–110	0–87	32–128	0–132	41–281
Valine	11–68	0–29	tr–60	0–50	0–98

Amino acid	Adult		Amino acid	Adult	
	mg/d	mg/g of creatinine		mg/d	mg/g of creatinine
Alanine	9–29	15–78	Leucine	3–70	tr–51
α-Aminoadipic acid	4–55	tr–43	Lysine	54–257	24–570
α-Amino-*n*-butyric acid	2–10	2–10	Methionine	1–28	tr–18
Asparagine	31–83	tr–171	1-Methylhistidine	tr–23	tr–93
Aspartic acid	2–20	13–95	3-Methylhistidine	3–9	tr–17
β-Alanine	tr–2	tr–11	Ornithine	tr–7	tr–110
β-Aminoisobutyric acid	tr–85	tr–126	Phenylalanine	6–30	tr–33
Cystine, ½	8–42	tr–18	Proline	tr	0–49
Glutamic acid	4–19	13–90	Sarcosine	6–41	tr–50
Glutamine	61–205	52–540	Serine	28–1590	21–186
Glycine	46–258	50–326	Taurine	18.5–168	tr–478
Histidine	14–31	12–187	Threonine	12–71	15–81
Isoleucine	2–24	tr–19	Tryptophane	5–39	tr–30
			Tyrosine	12–55	tr–65
			Valine	4–13	tr–22

tr, trace amount.

The separation and quantitation of amino acids from biological fluids requires sophisticated ion-exchange chromatography and detection of the free amino group with ninhydrin. For practical reasons, this technology is available only in automated amino acid analyzers from a few manufacturers (Beckman, Technicon, and Durrum are the major suppliers). All of the analyzers perform adequately and give satisfactory separation of the amino acids in physiologic fluids, with a reproducibility of $\pm 5\%$. The volume of sample required varies from 20 μL to 1.0 mL, depending upon instrumentation.

Plasma samples should be deproteinized soon after collection and stored frozen until analyzed. Storage for long periods may alter the amino acid profile; a decrease in glutamine and cystine concentration and an increase in glutamic acid are the primary alterations.

Interpreting amino acid values obtained from children with acute liver disease or receiving parenteral hyperalimentation is difficult. In both instances many of the amino acids may be strikingly increased, in a pattern that is not consistent with a specific disorder of amino acid metabolism.

Cerebrospinal Fluid

The concentration of most amino acids in CSF is approximately one-tenth of that in plasma. The predominant amino acid in CSF, glutamine, has a concentration of approximately 0.50 mmol/L, about the same as in plasma. Proline and cystine are usually not detectable.

Quantitation of amino acids in CSF is usually not necessary for establishing a diagnosis of an inborn error of amino acid metabolism, except for non-ketotic hyperglycinemia, in which the concentration of glycine is three- to fivefold greater than normal. Documentation of an increased CSF glycine assists in distinguishing this disorder from other causes of hyperglycinemia, in which the plasma glycine concentration may be increased but the concentration in CSF is normal.

Urine

The concentration of amino acids in urine is extremely variable, and considerable experience and knowledge of amino acid metabolism are required to interpret data obtained only from urine. In my opinion, the qualitative evaluation of amino acids in urine by two-dimensional paper or thin-layer chromatography is of more practical value than obtaining quantitative data. In all cases where an amino acid concentration is significantly increased in blood, there will also be a detectable increased excretion of the amino acid in urine.

The amino acids in greatest concentration in urine from healthy persons are glutamine, glycine, serine, taurine, and histidine. The exact pattern (and concentration) of components is dependent upon genetic factors, diet, age, state of health, and medications. Urine may contain many amino acids not normally detectable in plasma; β-aminoisobutyric acid or 3-methylhistidine, for example, are commonly present in urine because of a genetic enzyme polymorphism or because of dietary intake.

In children with inborn errors, urinary abnormalities are usually detectable, so that timed collections of urine are not necessary; any random sample of sufficient volume is adequate for evaluation. The urine should be collected and refrigerated (or frozen) and analyzed within 24–48 h. Bacterial contamination will distort the amino acid profile.

Disorders of renal tubular transport of amino acids (cystinuria, iminoglycinuria, etc.) will be detectable only by analyzing urine; these disorders are readily detectable by qualitative two-dimensional chromatography.

Finding increased amino acid concentrations in urine should lead one to evaluate the amino acids in plasma; a definitive diagnosis should eventually be documented by enzyme assay of the appropriate tissue. It is quite risky to establish a diagnosis of an inborn error of metabolism only upon the basis of data from urine.

1. Scriver, C. R., and Rosenberg, L. E., *Amino Acid Metabolism and Its Disorders*. W. B. Saunders Co., Philadelphia, PA, 1973.
2. Nyhan, W. L., Ed., *Heritable Disorders of Amino Acid Metabolism*. John Wiley & Sons, New York, NY, 1974.

Amino Acid Clearance

Specimen Tested:

P, S, U.

Laboratory Reporting

1.

Reference (Normal) Values:

Amino acid	Clearance, mL/min per 1.73 m² of body surface	Amino acid	Clearance, mL/min per 1.73 m² of body surface
Alanine	0.2–1.3	Leucine	0.2–0.9
α-Amino-*n*-butyric acid	1.5–5.6	Lysine	0.3–2.4
Arginine	0.15–1.2	Methionine	1.0.3.4
Aspartic acid	tr–8.8	Ornithine	0.2–0.8
Citrulline	0–0.6	Phenylalanine	0.3–2.3
Cystine, ½	1.0–1.4	Proline	0–0.3
Glutamic acid	0.08–2.4	Serine	1.2–3.4
Glycine	1.2–8.6	Taurine	9.9–26.2
Histidine	1.9–21.8	Tyrosine	0.8–3.3
Isoleucine	0.2–1.0	Valine	0.18–0.3

Sources of Reference (Normal) Values:

Scriver, C. R., and Davies, E., Endogenous renal clearance rates of free amino acids in pre-pubertal children. *Pediatrics* **36,** 592–598 (1965).

Analytical Method and Instrumentation:

Cation-exchange chromatography. Durrum (Dionex) 500 Amino Acid Analyzer.

Commentary—Garry M. Lum

Free amino acids are normally filtered by the glomerulus and reabsorbed by complex renal tubular transport mechanisms. There are many techniques for measuring amino acids, but automated ion-exchange chromatography provides the accuracy necessary to obtain clearance determinations. Children excrete more free amino acid than adults. The clearances vary for different age groups, and results and interpretations are available in the literature *(1,2)*. Abnormal aminoaciduria is helpful in the diagnosis of renal tubular disease (e.g., Fanconi syndrome) or of inborn errors of metabolism that result in excesses of certain amino acids in plasma or urine.

1. Woolf, L. I., and Norman, A. P., The urinary excretion of amino acids and sugars in early infancy. *J. Pediatr.* **50,** 271 (1957).
2. Scriver, C. R., and Davies, E., Endogenous renal clearance rates of free amino acids in pre-pubertal children. *Pediatrics* **36,** 592–598 (1965).

Delta-Aminolaevulinate (ALA) and Porphobilinogen

Specimen Tested:

U.

Laboratories Reporting:

2.

Reference (Normal) Values:

Child–adult:
    Lab. 1:   0–7 mg/d (0–32 μmol/d)
    Lab. 2:   (<40 μmol/L)

Note: Lab. 2 also determines porphobilinogen, and reports child to adult values at <9 μmol/L. (See also **Porphyrins.**)

Sources of Reference (Normal) Values:
Text ref. *1;* Bio-Rad Labs. Technical Bulletin, Richmond, CA.

Specimen Volume, Collection, and Preservation:
24-h U. **For Δ-ALA:** Acidify with tartaric acid crystals (excess). Store in dark. Loss is 2% in 72 h, and 6% in 2 wk at RT, but best stored in FR. **For porphobilinogen:** Do not store; analyze immediately.

Analytical Method:
Text ref. *2;* text ref. *4,* 1st ed., p 806; Bio-Rad test kit.

Instrumentation:
Beckman 25, Varian-Techtron 635 spectrophotometers.

Commentary—Roger L. Boeckx

Because circulating erythrocytes do not contain mitochondria and consequently do not display any ALA synthase (EC 2.3.1.37) activity, it is doubtful that inhibition of erythrocytic ALA dehydratase (ALAD; EC 4.2.1.24) is responsible for the increased plasma and urinary ALA observed in lead poisoning. Selander and Cramer *(1)* demonstrated an exponential increase in urinary ALA (ALAU) excretion with increasing blood lead contamination. However, increases in ALA concentration occur at blood lead concentrations lower than those associated with a decrease in blood hemoglobin values, so it seems doubtful that inhibition of ALAD, even at the site of erythropoiesis, is responsible for the high ALA concentrations seen in lead poisoning. In fact, lead may actually increase the activities of certain enzymes of the heme pathway. Lead can stimulate the formation of ALA in liver, in cultured liver cells, and in peripheral leukocytes. The signal for this increase in ALA synthase activity may be a decrease in heme synthesis, resulting from the decreased activity of heme synthetase *(2)*.

Regardless of the mechanism responsible for the increase of ALA concentrations in lead poisoning, the measurement of ALAU has long been considered a good screening test for lead poisoning, especially in the industrial setting *(3)*. Several analytical approaches have been described, but most laboratories use the method of Davis and Andelman *(4)*, which is based on the separation of ALA and porphobilinogen by ion-exchange chromatography. Both compounds can be quantitated from one urine sample.

Despite initial acceptance of ALAU as a screening test for lead poisoning, later reports showed that the procedure was not useful in screening children. Murphy and Lepow *(5)* showed that 50% of children with high blood lead concentrations had normal ALAU results. Conversely, 18 children with abnormal ALAU tests had normal blood lead values. The false-negative rate is even more surprising when one notes that the upper limit of normal for blood lead in these studies was 50 µg/dL. Had the present upper limit of normal blood lead (30 µg/dL) been applied, the test would be even more subject to false-negative results.

Almost simultaneously, two other reports presented similar findings. Specter et al. (6) found that there was no single value for ALAU that could be used to separate normal children from those with evidence of an excessive lead burden. Blumenthal et al. (7) performed a large study in New York, in which they correlated results for blood lead and ALAU in more than 600 children between 18 months and five years of age. They reported a false-negative rate of 33% and a false-positive rate of 39%, using the upper limits for blood lead of 60 µg/dL.

Although the measurement of ALAU may still serve a useful function in industrial medicine, it is clearly not sensitive enough to be used as a screening test in childhood.

Urinary excretion of ALA and porphobilinogen is increased in acute intermittent porphyria and in variegate porphyria. In both cases, a partial block in heme synthesis is thought to derepress ALA synthesis, with a concomitant increase in ALA and porphobilinogen concentrations in plasma and urine. In acute intermittent porphyria, there is a significant deficiency of uroporphorinogen I synthase (EC 4.3.1.8), the enzyme responsible for catalyzing the condensation of four molecules of porphobilinogen to produce uroporphorinogen I (8). In variegate porphyria, a partial enzyme block between protoporphorinogen and heme has been postulated (9).

Urinary ALA and porphobilinogen concentrations increase dramatically during attacks of acute intermittent porphyria. Porphobilinogen concentrations of 20–100 mg/L have been reported during acute attacks. In normal patients, porphobilinogen is not detectable in urine. During latency, ALA and porphobilinogen may be increased but can occasionally be normal. Their excretion is increased in variegate porphyria as well, but not to the extent seen in acute intermittent porphyria. Variegate porphyria is best detected by measuring stool and urine porphyrins. A large and continuous excretion of protoporphyrin and coproporphyrin in stool is usually seen in variegate porphyria.

1. Selander, S., and Cramer, K., Interrelationships between lead in blood, lead in urine, and ALA in urine during lead work. Br. J. Ind. Med. 27, 28–39 (1970).
2. Hammond, P. B., Exposure of humans to lead. Ann. Rev. Pharmacol. Toxicol. 17, 197–214 (1977).
3. Lahaye, D., Roosels, D., Bossiroy, J. M., and van Assche, F., The use of urinary excretion of delta-aminolevulinic acid as a criterion for lead absorption in industrial medicine and insurance medicine. Int. Arch. Occup. Environ. Health 39, 191–198 (1977).

4. Davis, J. R., and Andelman, S. L., Urinary delta-aminolevulinic acid (ALA) levels in lead poisoning: I. A modified method for the rapid determination of urinary delta-aminolevulinic acid using disposable ion-exchange chromatography columns. *Arch. Environ. Health* **15**, 53–59 (1967).
5. Murphy, Y., and Lepow, M. L., Comparison of delta-aminolevulinic acid levels in urine and blood levels for screening children for lead poisoning. *Conn. Med.* **35**, 488–492 (1971).
6. Specter, M. J., Guinee, V. F., and Davidow, B., The unsuitability of random urinary delta-aminolevulinic acid samples as a screening test for lead poisoning. *J. Pediatr.* **79**, 799–804 (1971).
7. Blumenthal, S., Davidow, B., Harris, D., and Oliver-Smith, F. A., Comparison between two diagnostic tests for lead poisoning. *Am. J. Public Health* **62**, 1060–1064 (1972).
8. Strand, L. J., Meyer, U. A., Felsher, B. F., Redeker, A. G., and Marver, H. S., Decreased red cell uroporphorinogen I synthetase activity in intermittent acute porphyria. *J. Clin. Invest.* **51**, 2530–2536 (1972).
9. Meyer, U. A., and Schmid, R., The porphyrias. In text ref. *11*, 4th ed., pp 1166–1200.

Delta-Aminolaevulinic Acid Dehydratase, ALAD
(EC 4.2.1.24; 5-aminolaevulinate hydro-lyase)

Specimen Tested:

B.

Laboratories Reporting:

4.

Reference (Normal) Values:

Lab. 1: Child, 0–2 yr: 42–122 arbitrary units/mL of erythrocytes per hour, at 38 °C

Lab. 2: 4–12 yr: range: 420–1160 arbitrary units (nmol of porphobilinogen produced/mL of erythrocytes per hour, at 37 °C); mean: 790

Lab. 3: Child: >600 arbitrary units (nmol of porphobilinogen produced/mL of erythrocytes per hour, at 37 °C)

Lab. 4: When blood lead is <30 μg/dL, ALAD is 10–54 arbitrary units/mL of erythrocytes per minute, at 37 °C. When blood lead is >60 μg/dL, ALAD is 5–19 arbitrary units/mL of erythrocytes per minute at 37 °C.

Sources of Reference (Normal) Values:

Lab. 1: a study made on 50 healthy children, ages 0–2 yr. **Lab. 2:** a study made on 105 elementary school children, ages 4–12 yr. **Lab. 3:** Bodlaender, P., Ulmer, D. D., and Vallee, B. L., Automated determination of δ-aminolevulinic acid dehydratase activity in human erythrocytes. *Anal. Biochem.* **58**, 500–510 (1974). **Lab. 4:** institutional.

Specimen Volume, Collection, and Preservation:

100 to 200 μL. Heparin anticoagulant. The specimen should be frozen on solid CO_2 without delay after collection, and kept at that tempera-

ture until analyzed (1–2 h). The specimen may lose 0–25% of its activity after storage at 4 °C for 24 h, and up to 85% after 24 h at RT. Stable at −80 °C.

Analytical Method:

Lab. 1: Burch, H. B., and Siegel, A. L., Improved method for measurement of delta-aminolevulinic acid dehydratase activity of human erythrocytes. *Clin. Chem.* **17,** 1038–1041 (1971). **Lab. 2:** Granick, S., Sassa, S., Granick, J. L., Levere, R. D., and Kappas, A., Assays for porphyrins, Δ-aminolevulinic acid dehydratase, and porphyrinogen synthetase in microliter samples of whole blood: Applications to metabolic defects involving the heme pathway. *Proc. Natl. Acad. Sci. USA* **69,** 2381–2385 (1978). **Lab. 3:** Bodlaender et al., *op. cit.* **Lab. 4:** Weissberg, J. B., Lipschutz, F., and Oski, F. A., δ-Aminolevulinic acid dehydratase activity in circulating blood cells. *N. Engl. J. Med.* **284,** 565–569 (1971).

Enzyme Data:

See references cited by each laboratory under *Analytical method,* above.

Instrumentation:

Spectrophotometers: Gilford 300-N, Stasar III; Bausch and Lomb Spectronic 100; Beckman 25 K.

Commentary—Roger L. Boeckx

The inhibition of ALAD is generally believed to increase both plasma and urine delta-aminolaevulinic acid (ALA) concentrations. ALAD can be measured in peripheral blood, but mammalian erythrocytes are devoid of the mitochondrial enzymes required for heme synthesis, and it is doubtful that the inhibition of erythrocytic ALAD by lead is responsible for increasing the ALA concentrations in blood and urine. Liver and brain ALAD are also inhibited by lead, but because ALAD is inhibited at lead concentrations much lower than those required to increase urinary ALA excretion, the body apparently has a considerable enzyme reserve. Therefore, the actual implications of ALAD inhibition remain unclear.

In any case, many workers have suggested that the assay of erythrocytic ALAD can serve as a sensitive indicator of excessive lead exposure. The first widely used assay for erythrocytic ALAD was described by Bonsignore et al. in 1965 *(1)*, and was based on the measurement of the porphobilinogen synthesized by the action of ALAD on its substrate, ALA. Sample volumes of 100 μL of blood or less can be used, making the test applicable for childhood screening in which fingerstick samples are used.

Granick et al. *(2,3)* modified this assay and further showed that the inhibition of ALAD by lead in vitro could be decreased by adding strong sulfhydryl reagents such as dithiothreitol to the assay systems. In fact, they proposed using the ratio of activated to non-activated ALAD as an indication of lead poisoning. This activation ratio correlates well with blood lead concentrations.

Most reported methods, whether manual or automated, are based on the methods of Bonsignore et al. *(1)* and Granick et al. *(2,3)*. The latter authors cautioned against the use of saponin as a hemolyzing agent, because some batches of it caused enzyme inhibition. Freezing and thawing, and the use of Triton X-100, have been suggested as alternatives.

Between 1970 and 1977, several authors suggested that ALAD activity was an indication of early, subclinical lead poisoning *(4-7)*. The effect of lead on ALAD activity is direct, immediate, and not dependent on the accumulation of metabolites; consequently, ALAD is useful not only in detecting chronic lead poisoning but also in detecting acute poisoning. Furthermore, ALAD activity is not affected by iron-deficiency anemia, the major interference with tests based on protoporphyrin accumulation.

The test does have some drawbacks. Most significantly, the enzyme is unstable, its activity decreasing rapidly with storage. Furthermore, Tomokuni *(5)* has reported that ALAD displays different pH optima, depending on whether the source of the enzyme is a normal or a lead-exposed individual.

The susceptibility of ALAD to sulfhydryl inhibition and the different pH optima observed are major obstacles to the routine use of this test. Although ALAD is probably the most sensitive indicator of lead exposure yet devised, it is this very sensitivity that hinders the test's usefulness. For blood lead concentrations of 70–80 μg/dL or less, an acceptable correlation exists; however, at concentrations of 80 μg/dL or higher, ALAD is maximally inhibited. At the other end of the scale, marked changes in ALAD activity can be observed with very low and apparently harmless exposures to lead.

1. Bonsignore, D., Calissano, P., and Cartaseqna, C., Un semplice metodo per la determinazione della amino-levulinicodeidratasi nel sanque: Compartamento dell'enzima nell'intossicasione saturina. *Med. Lav.* **56,** 199–205 (1965).
2. Granick, J. L., Sassa, S., Granick, S., Levere, R. D., and Kappas, A., Studies in lead poisoning. II. Correlation between the ratio of activated to inactivated δ-aminolevulinic acid dehydratase of whole blood and blood lead level. *Biochem. Med.* **8,** 139–159 (1973).
3. Granick, S., Sassa, S., Granick, J. L., Levere, R. D., and Kappas, A., Assays for porphyrins, Δ-aminolevulinic acid dehydratase, and porphyrinogen synthetase in microliter samples of whole blood: Applications to metabolic defects involving the heme pathway. *Proc. Natl. Acad. Sci. USA* **69,** 2381–2385 (1972).

4. Secchi, G., Erba, L., and Cambiaghi, G., Delta-aminolevulinic acid dehydratase activity of erythrocytes and liver tissue in man. *Arch. Environ. Health* **28**, 130–132 (1974).

5. Tomokuni, K., Δ-Aminolevulinic acid dehydratase test for lead exposure. *Arch. Environ. Health* **29**, 247–281 (1974).

6. Nieburg, P. I., Weiner, L. S., Oski, B. F., and Iski, B. F. A., Red blood cell δ-aminolevulinic acid dehydratase activity. *Am. J. Dis. Child.* **127**, 348–350 (1974).

7. Goldstein, D. H., Kneip, T. J., Rulon, V. P., and Cohen, N., Erythrocytic aminolevulinic acid dehydratase (ALAD) activity as a biologic parameter for determining exposure to lead. *J. Occup. Med.* **17**, 157–162 (1975).

Ammonia Nitrogen

Specimen Tested:

B, P.

Laboratories Reporting:

5.

Reference (Normal) Values:

	Plasma[a]			Blood[a]	
Age	**μg/dL**	**μmol/L**		**μg/dL**	**μmol/L**
0–2 wk	77–126[b]	55–90[b]			
"Newborn"[c]	to 290 (NH₃)	to 171	Venous:	90–150[d]	64–107[d]
	90–150	64–107		to 150[b]	to 107[b]
1 mo	28–77[b]	20–55[b]			
"Post-natal"	to 60	to 43		to 70[b]	to 50[b]
"Infant + child"	to 155 (NH₃)	to 91	Arterial:	to 80[d]	to 57[d]
"Adult"	to 90	to 64			

[a] Enzymic method, except where indicated.
[b] Ion-exchange method.
[c] Values are higher in premature and jaundiced newborns than in full-term nonjaundiced newborns.
[d] Protein-free filtrate + colorimetric method.

Sources of Reference (Normal) Values:

Institutional.

Analytical Methods:

Plasma: **Enzymic:** Da Fonseca-Wollheim, V. F., Direkte Plasmammoniabestimmung ohne Entweissung. *J. Clin. Chem. Clin. Biochem.* **11**, 426–431 (1973). Bio-Dynamics/*bmc* Reagent Set Ammonia. **Ion-Exchange resin:** Forman, D, T., Rapid determination of plasma ammonia by an ion-exchange technic. *Clin. Chem.* **10**, 497–508 (1964); Miller, G. E., and Rice, J. D., Jr., Determination of the concentration of ammonia nitrogen in plasma by means of a simple ion-exchange method. *Am. J. Clin. Pathol.* **39**, 97–103 (1964); Hyland Blood Ammonia Test Kit; phenolate–hypochlorite reaction; Kingsley, G. R., and Tager, H. S., Ion-exchange method for the determination of plasma ammonia nitrogen with the Berthelot reaction. *Stand. Methods Clin. Chem.* **6,** 115–126 (1970).

Blood: **Enzymic:** Kurahasi, K., Ishihara, A., and Vehara, H., Determination of ammonia in blood plasma by an ion-exchange method. *Clin. Chim. Acta* **42,** 141–146 (1972); SKI-EskaLab Ammonia Test. **Colorimetric:** McCullough, H., The determination of ammonia in whole blood by a direct colorimetric method. *Clin. Chim. Acta* **17,** 297–304 (1967).

Specimen Volume, Collection, and Preservation:

Blood from *all* sources used: skin-puncture, venous, arterial, 0.2 to 2.0 mL. Heparin alone (lithium or sodium) as anticoagulant. Transport in ice bath. P is stable for several hours in ice bath, for 7 d on solid CO_2. At RT, ammonia nitrogen values increase by 17 μg/L per minute. Blood ammonia determinations are generally treated as "stat" (emergency) procedures.

Instrumentation:

Gilford 2400, Stasar II, Zeiss, LKB 7400, SKI EskaLab Alpha spectrophotometers.

Commentary—Robert L. Murray

Ammonia can be measured in whole blood, serum, or urine by isolation and quantitation, or by direct measurement without separation. Three main problems in the selection of a method involve *(a)* the low concentration of ammonia in blood, requiring highly sensitive and specific methods; *(b)* the high concentration of protein and nonprotein amino and imino moieties, which potentially form in vitro ammonia; and *(c)* the possibility of contamination.

Isolation of the ammonia on a cation-exchange resin, followed by elution and quantitation *(1)*, when reduced to micro-scale, is highly dependent on the analyst's skill. Micro-adaptation of glutamate dehydrogenase enzymic methods *(2)*, both kinetic and endpoint, seems more promising in dealing with the problems listed above. Development of an ammonia electrode suitable for routine use on microsamples has not yet been successfully accomplished.

The ammonia concentration of blood increases rapidly on standing at room temperature because of the deamination of amides. Unfortunately, there is no suitable preservative to prevent this conversion, but it can be minimized if a protein-free filtrate is made promptly, or if the specimen is kept in ice water and analyzed within 30 min of collection.

Ammonia from protein catabolism is normally disposed of either by hepatic enzyme conversion to urea or, to a much lesser extent, by direct renal elimination. Blood ammonia concentration therefore increases during hepatic insufficiency. Blood ammonia also increases and urinary ammonia decreases in metabolic and respiratory alkalosis (because of renal retention), and in renal disease in which the distal tubules are damaged. High-protein diet, starvation, and metabolic respiratory acidosis increase the excretion of ammonia.

Blood ammonia concentrations are increased in Reye's syndrome. The concentration has been reported to be directly related to the level of consciousness and to survival *(3)*. A constant increased blood ammonia is seen in certain inherited diseases, such as familial protein intolerance, presumably because of the decreased absorption of arginine and ornithine in the gut, resulting in a depression of urea-cycle function *(4)*. A similar depression of urea-cycle function has been reported in hereditary ornithine transcarbamylase deficiency, resulting in blood ammonia exceeding 2500 μg/dL *(5)*.

The ammonia content of peripheral blood in the normal neonate is higher than in adults, probably because the ductus venosus, which bypasses the liver, does not close completely until about the tenth postnatal day. Thus, because part of the circulation is shunted around the liver, less ammonia is available for conversion to urea.

1. *Clinical Biochemistry: Principles and Methods,* H. C. Curtius and M. Roth, Eds. Walter de Gruyter, New York, NY, 1974, pp 1122–1124.
2. Text ref. *5,* 2nd ed., pp 1051–1053.
3. Glasgow, A. M., Cotton, R. B., Dhiensiri, K., and Kaen, K., Reye's syndrome. I. Blood ammonia and consideration of the nonhistologic diagnosis. *Am. J. Dis. Child.* **124,** 827–833 (1972).
4. Kato, T., Tanaka, E., and Horisawa, S., Hyperdibasicaminoaciduria and hyperammonemia in familial protein intolerance. *Am. J. Dis. Child.* **130,** 1340–1344 (1976).
5. LaBrecque, D. R., Latham, P. S., Riely, C. A., Hsia, Y. E., and Klatskin, G., Heritable urea cycle enzyme deficiency liver disease in 16 patients. *J. Pediatr.* **94,** 580–587 (1979).

Ammonium Ion

Specimen Tested:

U.

Laboratory Reporting:

1.

Reference (Normal) Values:

2–11.5 mo: 4.2–19.9 μmol/min per m^2 of body surface
13 mo–16 yr: 5.9–16.5

Sources of Normal Values:
Institutional.

Specimen Volume:
0.4 mL.

Analytical Method and Instrumentation:
Text ref. *2*, p 42; Folin, O., and Bell, R. D., Applications of a new reagent for the separation of ammonia. The colorimetric determination of ammonia in urine. *J. Biol. Chem.* **29**, 329 (1917); Zeiss spectrophotometer.

[*Ed. note:* For determining urinary ammonia with the Berthelot reaction, see Kaplan, A., Urea nitrogen and urinary ammonia. *Stand. Methods Clin. Chem.* **5**, 245–256 (1965).]

Amylase (EC 3.2.1.1; 1,4-α-D-glucanohydrolase)

Specimen Tested:
P, S, U, duodenal fluid.

Laboratories Reporting:
6.

Reference (Normal) Values:

P, S	Labs. 1, 2	Labs. 3, 4	Lab. 5	Lab. 6
Newborn, full-term, 0–5 d:	10–75 arbitrary units (about 20–140 U/L)			
Infant:	50–500 U/L			
Adolescent–adult:	600–1600 U/L	600–1600 U/L	450–2000 dye units/L	60–330 Close-Street units/L
U				
Adolescent		3000 U/h; 2-h collection	400–3300 dye units/L; 2-h collection	
Duodenal fluid:			150–1200 dye units/mL	

Sources of Reference (Normal) Values:
Lab. 1: an institutional study on 50 healthy full-term newborns. **Lab. 3:** Caraway, W. T., A stable starch substrate for the determination of amylase and other body fliuds. *Am. J. Clin. Pathol.* **32**, 97–99 (1959). **All other labs:** institutional.

Analytical Method:

Labs. 1, 2: Nephelometry; Zinterhofer, L., Wardlaw, S., Jatlow, P., and Seligson, D., Nephelometric determination of pancreatic enzymes. I. Amylase. *Clin. Chim. Acta* **43**, 5–12 (1943); Perkin-Elmer reagent kit. **Labs. 3, 4:** Caraway, *op. cit.;* Harleco Amylase reagent set. **Lab. 5:** Street, H. V., and Close, J. R., Determination of amylase activity in biological fluids. *Clin. Chim. Acta* **1**, 256–268 (1956). **Lab. 6:** Klein, B., Foreman, J. A., and Searcy, R. L., A new chromogenic substrate for the determination of serum amylase activity. *Clin. Chem.* **16**, 32–38 (1970); Roche Amylochrome.

Enzyme Data:

Wide variations in methods, substrate, buffer, and units; substrate pH and reaction temperature uniformly at 7.0 and 37 °C, respectively.

Instrumentation:

Turbidimetry: Perkin-Elmer Model 91 Amylase–Lipase Analyzer. **Colorimetry:** Gilford 2400, Stasar II, III, Beckman 25, Coleman Jr. II spectrophotometers.

Commentary—Paul L. Wolf

Practically no amylase activity is present in the neonate's serum. Measurable enzyme activity appears at approximately two months of age and increases slowly to adult values by the age of 12 months. The activity during the first year of life is from the salivary isoenzyme, the pancreatic isoenzyme increasing by one year of age *(1)*.

The usual differential diagnosis for an above-normal serum amylase in adults cannot be utilized in children. The leading causes for an increased serum amylase in a child would include salivary amylase from mumps parotitis, mumps, or coxsackie pancreatitis; release of mucosal amylase secondary to intestinal obstruction and (or) infarction; increased production and release of salivary amylase in diabetic ketoacidosis; and decreased excretion of amylase in chronic renal failure. Adult conditions such as ruptured ectopic pregnancy, macroamylasemia, and penetrating peptic ulcer into the pancreas are not applicable *(2)*.

1. Hadorn, B., Zoppi, G., Schmerling, D. H., Prader, A., McIntyre, I., and Anderson, C. M., Quantitative assessment of exocrine function in infants and children. *J. Pediatr.* **73**, 39–50 (1968).
2. Berk, J. E., Searcy, R. L., Wilding, P., Kizu, H., and Svoboda, A. C., Macroamylase: A new cause for elevated serum amylase activity. *J. Am. Med. Assoc.* **200**, 545 (1967).

See also discussion of amylase in Chapter 8.

Amylo-1,6-Glucosidase, Debranching Enzyme
(EC 3.2.1.33; dextrin 6-α-glucosidase)

Specimen Tested:

Leukocytes, liver, muscle.

Laboratories Reporting:

2.

Reference (Normal) Values:

	Lab. 1 **(method indicated in parentheses)**	**Lab. 2**
Liver:	About 200 Hers units *(a)* About 3–5 Huijing units *(b)*	>1.0 μmol/min per gram (wet weight) of liver
Muscle:	About 190 Hers units *(a)* About 3–5 Huijing units *(b)*	
Leukocytes:	3160 ± 125 cpm/10^8 cells *(c)*	

Sources of Reference (Normal) Values:

Lab. 1: *(a)* Van Hoof, F., and Hers, H. G., The subgroups of type 3 glycogenesis. *Eur. J. Biochem.* **2,** 265–270 (1967); *(b)* Huijing, F., Glycogen and enzymes of glycogen metabolism. In *Clinical Biochemistry, Principles and Methods*, H. C. Curtius, and M. Roth, Eds. de Gruyter, New York, NY, 1974, pp 1228–1229; *(c)* Williams, H. E., Kendig, E. M., and Field, J. B., Leukocyte debranching enzyme in glycogen storage disease. *J. Clin. Invest.* **42,** 656–660 (1963). **Lab. 2:** Text ref. *1.*

Specimen Volume, Collection, and Preservation:

Lab. 1: Biopsy, 20 to 50 mg of liver or muscle; 20 μL of heparinized blood. **Lab. 2:** 50 μL of tissue extract (10 g/L).

The enzyme is quite temperature-labile. Quick (or "snap")-freeze the tissue or separated leukocytes on foil placed on solid CO_2. Store at −70 °C.

Analytical Method:

Lab. 1: [C^{14}]glucose incorporation into glycogen: Hers, H. G., Verhue, W., and Van Hoof, F., The determination of amylo-1,6-glucosidase. *Eur. J. Biochem.* **2,** 257–264 (1967); Thomas, J. A., Schlender, K. K., and Larner, J., A rapid filter paper assay for UDP glucose–glycogen glucosyltransferase, including an improved biosynthesis of UDP-14C-glucose. *Anal. Biochem.* **25,** 486–489 (1968); Nelson, T. E., and Larner, J., A rapid micro assay method for amylo-1,6-glucosidase. *Anal. Biochem.* **33,** 87–101 (1970). Run controls with normal human leukocytes, and rat liver or muscle. **Lab. 2:** text ref. *2.*

Enzyme Data:

Lab. 1:
1. Enzyme unit definition: *(a)* Hers unit = 0.1% of counts added as glucose/h per gram of tissue, wet weight; *(b)* Huijing unit = nmol of glucose incorporated/min per gram of tissue, wet weight; leukocytes: cpm/10^8 cells.
2. Buffer pH: *(a)* potassium phosphate, 6.5; *(b)* potassium phosphate, 7.4.
3. Substrate: glycogen (oyster), Sigma Type II; [U-^{14}C]glucose.
4. Reaction temperature: 37 °C.
5. Temperature reported: 37 °C.

Instrumentation:
Lab. 1: Packard B-counter; thermostatically controlled shaking waterbath. **Lab. 2:** Beckman 25 spectrophotometer.

Androstenedione, Δ^4-A

Specimen Tested:

P, S.

Laboratories Reporting:

3.

Reference (Normal) Values:

		nmol/L (ng/dL)	
Sex	**Age**	**Labs. 1, 2**	**Lab. 3**
M	1–5 mo	<2.8 (80)	
(+F)	To 6 mo		<6.0
	4 mo–7 yr	<1.8 (50)	
	5 mo–adrenarche[a]	<1.6 (45)	
(+F)	1–10 yr		0.3–2.5
	8 yr–adult	Increasing relative to stage of puberty	
	Adolescent		1.8–5.3
	Adult	2.1–8.0 (60–230)	4.0–10.8
F	1–4 mo	<1.6 (45)	
	Birth to adrenarche[a]	<6 (45)[b]	
	8 yr–adult	Increasing relative to stage of puberty	
	Adolescent		2.5–5.4
	Adult	1.8–10.6 (50–330)	3.3–10.9

[a] At adrenarche, adrenal androgens start increasing in preparation for puberty. Changes occur as early as 7–8 yr in girls, and 1–2 yr later in boys. During adrenarche and puberty, androstenedione increases to adult values.

[b] Parker, L. N., Sack, J., Fisher, D. A., and Odell, W. D. [The adrenarche: prolactin, gonadotropins, adrenal androgens, and cortisol. *J. Clin. Endocrinol. Metab.* **46**, 396–401 (1978)], suggest that the normal range may be up to 3.3 nmol/L (95 ng/dL). Their *lower* limit, however, is about 2.1 nmol/L (60 ng/dL), so there may be some nonspecific interference with their method.

Sources of Reference (Normal) Values:

Forest, M. G., Sizonenko, P. C., Cathiard, A. M., and Bertrand, J., Hypophyso-gonadal function in humans during the first year of life. I. Evidence for testicular activity in early infancy. *J. Clin. Invest.* **53,** 819–828 (1974); Forest, M. G., Age-related response to plasma testosterone, Δ⁴-androstenedione, and cortisol to adrenocorticotropin in infants, children and adults. *J. Clin. Endocrinol. Metab.* **47,** 931–937 (1978); Korth-Schutz, S., Levine, L. S., and New, M. I., Serum androgens in normal prepubertal and pubertal children and in children with precocious adrenarche. *J. Clin. Endocrinol. Metab.* **42,** 117–124 (1976); Endocrine Sciences; Thorneycroft, I. H., Ribeiro, W. O., Stone, S. C., and Tillson, S. A., A radioimmunoassay of androstenedione. *Steroids* **21,** 111–122 (1973); institutional.

Specimen Volume, Collection, and Preservation; Patient Preparation:

0.2 to 1 mL of heparinized or EDTA-treated plasma. Fasting, A.M. (0800 hours) specimen preferred but not essential. Preserve in RR or FR.

Analytical Method:

RIA. **Lab. 1, 2:** Seegan, G., Chandler, D., Berg, G., and Mayes, D., A direct radioimmunoassay for plasma androstenedione. Endocrine Sciences Bulletin, modified, Tarzana, CA. **Lab. 3:** charcoal separation; [³H]androstenedione from Amersham; antiserum from Miles Labs.; direct assay without preliminary column separation.

Instrumentation:

Packard 2425, 3375 Scintillation Counter.

Commentary—Elizabeth K. Smith

Androstenedione is a major precursor steroid in the biosynthesis of testosterone and estrogens in the adrenal cortex, ovary, and testis. Androstenedione occupies a position just after 17-hydroxyprogesterone in the synthetic pathway, and is converted to testosterone in peripheral tissues. It is considered one of the major adrenal androgens, and is secreted in large amounts in congenital adrenal hyperplasia. In adult men and women a dramatic and similar increase in plasma concentrations occurs in response to corticotropin (ACTH) administration, with no sex difference *(1)*. Significant increases in response to ACTH also occur in infants and in boys in early puberty.

Reference (normal) values are age-related, with prepubertal children having low values. Values begin to increase at adrenarche before puberty, and continue to increase gradually through puberty to adult concentrations *(2)*. Korth-Schutz et al. *(3)* reported results related to stage of pubertal development (Tanner stages I–IV), demonstrating a progressive increase and higher values for females than males at all stages.

Tanner stage of puberty	Mean + SD, ng/dL	
	F	M
I		
<7 yr, based on bone age	18.2 ± 12.0	12.6 ± 11.5
>7 yr, based on bone age	36.7 ± 23.4	19.4 ± 14.5
II	59.3 ± 42.0	42.8 ± 22.7
III	68.4 ± 41.6	50.5 ± 20.2
IV	140 ± 56	103 ± 58

Ducharme et al. (4) found that androstenedione increased significantly between eight and 10 years of age in girls and between 10 and 12 years in boys. Values in adult women have a wider range than in men, with highest values during the follicular stage of the menstrual cycle.

Forest et al. (5) reported high values in cord blood: F 93 ± 38 ng/dL, M 85 ± 27 ng/dL. Slightly higher values for female than male infants persisted throughout the first year of life. In early infancy, up to four to six months, androstenedione values are higher than in the young prepubertal child, but by one year of age and until adrenarche, androstenedione in boys and girls usually is less than 45 ng/dL (3,5).

Plasma concentrations of androstenedione are markedly increased in congenital adrenal hyperplasia (CAH) (21-hydroxylase deficiency), and are suppressed to normal values with adequate glucocorticoid replacement therapy. In longitudinal studies of serum androgens (androstenedione, dehydroepiandrosterone, and testosterone), to evaluate adequacy of treatment in children with CAH, the single androgen that best reflected good or poor control was androstenedione (3). Cavallo et al. (6) also reported that plasma androstenedione correlated well with clinical control in either females or males, regardless of stage of puberty. Other advantages of androstenedione over 17-hydroxyprogesterone for monitoring therapy are the minimal diurnal variation, better correlation with urinary 17-ketosteroid excretion, and the fact that plasma concentrations are not affected immediately by a dose of glucocorticoid (6,7).

1. Forest, M. G., Age-related response of plasma testosterone, Δ4-androstenedione and cortisol to adrenocorticotropin in infants, children and adults. *J. Clin. Endocrinol. Metab.* **47**, 931–937 (1978).
2. Parker, L. N., Sack, J., Fisher, D. A., and Odell, W. D., The adrenarche: Prolactin, gonadotropins, adrenal androgens and cortisol. *J. Clin. Endocrinol. Metab.* **46**, 396–401 (1978).
3. Korth-Schutz, S., Virdis, R., Saenger, P., Chow, D. M., Levine, L. S., and

New, M. I., Serum androgens as a continuing index of adequacy of treatment of congenital adrenal hyperplasia. *J. Clin. Endocrinol. Metab.* **46,** 452–458 (1978).

4. Ducharme, J., Forest, M. G., dePeretti, E., Sempe, M., Collu, R., and Bertrand, J., Plasma adrenal and gonadal sex steroids in human development. *J. Clin. Endocrinol. Metab.* **42,** 468–476 (1976).
5. Forest, M. G., Sizonenko, P. C., Cathiard, A. M., and Bertrand, J., Hypophyso-gonadal function in humans during the first year of life. *J. Clin. Invest.* **53,** 819–828 (1974).
6. Cavallo, A., Corn, C., Bryan, G. T., and Meyer, W. J., III, The use of plasma androstenedione in monitoring therapy of patients with congenital adrenal hyperplasia. *J. Pediatr.* **95,** 33–37 (1979).
7. Meyer, W. J., III, Gutai, J. P., Keenan, B. S., Davis, G. R., Kowarski, A. A., and Migeon, C. J., A chronobiological approach to treatment of congenital adrenal hyperplasia. In *Congenital Adrenal Hyperplasia,* P. A. Lee, L. P. Plotnik, A. A. Kowarski, and C. J. Migeon, Eds. University Park Press, Baltimore, MD, 1977.

Antidiuretic Hormone (ADH)

Specimen Tested:

P.

Laboratory Reporting:

1.

Reference (Normal) Values:

	ADH, micro-int. units/mL	Osmolality, milli-osmoles/kg
Random hydration	0.4–5.3	287.6–289.4
Overnight dehydration (12 h)	—	289.5–292.1
Overnight dehydration (18 h)	—	292.5–294.3

Sources of Reference (Normal) Values:

Nichols Institute Assay Summaries, Jan., 1978; Oct., 1980.

Specimen Volume, Collection, and Preservation:

1.0 mL. EDTA anticoagulant. Avoid painful venipuncture, which may cause inappropriate release of ADH. Separate the plasma without delay after blood collection. Freeze the plasma promptly and store in FR until assayed.

Analytical Method:

Extraction with bentonite; RIA; double-antibody vs ^{125}I-labeled arginine vasopressin; Skowsky, W. R., Rosenbloom, A. A., and Fisher, D. A., Radioimmunoassay measurement of arginine vasopressin in serum: Development and application. *J. Clin. Endocrinol. Metab.* **38,** 278–287 (1974); determine plasma osmolality simultaneously.

Commentary—Joan H. and Peter J. Howanitz

The three major stimuli controlling release of antidiuretic hormone (ADH) (also called arginine vasopressin, AVP) are: *(a)* changes in osmolality of the blood, *(b)* alterations in blood volume, and *(c)* psychogenic stimuli. Under ordinary circumstances osmolality probably predominates in the regulation of ADH secretion *(1)*. Although concentrations of ADH vary with the state of hydration, large individual differences in the relationship of plasma ADH and osmolality occur in healthy adults, apparently due to differences in osmoreceptor threshold and (or) sensitivity *(2)*.

In healthy adults, a wide range of plasma ADH concentrations has been reported under basal conditions, as well as with hydration and water loading *(1–3)*. However, basal plasma ADH values in adults have usually been reported to be in the range of about 1–2 micro-int. unit/mL (1 micro-int. unit = 2.5 pg = 2.3 fmol); after 8 to 24 h of water deprivation, greater than 2 micro-int. units/mL; and with water loading, usually less than 1 micro-int. unit/mL *(1–3)*. For example, Robertson et al. found that recumbent normal subjects have a mean plasma ADH concentration of about 1 micro-int. unit/mL, with a mean plasma osmolality of 287 milli-osmoles/kg. In their subjects who were fluid-deprived, mean ADH concentrations were slightly greater than 2 micro-int. units/mL, with a mean plasma osmolality of 292 milli-osmoles/kg, while with water loading, mean ADH concentrations decreased to about 0.6 micro-int. units/mL with a mean plasma osmolality of 282 milli-osmoles/kg *(3,4)*.

Several reports have documented that plasma ADH concentrations are very high at birth, and that the ADH is probably of fetal origin *(5–8)*. Infants born by vaginal delivery have more ADH than those delivered by cesarean section *(5–8)*. Although high concentrations of ADH in cord blood have been attributed to the stress of delivery, they may also be due to release of the hormone during labor *(6,7)*. Recently, it has been suggested that high cord-blood ADH concentrations may be secondary to increases in intracranial pressure that occur during labor and delivery; mild degrees of hypoxia, however, could not be excluded as the cause of the ADH increase *(7)*. Polin et al. found no correlation between plasma ADH concentrations and umbilical artery pH, base excess, or infant's 1-min Apgar score *(8)*.

During the first day after birth, ADH concentrations rapidly decrease in both full-term and pre-term infants *(7)*. Under conditions of normal hydration, a wide range of plasma ADH values has been found in children, especially during the first few months of life. In a group of children between 14 days and 10 years of age, no correlation was found between plasma ADH concentration and age *(9)*.

The clinical use of ADH measurements has been limited, owing to a lack of sufficiently sensitive and simple assays for the hormone. Although bioassay techniques are very sensitive, only a limited number of samples can be processed routinely *(10)*. Radioimmunoassays for ADH have not been available widely and until recently have not demonstrated adequate sensitivity. Even with the most sensitive assays, the specimen requires extraction, to remove interfering substances in plasma *(4,10,11)*. Bioassay and immunoassay values are in close agreement under most conditions; however, with water deprivation, bioassays generally yield higher values *(3)*.

Because ADH values vary with the state of hydration, plasma osmolality should be measured concomitantly. Posture does not significantly affect ADH values except under conditions of water deprivation, when the hormone concentrations increase as the subject assumes an upright posture *(3)*. Venipuncture must be performed carefully, to avoid pain or other stress and a subsequent increase in plasma ADH concentration. Blood specimens for ADH should be chilled, centrifuged in the cold as soon as possible, and the plasma stored frozen at -20 °C until assay *(4,10,11)*. Even under these conditions of storage, some loss of ADH activity may occur *(4)*.

Because of the difficulties with and lack of availability of assays for ADH, abnormalities in water metabolism usually are studied by obtaining plasma and urine osmolalities under various states of hydration.

Decreased ADH secretion, which results in diabetes insipidus, may occur from a variety of causes, including head trauma, pituitary lesions, and inherited deficiency of the hormone. Nephrogenic diabetes insipidus (renal resistance to ADH) also may be inherited or may be associated with hypercalcemia, hypokalemia, or renal disease.

To distinguish diabetes insipidus from other polyuric states, several different types of water-deprivation tests are used. For example, in an overnight dehydration test, a normal individual after 8 h of water deprivation produces urine with an osmolality greater than 800 milli-osmoles/kg and has a plasma osmolality not greater than 294 milli-osmoles/kg *(1)*. When this test is performed in patients with diabetes insipidus, their urine osmolality is usually less than that of plasma and the plasma osmolality exceeds 300 milli-osmoles/kg.

In another type of water deprivation test, urine is collected hourly until a plateau in osmolality is reached. The plateau is defined as two and preferably three consecutive hourly samples with about equal osmolality. In normal subjects approximately 16 to 18 h may be necessary to reach a plateau, but patients with polyuria may require only 4 to 8 h *(12)*. The subsequent response of the patient to subcutaneous injection of aqueous ADH allows differentiation of the polyuric states (Table 1). Patients with severe or partial diabetes insipidus show increased urine osmolality with ADH injection. Before the dehydration test is undertaken, conditions such as diabetes mellitus, hypercalcemia, and hypokalemia must be ruled out.

Patients with diabetes insipidus have plasma ADH concentrations significantly lower than normal that fail to increase significantly

Table 1. *Response to Dehydration Test*

Clinical state	Mean osmolality at plateau, milli-osmoles/kg		% increase in urine osmolality after ADH injection
	Plasma	Urine	
Normal	290	800	<5
Severe diabetes insipidus	306	168	>50
Partial diabetes insipidus	294	438	>9
Nephrogenic diabetes insipidus	302–320 (range)	96–151 (range)	<50

Modified from Moses and Miller *(12)*.

after water restriction *(10)*. In patients with primary polydipsia or nephrogenic diabetes insipidus, the relationship of plasma ADH values to plasma osmolality is the same as in normal individuals *(1)*.

The syndrome of inappropriate antidiuretic hormone (SIADH) is an important entity that may occur in a variety of clinical situations, including pulmonary disease, adrenal insufficiency, and disorders of the central nervous system. Various drugs, including carbamazepine and vincristine, can also produce the clinical picture of SIADH *(13)*. The diagnosis can be suspected in any patient who has hyponatremia, low plasma osmolality, and continued renal excretion of sodium, but whose urine in not maximally dilute. Additional criteria for the diagnosis for SIADH include normal renal function, normal adrenal function, and absence of clinical evidence of volume depletion *(14)*.

In most patients with the clinical picture of SIADH, ADH concentrations in plasma are increased relative to plasma osmolality. However, except in patients with ectopic production of the hormone, the absolute concentration of ADH tends to be in the same range as in healthy individuals *(3)*.

1. Edwards, C. W. R., Vasopressin and oxytocin in health and disease. *Clin. Endocrinol. Metab.* **6,** 223–259 (1977).
2. Robertson, G. L., The regulation of vasopressin function in health and disease. *Recent Prog. Horm. Res.* **33,** 333–374 (1977).
3. Robertson, G. L., Vasopressin in osmotic regulation in man. *Annu. Rev. Med.* **25,** 315–322 (1974).
4. Robertson, G. L., Mahr, E. A., Athar, S., and Sinha, T., Development and clinical application of a new method for the radioimmunoassay of arginine vasopressin in human plasma. *J. Clin. Invest.* **52,** 2340–2352 (1973).
5. Hoppenstein, J. M., Miltenberger, F. W., and Moran, W. H., The increase in blood levels of vasopressin in infants during birth and surgical procedures. *Surg. Gynecol. Obstet.* **127,** 966–974 (1962).
6. Chard, T., Hundon, C. N., Edwards, C. W. R., and Boyd, N. R. H., Release of oxytocin and vasopressin by the human foetus during labour. *Nature* **234,** 352–354 (1971).

7. Hadeed, A. J., Leake, R. D., Weitzman, R. E., and Fisher, D. S., Possible mechanisms of high blood levels of vasopressin during the neonatal period. *J. Pediatr.* **94**, 805–808 (1979).
8. Polin, R. A., Husain, M. K., James, L. S., and Frantz, A. G., High vasopressin concentrations in human umbilical cord blood: Lack of correlation with stress. *J. Perinat. Med.* **5**, 114–119 (1977).
9. Chwalbinska-Moneta, J., Trzebinski, A., Kozlowski, S., and Wojnarowski, M., Plasma antidiuretic activity in children. *Acta Physiol. Pol.* **28**, 411–416 (1977).
10. Morton, J. J., Padfield, P. L., and Forsling, M. L., A radioimmunoassay for plasma arginine-vasopressin in man and dog: Application to physiological and pathological states. *J. Endocrinol.* **65**, 411–424 (1975).
11. Skowsky, W. R., Rosenbloom, A. A., and Fisher, D. A., Radioimmunoassay measurement of arginine vasopressin in serum: Development and application. *J. Clin. Endocrinol. Metab.* **38**, 278–287 (1974).
12. Moses, A. M., and Miller, M., Urine and plasma osmolality in differentiation of polyuric states. *Postgrad. Med.* **52**, 187–190 (1972).
13. Moses, A. M., Miller, M., and Streeten, D. H. P., Pathophysiologic and pharmacologic alterations in the release and action of ADH. *Metabolism* **25**, 697–721 (1976).
14. Bartter, F. C., and Schwartz, W. B., The syndrome of inappropriate secretion of antidiuretic hormone. *Am. J. Med.* **42**, 790–806 (1976).

Antithrombin III

Specimen Tested:

P.

Laboratory Reporting:

1.

Reference (Normal) Values:

Age	Percentage of mean obtained from pooled plasma of healthy adults	
	Functional	Immunochemical
Newborn, premature	20–50	20–50
full-term	30–90	30–70
0–6 mo	40–90	40–90
6 mo–adult	80–120	80–120

Sources of Reference (Normal) Values:

Institutional; Barnard, D. R., and Hathaway, W. E., Neonatal thrombosis. *Am. J. Pediatr. Hematol. Oncol.* **1**, 235–244 (1979).

Specimen Volume, Collection, and Preservation:

10 μL. Venous blood collected into 109 mmol/L citrate. (Heparin is under current evaluation.) Store in FR.

Analytical Method:

Chromogenic substrate S-2238 (functional); RID (immunochemical); Dunikoski, L. K., Jr., Chromogenic antithrombin III assay with a centrifugal analyzer. *Clin. Chem.* **25**, 1076 (1979), abstract; Ortho Antithrombin-III assay; Behring Diagnostics M-Partigen Antithrombin-III Kit.

Instrumentation:

Electro-Necleonics GEMSAEC.

Commentary—Leonard K. Dunikoski, Jr.

Antithrombin III (AT III) is an α_2-globulin, relative molecular mass 64 000, that inhibits the activity of thrombin and activated factors X, IX, XI, and XII. Adults with decreased AT III concentrations may have a predisposition to thrombosis and a reduced response to heparin anticoagulation. Until recently, AT III could be quantitated only by using clotting assays that presented difficult specimen-collection and preservation problems for the pediatric laboratory (syringe specimen with citrate anticoagulant, 9/1 ratio of blood to anticoagulant). Serum has been used by some investigators, but some AT III is nonreproducibly consumed during clotting, values being about 25% less in serum than in plasma. Immunochemical procedures for AT III make specimen collection simpler for pediatric studies, but immunoreactivity and functional activity do not necessarily correlate. Recent development of chromogenic and fluorogenic substrates has enabled the pediatric laboratory to perform functional AT III assays on very small specimens. Citrated plasma is still the most widely used sample, although heparinized plasma may be suitable with most techniques.

Reference (normal) values for AT III activity are expressed as a percentage of normal pooled adult plasma. Values are lowest in premature infants *(1)*, increase with gestational age, and reach adult values by about six months of life. In infants younger than six months, functional AT III activity may be significantly higher than its immunochemical reactivity *(2)*. There are no statistically significant sex differences. Despite the low AT III activity in premature or full-term infants, thrombosis is a relatively uncommon problem in the newborn. Prothrombin concentrations and many of the vitamin K-dependent factors are also very low at this age, so that possibly the two effects counteract each other.

AT III values are extremely low in cases of intravascular coagulation of whatever cause. The increased capillary permeability seen in respiratory distress syndrome also produces very low AT III values, making these infants hypercoagulable and more resistant to heparinization than prematures without respiratory distress syndrome *(1)*.

The use of chromogenic or fluorogenic substrates for AT III assay is especially appealing to the pediatric laboratory, owing to the excellent precision of the method and the small sample size required. Assays can be performed on almost any kinetic enzyme analyzer, but the centrifugal analyzers seem especially suitable (3).

1. Hathaway, W. E., Neumann, L. L., Borden, C. A., and Jacobson, L. J., Immunologic studies of antithrombin III in the newborn. *Thrombos. Haemostas.* **39,** 624–630 (1978).
2. Teger-Nilsson, A. C., Antithrombin III in infancy and childhood. *Acta Paediatr. Scand.* **64,** 624–628 (1975).
3. Dunikoski, L. K., Jr., Automated chromogenic antithrombin-III assay with a centrifugal analyzer. *Clin. Chem.* **25,** 1076 (1979). Abstract.

Note: Also see Chapter 10, **Specific Proteins in Pediatrics.**

Alpha₁-Antitrypsin

Specimen Tested:

S.

Laboratories Reporting:

2.

Reference (Normal) Values:

Age	α_1-**Antitrypsin, mg/dL**
1–8 wk	127–404
3–4 mo	152–329
5–6 mo	151–321
7–9 mo	145–362
10–12 mo	146–347
13–18 mo	160–342
19–24 mo	191–382
2–4 yr	165–366
5–7 yr	148–394
8–10 yr	174–380
11–15 yr	184–345

Sources of Reference (Normal) Values:

Geiger, H., and Hoffmann, P., Quantitative immunological determination of 16 different serum proteins in 260 normal, 0 to 15-years-old children. *Z. Kinderheilk.* **109,** 22–40 (1970).

Specimen Volume, Collection, and Preservation:

5 µL. If not analyzed immediately, the specimen should be stored in RR or FR.

Analytical Method:

RID; Mancini, G., Carbonara, A. O., and Heremans, J. F., Immuno-chemical quantitation of antigens by single radial immuno-diffusion. *Int. J. Immunochem.* **2,** 235–254 (1965); Calbiochem-Behring M-Parti-gen α_1-antitrypsin RID Plates.

*   *   *

Laboratory Reporting:

1.

Reference (Normal) Values:

	Pi (protease inhibitor) typing
75% of normal[a]:	probably M type
55–75%:	possible MZ type
30–50%:	possible SZ type
40%:	probably Z type

[a] Sera of 1200 normals pooled to provide a calibration material, and assigned an activity of 100%.

Sources of Reference (Normal) Values:

Institutional.

Specimen Volume:

10 μL.

Analytical Method:

Laurell, C. B., Electroimmunoassay. *Scand. J. Clin. Lab. Invest.* **29,** Suppl. 124, 21–37 (1972); antiserum, Atlantic Antibodies; agarose, Marine Colloids, Inc.

*   *   *

Laboratory Reporting:

1.

Reference (Normal) Values:

3 yr–adult: 200–400 mg/dL

Sources of Reference (Normal) Values:

Laurell, C. B., Quantitative estimations of proteins by electrophoresis in agarose gel containing antibodies. *Anal. Biochem.* **15,** 45–52 (1966); Merrill, D. A., Hartley, T. F., and Claman, H. N., Electroimmunodiffusion (EID): A simple, rapid method for quantitation of immunoglobulins in diluted biological fluids. *J. Lab. Clin. Med.* **69,** 151–159 (1967).

Specimen Volume:

0.5 mL.

Analytical Method:

Sternberg, J. C., A rare nephelometer for measuring specific proteins by immunoprecipitin reactions. *Clin. Chem.* **23**, 1456–1464 (1977); Beckman Human AAT Reagent Test Kit.

Instrumentation:

Beckman Immunochemistry System 662400.

Commentary—Leonard K. Dunikoski, Jr.

α_1-Antitrypsin, a glycoprotein synthesized in the liver, accounts for almost 90% of the plasma protein migrating in the α_1-fraction of cellulose acetate or agarose gel electrophoresis. It has a potent antiprotease activity, inhibiting trypsin, chymotrypsin, collagenase, elastase, plasmin, and thrombin. The normal half-life is 5 to 6 d.

Concentrations of α_1-antitrypsin may be determined by a variety of immunochemical procedures, including radial immunodiffusion, electroimmunodiffusion, and nephelometry. Most procedures require a very small sample, typically 5 to 20 μL, and are rapidly performed. Recent data suggest that semi-automated nephelometers with automated pipettor/dispensers are capable of significantly better precision than manual methods. Any of the common quantitative procedures are potentially capable of indicating a genetic α_1-antitrypsin deficiency if the limitations of quantitation are understood.

Early studies *(1)* indicated a trimodal distribution of serum α_1-antitrypsin concentration: normal, low (10% of normal), and intermediate (60% of normal). These studies confirmed an autosomal recessive genetic inheritance of α_1-antitrypsin deficiency in homozygotes (low concentrations). However, later investigations demonstrated that at least 24 co-dominant alleles exist, with each allele contributing to the assayed antitrypsin activity. These alleles have been termed Pi alleles ("protease inhibitor"), and identification of the polymorphic variants may be required in conjunction with or in place of immunochemical quantitation. This procedure (Pi typing) involves starch-gel electrophoresis followed by crossed agarose electrophoresis *(2)*, isoelectric focusing *(3)*, or immunofixation *(4)*.

The importance of measuring α_1-antitrypsin lies in its physiologic role as a protease inhibitor. Trypsin, for example, is present in leukocyte lysosomes, and release of trypsin during inflammation or necrosis can cause serious autodigestion of protein. Autodigestion of human lung tissue has been clearly demonstrated *(5)*, as has the physiological role of α_1-antitrypsin in inhibiting proteases. Frequency of homozygous α_1-antitrypsin deficiency has been estimated at about 1:1500 (6), and of the heterozygous form as high as 1:20. The homozygous form presents clinically as a severe degenerative chronic obstructive pulmonary disease, appearing in young adults (20 to 30 years old). Many of these patients have a concomitant peptic ulcer disease, which may also be related to lack of protease inhibition. The heterozygous form of α_1-antitrypsin deficiency appears to cause increased susceptibility to inhaled environmental pollutants, with clinical consequences occurring at a later age than for homozygotes.

In pediatrics, 50 to 30% of infantile cholestatic jaundice has been associated with α_1-antitrypsin deficiency. Some patients exhibit mild liver disease initially, with complications of cirrhosis often developing in the first decade (7); other infants progress to hepatic decompensation, ascites, and hepatic failure within months (7). Hepatic complications may be related to an impairment in the release of hepatic α_1-antitrypsin, or to alternation in the carbohydrate and sialic acid residues. Diagnosis is established by quantitating α_1-antitrypsin, often after the observation of decreased α_1-staining in protein electrophoresis. Attempts to use phenobarbital or steroids to increase the release from hepatocytes have been unsuccessful.

α_1-Antitrypsin is one of the acute-phase proteins that may be increased nonspecifically due to numerous diseases, especially inflammation or tissue necrosis. Such increases are related to increased synthesis, can be detected as early as 12 to 24 h after onset, and usually peak within 72 to 96 h. These acute-phase reactions may hide α_1-antitrypsin deficiency if not recognized by the physician or the laboratory. Evaluation of other acute-phase proteins (ceruloplasmin, C-reactive protein, haptoglobin, etc.) may clarify this possibility.

1. Daniels, J. C., Abnormalities of protease inhibitors. In *Serum Protein Abnormalities*, S. E. Ritzmann and J. C. Daniels, Eds. Little Brown and Co., Boston, MA, 1975, pp 243–264.
2. Talamo, R. C., Langley, C. E., Levine, B. W., and Kazemi, H., Genetic vs. quantitative analysis of serum alpha-1-antitrypsin. *N. Engl. J. Med.* **287**, 1067–1069 (1972).
3. Guenter, C. A., Welch, M. H., Russell, T. R., Hyde, R. M., and Hammarsten, J. F., The pattern of lung disease associated with alpha-1-antitrypsin deficiency. *Arch. Intern. Med.* **122**, 254–257 (1968).
4. Ritchie, R. F., and Smith, R., Immunofixation II: Application to typing of α_1-antitrypsin at acid pH. *Clin. Chem.* **22**, 1735–1737 (1976).
5. Lieberman, J., and Gawad, M., Inhibitors and activators of leukocytic proteases in purulent sputum. Digestion of human lung and inhibition by alpha-1-antitrypsin. *J. Lab. Clin. Med.* **77**, 713–727 (1971).
6. Sveger, T., Liver disease in alpha-1-antitrypsin deficiency detected by screening of 200 000 infants. *N. Engl. J. Med.* **294**, 1316–1321 (1976).
7. Watkins, J. B., Alpha-1-antitrypsin deficiency. In text ref. *17*, 11th ed., pp 1126–1127.

Note: Also see Chapter 10, **Specific Proteins in Pediatrics.**

Arsenic

Specimen Tested:

U.

Laboratory Reporting:

1.

Reference (Normal) Values:

0–30 μg/d

Sources of Reference (Normal) Values:

Institutional.

Specimen Volume, Collection, and Preservation:

50 mL. 24-h U collected into an acid-washed container.

Analytical Method:

Sunshine, I., CRC manual of *Analytical Toxicology*, The Chemical Rubber Co., Cleveland, OH, 1971, p 32; Ratliff, C. R., Hall, F. F., and Culp, T. W., The colorimetric determination of arsenic in biological materials. *Clin. Chem.* **18,** 717 (1972), abstract.

Instrumentation:

Zeiss spectrophotometer.

Commentary—M. J. Levitt

Arsenic is measured to detect or document chronic exposure or acute poisoning. Amounts in urine of asymptomatic individuals are <50–100 μg/L. A potentially fatal dose of arsenic is 1–2 mg/kg of body weight *(1)*.

Arsenic is usually semiquantitatively and quantitatively measured by toxicology laboratories after acid digestion of body fluids or tissues. The arsenic is converted to volatile arsine (AsH_3), which is then detected with mercuric bromide, or measured by its reduction of silver nitrate *(2)*. The Reinsch test is still commonly used as a screening test for arsenic and other heavy metals. After an acidified sample of urine is boiled with copper wire, a positive result is indicated by discoloration of the copper *(2)*.

1. Text ref. 5.
2. Stolman, A., In *Toxicology—Mechanisms and Analytical Methods*, **2,** C. P. Stewart and A. Stolman, Eds. Academic Press, New York, NY, 1961, pp 640–643.

Arylsulphatase, Arylsulphatase A[1]
(EC 3.1.6.1; aryl-sulphate sulphohydrolase)

Specimen Tested:

Leukocytes.

Laboratories Reporting:

2.

Reference (Normal) Values:

Arbitrary units	
Lab. 1	**Lab. 2**
51.0–214.8; mean = 109.2; SD = 37	(a) 44–288; mean = 135 (b) 65–139; mean = 101

Sources of Reference (Normal) Values:

Institutional; Percy, A. K., and Brady, R. O., Metachromatic leukodystrophy: Diagnosis with samples of venous blood. *Science* **161**, 594–595 (1968).

Analytical Method:

Percy and Brady, *op. cit.*

Specimen Volume, Collection, and Preservation:

10 mL. Venous or arterial heparinized whole blood. Use 5 to 50 μL of leukocytes. Blood should be put on ice and leukocyte pellets prepared as soon as possible.

Enzyme Data:

1. Enzyme unit definition: 1 arbitrary unit = 1 nmol of p-nitrocatechol released per hour per milligram of leukocyte protein.
2. Buffer, pH: acetate/phosphate/NaCl, 5.0.
3. Substrate: p-nitrocatechol sulfate, dipotassium.
4. Reaction temperature: 37 °C.
5. Temperature reported: 37 °C.

Instrumentation:

Varian 635 spectrophotometer.

Note: See Appendix 4, **General Comments on Leukocyte Preparation.**

---

[1] Arylsulphatase is a generic name for a group of enzymes. Arylsulphatase A activity resides principally in leukocytes of the granulocytic series. A leukocyte and differential count must be performed to detect changes in sulphatase activity that may be due to changes in leukocyte proportions (granulocyte/lymphocyte).

Ascorbic Acid (Vitamin C)

Specimen Tested:

P, S, U.

Laboratories Reporting:

3.

Reference (Normal) Values:

P, S: 0.2–2.0 mg/dL (11.4–113.6 μmol/L); > 0.5 ($>$28.4)
U: $>$5% of an oral loading dose of 20 mg/kg of body weight per day; $<$1%
  in scurvy

Sources of Reference (Normal) Values:

Institutional; text ref. *4*, 1st ed., p 715; text ref. *2*, p 48.

Specimen Volume, Collection, and Preservation:

0.4 to 2.0 mL, venous. Use heparin as anticoagulant of choice, but
EDTA (K_3) may also be used (1.5 mg/mL). Separate P or S without
delay. Oxalic acid, 20 mg/mL of P, has been used to stabilize ascorbic
acid at RT, but samples are best stored in ice or FR.

Analytical Method:

Roe, J. H., and Kuether, C. A., The determination of ascorbic acid
in whole blood and urine through the 2,4-dinitrophenylhydrazine
derivative of dehydroascorbic acid. *J. Biol. Chem.* **147,** 399–407 (1943);
text ref. *4;* Farmer, C. J., and Abt, A. F., Determination of reduced
ascorbic acid in small amounts of blood. *Proc. Soc. Exp. Biol. Med.*
34, 146 (1936); text ref. *3*, pp 162–165.

Instrumentation:

Gilford Stasar III, Ziess spectrophotometers.

Commentary—S. Meites

Water-soluble vitamins, including ascorbic acid, are present in
higher concentrations in fetal blood than in blood from the mother
(1). Premature newborns not receiving an adequate intake of vitamin
C metabolize tyrosine and phenylalanine imperfectly, with loss of
intermediate products into the urine. Because the concentration in
plasma varies with dietary intake, several determinations are required to assess nutritional status. Infants with diseases associated
with ascorbic acid deficiency may have plasma concentrations from
0.0 to 0.3 mg/dL *(2,3)*.

Of the three laboratories reporting here, none emphasizes the use
of capillary specimens, probably reflecting the infrequency of requests
for the vitamin determination. Further information on analytical

methods and the stability of collected specimens is available in text ref. *4*, pp 1393–1398, and text ref. *3*, pp 162–165.

1. Nesbitt, R. E. L., Jr., Perinatal development. In text ref. *10*, p 129.
2. Text ref. *8*, pp 658–659.
3. Sauberlich, H., Goad, W. C., Skala, J. H., and Waring, P. P., Procedure for mechanized (continuous-flow) measurement of serum ascorbic acid (vitamin C). *Clin. Chem.* **22,** 105–110 (1976). Proposed Selected Method.

Aspartate Aminotransferase AST (EC 2.6.1.1; L-aspartate:2-oxoglutarate aminotransferase)

Specimen Tested:

P, S.

Laboratories Reporting:

7.

Reference (Normal) Values:

		95th percentiles, U/L[a]	
Age	**U/L**	**M**	**F**
Cord(S)	22.0–37.8		
Up to 0.99 yr		67	67
0–2 yr	20–55		
Newborn	14–70; 18–74; 3 × adult		
6 wk–18 mo	13–64		
Infant	up to 67		
1.00–2.99 yr		30	30
18 mo–5 yr	16–46		
2–5 yr	20–50		
3.00–4.99 yr		28	26
5.00–7.99 yr		28	26
5–8 yr	20–45		
5–11 yr	10–41		
8.00–10.99 yr		24	27
8–12 yr	15–40		
Older children	10–30		
11.00–12.99 yr		22	23
11–16 yr	7–34		
12–14 yr	15–35		
13.00–14.99 yr		20	22
14–16 yr	15–30		
15.00–16.99 yr		19	23
16 yr–adult	10–27		
17.00 yr and over		23	24
Adult	0–40; 5–40; 8–40		
M	8–46		
F	7–34		

[a] Percentile values from one institution.

Sources of Reference (Normal) Values:

Institutional; text ref. 2, p 315; Cherian, A. G., and Hill, J. G., Age dependence of serum enzymatic activities (alkaline phosphatase, aspartate aminotransferase, and creatine kinase) in healthy children and adolescents. *Am. J. Clin. Pathol.* **70**, 783–789 (1978); Cheng, M. H., Lipsey, A. I., Blanco, V., Wong, H. T., and Spiro, S. H., Microchemical analysis for 13 constituents of plasma from healthy children. *Clin. Chem.* **25**, 692–698 (1979); a study of data obtained on the Technicon SMAC analytical system, with the charts of 450 pediatric patients examined to exclude evidence of active infectious or inflammatory disease, malignancy, and anemia.

Specimen Volume, Collection, and Preservation:

5 to 100 μL (except for Technicon methods: 0.47 mL). Only heparin (lithium or ammonium) used as anticoagulant. Specimen is stable 3 to 4 d at RT (claims for as long as 1 to 3 wk), 7 to 10 d in RR, 6 mo in FR. Avoid hemolysis, which increases the activity values determined. Turbidity and icterus may interfere.

Analytical Method:

All methods list as a basis: Henry, R. J., Chiamori, N., Golub, O. J., and Berkman, S., Revised spectrophotometric methods for the determination of glutamic–oxalacetic transaminase, glutamic–pyruvic transaminase and lactic acid dehydrogenase. *Am. J. Clin. Pathol.* **34**, 381–398 (1960). Other references are: Rodgerson, D. O., and Osberg, I. M., Sources of error in spectrophotometric measurement of aspartate aminotransferase and alanine aminotransferase activities in serum. *Clin. Chem.* **20**, 43–50 (1973); Kessler, G., Rush, R., Leon, L., Delea, A., and Cupiola, R., Automated 340 nm measurement of SGOT, SGPT, and LDH. In *Advances in Automated Analysis*, **1**, Technicon International Congress, 1970, Thurman Associates, Miami, FL, 1971, pp 67–74; Kessler, G., Morgenstern, S., Snyder, L., and Varady, R., Improved point assays for ALT and AST in serum using the Technicon SMAC high-speed, computer-controlled biochemical analyzer to eliminate the common errors found in enzyme analysis. *Ninth International Congress on Clinical Chemistry*, Toronto, Canada, 1975; Amador, E., and Wacker, W. E. C., Serum glutamic–oxaloacetic transaminase activity. A new modification and an analytical assessment of current assay technics. *Clin. Chem.* **8**, 343–350 (1962); Bio-Dynamics/*bmc* kit no. 15923; Abbott A-Gent SGO-T; Technicon.

Enzyme Data:

1. Enzyme unit definition: 1 IUB unit (U) = enzyme activity transforming 1 μmol of aspartate to 1 μmol of oxaloacetate per minute.
2. Buffer, pH: phosphate buffer, 7.4.

3. Substrate, pH: L-aspartate and α-ketoglutarate, 7.4.
4. Reaction temperature: 37 °C (6 labs.); 30 °C (2 labs.).
5. Temperature reported: 37 °C (5 labs.); 30 °C (3 labs.).

Instrumentation:

Electro-Nucleonics GEMSAEC; Beckman TR Enzyme Analyzer; Abbott ABA-100 Bichromatic Analyzer; Technicon SMA II and SMAC; Union Carbide CentrifiChem.

*   *   *

Laboratory Reporting:

1.

Reference (Normal) Values:

<1 yr	20–110 U/L
1–3 yr	13–65
3–16 yr	7–50

Sources of Reference (Normal) Values:

Institutional.

Analytical Method:

Bio-Dynamics/*bmc* kit.

Commentary—Paul L. Wolf

Aspartate aminotransferase (AST; formerly called glutamic–oxaloacetic transaminase, GOT) is a ubiquitous enzyme found in many tissues including the liver, heart, skeletal muscle, smooth muscle, kidney, pancreas, brain, erythrocyte, and skin. Freer recently studied 69 newborns and found a normal range of 7–62 U/L (1). Kove also found that newborns have greater AST values than normal adults, declining to adult activities by three months (2), but King and Morris (3) did not identify this higher neonatal activity. The higher AST activity in neonatal blood has been attributed to seepage from the neonate's hepatocytes, which, being immature, have more permeable membranes. Increased AST in neonates may also be the result of increased synthesis, physiologic hemolysis of erythrocytes, skeletal muscle trauma during birth, or a minor amount contributed from the mother's skeletal muscle and uterus during labor.

Freer also found that alanine aminotransferase (ALT) ranged from 6 to 62 U/L in 69 normal neonates. Again, this has not been confirmed by King and Morris. The reasons for a higher normal range for ALT in newborns are similar to those cited for AST (see also **Alanine Aminotransferase**).

The usual pathologic cause for an increase in serum AST and ALT in infants is hepatic disease, especially viral or giant cell hepatitis. Cholestasis will also result in serum increases in AST and ALT, because both enzymes are regurgitated from bile into the blood circulation in connection with ultra- or extrahepatic obstructive jaundice caused by neoplastic infiltrates or biliary atresia. Increased hepatocyte synthesis of AST and ALT occurs in cholestasis as a result of increased pressure in the biliary system. It is important to assess the quantity of AST and ALT in hepatic disease because the highest values are associated with viral hepatitis or toxic hepatitis. Rarely, hepatitis with marked hepatic necrosis may not present with increased enzyme activities because of exhaustion of enzyme from the cells.

In addition to hepatic disease, other conditions may cause an increase in serum AST or ALT: myocardial damage, rhabdomyolysis, myositis, muscular dystrophy, renal infarction, acute pancreatitis, or burns. Cerebral damage increases the AST in CSF, but the blood–brain barrier prevents an increase in the enzyme's activity in serum.

The ratio of AST to ALT is important in hepatic disease. A ratio greater than 1 usually is associated with serious damage—AST is present in hepatic cell microsomes and mitochondria, in contrast to ALT, which is present only in microsomes. Thus, inflammatory liver lesions cause ALT activity to exceed AST, whereas necrosis causes a higher AST activity than ALT *(4)*.

Finally, it is important to understand the causes for a lower than normal AST or ALT. Both aminotransferases require pyridoxal phosphate as a cofactor. If vitamin B_6 is decreased, AST and ALT are decreased too. Decreased vitamin B_6 occurs in pregnancy, malnutrition, and chronic renal failure. An inhibitor of AST may also be produced in chronic renal failure *(5,6)*.

1. Freer, D. E., Statland, B. E., Johnson, M., and Felton, H., Reference values for selected enzyme activities and protein concentrations in serum and plasma derived from cord-blood specimens. *Clin. Chem.* **25,** 565–569 (1979).
2. Kove, S., Patterns of serum transaminase activity—diagnostic aid in neonatal jaundice. *J. Pediatr.* **57,** 802–805 (1960).
3. King, J., and Morris, M. B., Serum enzyme activity in the normal newborn infant. *Arch. Dis. Child.* **36,** 604–609 (1961).
4. DeRitis, F., Coltorti, M., and Giusti, G., Diagnostic value and pathogenic significance of transaminase activity changes in viral hepatitis. *Minerva Med.* **47,** 167–171 (1956).
5. Wolf, P. L., Williams, D., Coplon, N., and Coulson, A., Low aspartate transaminase activity in serum of patients undergoing chronic hemodialysis. *Clin. Chem.* **18,** 567–568 (1972).
6. Cohen, G. A., Goffinet, J. A., Donabedian, R. K., and Conn, H. O., Observations on decreased serum glutamic oxalacetic transaminase (SGOT) activity in azotemic patients. *Ann. Intern. Med.* **84,** 275–280 (1976).

Bile Acids, Total

Specimen Tested:
Bile.

Laboratory Reporting:
1.

Reference (Normal) Values:
Adult: 20–40 μmol/L

Sources of Reference (Normal) Values:
Bergmeyer, H. U., Ed., *Methods of Enzymatic Analysis,* **4,** 2nd English ed. Academic Press, Inc., New York, NY, 1974, p 1886.

Specimen Volume:
20 μL.

Analytical Method:
Enzymic; Bergmeyer, *op. cit.*

Instrumentation:
Beckman 25 K Spectrophotometer.

Bilirubin

Specimen Tested:
P, S.

Laboratories Reporting:
6.

Reference (Normal) Values:
Cord S: up to 2.8 mg/dL (48 μmol/L)

mg/dL (μmol/L)		
Infants:	**Premature, total**	**Full-term, total**
24 h	1–6 (17–103)	2–6 (34–103)
48 h	6–8 (103–137)	6–7 (103–120)
3–5 d	10–12 (171–205)	4–6 (68–103)

1 mo–adult: up to 1.5 mg/dL (26 μmol/L) of total bilirubin; up to 0.5 mg/dL (9 μmol/L) of conjugated bilirubin.

Sources of Reference (Normal) values:

Institutional; Routh, J. I., Liver function. In Text ref. 5, 2nd ed., p 1040; Cheng, M. H., Lipsey, A. I., Blanco, V., Wong, H. T., and Spiro, S. H., Microchemical analysis for 13 constituents of plasma from healthy children. *Clin. Chem.* **25,** 692–698 (1979); Arias, I. M., Gartner, L., Furman, M., and Wolfson, S., Studies of the effect of several drugs on hepatic glucuronide formation in newborn rats and humans. *Ann. N.Y. Acad. Sci.* **111,** 274–280 (1963).

Specimen Volume, Collection, and Preservation:

10 to 100 μL. Only heparin (lithium or ammonium) is used as anticoagulant. Protect specimen from light (blue opaque collecting tube is helpful). Store in total darkness. May be stable for 1 d in RR. Avoid hemolysis and lipemia.

Analytical Methods:

All methods involve a diazo reaction for total bilirubin, with variation primarily in the "accelerators" used and in whether the final azobilirubin color is read in alkaline or acid medium. Direct-reacting bilirubin is measured in aqueous medium in the absence of the accelerator.

Alkaline medium: Jendrassik, L., and Grof, P., Vereinfachte photometrische Methoden zur Bestimmung des Blutbilirubins. *Biochem. Z.* **297,** 81–89 (1938); Nosslin, B., The direct diazo reaction of bile pigments in serum. *Scand. J. Clin. Lab. Invest.* **12,** Suppl. 49, 1–176 (1960); Gambino, S. R., Bilirubin (modified Jendrassik and Grof)—provisional. *Stand. Methods Clin. Chem,* **5,** 55–64 (1965); Doumas, B. T., Perry, B. W., Sasse, E. A., and Straumfjord, J. V., Jr., Standardization in bilirubin assay: Evaluation of selected methods and stability of bilirubin solutions. *Clin. Chem.* **19,** 984–993 (1973).

Acid medium: Rand, R. N., and di Pasqua, A., A new diazo method for the determination of bilirubin. *Clin. Chem.* **8,** 570–578 (1962); Meites, S., and Hogg, C. K., Studies on the use of the van den Bergh reagent for determination of serum bilirubin. *Clin. Chem.* **5,** 470–478 (1959); Meites, S., and Traubert, J. W., Use of bilirubin standards. *Clin. Chem.* **11,** 691–699 (1965); Lathe, G. H., and Ruthven, C. R. J., Factors affecting the rate of coupling of bilirubin and conjugated bilirubin in the van den Bergh reaction. *J. Clin. Pathol.* **11,** 155–161 (1958).

Additional recommended reference: Schmid, R., Jaundice and bilirubin metabolism. *Arch. Intern. Med.* **101,** 669–674 (1958). (Also see *Instrumentation* for additional analytical methods.)

Instrumentation and Kits:

Greiner Selective Analyzer II; Stasar III spectrophotometer; American Monitor Jendrassik Bilirubin; Abbott ABA-100 Bichromatic Analyzer; Electro-Nucleonics Gemeni centrifugal analyzer; Technicon

SMA II. **Backup and stats:** American Optical Co. Bilirubinometer; Evans, R. T., and Holton, J. B., An assessment of a bilirubinometer. *Ann. Clin. Biochem.* **7,** 104–106 (1970); Levkoff, A. H., Westphal, M. C., and Finklea, J. F., Evaluation of a direct reading spectrophotometer for neonatal bilirubinometry. *Am. J. Clin. Pathol.* **54,** 562–565 (1970). **Direct spectrophotometry:** Beckman 25 spectrophotometer; Meites, S., and Hogg, C. K., Direct spectrophotometry of total serum bilirubin in the newborn. *Clin. Chem.* **6,** 421–428 (1960).

*   *   *

Laboratory Reporting:

1.

Reference (Normal) Values:

Peak bilirubin values during newborn period

Birth weight, g	< 2000	2001–2500	> 2500
No. of babies	379	1428	18 488
Total bilirubin concn., mg/dL (μmol/L)	*Percentage of babies exceeding this value*		
> 20.0 (342)	8.2	2.6	0.8
> 18.0 (308)	13.5	4.6	1.5
> 16.0 (274)	20.3	7.6	2.6
> 14.0 (239)	33.0	12.0	4.4
> 11.0 (188)	53.8	23.0	9.3
> 8.0 (137)	77.0	45.4	26.1

Sources of Reference (Normal) Values:

Boggs, T. R., Jr., Hardy, J. B., and Frazier, T. M., Correlation of neonatal serum total bilirubin concentrations and developmental status at age eight months. *J. Pediatr.* **71,** 553–560 (1967); institutional.

Commentary—T. A. Blumenfeld

The major reason for measuring bilirubin in the newborn is to distinguish physiological from nonphysiological (pathological) hyperbilirubinemia. If therapeutic means are not undertaken to lower nonphysiological concentrations of bilirubin, bilirubin encephalopathy may result. The criteria for nonphysiological (pathological) jaundice are:

1. Jaundice in the first 24 h of life.
2. Serum bilirubin increasing at a rate > 5 mg/dL per day.
3. Serum bilirubin exceeding 12 mg/dL in full-term infants.
4. Serum bilirubin exceeding 15 mg/dL in pre-term infants.
5. Persistence of jaundice after the first week of life.
6. Value for direct-reacting bilirubin exceeding 1.5 mg/dL at any time.

Physiological jaundice may be due to abnormal hepatic uptake of bilirubin, abnormal bilirubin conjugation, or abnormal bilirubin excretion. Specific reasons for these abnormalities are:

1. *Abnormal liver cell uptake of bilirubin.* In fetal and neonatal life, subnormal amounts of receptor carrier proteins (Y and Z) that bind bilirubin are present in liver cytosol.

2. *Conjugation.* Conjugated bilirubin is bilirubin that is conjugated with glucuronic acid. It is produced from uridine diphosphate glucuronic acid (UDPGA) and unconjugated bilirubin in the presence of the enzyme UDPglucuronosyltransferase (EC 2.4.1.17). This enzyme is deficient in the fetus and in the first week of life. UDPGA is produced from uridine diphosphate glucose (UDPglucose) in the presence of the enzyme UDPglucose dehydrogenase (EC 1.1.1.22), which is deficient in newborns. UDPglucose is produced from nucleotides that may be deficient in the newborn. Also necessary for its formation is an adequate supply of glucose, which may also be deficient in certain conditions in the newborn.

3. *Bilirubin excretion.* In the normal adult, conjugated bilirubin is excreted from the gall bladder into the small bowel and metabolized to urobilinogen by bacterial flora. Urobilinogen may be excreted in the feces and (or) reabsorbed from the gastrointestinal tract and excreted by the liver into bile and (or) excreted by the kidney into the urine. In the fetus and infant, conjugated bilirubin, after reaching the gut, is not metabolized by bacteria because no bacterial flora are present at that time. However, in the lumen of the newborn's bowel, the enzyme β-glucuronidase (EC 3.2.1.31) deconjugates bilirubin, producing unconjugated bilirubin, which may be reabsorbed into the blood or excreted into the feces. Meconium contains relatively large amounts of deconjugated bilirubin as a result of the action of β-glucuronidase. Meconium contains five- to 10-fold the amount of bilirubin produced daily by the normal newborn; if meconium passage is delayed, a great increase in the bilirubin load will occur.

Thus, physiological jaundice is a result of abnormal cellular uptake, abnormal conjugation, and abnormal excretion of bilirubin—a combination unique to the newborn period.

Unconjugated serum bilirubin exceeding 12 mg/dL during neonatal life is toxic to neuronal tissue and can result in bilirubin encephalopathy. The exact mechanism of in vivo bilirubin toxicity is not known. In vitro studies show that bilirubin can depress cell respiration, uncouple oxidative phosphorylation, increase glycolysis, and impair protein synthesis. Bilirubin is known to have a very high surface activity and will concentrate at monolayers of protein and fatty acids. This surface activity could reduce the biological activity of plasma membranes and result in cell death.

In its severest clinical form, bilirubin encephalopathology is known as "kernicterus" (*Ger.*, "nuclear jaundice") because bilirubin is deposited in injured neurons, characteristically the basal ganglia, hippocampus, cerebellum, and nuclei of the floor of the fourth ventricle. Clinically, kernicterus is manifested in severely jaundiced term infants on the third to sixth day of extrauterine life. Those who survive have cerebral palsy. In premature infants, a history of fetal distress and asphyxia is common, and it is not clear whether this circumstance makes neuronal tissues more sensitive to bilirubin or whether nonspecific precipitation of bilirubin in previously asphyxiated cells results in the bilirubin staining reported in prematures with bilirubin concentrations of less than 12 mg/dL. These infants often have severe acidemia, which may be associated with a shift of bilirubin from an extracellular to an intracellular location.

1. Odell, G. B., Neonatal jaundice. In *Progress in Liver Disease,* H. Popper and F. Schaffner, Eds. Grune and Stratton, New York, NY, 1976.

Note: See also Chapter 6, **Free Bilirubin.**

Body Water

Specimen Tested:

B, P.

Laboratory Reporting:

1.

Reference (Normal) Values:

	% of body weight		
Age	**Total body water**	**Extracellular**	**Intracellular**
0–11 d	77.8 (69–84)	42.0 (34–53)	34.6 (28–40)
11 d–6 mo	72.4 (63–83)	34.6 (28–57)	38.8 (20–47)
6 mo–2 yr	59.8 (52–72)	26.6 (20–30)	34.8 (28–38)
2–7 yr	63.4 (55–73)	25.0 (21–30)	40.4 (31–53)
7–16 yr	58.2 (50–64)	20.5 (18–26)	46.7

Sources of Reference (Normal) Values:

Institutional.

Specimen Volume:

1.0 mL, venous.

Analytical Method:

Deuterium oxide; Thornton, V., and Condon, F. E., Infrared spectrophotometric determination of deuterum oxide in water. *Anal. Chem.* **22,** 690 (1950); Turner, M. D., Neely, W. A., and Hardy, J. D., Rapid determination of deuterium oxide in biological fluids. *J. Appl. Physiol.* **15,** 309 (1960).

Instrumentation:

Zeiss spectrophotometer.

Commentary—John F. Connelly

Total body water may be estimated by measuring the concentration of deuterium oxide (D_2O) in plasma water 3 h after oral or intravenous administration of D_2O after an overnight fast. To measure extracellular water, several methods have been described (1), but one that is favored is to administer sodium bromide simultaneously with D_2O and measure plasma bromide concentration in the same blood specimen. The extracellular volume is estimated by making an appropriate correction to the calculated bromide space (2).

Neither of these tests is performed widely in hospital clinical chemistry laboratories. D_2O is expensive, the methods are often difficult, and special equipment is needed. Because of its relative ease of operation, infrared spectrophotometry has been favored by some for measurement of D_2O (3).

Total body water and extracellular water are expressed as percentages of body weight for different age groups (4). In infancy the total body water drops from 75% of body weight at birth to 60% one year later, the result of a relative decrease in extracellular water as a consequence of intense cellular growth (5). Male infants show a greater water content than females (6). The percentage of water relative to body weight also depends on the amount of fat, which is relatively anhydrous.

Cheek et al. (7) studied the relationship between total body water and height and weight in 40 normal boys and girls between the ages of one month and 16 years. They found that although there was a linear relationship between weight and total body water, multivariate equations incorporating height and weight gave a better prediction of total body water than weight alone.

Behrendt (1) gives an excellent discussion of body water, with tables of the variation in size of fluid compartments with age.

1. Text ref. *9*, pp 244–255.
2. Graystone, J. E., In *Human Growth*, D. B. Cheek, Ed. Lea and Febiger, Philadelphia, PA, 1968, pp 668–673.
3. Text ref. *2*, pp 123–125.
4. Friis-Hansen, B., Changes in body water compartments during growth. *Acta Pediatr.* **46**, Suppl. 110, 1–68 (1957).
5. Cheek, D. B., Observations of total body chloride in children. *Pediatrics* **14**, 5–10 (1954).
6. Owen, G. M., Filer, L. J., Jr., Maresh, M., and Fomon, S., Body composition of the infant. In text ref. *10*, p 249.
7. Cheek, D. B., Mellitz, D., and Elliott, D., Body water, height and weight during growth in normal children. *Am. J. Dis. Child.* **112**, 312–317 (1966).

Calcitonin

Specimen Tested:

S.

Laboratory Reporting:

1.

Reference (Normal) Values:

Adult: < 400 pg/mL

Sources of Reference (Normal) Values:

Radioimmunoassay Manual, 4th ed. Nichols Institute, San Pedro, CA, 1977, p 199.

Specimen Volume, Collection, and Preservation; Patient Preparation:

100 mL, venous. Obtain fasting, A.M. sample. Place blood in chilled tube. Centrifuge in refrigerated centrifuge. Remove serum and freeze without delay. Store in FR before assay.

Analytical Method:

RIA: double-antibody, ^{125}I-labeled calcitonin.

Commentary—Joan A. and Peter J. Howanitz

Although calcitonin has been studied extensively, there is considerable controversy regarding basal values in humans. Some authors report values of less than 100 pg/mL *(1–3)*; others report the normal reference interval as up to 400 pg/mL *(4,5)*. In all assays a significant number of normal subjects have undetectable calcitonin concentrations in their serum.

The discrepancies in reference intervals may be related not only to differing antibody specificities, but also to heterogeneity of plasma calcitonin forms. Metabolic precursors of calcitonin (a procalcitonin and probably a pre-procalcitonin) have been described, and aggregations of these heterogeneic forms with themselves and with other proteins may occur in serum *(6)*. Another contribution to the discrepancy between reference intervals may be nonspecific effects of the patient's serum on the assays. Because calcitonin exhibits a diurnal variation *(2)*, a fasting morning sample is recommended. Specimens collected with either EDTA or Trasylol *(7)* give less-consistent assay results than serum specimens allowed to clot at room temperature. If the specimen is centrifuged in the cold and stored at −20 °C, there is no significant loss of calcitonin activity for at least three months.

Despite quantitative differences, there are some similarities among results from different laboratories.

In cord blood of full-term infants, calcitonin is high *(8)*, but premature infants may have even higher calcitonin concentrations than full-term infants *(9)*. In newborn full-term infants, there is a steady increase in calcitonin, peaking at about three- to fourfold normal values between 13 and 36 h after birth. Thereafter, calcitonin concentration progressively decreases but still remains slightly increased between 72 and 96 h after birth. Hypocalcemic infants have slightly higher concentrations of serum calcitonin than their normocalcemic counterparts at the same gestational age. Older children have not been studied extensively, but in a group within the age range of six to 12 years, almost one-fourth had calcitonin values exceeding the adult reference interval *(10)*; in this small group, calcitonin concentrations increased slowly with age.

The major use of calcitonin assays is in the diagnosis of medullary carcinoma of the thyroid, which is inherited as an autosomal dominant trait. This carcinoma can be diagnosed in most patients by the finding of an increased concentration of plasma calcitonin under basal fasting conditions. However, a certain percentage of patients with this tumor, many of whom have early stages of C-cell neoplasia, have base concentrations of the hormone that are indistinguishable from normal. Because the patients with early lesions are the most amenable to surgical care, it is important to identify this group. Thus provocative testing is used to identify patients who are suspected of having medullary carcinoma of the thyroid but who have normal basal values of calcitonin. Several agents have been shown to cause a hyper-response of calcitonin secretion in patients with C-cell neoplasia; pentagastrin and calcium infusions are commonly used *(11)*. If one of these stimulating agents fails to elicit a response in a patient suspected of having medullary carcinoma of the thyroid, an alternative procedure should be used before excluding the diagnosis.

Increased calcitonin concentrations may occur in conditions other than this carcinoma; e.g., several other tumors produce the same effect *(12)*. In addition, chronic renal disease, chronic hypercalcemia, and acute pancreatitis *(13)* reportedly increase calcitonin.

1. Heath, H., and Sizemore, G. W., Plasma calcitonin in normal man. *J. Clin. Invest.* **60**, 1135–1140 (1977).
2. Hillyard, C. J., Cooke, T. J. C., Coombes, R. C., Evans, I. M. A., and MacIntyre, I., Normal plasma calcitonin: Circadian variation and response to stimuli. *Clin. Endocrinol.* **6**, 291–298 (1977).
3. Parthemore, J. G., and Deftos, L. J., Calcitonin secretion in normal human subjects. *J. Clin. Endocrinol. Metab.* **47**, 184–188 (1978).
4. Vora, N. M., Williams, G. A., Hargis, G. K., Bowser, E. N., Kawahara, W., Jackson, B. L., Henderson, W. J., and Kukreja, S. C., Comparative effect of calcium and of the adrenergic system of calcitonin secretion in man. *J. Clin. Endocrinol. Metab.* **46**, 567–571 (1978).

5. Tashijan, A. H., Wolfe, H. J., and Voelkel, E. F., Human calcitonin. *Am. J. Med.* **56,** 840–849 (1974).
6. Deftos, L. J., Calcitonin in clinical medicine. *Adv. Intern. Med.* **23,** 159–193 (1978).
7. Rojanasathit, S., and Haddad, J. G., Human calcitonin radioimmunoassay: Characterization and application. *Clin. Chim. Acta* **78,** 425–437 (1977).
8. Samaan, N. A., Hill, C. S., Beceiro, J. R., and Schultz, P. N., Immunoreactive calcitonin in medullary carcinoma of the thyroid and in maternal and cord serum. *J. Lab. Clin. Med.* **81,** 671–681 (1973).
9. Dirksen, H. C., and Anast, C. S., Interrelationship of serum immunoreactive calcitonin and serum calcium in newborn infants. *Pediatr. Res.* **10,** 408 (1979). Abstract 642.
10. Shainkin-Kerstenbaum, R., Funkenstein, B., Conforti, A., Shani, S., and Berlyne, G., Serum calcitonin and blood mineral interrelationships in normal children aged six to twelve years. *Pediatr. Res.* **11,** 112–116 (1977).
11. Hillyard, C. J., Stevenson, J. C., and MacIntyre, I., Relative deficiency of plasma calcitonin in normal women. *Lancet* **i,** 961–962 (1978).
12. Wells, S. A., Baylin, S. B., Linehan, W. M., Farrell, R. E., Cox, E. B., and Cooper, C. W., Provocative agents and the diagnosis of medullary carcinoma and the thyroid gland. *Ann. Surg.* **188,** 139–141 (1978).
13. Schwartz, K. E., Wolfsen, A. R., Forster, B., and Odell, W. D., Calcitonin in nonthyroidal cancer. *J. Clin. Endocrinol. Metab.* **49,** 438–444 (1979).
14. Gillquist, J., Larsson, J., and Sjodahl, R., Serum calcitonin in acute pancreatitis in man. *Scand. J. Gastroenterol.* **12,** 21–25 (1977).

Calcium

Ionized Calcium

Specimen Tested:

P, S.

Laboratories Reporting:

2.

Reference (Normal) Values:

Child > 1 mo–adult:
    Calculated[a]: 4.1–5.4 mg/dL (1.02–1.35 mmol/L)
    Determined: 4.4–5.4 (1.10–1.35)

[a] Values obtained depend on established normal range for total serum calcium. This calculated ionized calcium has been surprisingly useful. All Ca values out of the normal range (frequent in the premature newborn) are reported with the calculated ionized calcium, the total protein, and albumin. Current instrumentation for measuring ionized calcium directly is impractical because of excessive specimen volume requirement.

Sources of Reference (Normal) Values:

Institutional.

Specimen Volume:

150 to 200 µL, venous.

Analytical Method:

Calculated: Pottgen, P., and Davis, E. R., Why measure total serum calcium? *Clin. Chem.* **22**, 1756–1757 (1976). **Determined:** Calcium-selective electrode, Orion Research, Inc.

Total Calcium

Specimen Tested:

P, S.

Laboratories Reporting:

8.

Reference (Normal) Values:

Age	Calcium, mg/dL (mmol/L)	
	Lower range	Upper range
Cord, S	9.0 (2.25)	11.5 (2.87)
Newborn		
Premature, 0–1 wk	6.0–7.0 (1.50–1.75)	9.0–10.0 (2.25–2.50)
Full-term, 0–1 wk	7.0–8.0 (1.75–2.00)	10.0–12.0 (2.50–2.99)
To 2 yr	8.8 (2.20)	11.2 (2.79)
Infant–adult	8.5–9.6[a] (2.12–2.40)	10.9[b]–11.0 (2.72–2.74)
2–16 yr	8.6 (2.15)	11.0 (2.74)
16 yr–adult	9.0 (2.25)	11.0 (2.74)

[a] 5th percentile.
[b] 95th percentile.

Sources of Reference (Normal) Values:

Meites, S., Total plasma calcium in the newborn. *Crit. Rev. Clin. Lab. Sci.* **6,** 1–18 (1975); Cherian, A. G., and Hill, J. G., Percentile estimation of reference values for fourteen chemical constituents in sera of children and adolescents. *Am. J. Clin. Pathol.* **69**, 24–31 (1978); Cheng, M. H., Lipsey, A. I., Blanco, V., Wong, H. T., and Spiro, S. H., Microchemical analysis for 13 constituents of plasma from healthy children. *Clin. Chem.* **25**, 692–696 (1979); institutional; text ref. *9*, p 180; Colletti, R. B., Pan, M. W., Smith, E. W. P., and Genel, M., Detection of hypocalcemia in susceptible neonates—the Q-oTc interval. *N. Engl. J. Med.* **290**, 931–935 (1974).

Specimen Volume, Collection, and Preservation:

5 to 200 µL. Heparin anticoagulant only. Stable. "Old" serum may cause precipitation of calcium with denatured protein or fatty acids.

Analytical Method:

Most use a dye-binding method with *o*-cresolphthalein complexone: Gitelman, H. J., An improved automated procedure for the determination of calcium in biological specimens. *Anal. Biochem.* **18,** 520–531 (1967); Dow Diagnostics Calcium Reagent Set; Baginski, E. S., Marie, S. S., Clark, W. L., and Zak, B., Direct microdetermination of serum calcium. *Clin. Chim. Acta* **46,** 46–54 (1973); Technicon SMA-II adaption.

Other methods: Gindler, E. M., and King, J. D., Rapid colorimetric determination of calcium in biological fluids with methylthymol blue. *Am. J. Clin. Pathol.* **58,** 376–382 (1972); Pierce Chemical Co., Calcium Rapid Stat Kit (manual); Zettner, A., and Seligson, D., Application of atomic absorption spectrophotometry in the determination of calcium in serum. *Clin. Chem.* **10,** 869–890 (1964); Willis, J. B., Determination of calcium and magnesium in urine by atomic absorption spectroscopy. *Anal. Chem.* **33,** 556 (1961); Pybus, J., Determination of calcium and magnesium in serum and urine by atomic absorption spectrophotometry. *Clin. Chim. Acta* **23,** 309–317 (1969).

Instrumentation:

Colorimetric procedures: Greiner Selective Analyzer II, Abbott ABA-100 Bichromatic Analyzer; Technicon SMA-II: Gilford Stasar II spectrophotometer. **Others:** Instrumentation Laboratory Atomic Absorption Spectrophotometer Model 251; Perkin-Elmer Atomic Absorption Spectrophotometer Model 290.

*   *   *

Laboratory Reporting:

1.

Reference (Normal) Values:

Age	No.	Calcium, mg/dL (mmol/L)
Newborn	24	6.3–11.9 (1.57–2.97)
6 wk–18 mo	40	8.9–11.3 (2.22–2.82)
18 mo–15 yr	366	9.0–10.8 (2.25–2.69)
16 yr	19	8.4–10.8 (2.10–2.69)
Adult	150	8.4–10.0 (2.10–2.50)

Sources of Reference (Normal) Values:

A retrospective study of data from patients selected to exclude active infectious, inflammatory disease, malignancy, and anemia.

Analytical Method, Instrumentation:

o-Cresolphthalein complexone method with Technicon SMAC system; Gitelman, *op. cit.;* Kessler, G., and Wolfman, M., An automated procedure for the determination of calcium and phosphorus. *Clin. Chem.* **10,** 686–703 (1964).

Urinary Calcium

Specimen Tested:

U.

Laboratories Reporting:

3.

Reference (Normal) Values:

4–12 yr: 2.0–4.0 mmol/d
Adult: up to 0.21 mmol/kg of body weight per day

Sources of Reference (Normal) Values:

Institutional; Paunier, L., Borgeaud, M., and Wyss, M., Urinary excretion of magnesium and calcium in normal children. *Helv. Paediatr. Acta* **25,** 577–584 (1970).

Specimen Volume, Collection, and Preservation; Patient Preparation:

20 to 25 µL. Urinary excretion of calcium varies greatly with its intake. Results are significant, provided the patient is placed on a low-calcium, neutral-ash diet and a 24-h urine is collected.

Analytical Method, Instrumentation:

See *Total Calcium.*

Commentary—M. J. Levitt

Values for total calcium in serum and plasma vary markedly during the perinatal period. The high incidence of hypocalcemia in the first two to three days of postnatal life (neonatal tetany) may be the result of conditions originating months before in the womb.

At about four months of gestation, fetal plasma calcium concentrations begin to surpass maternal plasma calcium values (1). This gradient may be maintained by a calcium pump in the placenta (2). Another possibility is that some form of maternal parathyroid hormone could cross the placenta and create functional hyperparathyroidism in the fetus (2). This situation could occur even if there were no maternal hyperparathyroidism, if the postulated hormone fragment were more active in the fetus than in the mother. Whatever the cause may be, the difference between maternal and fetal plasma calcium concentrations bears no obvious relation to the absolute concentration of circulating calcium in the mother (1).

Towards the end of pregnancy, serum calcium values in the mother tend to decline. This decline is less marked in diabetic than in healthy mothers, even when fluids are administered (3). Diabetics may have relative hyperparathyroidism, compared with healthy mothers (3).

Plasma calcium concentrations in the newborn are at the adult value of about 4.5–5.5 mEq/L (2.25–2.75 mmol/L), but may decline in two to three days to hypocalcemic values of 3 or 4 mEq/L (1.5–2.0 mmol/L) or less. Inability to maintain calcium homeostasis during this period suggests inadequate control by parathyroid hormone. One possibility is that fetal hypercalcemia results in secondary hypoparathyroidism extending into the neonatal period (2).

Plasma calcium concentrations at birth are lower in premature than in full-term infants (1). Prematurity alone, however, is not a sufficient cause for neonatal hypocalcemia. Neonates are predisposed to plasma calcium values below 4 mEq/L (2 mmol/L) if asphyxia, shock, acidosis, respiratory distress, or maternal diabetes occurs (4). These factors may cause sluggish parathyroid response to hypocalcemia, impaired kidney response to parathyroid hormone, or both (4). Diabetes in the mother may be a contributory factor in that relative material hyperparathyroidism could lead to neonatal hypoparathyroidism (3).

Neonatal serum calcium concentrations do not correlate with serum magnesium concentrations, gravidity, age of mother, length of labor, or sex of the infant (3). Most studies also find no correlation with race, although in one study serum calcium values were higher in Negroes than in Caucasians during at least the first four days of postnatal life (3,5).

Diet evidently is not a significant factor in early neonatal hypocalcemia, because feeding does not prevent convulsions associated with low serum calcium values two to three days postnatally. However, serum calcium values at four to seven days can be affected by diet (1,6). Feeding with cow's milk, which has a lower calcium/phosphorus ratio than human milk, can cause decreased serum calcium values (6).

Normal adult values for serum calcium are not reached again until about two weeks in full-term infants, or four weeks or more in premature infants (1,7). These intervals may reflect the time required for maturation of the parathyroid glands or kidneys in the two groups of infants.

Exchange transfusions with acid–citrate–dextrose-treated blood and calcium gluconate can result in hypercalcemia. Total plasma calcium in one study went from 4.2 to 5.3 mEq/L (2.1 to 2.65 mmol/L) after transfusions in sick newborn infants (7).

Atomic absorption spectrometry is the preferred method for measurement of calcium, but is not convenient for around-the-clock operation *(8)*. Complexometric techniques for measuring calcium are well suited to the needs of a pediatric laboratory; they are simple to perform and require only ultramicro volumes of samples. Instruments are now available that automatically titrate the sample, measure the fluorescence in the reaction chamber, and display the resulting calcium value. Interference by magnesium is avoided by titrating at high pH; however, interference by abnormally high amounts of either hemoglobin or bilirubin can result in falsely low calcium values *(9)*. Contamination of glassware with calcium can be a source of significant error in any method for measuring calcium *(10)*.

Ionized Calcium

Ionized calcium is measured in serum or plasma to determine the fraction of total calcium that is thought to be metabolically active.

Ionized calcium concentrations in the neonate's serum at birth exceed those in the mother's serum, as is also the case for total calcium concentrations *(2,7)*. Values for the neonate are 2.4–2.5 mEq/L (1.2–1.25 mmol/L); the average maternal value is 2.0 mEq/L (1.0 mmol/L) *(2,7)*. Values exceeding the adult value occur more frequently in prematures of less than 36 weeks' gestation *(2)*.

During the first three days of postnatal life, values for ionized calcium in serum decrease like those for total calcium, reaching a minimum in two to three days of 1.0–1.5 mEq/L (0.5–0.75 mmol/L) *(2,7)*. Concentrations in serum then increase in one to two weeks to 1.8–2.3 mEq/L (0.9–1.65 mmol/L), values characteristic of older children and adults *(7)*. The changes occurring during this two-week period are presumably due to the same factors mentioned for the homeostatic mechanisms of total calcium.

During the early neonatal period, values for ionized and total calcium in serum correlate poorly. Calcium ion concentrations of less than 1.4 mEq/L (0.7 mmol/L) can be correlated with total calcium values of less than 3.0 mEq/L (1.5 mmol/L) in only about 80% of the infants *(7)*. Predictions of values for ionized calcium from those for total calcium can be in error by as much as 0.7 mEq/L (0.35 mmol/L) *(2)*. This poor correlation may result from the fact that premature infants tend to have serum ionized calcium concentrations equal to those in full-term infants, even though their total calcium values are lower than in full-term infants *(4)*. Values for ionized calcium below 1.8 mEq/L (0.9 mmol/L) are found in both premature and full-term infants with a history of asphyxia, shock, acidosis, respiratory distress, or maternal diabetes. Values below 1.8 mEq/L (0.9 mmol/L) are seldom found in infants who have survived other complications of pregnancy, even if they are born prematurely *(4)*.

Serum ionized calcium concentration can be decreased 0.1–0.2 mEq/L (0.05–0.1 mmol/L) by the administration of sodium bicarbonate to infants *(7)*. Because this effect is correlated with a significant and simultaneous increase in pH, it probably results from the binding of calcium ion to the additional proteinate ion liberated as a result of the pH change.

Serum calcium ion concentration in infants can be decreased markedly, from normal values of 1.8–2.3 mEq/L (0.9–1.15 mmol/L) to values of less than 1.0 mEq/L (0.5 mmol/L) by means of exchange transfusion, even if calcium gluconate is also administered to increase the total circulating calcium *(7)*. Apparently the calcium ion contributed by gluconate is not sufficient to replace the calcium ion bound to the citrate ion introduced in acid–citrate–dextrose-treated blood.

The value of measuring serum or plasma ionized calcium concentration in the neonate is supported by its correlation with electrocardiographic changes *(4)*.

Ionized calcium in plasma or serum is measured with an ion-selective electrode. Procedures have been established for performing this test on capillary blood from infants *(11)*, but the test is not commonly used by the laboratories reporting here.

1. Meites, S., Normal total plasma calcium in the newborn. *CRC Crit. Rev. Clin. Lab. Sci.* **6**, 1–18 (1975).
2. Tsang, R. C., Chen, I. W., Friedman, M. A., and Chen, I., Neonatal parathyroid function: Role of gestational age and postnatal age. *J. Pediatr.* **83**, 728–738 (1973).
3. Tsang, R. C., Kleinman, L. I., Sutherland, J. M., and Light, I. J., Hypocalcemia in infants of diabetic mothers. *J. Pediatr.* **80**, 384–395 (1972).
4. Colletti, R. B., Pan, M. W., Smith, E. W. P., and Genel, M., Detection of hypocalcemia in susceptible neonates; the Q-oTc interval. *N. Engl. J. Med.* **290**, 931–935 (1974).
5. de Baare, L., Lewis, J., and Sing, H., Ultramicroscale determination of clinical chemical values for blood during the first four days of postnatal life. *Clin. Chem.* **21**, 746–750 (1975).
6. Editorial, Neonatal calcium, magnesium and phosphorus homeostasis. *Lancet* **i**, 155–156 (1974).
7. Raade, I. C., Parkinson, D. K., Höffken, B., Appiah, K. E., and Hanley, W. B., Calcium ion activity in the sick neonate: Effect of bicarbonate administration and exchange transfusion. *Pediatr. Res.* **6**, 43–49 (1972).
8. Cali, J. P., Bowers, G. N., Jr., and Young, D. S., A Reference Method for the determination of total calcium in serum. *Clin. Chem.* **19**, 1208–1213 (1973).
9. Weissman, E. B., Pragay, D. A., and Bishop, C., Evaluation of the Corning 940 calcium titrator for use with serum and urine. *Clin. Chem.* **21**, 264–267 (1975).
10. Pragay, D. A., Howard, S. F., and Chilcote, M. E., Inorganic ion contaminations in Vacutainer Tubes and micropipets used for blood collection. *Clin. Chem.* **17**, 350–351 (1971).
11. Raade, I. C., Höffken, B., Parkinson, D. K., Sheepers, J., and Luckham, A., Practical aspects of a measurement technique for calcium ion activity in plasma. *Clin. Chem.* **17**, 1002–1006 (1971).

Carbamazepine (Tegretol)

Specimen Tested:

P, S.

Laboratories Reporting:

4.

Reference (Normal) Values:

Suggested therapeutic concentration, mg/L			
Lab. 1	**Lab. 2**	**Lab. 3**	**Lab. 4**
8–12	4–10	4–8	4–8
		(variable)	

Note: Toxic at 15 mg/L. Time needed to reach steady state: 7 d. Draw blood before administering dose.

Sources of Reference (Normal) Values:

Institutional; Kutt, H., and Penry, J. K., Usefulness of blood levels of antiepileptic drugs. *Arch. Neurol.* **31,** 283–288 (1974).

Specimen Volume, Collection, and Preservation:

5 to 50 µL. Heparin anticoagulant. Specimens should not be grossly icteric, lipemic, or hemolyzed. Store in FR for prolonged periods, or for 2 d in RR.

Analytical Method:

Three labs.: EMIT (homogenous enzyme immunoassay), Syva Co.; Kananen, G., Osiewicz, J. R., and Sunshine, I., Barbiturate analysis— a current assessment. *J. Chromatogr. Sci.* **10,** 283–287 (1972). **One lab:** HPLC; Soldin, S. J., and Hill, J. G., A rapid micromethod for measuring anticonvulsant drugs in serum by high-performance liquid chromatography. *Clin. Chem.* **22,** 856–859 (1976).

Instrumentation:

EMIT systems: Bausch and Lomb Spectronic 710, with thermally regulated flow cell, timer, printer, semi-automatic pipetter–dilutor, conical bottom disposable beakers (also see report on **Phenobarbital**); Abbott ABA-100. **HPLC:** Waters ALC/GPC—204/6000 A, with a Perkin-Elmer LC 55 Variable Wavelength spectrophotometer.

Commentary—Peter J. and Joan H. Howanitz

Carbamazepine ("Tegretol"), alone or in combination with other drugs, is used for focal and major generalized seizures (grand mal), partial seizures with complex symptomatology (psychomotor seizures), and trigeminal neuralgia. In healthy volunteers, gastrointestinal absorption of the drug is rather slow, peak serum concentrations usually being attained 6 h or more after an oral dose (1). Peak serum concentrations occur earlier and are significantly higher with the syrup than with the tablet form (2). Up to 15% of an ingested dose may be found in some form in the feces, indicating that carbamazepine absorption is not complete.

Carbamazepine is metabolized extensively in the liver; less than 1% of the native drug appears in urine unchanged. One metabolite, a 10,11-epoxide, is found in serum in a concentration of about 10% that of the native drug. This metabolite has nearly as much anticonvulsant activity as the parent drug (3), but little is known of its relationship to or importance in seizure control in humans. The 10,11-epoxide is found in relatively lower concentrations in children than in adults, probably because children may have a slightly increased ability to oxidize the parent drug (4). The half-life of carbamazepine during chronic dosing in adults and children is almost equivalent, about 18 h; after a single initial dose, the half-life of carbamazepine in adults is 36 h. The difference in half-life between acute and chronic dosing probably is due to auto-induction of drug metabolism, which occurs after chronic treatment with carbamazepine (5). The half-life also is short in infants whose mothers have taken the drug during pregnancy. In children, auto-induction of drug metabolism is manifested fully after one month of carbamazepine treatment (6).

During the 10 to 24 h after ingestion, carbamazepine concentrations in serum show very little variation (1). Salivary and free drug concentrations are about one-fourth of total serum concentrations (1,2,7). The drug is not displaced from its binding to albumin by aspirin, phenytoin, ethosuximide, or phenobarbital. Very little correlation has been found between dose and serum concentration of carbamazepine in adults and children, whether they are treated with carbamazepine alone or in combination with other anticonvulsants (1,4). Therapeutic amounts are defined poorly; however, serum concentrations of carbamazepine exceeding 4 μg/mL generally correlate with seizure control (8). In a well-controlled study, serum concentrations of 8 to 12 μg/mL produce optimum seizure control with fewest side effects (9), but few patients were studied. In other studies, therapeutic ranges reported include 4 to 8 μg/mL (10), 6 to 12 μg/mL (11), and 4.25 to 11.8 μg/mL (7). Although some patients can tolerate high doses of carbamazepine without side effects, serum concentrations exceeding 16 μg/mL have not been associated with increased anticonvulsant efficacy. In addition, in at least one case, paradoxical intoxication has been reported with high doses of the drug. Meinardi (12) has predicted that 50% of the patients with serum concentrations of 8.5 to 10 μg/mL will experience side effects; data are still incomplete, however. Side effects rarely appear at concentrations less than

6 μg/mL, and values exceeding 10 μg/mL may be associated with intoxication.

The major side effects of carbamazepine are diplopia, drowsiness, and leukopenia. Idiosyncratic hematologic side effects are rare and usually disappear with discontinuance of the drug (13). Other side effects that appear during initiation of therapy usually disappear with further therapy. Several of the side effects of carbamazepine are similar to those of phenytoin, and seem to be additive in some carbamazepine-treated patients who have high phenytoin concentrations (14). In three brain-damaged children, one of whom had a therapeutic concentration of phenytoin, dystonia was associated with carbamazepine administration (15). Inappropriate antidiuretic hormone secretion has been observed in elderly patients during carbamazepine treatment; in one patient, this has been reversed with concomitant phenytoin therapy (16).

In a woman who came to delivery, serum carbamazepine values were slightly higher than those in cord serum. Carbamazepine concentration in breast milk of this mother were less than one-half of that in her serum (17).

1. Morselli, P. L., Carbamazepine: Absorption, distribution, and excretion. *Adv. Neurol.* **11,** 279–293 (1975).
2. Wada, J. A., Troupin, A. S., Friel, P., Remick, R., Leal, K., and Pearmain, J., Pharmacokinetic comparison of tablet and suspension dosage forms of carbamazepine. *Epilepsia* **19,** 251–255 (1978).
3. Frigerio, A., and Morselli, P. L., Carbamazepine: Biotransformation. *Adv. Neurol.* **11,** 296–308 (1975).
4. Rane, A., Hojer, B., and Wilson, J. T., Kinetics of carbamazepine and its 10,11-epoxide metabolite in children. *Clin. Pharmacol. Ther.* **19,** 276–283 (1976).
5. Eichelbaum, M., Ekbom, K., Bertilsson, L., Ringberger, V. A., and Rane, A., Plasma kinetics of carbamazepine and its epoxide metabolite in man after single and multiple doses. *Eur. J. Clin. Pharmacol.* **8,** 337–341 (1975).
6. Bertilsson, L., Hojer, B., Tybring, G., Osterloh, J., and Rane, A., Autoinduction of carbamazepine metabolism in children examined by a stable isotope technique. *Clin. Pharmacol. Ther.* **27,** 83–88 (1980).
7. Rylance, G. W., Butcher, G. M., and Moreland, T., Saliva carbamazepine levels in children. *Br. Med. J.* **ii,** 1481 (1977).
8. Kutt, H., and Penry, J. K., Usefulness of blood levels of antiepileptic drugs. *Arch. Neurol.* **31,** 283–288 (1974).
9. Troupin, A., Ojemann, L. M., Halpern, L., Dodrill, C., Wilkus, R., Friel, P., and Feigl, P., Carbamazepine—a double-blind comparison with phenytoin. *Neurology* **27,** 511–519 (1977).
10. Low, N. L., and Pellock, J. M., Seizure disorder. *Pract. Pediatr.* **4,** 1–39 (1976).
11. Eadie, M. J., Plasma level monitoring of anticonvulsants. *Clin. Pharmacol. Kinet.* **1,** 52–66 (1976).
12. Meinardi, H., Carbamazepine. In *Antiepileptic Drugs,* D. M. Woodbury, J. K. Penry, and R. P. Schmidt, Eds. Raven Press, New York, NY, 1972, pp 487–496.
13. Pisciotta, A. V., Hematologic toxicity of carbamazepine. *Adv. Neurol.* **11,** 355–368 (1975).

14. Kutt, H., Solomon, G., Wasterlain, C., Peterson, H., Louis, S., and Carruthers, R., Carbamazepine in difficult to control epileptic out-patients. *Acta Neurol. Scand. Suppl.* **60,** 27–32 (1975).
15. Crosley, C. J., and Swender, P. T., Dystonia associated with carbamazepine administration: Experience in brain-damaged children. *Pediatrics* **63,** 612–615 (1979).
16. Sordillo, P., Sagransky, D. M., Mercado, R., and Michelis, M. F., Carbamazepine-induced syndrome of inappropriate antidiuretic hormone secretion. *Arch. Intern. Med.* **138,** 299–301 (1971).
17. Niebyl, J. R., Blake, D. A., Freeman, J. M., and Luff, R. D., Carbamazepine levels in pregnancy and lactation. *Obstet. Gynecol.* **53,** 139–140 (1979).

Carboxyhemoglobin (Carbon Monoxide)

Specimen Tested:

B.

Laboratories Reporting:

2.

Reference (Normal) Values:

Newborn (nonsmoking mother): about 1% (<5%) of total Hb

Sources of Reference (Normal) Values:

Institutional.

Analytical Method:

Text ref. 2, p 182.

Instrumentation:

Beckman 25K spectrophotometer.

Commentary—T. A. Blumenfeld

The major effect of carbon monoxide (CO) depends upon its capacity to impair oxygen transport through two mechanisms: *(a)* The affinity of hemoglobin for CO is 210-fold greater than for oxygen. Thus, a very small quantity of CO can reversibly inactivate a substantial proportion of the oxygen-carrying capacity of the blood. *(b)* CO has a conformational effect on hemoglobin, resulting in an increase in oxygen affinity. This means that it requires an even lower p_{O_2} to remove the remaining oxygen from the hemoglobin, thereby exacerbating the anoxic effect of CO at the cellular level.

In general, the signs and symptoms of acute CO toxicity reflect the proportion of hemoglobin combined with CO, a function of the concentration of CO in the air and the duration of exposure. The effect of CO is intensified at higher altitudes.

Healthy persons exposed to various concentrations of CO for an hour do not experience definite symptoms, unless the concentrations of the gas in the blood reach 26 to 30% of saturation; however, in chronic poisoning, especially in children, serious symptoms may occur with lower CO concentrations (1).

Smoking may significantly increase blood CO concentrations (2).

Seventy to ninety percent of hemoglobin in the fetus and newborn is fetal hemoglobin. This hemoglobin type predominates through the first week of postnatal life and is gradually replaced by adult-type hemoglobin. A functional difference between fetal and adult hemoglobin is the inability of fetal hemoglobin to interact with low-molecular-mass phosphorylated compounds in erythrocytes to produce altered oxygen-binding properties of hemoglobin. When adult-type hemoglobin combines with 2,3-diphosphoglycerate, there is a marked decrease in the affinity of the hemoglobin for oxygen. Fetal hemoglobin undergoes virtually no such interaction. Because of this difference in adult and fetal hemoglobin, there is a leftward shift of the oxygen dissociation curve in fetal blood as compared with adult blood; i.e., the fetal blood has a relatively greater affinity for oxygen. As a consequence, release of oxygen to the tissues is impeded.

In newborns of smoking mothers, as much as 9.6% of the hemoglobin in cord blood is saturated with CO (3). Thus, in the normal newborn with a high percentage of fetal hemoglobin, the oxygen-dissociation curve is shifted to the left of that of the adult, and with the addition of CO from a mother who smokes, the problem of increased oxygen affinity may complicate any respiratory disorders that occur shortly after birth.

1. Text ref. *18.*
2. Goldsmith, J. R., and Landaw, S. A., Carbon monoxide and human health. *Science* **162.** 1352–1359 (1968).
3. Haddon, W., Jr., Nesbitt, R. E., and Garcia, R., Smoking and pregnancy: Carbon monoxide in blood during gestation and at term. *Obstet. Gynecol.* **18,** 262–267 (1961).

Carotenes (Carotinoids)

Specimen Tested:

P, S.

Laboratories Reporting:

4.

Reference (Normal) Values:

	mg/dL (μmol/L)
0–6 mo[a]	0–40 (0–0.75)
6 mo–adult	40–180 (0.75–3.4)
Child	50–100 (0.93–1.9)
>3 yr	100–150 (1.9–2.8)
Adult	100–150 (1.9–2.8)

[a] Values as high as 70 mg/dL (1.30 μmol/L) are reported at birth, increasing to 340 mg/dL (6.3 μmol/L) at 1 yr. See *Patient preparation*, below.

Sources of Reference (Normal) Values:

Institutional; text ref. 2, p. 355.

Specimen Volume, Collection, and Preservation; Patient Preparation:

80 μL to 0.6 mL. Heparin anticoagulant. Patient must be fasting, and receive no vitamin supplement or foods containing vitamin A or carotene for 24 h before testing in the case of the younger age group (0–6 mo), 48 h in the case of the older group (older than 6 mo). Serum should not be exposed to light. It may be stored for 4 d in the FR.

Analytical Method:

Bessey, O. A., Lowry, O. H., Brock, M. J., and Lopez, J. A., The determination of vitamin A and carotene in small quantities of blood serum. *J. Biol. Chem.* **166**, 177–188 (1946); Neeld, J. D., Jr., and Pearson, W. N., Macro and micromethod for the determination of serum vitamin A using trifluoroacetic acid. *J. Nutr.* **79**, 454 (1963); Van Steveninck, J., and DeGoeij, A.F.P.M., Determination of vitamin A in blood plasma of patients with carotenemia. *Clin. Chim. Acta* **49**, 61–64 (1973).

Instrumentation:

Carl Zeiss PMQ II, Beckman 25, Gilford 200 spectrophotometers.

Note: See **Vitamin A** Commentary.

Catecholamines (Norepinephrine, Epinephrine)

Specimen Tested:

U.

Laboratories Reporting:

4.

Reference (Normal) Values:

	Catecholamines excreted daily, μg (nmol)		
Age, yr	**Total**[a]	**Norepinephrine**	**Epinephrine**
<1	up to 20	5.4–15.9 (32–94)	0.1–4.3 (0.5–23.5)
1–5	up to 40	8.1–30.8 (48–182)	0.8–9.1 (4.4–49.1)
6–15	up to 80	19.0–71.1 (112–421)	1.3–10.5 (7.1–82)
>15	up to 100	34.4–87.0 (203–514)	3.5–13.2 (19.1–72.1)
Adult	up to 270		

[a] One lab reports total as <1.0 mmol/mol of creatinine.

Sources of Reference (Normal) Values:

Institutional; Voorhess, M. L., Urinary catecholamine excretion by healthy children. 1. Daily excretion of dopamine, norepinephrine, epinephrine, and 3-methoxy-4-hydroxymandelic acid. *Pediatrics* **39,** 252–257 (1967); Bio-Rad Labs. Instruction Manual, Richmond, CA, 1977, p 11; Weetman, R. M., Rider, P. S., Oei, T. O., Hempel, J. S., and Baehner, R. L., Effect of diet on urinary excretion of VMA, HVA, metanephrine and total free catecholamine in normal preschool children. *J. Pediatr.* **88,** 46–50 (1976).

Specimen Volume, Collection, and Preservation; Patient Preparation:

Aliquot of 24-h U collection. Collect urine into bottle containing 15 mL of 6 mol/L hydrochloric acid (concentrated HCl diluted with equal volume of H_2O); for adults, use 30 mL of acid solution. Refrigerate urine during collection. Urine stored in RR may be stable for 3 d (some claim that HCl-treated urine may be stable for several days at RT). Patients should preferably not be receiving any drugs, especially antihypertensive agents such as Aldomet, for 72 h before collection of urine.

Analytical Method:

Routh, J. I., Bannow, R. E., Fincham, R. W., and Stoll, J. L., Excretion of L-dopa and its metabolites in urine in Parkinson's disease patients receiving L-dopa therapy. *Clin. Chem.* **17,** 867–871 (1971); Bio-Rad Lab. Catecholamine Reagent kit; Crout, J. R., Catecholamines in urine. *Stand. Methods Clin. Chem.* **3,** 62–80 (1961); Hathaway, P., Jakoi, L., Troyer, W. G., Jr., and Bogdonoff, M. D., A method for semiautomatic differential analysis of urinary catecholamines. *Anal. Biochem.* **20,** 466–476 (1967); modification of method by Bell, Horrocks, and Varley, in Varley, H., *Practical Clinical Biochemistry*, 2nd ed. Interscience Publishers Inc., New York, NY, 1958.

Instrumentation:

Farrand Mark I and Aminco Bowman spectrofluorometers; Turner Model III fluorometer.

Commentary—Michael A. Pesce

The catecholamines norepinephrine and epinephrine are biogenic amines that contain two hydroxy groups attached to a benzene ring; they are derived from the amino acid tyrosine. Norepinephrine, synthesized primarily in the sympathetic nerve endings and to a lesser extent in the adrenal medulla, is stored in the sympathetic nerve endings. Epinephrine is synthesized and stored in the chromaffin cells of the adrenal medulla. Norepinephrine and epinephrine are released in response to stress. Almost all of the norepinephrine and epinephrine released is metabolized. Small amounts are excreted in the urine, either conjugated as the sulfate or glucuronide or in the free form. The total catecholamine content of urine (free and conjugated) is usually determined fluorometrically by the trihydroxyindole method. An internal standard must be added to the urine to account for quenching.

Catecholamines are unstable in urine at alkaline pH. A 24-h urine should be collected in a bottle containing 15 mL of 6 mol/L HCl and the urine kept refrigerated during the 24-h collection. In urine collected at a pH of less than 3 and stored at 4 °C, the catecholamines are stable for at least one week.

There is a diurnal variation in catecholamine excretion (1). Urine collected from 0800 to 2000 hours shows a greater excretion of catecholamines than does the urine collected from 2000 to 0800 hours. Diet does not affect the excretion of free catecholamines (1); children ingesting vanilla ice cream, vanillin, and bananas showed no increase in their urinary amounts of free catecholamines. Drugs, however, can alter the urinary catecholamine excretion (2), so the patient should not be receiving medication before collection of the urine. The normal urinary contents of catecholamines (expressed as µg/24 h) are lower in children than in adults (3), but increase with age and reach adult values between the ages of 10 and 16 years.

Neuroblastoma and pheochromocytoma are pathological disorders associated with abnormal excretion of urinary catecholamines and their metabolites. Neuroblastoma is a malignant neoplasm that can appear at any time from birth to six years of age, with a peak incidence before the age of three. The rate of occurrence is about 1:10 000 births, with a slight preponderance in boys. Neuroblastoma should be suspected on finding a mass in the abdomen and increased amounts of catecholamines and their metabolites in urine. Pheochromocytomas are rare tumors; they usually originate from the chromaffin cells in the adrenal medulla and are usually benign. Over a span of 50 years, only 100 cases of pheochromocytoma (11 children and 89 adults) were reported at Columbia–Presbyterian Medical Center (4). Malignant pheochromocytoma was detected in only one child and six adults (4). Pheochromocytoma should be considered when the patient exhibits chronic hypertension with high urinary amounts of catecholamines and their metabolites.

In both neuroblastoma and pheochromocytoma the catecholamine content returns to normal when the tumor is surgically removed. Urinary catecholamines should therefore be monitored to determine whether all of the functioning tumor has been removed. Persistant increased amounts of urinary catecholamines indicate the presence of residual tumors. Above-normal urinary catecholamines are also observed in patients with progressive muscular dystrophy or myasthenia gravis and in individuals undergoing vigorous exercise before urine collection.

1. Weetman, R. M., Rider, P. S., Oei, T. O., Hempel, J. S., and Baehner, R. L., Effect of diet on urinary excretion of VMA, HVA, metanephrine and total free catecholamine in normal preschool children. *J. Pediatr.* **88,** 46–50 (1976).
2. Young, D. S., Pestaner, L. C., and Gibberman, V., Effects of drugs on clinical laboratory tests. *Clin. Chem.* **21,** 275D–276D (1975).
3. De Schaepdryver, A. F., Hooft, C., Delbeke, M. J., and Van den Noortgaete, M., Urinary catecholamines and metabolites in children. *J. Pediatr.* **93,** 266–268 (1978).
4. Melicow, M. M., One hundred cases of phenochromocytoma (107 tumors) at the Columbia Presbyterian Medical Center, 1926–1976. *Cancer* **40,** 1987–2004 (1977).

Note: See also Commentary for **Metanephrines.**

Ceruloplasmin

Specimen Tested:

P, S.

Laboratories Reporting:

2.

Reference (Normal) Values:

Child: 20–40 mg/dL; 21–43

Sources of Reference (Normal) Values:

Institutional.

Specimen Volume:

50 to 200 μL. Unstable at RT. Stable for 2 to 14 d in RR, 2 wk in FR.

Analytical Method:

Ravin, H. A., An improved colorimetric enzymatic assay of ceruloplasmin. *J. Lab. Clin. Med.* **58,** 161–168 (1961); Scheinberg, I. H., Harris,

R. S., Morell, A. G., and Dubin, D., Some aspects of the relation of ceruloplasmin to Wilson's disease. *Neurology* **8,** Suppl. 1, 44–51 (1958).

Instrumentation:

Beckman 25 and Carl Zeiss PMQ II spectrophotometers.

Note: See Commentary on **Copper.**

Chloramphenicol

Specimen Tested:

S.

Laboratory Reporting:

1.

Reference (Normal) Values:

Therapeutic range: the trough serum concentration should be maintained between 5 and 25 mg/L. Severe hematologic toxicity may appear at trough values exceeding 25 mg/L.

Sources of Reference (Normal) Values:

Yunis, A. A., Chloramphenicol toxicity. In *Blood Disorders due to Drugs and Other Agents,* R. H. Girdwood, Ed. Excerpta Medica, Amsterdam, 1973, pp 107–126; McCurdy, P. R., Plasma concentration of chloramphenicol and bone marrow suppression. *Blood* **21,** 363–372 (1963); Scott, J. L., Finegold, S. M., Belkin, G. A., and Lawrence, J. L., A controlled double-blind study of hematologic toxicity of chloramphenicol. *N. Engl. J. Med.* **272,** 1137–1142 (1965).

Specimen Volume, Collection, and Preservation; Patient Preparation:

0.5 to 1 mL. Use no preservatives. Separate serum rapidly, and store at once in FR. Samples should be drawn just before the next dose. Steady state is generally reached within one day. A longer waiting period may be required for patients with liver disease.

Analytical Method and Instrumentation:

HPLC; Milton Roy Co., Laboratory Data Control Division Constametric I pump/Spectromonitor I; Waters Assoc. column, 25 cm μBondapak C_{18}; Rheodyne injector valve.

Chloride

In Cerebrospinal Fluid

Laboratories Reporting:
3.

Reference (Normal) Values:
Child–adult: 120–128 mmol/L; 122–132 mmol/L

Source of Reference (Normal) Values:
Institutional; text ref. 2, p 89.

Specimen Volume, Analytical Method, Instrumentation:
Same as for P, S (next section).

Commentary—J. Gilbert Hill

The fact that only three laboratories participating in this project report normal values for chloride in cerebrospinal fluid indicates the low esteem to which this test has fallen. At one time regarded as useful in the diagnosis of tuberculosis meningitis, this measurement is now held to merely reflect plasma chloride and has no special significance in tubercular meningitis.

Chloride estimation in CSF is of no value as a diagnostic aid *(1)*.

1. Zilva, J. F., and Pannal, P. R., *Clinical Chemistry in Diagnosis and Treatment.* Year Book Medical Publishers, Chicago, IL, 1972.

In Blood

Specimen Tested:
P, S.

Laboratories Reporting:
4.

Reference (Normal) Values:

Cord, S:	105–113 mmol/L
Newborn:	96–106
Child–adult:	95–105
	100–109 (5th–95th percentiles)

Source of Reference (Normal) Values:

Institutional; text ref. *2*, p 89; Cherian, A. G., and Hill, J. G., Percentile estimates of reference values for fourteen chemical constituents in sera of children and adolescents. *Am. J. Clin. Pathol.* **69**, 24–31 (1978).

Specimen Volume, Collection, and Preservation:

8 to 20 μL. Heparin anticoagulant. Stable for 1 wk at RT or in RR, for months in FR.

Analytical Method:

Cotlove, E., Determination of chloride in biological materials. In *Methods of Biochemical Analysis,* **12**, D. Glick, Ed. Interscience, New York, NY, 1964, pp 277–293; Cotlove, E., Chloride. *Stand. Methods Clin. Chem.* **3**, 81–92 (1961); Cotlove, E., Trantham, H. V., and Bowman, R. L., An instrument for rapid, accurate, and sensitive titration of chloride in biologic samples. *J. Lab. Clin. Med.* **51**, 461–468 (1958); Sternberg, J. C., Buzza, E., and Lillig, J., Simultaneous electrochemical determination of total CO_2 and chloride. 9th International Congress on Clinical Chemistry Procedures, 1975; mercuric thiocyanate–ferric nitrate method (Technicon, Greiner).

Instrumentation:

Beckman CO_2/Cl Analyzer, with Beckman Blue Tip or Sherwood Lancer pipetter; Beckman Astra 8; Greiner Selective Analyzer II (1 lab.); Technicon SMA II (1 lab.).

In Urine

Laboratories Reporting:

3.

Reference (Normal) Values:

Infant: 1.7–8.5 mmol/d
Child: 17–34
Adult: 140–240; 110–250

Sources of Reference (Normal) Values:

Institutional; text ref. *9*, p 224.

Specimen Volume, Collection, and Preservation:

Aliquot of 24-h collection. Stable 45 d at RT without preservation.

Analytical Method, Instrumentation:

Same as for P, S (previous section).

Cholesterol, Total

Specimen Tested:

P, S.

Laboratories Reporting:

7.

Reference (Normal) Values:

	Cholesterol, mg/dL (mmol/L)	
Age	**Lower limit**	**Upper limit**
Cord blood, S		
Premature	47 (1.3)	98 (2.5)
Full-term	45 (1.2)	98 (2.5)
Newborn	45–50 (1.2–1.3)	100–167 (2.6–4.3)
3 d–1 yr	65–69 (1.7–1.8)	120–175 (3.1–4.6)
<2 mo	80 (2.1)	160 (4.1)
<3 mo		up to 175 (4.6)
4 mo–11 mo		up to 195 (5.1)
1–4 yr		up to 210 (5.4)
1–20 yr	95 (2.5)	195 (5.1)
2–14 yr	138 (3.6)	242 (6.3)
5–14 yr		up to 220 (5.7)
Child	120 (3.1)	230 (5.9)
19 yr and less	120 (3.1)	210 (5.4)
Adult	120 (3.1)	230 (5.9)
20–29 yr	120 (3.1)	240 (6.2)
30–39 yr	140 (3.6)	270 (7.0)
40–49 yr	150 (3.9)	310 (8.0)
50–59 yr	160 (4.1)	330 (8.5)

Sources of Reference (Normal) Values:

Institutional; Cheng, M. H., Lipsey, A. I., Blanco, V., Wong, H. T., and Spiro, S. H., Microchemical analysis for 13 constituents of plasma from healthy children. *Clin. Chem.* **25**, 692–698 (1979); Chase, H. P., O'Quin, R. J., and O'Brien, D., Screening for hyperlipidemia in childhood. *J. Am. Med. Assoc.* **230**, 1535–1537 (1974).

Specimen Volume, Collection, and Preservation; Patient Preparation:

Generally 5 to 10 µL. Heparin anticoagulant. Fasting sample preferred. Stable up to 7 d at RT and in RR. Avoid lipemia.

Analytical Method:

All seven labs. used enzymic method: Allain, C. C., Poon, L. S., Chan, C. S. G., Richmond, W., and Fu, P. C., Enzymatic determination of total serum cholesterol. *Clin. Chem.* **20**, 470–475 (1974); Bio-Dynamics/*bmc* Enzymatic Cholesterol kit; Abbott A-Gent kit; Electro-Nucleonics Gemeni Cholesterol kit; Pesce, M. A., and Bodourian, S. H., Enzymatic rate method for measuring cholesterol in serum. *Clin. Chem.* **22,** 2042–2045 (1976); Flegg, H. M., An investigation of the determination of serum cholesterol by an enzymatic method. *Ann. Clin. Biochem.* **10,** 79–84 (1973).

Instrumentation:

Abbott ABA-100 Bichromatic Analyzer; Gilford 3500 spectrophotometer; Electro-Nucleonics GEMSAEC, Gemeni; Union Carbide Centrifi-Chem Centrifugal Analyzer System 400.

*   *   *

Laboratory Reporting:

1.

Reference (Normal) Values:

| Age, yr | Cholesterol, mg/dL (mmol/L) | |
	White	Black
F:		
6–7	116–200 (2.98–5.20)	96–220 (2.48–5.69)
8–9	118–198 (3.04–5.12)	114–230 (2.92–5.95)
10–11	102–226 (2.64–5.84)	117–225 (3.01–5.82)
12–13	112–208 (2.86–5.38)	91–243 (2.33–6.28)
14–15	97–213 (2.51–5.51)	112–200 (2.86–5.17)
16–17	107–203 (2.74–5.25)	107–183 (2.74–4.76)
M:		
6–7	129–193 (3.37–4.99)	138–198 (3.56–5.12)
8–9	120–204 (3.10–5.28)	132–220 (3.44–5.69)
10–11	111–211 (2.83–5.46)	116–204 (2.98–5.28)
12–13	111–211 (2.83–5.46)	118–218 (3.04–5.64)
14–15	109–193 (2.78–4.99)	130–202 (3.40–5.22)
16–17	111–207 (2.83–5.35)	104–200 (2.68–5.17)

Sources of Reference (Normal) Values:

Morrison, J. A., deGroot, I., Edwards, B. K., Kelly, K. A., Mellies, M. J., Khoury, P., and Glueck, C. J., Lipids and lipoproteins in 927 school children, ages 6 to 17 years. *Pediatrics* **62,** 990–995 (1978).

Specimen Volume, Collection, and Preservation; Patient Preparation:

0.5 mL. Blood collected into Na_2 EDTA. Specimen refrigerated at all stages. Patient fasted 12–16 h.

Analytical Method:

Automated Liebermann–Burchard, with isopropanol extraction; Manual of Laboratory Operations, Lipid Research Clinics Program. I. *Lipid and Lipoprotein Analysis.* DHEW Publication No. (NIH) 75–628. Bethesda, MD, 1974.

Instrumentation:

Technicon AutoAnalyzer II.

*   *   *

Laboratory Reporting:

1.

Reference (Normal) Values:

Age	No.	Cholesterol, mg/dL (mmol/L)
Newborn	24	70–202 (1.80–5.22)
6 wk–18 mo	39	81–184 (2.12–4.76)
18 mo–4 yr	67	101–196 (2.62–5.07)
4–8 yr	86	104–218 (2.68–5.64)
8–15 yr	180	115–221 (2.95–5.72)
15–16 yr	46	100–192 (2.60–4.97)
Adult	150	120–277 (3.10–7.16)

Sources of Reference (Normal) Values:

Institutional: a retrospective study of patients' charts. Excluded were patients with active infectious, inflammatory disease, malignancy, and anemia. Adults include men and women from 20 to more than 60 years old, who were fasted 12 to 14 h before the test.

Specimen Volume, Collection, and Preservation:

0.47 mL. Specimens were collected into Becton-Dickinson SST, and Technicon Sera-Clear serum separators were used. Hemolyzed samples were rejected, except for newborns. Samples were separated within 1 h of collection and stored at 4 °C until analyzed.

Analytical Method and Instrumentation:

Modified Liebermann–Burchard; Levine, J., Morgenstern, S., and Vlastelica, D., A direct Liebermann–Burchard method for cholesterol. In *Automation in Analytical Chemistry* (Technicon Symposia, 1967), Mediad Inc., White Plains, NY, 1968, pp 25–28; Huang, C., Chen, C. P., Wefler, V., and Raftery, A., A stable reagent for the Liebermann–Burchard reaction; application to rapid serum cholesterol determination. *Anal. Chem.* **33**, 1405–1407 (1961); Technicon SMAC.

<h3 style="text-align:center">Commentary—Michael A. Pesce</h3>

Cholesterol is measured in children to predict coronary heart disease so that preventive measures can be initiated. There are conflicting reports as to the "normal" serum cholesterol values in black and white neonates. One study (1) reported that there was no difference in cholesterol concentrations with respect to race and sex; mean cholesterol was 72 mg/dL. In another study (2) white neonates were reported to have higher cholesterol values than black neonates, and white girls had higher cholesterol values than white boys. The upper limit of normal for cholesterol in cord blood is about 100 mg/dL. Cholesterol concentrations rapidly increase and by one year reach a mean of 135 (SD 19 mg/dL). For ages 2.5 to 11 years there is very little difference in cholesterol in blacks and whites with respect to race and sex, concentrations ranging between 125 and 204 mg/dL. From ages 12 to 16, cholesterol decreases, but then increases at age 17. From ages six to 17, cholesterol is slightly higher in blacks than in whites, but the difference is not clinically significant (3).

In the enzymic assays for measuring cholesterol in serum, cholesterol esterase is used to hydrolyze cholesterol esters and cholesterol oxidase to oxidize cholesterol to cholest-4-en-3-one and hydrogen peroxide. The cholesterol is usually quantitated by reaction of hydrogen peroxide to form a quinoneimine product, which is measured spectrophotometrically. A review of several commercially available reagent kits for measuring cholesterol through this reaction indicated that 10 mg of bilirubin per deciliter and lipemic serum produced negative interferences (4). Ascorbic acid at concentrations of 5.0 mg/dL decreased cholesterol values by about 10%. Uric acid up to 20 mg/dL, hemoglobin at 100 mg/dL, and the drugs clofibrate, phenobarbital, Ketochol, and Ovral-28 did not interfere with this procedure. Serum cholesterol values in blood obtained from fasting and nonfasting children are reported to be not significantly different (3); therefore, cholesterol can be measured in unselected blood samples.

1. Glueck, C. J., Gartside, P. S., Tsang, R. C., Mellies, M., and Steiner, P. M., Black–white similarities in cord blood lipids and lipoproteins. *Metabolism* **26,** 347–350 (1977).
2. Frerichs, R. R., Srinivasan, S. R., Webber, L. S., Rieth, M. C., and Berenson, G. S., Serum lipids and lipoproteins at birth in a biracial population: The Bogalusa heart study. *Pediatr. Res.* **12,** 858–863 (1978).
3. deGroot, I., Morrison, J. A., Kelly, K. A., Rauh, J. S., Mellies, M. J., Edwards, B. K., and Glueck, C. J., Lipids in school children 6 to 17 years of age: Upper normal limits. *Pediatrics* **60,** 437–443 (1977).
4. Pesce, M. A., and Bodourian, S. H., Interference with the enzymic measurement of cholesterol in serum by use of five reagent kits. *Clin. Chem.* **23,** 757–760 (1977).

Cholinesterase, Pseudocholinesterase
(EC 3.1.1.8; acylcholine acylhydrolase)

Specimen Tested:

P, S.

Laboratory Reporting:

1.

Reference (Normal) Values:

Child, M: 2.2–5.3 kU/L
        F: 2.1–5.1

Sources of Reference (Normal) Values:

Garry, P. J., A manual and automated procedure for measuring serum cholinesterase activity and identifying enzyme variants. *Clin.
Chem.* **17,** 192–198 (1971); Garry, P. J., Owen, G. M., and Lubin,
A. H., Identification of serum cholinesterase fluoride variants by differential inhibition in Tris and phosphate buffers. *Clin. Chem.* **18,**
105–109 (1972).

Specimen Volume, Collection, and Preservation:

25 µL. Heparin anticoagulant. Specimen stable up to 3 d at RT, 17
d in RR, indefinitely in FR.

Analytical Method:

Garry, *op. cit.,* modified to use freshly prepared rather than lyophilized reagents.

Enzyme Data:

1. Enzyme unit definition: 1 IUB unit (U) = 1 µmol of substrate
   hydrolyzed per minute.
2. Buffer, pH: Tris and phosphate, 7.4.
3. Substrate; pH: butyrylthiocholine, 7.4.
4. Reaction temperature: 25 °C.
5. Temperature reported: 25 °C.

Instrumentation:

Beckman DBG spectrophotometer.

*   *   *

Laboratory Reporting:

1.

Reference (Normal) Values:

Newborn, full-term, 0–5 d: 0–20.2 arbitrary units (DuPont)
Adult: 7–19

Sources of Reference (Normal) Values:

Institutional study: sera were obtained from 50 full-term, apparently
healthy newborns, 0–5 d.

Specimen Volume, Collection, and Preservation:

30 µL. Specimens collected into unheparinized plastic microcentrifuge tubes. Serum is stable at RT up to 24 h, up to 60 d in RR.

Analytical Method and Instrumentation:

DuPont *aca*, using the coupled oxidation–reduction indicator of Gal, E. M., and Roth, E. [Spectrophotometric methods for determination of cholinesterase activity. *Clin. Chim. Acta* **2**, 316–326 (1957)], and butyrylthiocholine substrate.

Enzyme Data:

The DuPont unit is not defined in the literature supplied. Reaction and reporting temperatures are both at 37 °C.

Commentary—J. Gilbert Hill

In an attempt to clarify the sometimes confusing nomenclature in this field, the International Union of Biochemistry has officially recognized two enzymes in the cholinesterase family: one has the formal name acetylcholine acetylhydrolase, the trivial name acetylcholinesterase, and the EC number 3.1.1.7; the other has the formal name acylcholine acylhydrolase, the trivial name cholinesterase, and the EC number 3.1.1.8. Because the latter enzyme has the ability to catalyze the hydrolysis of various choline esters in addition to acetylcholine, it has also been called pseudocholinesterase. However, this nomenclature is now less favored, and to avoid ambiguity, only the names acetylcholinesterase and cholinesterase are recommended for referring to these two enzymes.

Acetylcholinesterase occurs in erythrocytes, and at the neuromuscular junction, where it has a well-defined physiological role at the motor end-plate. In contrast, cholinesterase is present in plasma and many other tissues, but not in erythrocytes. The physiological role of cholinesterase is uncertain, but it may be somewhat protective, by hydrolyzing choline esters that could inhibit acetylcholinesterase.

In the usual practice of clinical chemistry, there appears to be no indication for the measurement of acetylcholinesterase; the remainder of these remarks refer primarily to cholinesterase.

Much conflicting information is available about variations with age in the cholinesterase concentration in plasma, but the general picture appears to be that concentrations are low at birth and for the first six months of life, increase to values 30 to 50% above adult values until about age five years, then gradually decrease until adult concentrations are reached at puberty. Because the population reference range is much wider than the reference range for an individual, interpretation of a result may require knowledge of a previous cholinesterase value for the individual being tested.

There are three potential applications for the measurement of cholinesterase: *(a)* assessment of liver function, *(b)* monitoring of exposure to organophosphate pesticides, and *(c)* identification of hypersensitivity to succinylcholine.

Liver Function

Because cholinesterase is synthesized in the liver, the concentration of cholinesterase in plasma has been used as an index of liver function. However, the plasma value can be affected by such a large number of different hepatic and nonhepatic diseases that its use as a liver-function test is quite limited.

Organophosphate Pesticides

Both cholinesterase and acetylcholinesterase are irreversibly inhibited by organophosphate pesticides, so that either plasma cholinesterase or erythrocyte acetylcholinesterase may be used to monitor exposure. However, plasma cholinesterase is usually preferred; this enzyme is somewhat more stable than acetylcholinesterase and the procedure for its measurement is more precise. Ideally, industrial and agricultural workers who may be exposed to organophosphates should have plasma cholinesterase measured before exposure and at frequent intervals during exposure, because more significance can be placed on changes in results than on any single value. Unfortunately, baseline values are rarely available for children thought to have been exposed to these chemicals, and interpretation of results is difficult. After contact with organophosphate ceases, plasma cholinesterase values can be expected to return to normal in approximately six weeks, depending on the degree of depression of enzyme activity. Erythrocyte acetylcholinesterase activity requires about four months to return to normal.

Succinylcholine Sensitivity

Succinylcholine (suxamethonium, Anectine, Scoline) is a short-acting muscle relaxant used widely in anaesthesia since 1951. The drug acts by competing with acetylcholine for the cholinergic receptors at the neuromuscular junction, thus depolarizing the motor end-plate and preventing muscular contraction. In most individuals the period of muscle relaxation ends after 3–5 min when the drug has been destroyed by cholinesterase. In some individuals the drug action persists for hours, and the prolonged apnea resulting from paralysis of respiratory muscles requires assisted ventilation until spontaneous respiration returns.

Succinylcholine sensitivity may occur in individuals who have below-normal values of normal plasma cholinesterase, or whose plasma cholinesterase has less hydrolyzing activity because of variations in molecular structure. These genetic variations have been extensively investigated, and it is now possible to predict the sensitivity of an individual to succinylcholine through appropriate laboratory studies (degree of inhibition of enzyme activity by dibucaine and fluoride). Although extensive population screening is not recommended, any individual who has experienced a period of prolonged apnea after the administration of succinylcholine should be investigated. The plasma sample for use in the investigation should not be collected during the period of apnea, to avoid interference due to succinylcholine still in circulation. If the investigation reveals a cholinesterase variant, the sensitive individual's family should be phenotyped to identify those at risk. It is essential to emphasize that the penalty for possessing a genetic variant of cholinesterase is limited to sensitivity to an external pharmacologic agent, and is not associated with any other known abnormality.

1. Silk, E., King, J., and Whittaker, M., Assay of cholinesterase in clinical chemistry. *Ann. Clin. Biochem.* **16,** 57–75 (1979).
2. Whittaker, M., Plasma cholinesterase variants and the anaesthetist. *Anaesthesia* **35,** 174–197 (1980).

Commentary—Paul L. Wolf

Cholinesterase hydrolyzes choline esters. True acetylcholinesterase (EC 3.1.1.7) is found in erythrocytes and in nervous tissue, while pseudocholinesterase is found primarily in the liver, small intestinal mucosa, and pancreas.

The cholinesterase activity in cord blood is approximately two-thirds of the activity in normal adult serum. Activity in the serum of the neonate is approximately 20% greater than adult serum activity and returns to adult values by the age of three years. The increased activity may be related to physiologic hemolysis in the newborn and an increased rate of enzyme synthesis in hepatic cells *(1)*.

The three major clinical applications for assessing cholinesterase are the identification of hepatic disease, of organic phosphorus insecticide poisoning, and of sensitivity to suxamethonium (succinylcholine).

Serum albumin is an excellent index to the synthesis function of the liver, but pseudocholinesterase, also produced by the liver, is a more sensitive test of this. Thus, pseudocholinesterase activities are useful in evaluating prognosis in children with hepatitis and cirrhosis. Benign obstructive disease does not decrease pseudocholinesterase activity, but obstructive jaundice due to metastatic disease does. Decreased pseudocholinesterase activity may also occur in children with nonhepatic conditions, especially in hereditary deficiency, severe malnutrition, diabetic ketoacidosis, and acute infections. Children with the nephrotic syndrome usually demonstrate increased activity. The rates of synthesis of albumin and pseudocholinesterase increase in nephrosis, with a marked decrease of serum albumin because of proteinuria *(2)*.

Exposure to organic phosphorus insecticides causes paralysis, with a prominent decrease in cholinesterase from erythrocytes, the nervous system, and serum.

The regular determination of the erythrocyte enzyme is an important procedure to identify the early toxic effects of these insecticides. When the erythrocyte activity decreases to 25% of pre-exposure values, clinical illness occurs. A 40% decrease is dangerous, and a 60% decrease is a mandatory indication to transfer the affected child to another environment.

Children with severe hepatic disease that results in depressed pseudocholinesterase activity may sustain an "overdose"-prolonged apnea if they receive succinylcholine during the course of anesthesia. Apnea during anesthesia with succinylcholine may also occur if there is a hereditary enzyme deficiency.

1. Takeda, I., Study on the active value of serum cholinesterase in children. *Acta Paediatr. Jpn.* **2**, 44 (1959).
2. Vorhaus, L. J., and Kark, R. M., Serum cholinesterase in health and disease. *Am. J. Med.* **14**, 707–719 (1953).

Chymotrypsin (EC 3.4.21.1)

In Intestinal Juice

Laboratory Reporting:

1.

Reference (Normal) Values:

245–275 µg/mL.

Source of Reference (Normal) Values:

Text ref. *1.*

Volume of Specimen:

1.0 mL.

Analytical Method:

Schwert, G. W., and Takenaka, Y., A spectrophotometric determination of trypsin and chymotrypsin. *Biochim. Biophys. Acta* **16**, 570–575 (1955); Worthington "Determatube."

Instrumentation:

Beckman Model DU spectrophotometer.

In Feces

Laboratory Reporting:

1.

Reference (Normal) Values:

30–750 U/g

Sources of Reference (Normal) Values:

Institutional.

Analytical Method:

Dyck, W. P., Titrimetric measurements of fecal trypsin and chymotrypsin in cystic fibrosis with pancreatic exocrine insufficiency. *Am. J. Dig. Dis.* **12,** 310–317 (1967).

Enzyme Data:

1. Enzyme unit definition: 1 IUB unit (U) = enzyme activity leading to the hydrolysis of 1 μmol of substrate per minute.
2. Substrate: *N*-acetyl-L-tyrosine ethyl ester.
3. Reaction temperature: 37 °C.
4. Reported temperature: 37 °C.

Instrumentation:

Metrohm E 300 B pH meter, E 473 Impulsomat, Dosimat, and recorder.

Commentary—K. W. Schmitt

Chymotrypsin and trypsin activities are measured in duodenal fluid or feces to indicate functioning pancreatic acinar cells. These measurements are best made after stimulating the cells with secretin and pancreozymin *(1–3)*. Values for duodenal trypsin activity after such stimulation vary in premature infants and in infants less than one month old *(1)*. Premature infants have higher concentrations than full-term infants. Both the premature and full-term infant have usual post-stimulation values by about one month *(1)*. Similar studies with chymotrypsin have not been done. Post-stimulation values are normal a few weeks after birth *(2)*.

Fecal trypsin activity can be estimated for children younger than one year by methods in which gelatin is used as substrate. Characteristic of this age group is the rapid transit of trypsin through the colon, preventing enzyme alteration. The stool should be cultured, because *Proteus* sp. can also digest gelatin, giving a falsely positive result; alternatively, a specific trypsin inhibitor may be added as a control for specificity.

Fresh stool specimens are recommended for the titrimetric measurement of fecal trypsin and chymotrypsin activity. No consistent loss on storage of specimens for the assay of trypsin or chymotrypsin has been observed under various storage conditions (RT, RR, FR), or with antibiotic therapy. Variations by as much as 50% may ensue on short storage, or there may be no change during several weeks. Because activities in feces can be measured by the time the infant is four days old, pancreatic insufficiency can be assessed by the end of the first week. Measurement of fecal chymotrypsin is a more sensitive index of pancreatic function than trypsin. At best, both are semiquantitative assessments of pancreatic enzyme secretion, their stability being influenced by bile, bacterial flora, mobility, and factors that may lead to binding to intestinal debris (4,5).

1. Zoppi, G., Andreotti, G., Pajno-Ferrara, F., Njai, D. M., and Gaburro, D., Exocrine pancreas function in premature and full-term neonates. *Pediatr. Res.* **6,** 880–886 (1972).
2. Hadorn, B., Zoppi, G., Shmerling, D. H., Prader, A., McIntyre, I., and Anderson, C. M., Quantitative assessment of exocrine pancreatic function in infants and children. *J. Pediatr.* **73,** 39–50 (1968).
3. Hadorn, B., Johansen, P. G., and Anderson, C. M., Pancreozymin secretion test of exocrine pancreatic function in cystic fibrosis and the significance of the results for the pathogenesis of the disease. *Can. Med. Assoc. J.* **98,** 377–384 (1968).
4. Barbero, G. J., Sibinga, M. S., Marino, J. M., and Seibel, R., Stool trypsin and chymotrypsin. *Am. J. Dis. Child.* **112,** 536–540 (1966).
5. Dyck, W. P., Titrimetric measurements, fecal trypsin and chymotrypsin in cystic fibrosis with pancreatic exocrine insufficiency. *Am. J. Dig. Dis.* **12,** 310–317 (1967).

Note: See also Chapter 8, **Laboratory Tests in Pediatric Gastroenterology.**

Complement, B₁C (C3)

Specimen Tested:
S.

Laboratories Reporting:
3.

Reference (Normal) Values:

Age	C3, mg/dL	Age	C3, mg/dL
Cord blood	52–166	1 yr–adult[a]	90–203
2–7 d	59–169	2–5 yr	76–182
1–5 mo	65–172	5–9 yr	79–188
6 mo–2 yr	71–177	9–14 yr	82–195

[a] Report by one lab.

Sources of Reference (Normal) Values:

Norman, M. E., Gall, E. P., Taylor, A., Laster, L., and Nilsson, U. R., Serum complement profiles in infants and children. *J. Pediatr.* **87**, 912–916 (1975); Laurell, C. B., Quantitative estimations of proteins by electrophoresis in agarose gel containing antibodies. *Anal. Biochem.* **15**, 45–52 (1966); Merrill, D. A., Hartley, T. F., and Claman, H. N., Electroimmunodiffusion (EID): A simple, rapid method for quantitation of immunoglobulins in diluted biological fluids. *J. Lab. Clin. Med.* **69**, 151–159 (1967).

Specimen Volume, Collection, and Preservation:

10 µL (Labs. 1, 2) for RID; 100 µL (Lab. 3) for nephelometric method. Allow blood specimen to clot for about 1 h; centrifuge and separate serum within 2 h of collection. Refrigerate if tested within 24 h, or store in FR until used.

Analytical Method and Instrumentation:

Labs. 1 and 2: RID; Mancini, G., Carbonara, A. O., and Heremans, J. F., Immunochemical quantitation of antigens by single radial immuno-diffusion. *Int. J. Immunochem.* **2**, 235–254 (1965); Hyland Human Complement C3 Radial Immunodiffusion Test, Immuno-Plate. **Lab. 3:** Kinetic nephelometric immunoprecipitin reaction. Sternberg, J. C., A rate nephelometer for measuring specific proteins by immunoprecipitin reactions. *Clin. Chem.* **23**, 1456–1464 (1977); Beckman Human C3 Reagent Test Kit; Beckman Immunochemistry Analyzer.

Commentary—Gregory J. Buffone

For measuring complement activity, either individual components or total hemolytic complement specimens may be collected by skin puncture or venipuncture and handled at 4 °C. Immunochemical methods such as gel diffusion, light scattering, and RIA can give different results, owing to technique differences, antibody specificity, and the material used for standardization *(1,2)*. The potential introduction of monoclonal antibodies as reagents may reduce variability from antibody specificity as well as improve analytical performance of many immunochemical methods. In any case, comparison of reference limits between laboratories ideally should include not only the method but also specific reagents, i.e., antiserum and calibrators.

Changes in C3 and C4 concentrations in various disease states are listed in Chapter 10, Table 3.

Simple immunochemical methods are often not sufficient to provide complete information for diagnostic purposes. It is often necessary to demonstrate that complement split products are present in vivo, to document complement activation.

1. Buffone, G. J., and Lewis, S. A., Effect of analytical factors on immuno-chemical reference limits for complement components C3 in serum of pediatric reference population. *Clin. Chem.* **23,** 994–999 (1977).
2. Buffone, G. J., Brett, E. M., Lewis, S. A., Iosefsohn, M., and Hicks, J. M., Limitations of immunochemical measurement of ceruloplasmin. *Clin. Chem.* **25,** 749–751 (1979).

Note: See also Chapter 10, **Specific Proteins in Pediatrics.**

Complement, C4

Specimen Tested:
S.

Laboratory Reporting:
1.

Reference (Normal) Values:
Child: 20–40 mg/dL

Sources of Reference (Normal) Values:
Institutional.

Specimen Volume:
10 μL.

Analytical Method and Instrumentation:
RID. Behring Diagnostics Tri-Partigen plates.

Note: See Commentary for **Complement C3.**

Complement, Total Hemolytic (CH$_{50}$)

Specimen Tested:
S.

Laboratory Reporting:
1.

Reference (Normal) Values:
All ages: 25–45 CH$_{50}$ units/mL

Sources of Reference (Normal) Values:
Institutional.

Specimen Volume, Collection, and Preservation:

0.25 mL, venous. Blood allowed to stand clotted for 15 to 30 min at RT, centrifuged at 4 °C, then either assayed immediately or stored at −70 °C.

Analytical Method and Instrumentation:

Gewurz, H., and Suyehyra, L. A., Complement. In *Manual of Clinical Immunology*, N. R. Rose, and H. Friedman, Eds., American Society for Microbiology, Washington, DC, 1976, p 36; Beckman DB spectrophotometer.

Copper

Specimen Tested:

Liver, P, S, U.

Laboratories Reporting:

3.

Reference (Normal) Values:

Age	Copper (P,S), μg/dL (μmol/L)	Age	Copper (P,S), μg/dL (μmol/L)
Cord	26–32 (4.1–5.0)	2 yr	95–186 (14.9–29.3)
Newborn	26–32 (4.1–5.0)	5–17 yr	94–234 (14.2–36.8)
1 mo	73–93 (11.5–14.6)	6 yr	87–174 (13.7–27.4)
2 mo	59–69 (9.3–10.9)	10 yr	72–162 (11.3–25.5)
6 mo	<70 (<11.0)	Adult	70–118 (11.0–18.6)
6 mo–5 yr	27–153 (4.2–24.1)		69–150 (10.9–23.6)
Child	67–147 (10.5–23.1)		

U: up to 30 μg/dL (4.7 μmol/L); <40 (<6.3)
Liver: <20 μg/g of wet tissue (<3.1 μmol/g)

Sources of Reference (Normal) Values:

Institutional; Sass-Kortsak, A., Copper metabolism. *Adv. Clin. Chem.* **8,** 1–67 (1965); Henkin, R. I., Schulman, J. D., Schulman, C. B., and Bronzert, D. A., Changes in total non-diffusible and diffusible plasma zinc and copper during infancy. *J. Pediatr.* **82,** 831–837 (1973); text ref. *2,* p 105.

Specimen Volume, Collection, and Preservation:

25 μL for atomic absorption to 1.5 mL for colorimetry. P, S presumably stable at RT, 2 wk in RR. After collecting 24-h urine specimen, add 10 mL of glacial acetic acid to stabilize for up to 11 d at RT.

Analytical Method:

Atomic absorption spectrometry: Evenson, M. A., and Warren, B. L., Determination of serum copper by atomic absorption, with use of the graphite cuvette. *Clin. Chem.* **21,** 619–625 (1975); Walshe, J. M., The physiology of copper in man and its relation to Wilson's disease. *Brain* **90,** 149–176 (1967); Olson, A. D., *At. Absorpt. Newsl.* **7,** 4 (1968). **Colorimetry:** Eden, A., and Green, H. H., Micro-determination of copper in biological material. *Biochem. J.* **34,** 1202 (1940). **Other information:** Reinhold, J. G., Trace elements—a selective survey. *Clin. Chem.* **21,** 476–500 (1975); Piper, K. G., and Higgins, G., Estimation of trace metals in biological material by atomic absorption spectrophotometry. *Proc. Assoc. Clin. Biochem.* **4,** 190–200 (1967).

Instrumentation:

Atomic absorption spectrometry: Varian Techtron A-175, Perkin-Elmer 360 (+2100 HGA Controller and Furnace) atomic absorption spectrophotometers; Oxford sampler and dispenser. **Colorimetry:** Carl Zeiss PMQ II spectrophotometer.

Commentary—M. J. Levitt

Copper is generally measured when Wilson's disease is suspected. This recessive genetic disease is characterized by low circulating concentrations of ceruloplasmin, the α_2-globulin to which about 98% of the circulating copper is bound. A deficiency of ceruloplasmin allows copper to escape readily from the circulation, resulting in high amounts in the urine and deposition in the liver, brain, and cornea.

Newborn infants without Wilson's disease may exhibit abnormally low serum ceruloplasmin concentrations (<20 µg/dL) and abnormally increased hepatic copper concentrations (>250 µg/g). This situation is self-correcting in about six months and has no apparent pathological sequelae *(1)*. It may be that these individuals have delayed maturation of the biosynthetic pathways leading to ceruloplasmin *(q.v.)*.

Victims of Wilson's disease are probably born with deficient concentrations of ceruloplasmin, yet symptoms may not be detected for six months or recognized for much longer *(1)*. Apparently, six months or longer is required for copper to be deposited in tissues before manifestations of the disease appear. In children more than six months old, Wilson's disease is suggested by the presence of a serum ceruloplasmin concentration of <20 µg/dL and a urinary copper excretion exceeding 100 µg/24 h. Confirmation of a diagnosis of homozygous Wilson's disease requires an hepatic copper concentration exceeding 100 µg/g of dry tissue *(1)*.

Atomic absorption spectrometry is the preferred method for measuring copper in biological specimens *(2)*.

1. Sternlieb, I., and Scheinberg, I. H., Prevention of Wilson's disease in asymptomatic patients. *N. Engl. J. Med.* **278,** 352–359 (1968).
2. Evenson, M. A., and Anderson, C. T., Jr., Ultramicro analysis for copper, cadmium, and zinc in human liver tissue by use of atomic absorption spectrophotometry and the heated graphite tube atomizer. *Clin. Chem.* **21,** 537–543 (1975).

Cortisol

Specimen Tested:

P, S.

Laboratories Reporting:

4.

Reference (Normal) Values:

Time of sampling	Cortisol, μg/dL (nmol/L)	
	Lower values	**Upper values**
0800 hours	5–7 (138–193)	20–27 (550–740)
1400 hours	1 (28); <50% of 0800 value in 88% of cases	11 (300)
1600–2000 hours	2–5 (55–138); 50% of baseline	9–15 (248–410)
After corticotropin:	>18 (500) 60 min after Cortosyn, or 2–3 × baseline	
After dexamethasone:	5 (138) or less; (<100)	

Sources of Reference (Normal) Values:

Institutional; experience with 10 healthy children and 15 healthy adults; Ellis, G., and Morris, R., A one-tube micromethod for radioimmunoassay of plasma cortisol. *Clin. Chem.* **24,** 1954–1957 (1978); Foster, L. B., and Dunn, R. T., Single-antibody technique for radioimmunoassay of cortisol in unextracted serum or plasma. *Clin. Chem.* **20,** 365–368 (1974).

Specimen Volume, Collection, and Preservation:

10 to 100 μL. Heparin anticoagulant. Baseline value collected between 0700 and 0900 hours. Store P, S in FR.

Analytical Method:

RIA: Ellis and Morris, *op. cit.;* Bulletin, CORTISOL [125I] Radioimmunoassay Kit, New England Nuclear, 1979; Rolleri, E., Zannino, M., Orlandini, S., and Malvano, R., Direct radioimmunoassay of plasma cortisol. *Clin. Chim. Acta* **66,** 319 (1976); Beckman Solid Phase Cortisol; Diagnostics Products Corp. [125]I Cortisol-Premix Radioassay kit.

Instrumentation:

Liquid scintillation counters: Packard Model 5110; Nuclear Chicago; LKB Model 80000.

Commentary—Elizabeth K. Smith

The concentration of cortisol in plasma or serum attains adult values by the end of the first week of postnatal life and thereafter does not vary with age. No sex-related difference has been demonstrated. In the healthy newborn infant a transient increase occurs immediately after delivery, declines at 12–48 h to a value less than for cord blood, and finally increases to stabilize at adult values by about one week of age *(1).* Umbilical cord blood contains more cortisone than cortisol, but the concentration decreases in a short time to approximately one-fourth that of cortisol. Plasma cortisol concentrations in the healthy premature infant are similar to those of full-term infants. However, in the premature infant with respiratory distress syndrome, concentrations are significantly increased, being greater the shorter the gestational age *(2).*

Plasma cortisol concentration varies, showing episodic secretion throughout the 24 h as well as a daily circadian rhythm. The concentration peaks between 0700 and 0900 hours; lowest values occur in early evening. The concentration increases after a meal and also after exercise *(3);* therefore, blood for cortisol assay should be drawn between 0700 and 0900 hours from a fasting patient.

Cortisol concentration in plasma may be increased in stress, such as may result from surgery, severe illness, anesthesia, a severe struggle in obtaining the blood sample, or even the emotional stress of hospitalization. Cortisol concentration is low in Addison's disease and low or low normal in adrenal cortex hypofunction secondary to hypopituitarism. Values are increased in Cushing's syndrome, and diurnal variation is absent. If Cushing's syndrome is caused by a tumor, cortisol values are not suppressible with high-dose dexamethasone. A single cortisol value has limited usefulness. More diagnostic information may be obtained from appropriate function tests, i.e., after corticotropin (ACTH), metyrapone, or dexamethasone. The response to ACTH is significantly greater in the one- to four-month-old infant than at any later age, with postadministration values of 253 ± 129 vs 64 ± 17 μg/dL *(4).*

Reference values vary with specificity of the assay method. Higher values are obtained with the Mattingly fluorometric method than with modifications involving prior extraction of plasma with CCl_4. Also, simple competitive protein-binding (Murphy) methods for total corticosteroids, sometimes reported as "cortisol," give results significantly higher than those obtained with methods specific for cortisol, such as competitive protein-binding after chromatography, or RIA. Because of the complex blood-steroid pattern in newborns, a nonspecific method is not reliable for measuring cortisol concentration (2). Highly sensitive methods (e.g., RIA) permit use of skin-puncture blood. Many RIA methods and kits now available involve antibodies developed against cortisol bound to protein, thus permitting use of ^{125}I-labeled cortisol, a gamma counter, and as little as 10 μL of plasma or serum to determine cortisol.

Blood must be processed promptly, with plasma or serum separated from the cells and stored in the cold or frozen. Several drugs interfere with the assay, especially with the fluorometric and the older Porter–Silber methods. Other drugs, such as the therapeutic anti-inflammatory corticosteroids, produce physiological effects that alter concentrations in the blood and interfere with interpretation of results. Estrogens, the contraceptive "pill," and pregnancy increase transcortin, the circulating cortisol-binding globulin, and increase cortisol concentrations above normal values.

1. Seely, J. R., The fetal and neonatal adrenal cortex. In text ref. 7, vol. **1**, p 238.
2. Klein, G. P., Braden, M., Giroud, C. J. P., and Arato, J. S., Quantitative measurement and significance of five plasma corticosteroids during the perinatal period. *J. Clin. Endocrinol. Metab.* **36**, 944–950 (1973).
3. Brandenberg, G., and Follenius, M., Influence of timing and intensity of muscular exercise on temporal patterns of plasma cortisol levels. *J. Clin. Endocrinol. Metab.* **40**, 845–849 (1975).
4. Forest, M. G., Age-related response of plasma testosterone, Δ^4-androstenedione and cortisol to adrenocorticotropin in infants, children and adults. *J. Clin. Endocrinol. Metab.* **47**, 931–936 (1978).

Free Cortisol

Specimen Tested:

U.

Laboratories Reporting:

3.

Reference (Normal) Values:

	Daily excretion of free cortisol	
Age	**μg (nmol)**	**$\mu g/g$ creatinine (nmol/g)**
4 mo–10 yr	2–27 (5.5–74)	35–176 (97–486)
11–20 yr	1–55 (2.8–152)	1–44 (2.8–121)
Child < 16 yr	(10–160)	
Adult	18–98 (50–270)	13–60 (36–166)

Sources of Reference (Normal) Values:

Institutional; Juselius, R. E., and Kenny, F. M., Urinary free cortisol excretion during growth and aging; correlation with cortisol production rate and 17-hydroxycorticosteroid excretion. *Metabolism* **23**, 847–852 (1974).

Specimen Volume, Collection, and Preservation:

0.5 to 2 mL. 24-h U collection over 1 g of boric acid.

Analytical Method and Instrumentation:

As in **Cortisol** (P, S).

Commentary—Elizabeth K. Smith

Because free cortisol in plasma, unbound to transcortin, is not readily measurable on a routine basis, an indirect approach is used, the determination of free cortisol in urine. This measurement is based on the principle that only the unbound and unconjugated fraction of plasma cortisol is filtered through the glomeruli. Because glomerular filtration and tubular reabsorption are passive and thus concentration-dependent, urinary free cortisol is directly related to plasma free cortisol. Availability of RIA methods has made determination of urinary free cortisol a relatively simple procedure.

Excretion of free cortisol in urine exhibits a diurnal rhythm paralleling the changes in plasma cortisol; therefore, measurement should be made on a 24-h urine collection. The circadian rhythm in cortisol secretion is established in early infancy. A sleep–wake rhythm has been demonstrated in one-year-old infants [1], with the cortisol excretion rate significantly higher during waking periods than in sleep.

The output of free cortisol in the urine increases with age until approximately 20 years, after which it is relatively constant [2]. When expressed in relationship to creatinine excretion, however, the highest values occur in young children, values in the 11- to 20-year-old group being slightly less than in adults. No sex-related difference has been reported.

Franks [3] reported a mean value of 41 ± 23 μg/24 h in 30 normal children, with lower values (both absolute and relative to surface area) in children who were obese, and higher values in children who were "stressed" with a variety of illnesses. Because the concentration of free cortisol in urine is increased in adrenocortical hyperfunction (Cushing's syndrome) but not in simple obesity, the measurement of urinary free cortisol is a useful test in the differential diagnosis of Cushing's syndrome in obese children and adolescents.

1. Tennes, K., and Vernadakis, A., Cortisol excretion levels and daytime sleep in one-year-old infants. *J. Clin. Endocrinol Metab.* **44**, 175–179 (1977).

2. Juselius, R. E., and Kenny, F. M., Urinary free cortisol excretion during growth and aging: Correlation with cortisol production rate and 17-hydroxycorticosteroid excretion. *Metabolism* **23,** 849–852 (1974).
3. Franks, R. C., Urinary 17-hydroxycorticosteroid and cortisol excretion in childhood. *J. Clin. Endocrinol. Metab.* **36,** 702–705 (1973).

Creatine Kinase (EC 2.7.3.2; ATP:creatine phosphotransferase)

Specimen Tested:

P, S.

Laboratory Reporting:

1.

Reference (Normal) Values:

Age	Upper 95th percentile values, U/L	
	M	F
1 d	600	500
2–10 d	440	440
11–364 d	170	170
1.00–4.99 yr	109	100
5.00–6.99 yr	109	100
7.00–8.99 yr	103	85
9.00–10.99 yr	109	88
11.00–12.99 yr	108	85
13.00–14.99 yr	129	85
15.00–16.99 yr	247	74
17.00–18.99 yr	190	68

Sources of Reference (Normal) Values:

For ages to 4.99 yr: Bodensteiner, J. B., and Zellweger, H., Creatine phosphokinase in normal neonates and young adults. *J. Lab. Clin. Med.* **77,** 853–858 (1971); Zellweger, H., Hanson, J. W., and Markowitz, E., Age and sex-dependent differences of serum enzymes in normal controls. In *Muscle Diseases*, J. N. Walton, N. Canal, and G. Scarlato, Eds. Proc. International Symposium, Milan, Italy, 1969, pp 445–449. Modifications were made to convert units at 30 °C and to make results compatible with data for patients five years and older. **For ages 5.00 yr and older:** Cherian, A. G., and Hill, J. G., Age dependence of serum enzymatic activities (alkaline phosphatase, aspartate aminotransferase, and creatine kinase) in healthy children and adolescents. *Am. J. Clin. Pathol.* **70,** 783–789 (1978).

Specimen Volume, Collection, and Preservation:

50 μL. Separate serum immediately. For plasma, *only* heparin anti-

coagulant may be used. Bright light may be harmful. Do not predilute specimens before assay. Excessive hemolysis must be avoided. Stability at RT not established. Stable in RR 1 to 10 d, longer in FR.

Analytical Method:

Bio-Dynamics/*bmc* kit 15926; Oliver, I. T., A spectrophotometric method for the determination of creatine phosphokinase and myokinase. *Biochem. J.* **61,** 116–122 (1955); Rosalki, S. B., An improved procedure for serum creatine phosphokinase determination. *J. Lab. Clin. Med.* **69,** 696–705 (1967); Szasz, G., Busch, E. W., and Farohs, H. B., Serum-Kreatin Kinase. 1. Methodische Erfahrungen und Normalwerte mit einem handelsüblichen Test. *Dtsch. Med. Wochenschr.* **95,** 829–839 (1970).

Enzyme Data:

1. Enzyme unit definition: 1 IUB unit (U) = the amount of enzyme that will transform 1 μmol of substrate per minute under the conditions listed.
2. Buffer system, pH: triethanolamine, 7.0.
3. Substrate: creatine phosphate.
4. Reaction temperature: 30 °C.
5. Temperature reported: 30 °C.

Instrumentation:

Electro-Nucleonics Inc. GEMSAEC.

*　　　*　　　*

Laboratories Reporting:

5.

Reference (Normal) Values:

	U/L				
Analytical details	**Cord blood**	**Newborn**	**3 wk– 3 mo**	**Child**	**Adult**
Beckman kit, Rosalki method; piperazinedi-ethanesulfonic acid, pH 6.8, 37 °C		40–474			M: 30–210 F: 20–128
Worthington kit, Rosal-ki method; imidazole acetate, pH 6.7, 30 °C	50–387				
Abbott A-Gent kit; (morpholino)ethanesul-fonic acid, pH 6.15, 37 °C			3–5 × A	to 2 × A to 1.5 × A; 4–75 U (30 °C)	36–188

A, adult values.

Sources of Reference (Normal) Values:

Institutional; Sitzmann, F. C., Die enzymdiagnostik Erkrankungen im Kindesalter. *Arch. Kinderheilk. Beih.* **57,** 1–59 (1968)

Specimen Volume, Collection, and Preservation:

5 to 50 μL. See preceding report for collection and preservation.

Analytical Method:

Beckman kit (Rosalki, *op. cit.*); Worthington Statzyme (Rosalki, *op. cit.*); Bio-Dynamics/*bmc;* Forster, G., Bernt, E., and Bergmeyer, H. U., Creatine kinase. In *Methods of Enzymatic Analysis,* **2,** H. U. Bergmeyer, Ed., 2nd English ed. Academic Press, New York, NY 1974, p 784; Oliver, *op. cit.;* Abbott A-Gent kit.

Instrumentation:

Abbott ABA-100 Bichromatic Analyzer; Beckman TR Enzyme Analyzer; Union Carbide CentrifiChem; American Instrument Co. Rotochem; Electro-Nucleonics GEMSAEC.

Commentary—Paul A. Wolf

Neonatal creatine kinase (CK) values exceed adult values, and all three isoenzymes are present in neonatal serum. Freer et al. found that in 38 plasma samples 21 had the CK-BB band and three were positive for CK-MB. Two of 20 serum specimens were positive for CK-BB, and one contained CK-MB *(1).* CK in specimens drawn a few hours after delivery is significantly higher in infants delivered vaginally than in those delivered by cesarean section. The increase in CK occurs within 24 h after delivery and is caused by the skeletal muscle trauma of delivery. The MM and MB isoenzymes are derived from the trauma to the skeletal muscle of the infant; the MB is also derived from the CK-MB of the placenta, and the CK-MM from contraction of the mother's skeletal muscle during labor. CK-BB is derived from the placenta and the smooth muscle of the uterus *(2).* Cord blood CK-BB is an excellent source for quality-control serum for routine CK isoenzyme determination.

Pathologic increases of CK in children are usually associated with only a few conditions. It is unusual, for instance, for children to develop myocardial infarction. Thus high serum CK activity in children usually is associated with muscular dystrophy, polymyositis, dermatomyositis, or rhabdomyolysis. A central or peripheral nervous system lesion may also lead to an increase in serum CK. Skeletal muscle lesions can increase CK-MM and CK-BB.

1. Freer, D. E., Statland, B. E., Johnson, M., and Felton, H., Reference values

for selected enzyme activities and protein concentrations in serum and plasma derived from cord-blood specimens. *Clin. Chem.* **25,** 565–569 (1979).

2. Bodensteiner, J. B., and Zellweger, H., Creatine phosphokinase in normal neonates and young infants. *J. Lab. Clin. Med.* **77,** 853–858 (1971).

Commentary—Michael A. Pesce

The enzyme creatine kinase (CK) catalyzes the reversible phosphorylation of creatine to creatine phosphate. CK is composed of three isoenzymes, each of which is a dimer composed of the subunits designated M for muscle and B for brain. These subunits are combined into three possible dimers: BB, MB, and MM, corresponding to CK-1, CK-2, and CK-3, respectively. The BB isoenzyme migrates fastest in electrophoresis and is found closest to the anode; the MM isoenzyme migrates slowest, and the MB isoenzyme migrates about halfway between the MM and BB fraction. CK-1 is found predominantly in the brain, with lesser amounts in the lung, thyroid, intestine, kidney, prostate, and uterus. CK-2 is found mainly in heart muscle with smaller amounts in the lung, diaphragm, tongue, prostate, and uterus. CK-3 is found primarily in the skeletal and heart muscles. In relation to electrophoresis of serum proteins, the CK-1 fraction migrates in the prealbumin region, the CK-2 fraction in the α_2-globulin region, and the CK-3 fraction in the γ-globulin region.

Normal serum usually contains only CK-3. CK isoenzymes can aid in the diagnosis of myocardial infarction because CK-2 appears in serum about 4 to 8 h after chest pain and usually reaches a peak activity after 24 h. The presence of CK-2 in serum is not entirely specific for heart muscle, being also observed in the serum of patients with polymyositis, Duchenne's muscular dystrophy, dermatomyositis, myoglobinuria, Rocky Mountain spotted fever, and Reye's syndrome. However, the presence in serum of abnormal amounts of CK-2, in combination with a "flipped" lactate dehydrogenase pattern (LD 1 > 2) and the proper clinical setting, is diagnostic of myocardial infarction. The CK-1 fraction in serum is observed in Reye's syndrome, prostate cancer, acute brain injury, and intestinal infarction.

CK isoenzymes are usually determined by either electrophoresis or ion-exchange chromatography. CK-1 and CK-2 have been reported in the plasma of some neonates *(1)*. A hemolyzed specimen will not affect the isoenzyme pattern because CK is not present in erythrocytes. Serum can be stored at 4 °C for two days without an appreciable change in the isoenzyme pattern.

1. Freer, D. E., Statland, B. E., Johnson, M., and Felton, H., Reference values for selected enzyme activities and protein concentrations in serum and plasma derived from cord-blood specimens. *Clin. Chem.* **25,** 565–569 (1979).

Creatinine

Specimen Tested:

P, S.

Laboratories Reporting:

6.

Reference (Normal) Values:

Lower limits from birth to 17 yr: 0.3 mg/dL or less (26.5 μmol/L) for M and F. Upper limits gradually increase during this period from 0.5 to 1.2 mg/dL (44–106 μmol/L), with F lagging behind M by about 0.1 mg/dL (8.8 μmol/L).

Age, yr	Upper limits, mg/dL (μmol/L)	
	M	**F**
1	0.6 (53)	0.5 (44)
2–3	0.7 (62)	0.6 (53)
4–7	0.8 (71)	0.7 (62)
8–10	0.9 (80)	0.8 (71)
11–12	1.0 (88)	0.9 (80)
13–17	1.2 (106)	1.1 (97)
18–20	1.3 (115)	1.1 (97)

Adult, M + F: 0.5–1.2 (44–106); 0.5–1.4 (44–124)

Source of Reference Values:

Institutional; Hood, L., and Smith, E. K., A study made on 115 children, age 1 mo to 17 yr, and 22 young adults (to be published); Schwartz, G. J., Haycock, G. B., and Spitzer, A., Plasma creatinine and urea concentration in children: Normal values for age and sex. *J. Pediatr.* **88,** 828–830 (1976); Novak, L. P., Age and sex differences in body density and creatinine excretion of high school children. *Ann. N.Y. Acad. Sci.* **110,** 545–577 (1963); Clark, L. C., Thompson, H. L., Beck, E. I., and Jacobson, W., Excretion of creatine and creatinine by children. *Am. J. Dis. Child.* **81,** 774–783 (1951); Barratt, T. M., and Chantler, C., Clinical assessment of renal function. In *Pediatric Nephrology*, M. I. Rubin and T. M. Barratt, Eds. Williams and Wilkins Co., Baltimore, MD, 1975, pp 60–62; Greenhill, A., and Gruskin, A. B., Laboratory evaluation of renal function. *Pediatr. Clin. North Am.* **23,** 673–674 (1976).

Specimen Volume, Collection, and Preservation:

25 to 100 μL, generally. Only heparin anticoagulant reported. Stability of 4 to 7 d at RT is claimed; however, most recommend that samples be stored in FR.

Analytical Method:

All methods reported are based on the alkaline picrate (Jaffé) reaction. Specificity is improved by use of a "kinetic" method, or by prior adsorption of creatinine onto Lloyd's reagent. Osberg, I. M., and Hammond, K. B., A solution to the bilirubin interference problem with the kinetic Jaffé method for serum creatinine. *Clin. Chem.* **24,** 1196–1197 (1978); Fabiny, D. L., and Ertingshausen, G., Automated reaction-rate method for determination of serum creatinine with the CentrifiChem. *Clin. Chem.* **17,** 696–700 (1971); Heinegärd, D., and Tiderström, G., Determination of serum creatinine by a direct colorimetric method. *Clin. Chim. Acta* **43,** 305–310 (1973); Beckman Creatinine Reagent kit.

Instrumentation:

Beckman Creatinine Analyzer 2, Astra-8; Electro-Nucleonics Gemeni; Union Carbide CentrifiChem; Technicon AutoAnalyzer.

*　　*　　*

Laboratory Reporting:

1.

Reference (Normal) Values:

Age, yr	Sex	Percentile estimates, mg/dL (µmol/L)	
		5th	95th
4–5	F	0.4 (35)	0.7 (62)
4–6	M	0.4 (35)	0.7 (62)
6–9	F	0.5 (44)	0.8 (71)
7–9	M	0.5 (44)	0.8 (71)
10–11	M	0.6 (53)	0.9 (80)
10–14	F	0.6 (53)	0.9 (80)
12–14	M	0.7 (62)	1.0 (88)
15–17	M	0.8 (71)	1.1 (97)
15–18	F	0.7 (62)	1.0 (88)
18–20	M	0.9 (80)	1.2 (106)
19–20	F	0.8 (71)	1.1 (97)

Sources of Reference (Normal) Values:

Cherian, A. G., and Hill, J. G., Percentile estimates of reference values for fourteen chemical constituents in sera of children and adolescents. *Am. J. Clin. Pathol.* **69,** 24–31 (1978).

Specimen Volume, Collection, and Preservation:

120 µL. See preceding report for collection and preservation.

Analytical Method and Instrumentation:
Kinetic alkaline picrate; Greiner Selective Analyzer II.

Commentary—Robert L. Murray

Creatinine is most commonly analyzed with alkaline picrate, the Jaffé reaction. The precise mechanism of this reaction is not well understood, although it is known to be relatively nonspecific, producing chromogens with such noncreatinine compounds as acetoacetate, ascorbic acid, fructose, hemoglobin, oxaloacetate, and pyruvate (1). Enzymic methods based on creatinase-mediated hydrolysis have been reported (2); at present, however, these are tedious and have low analytical sensitivity, thus limiting their applicability. The specificity of the Jaffé reaction can be improved by removal of noncreatinine chromogens with Lloyd's reagent. Interference can also be reduced but not eliminated by measurement of the rate of chromogen formation, noncreatinine compounds reacting at slower rates than creatinine under the analytical conditions chosen. Bilirubin reportedly depresses the creatinine result significantly, although the extent of this effect remains open to debate (3,4). Unless minimized, this is a potential source of error in analysis of icteric neonatal specimens.

Creatinine, the waste product of creatine metabolism, is eliminated by the kidneys. Unlike urea, it is not reabsorbed and is only minimally secreted by the tubules. Thus, its clearance by the kidneys approximates the glomerular filtration rate. Fenner et al. reported that glomerular filtration rates in pre-term neonates are less than in full-term neonates; renal maturation, moreover, appears to be sudden in onset rather than gradual (5). Sertel and Scopes report that creatinine clearance doubles in the first six days of life in the normal neonate (6).

The difficulty in collecting complete 24-h urine specimens from children and neonates and the large relative error introduced by even small losses render creatinine clearance measurements subject to question. Consequently, Szelid and Méhes have developed a nomogram for the calculation of creatinine clearance, based on plasma creatinine and the child's height (7):

$$0.43 \times \text{height (cm)/plasma creatinine (mg/dL)} = \text{creatinine clearance}$$

Using this nomogram, they have published expected clearances for children through the age of 14 years (Table 1).

On the basis of findings in 1398 healthy children, Schwartz et al. have developed expected ranges for plasma creatinine concentrations through the age of 17 years (Table 1) (8); although these latter data are separated by sex, no statistically significant difference in the

Table 1. Expected Mean Creatinine Clearance (7) and Plasma Creatinine Range (8) in Children

Age, yr	Mean creatinine clearance, mL/min per 1.73 m² of body surface	Plasma creatinine, mg/dL (mean ± 2 SD)	
		F	M
0–1	72		
1	45	0.25–0.45	0.21–0.61
2	55	0.31–0.59	0.19–0.67
3	60	0.26–0.58	0.24–0.68
4	71	0.23–0.71	0.23–0.67
5	73	0.24–0.68	0.28–0.72
6	64	0.26–0.70	0.28–0.76
7	67	0.29–0.77	0.26–0.82
8	72	0.31–0.75	0.25–0.89
9	83	0.33–0.77	0.27–0.91
10	89	0.29–0.81	0.17–1.05
11	92	0.34–0.86	0.34–0.90
12	109	0.33–0.85	0.33–0.97
13–14	86		
13		0.34–0.90	0.26–1.10
14		0.39–0.91	0.24–1.20
15		0.23–1.11	0.32–1.20
16		0.35–0.95	0.28–1.20
17		0.30–1.10	0.44–1.16

plasma creatinine concentrations was found between boys and girls in these age groups.

1. Young, D. S., Pestaner, L. C., and Gibberman, V., Effects of drugs on clinical laboratory tests. *Clin. Chem.* **21**, 1D-432D (1975).
2. Moss, G. A., Bondar, R. J. L., and Buzzelli, D. M., Kinetic enzymatic method for determining serum creatinine. *Clin. Chem.* **21**, 1422–1426 (1975).
3. Soldin, S. J., Henderson, L., and Hill, J. G., The effect of bilirubin and ketones on reaction rate methods for the measurement of creatinine. *Clin. Biochem.* **11**, 82–86 (1978).
4. Osberg, I. M., and Hammond, K. B., A solution to the problem of bilirubin interference with the kinetic Jaffé method for serum creatinine. *Clin. Chem.* **24**, 1196–1197 (1978).
5. Fenner, A., Lange, G. U., Mönkemeier, D., and Ohlenroth, G., Creatinine levels in first urines of male preterm and term infants. *J. Perinat. Med.* **2**, 185–188 (1974).
6. Sertel, H., and Scopes, J., Rates of creatinine clearance in babies less than one week of age. *Arch. Dis. Child.* **48**, 717–720 (1973).
7. Szelid, Z., and Méhes, K., Estimation of glomerular filtration rate from plasma creatinine concentration in children of various ages. *Arch. Dis. Child.* **52**, 669–670 (1977). Letter.
8. Schwartz, G. J., Haycock, G. B., Chir, B., and Spitzer, A., Plasma creatinine and urea concentration in children: Normal values for age and sex. *J. Pediatr.* **88**, 828–830 (1976).

Creatinine Clearance, Coefficients and Output

Specimen Tested:

U (P, S).

Laboratories Reporting:

5.

Reference (Normal) Values:

Age	Daily clearance Coefficient, mg/kg of body weight	Output, mL	Age		Daily clearance Coefficient, mg/kg of body weight	Output, mL
Newborn	8–13	19–51	7–15 yr,	M	5.2–41.0	
Premature	8.1–15.0			F	11.5–29.1	
Full-term	10.4–19.7		10–12 yr,	M		315–1305
1 mo–1 yr	2.0–22	25–150		F		325–1150
Up to 2 yr	5–15		10–15 yr		9.6–31.0	
1–5 yr	5.6–24.0	70–300	10–17 yr		8–26	
1.5–7 yr	10.0–15.0		13–16 yr,	M		500–1675
3–6 yr		100–580		F		665–1305
3–10 yr	14–24	100–600	17–20 yr,	M	20–28	1175–2000
5–10 yr	9.6–31.0	175–835		F	18–26	885–1545
7–9 yr			Adult,	M	21–30	1385–2300
				F	16–23	715–1615

Age	Clearance, per m^2 of body surface mL/min	L/d
Newborn	40–60	33–54
6 mo	75	
1 yr and older	100	
Child, M		59–147
F		64–112
Adult, M		64–112
F		49–109

Source of Reference (Normal) Values:

Institutional; Novak, L. P., Age and sex differences in body density and creatinine excretion of high school children. *Ann. N. Y. Acad. Sci.* **110,** 545–577 (1963); Clark, L. C., Thompson, H. L., Beck, E. I., and Jacobson, W., Excretion of creatine and creatinine by children. *Am. J. Dis. Child.* **81,** 774–783 (1951); Smith, E. K., unpublished study of creatinine output in 137 healthy individuals: 15 newborns, 98 children aged 3–19 yr, and 24 adults aged 20–40 yr; Applegarth, D. A., Hardwick, D. F., and Ross, P. M., Creatinine excretion in children and the usefulness of creatinine equivalents in amino acid chromatography. *Clin. Chim. Acta* **22,** 131–134 (1968); Mabry, C. C., Roeckel, I. E., Gevedon, R. E., and Koepke, J. A., *Recent Advances in Pediatric Clinical Pathology.* Grune and Stratton, New York, NY, 1968, p 133.

Specimen Volume, Collection, and Preservation:

Analytical volume same as for plasma determinations. Urine should be kept on ice or in RR during collection, and stored in RR. There is a claim, however, that urine may be stored for 4 to 7 d at RT.

Analytical Method:

Same as for creatinine determinations in plasma. Also see Owen, J. A., Iggo, B., Scandrett, F. J., and Stewart, C. P., The determination of creatinine in plasma or serum, and in urine; a critical examination. *Biochem. J.* **58,** 426 (1954); Taussky, H. H., A procedure increasing the specificity of the Jaffé reaction for the determination of creatine and creatinine in urine and plasma. *Clin. Chim. Acta* **1,** 210 (1956); Taussky, H. H., A microcolorimetric determination of creatine in urine by the Jaffé reaction. *J. Biol. Chem.* **208,** 853–861 (1954).

Commentary—Garry M. Lum

Each day approximately 2% of muscle creatine is converted to creatinine, which is eliminated by renal excretion. Creatinine excretion is fairly constant from day to day, depending on renal factors and the steady state of muscle mass and metabolism. Although plasma creatinine increases from birth throughout childhood, serial measurements of serum creatinine can be very useful in assessing renal function and development.

The clearance of creatinine as an estimate of glomerular filtration rate is clinically applicable because plasma and urine concentrations are relatively stable. Although the renal tubules do secrete some creatinine, the resulting overestimation of glomerular filtration does not present serious clinical problems when viewed within a range of normal values. Determining creatinine clearance as opposed to simple measurement of the plasma concentration will eliminate error introduced by differences in muscle mass. However, a strictly timed collection of urine flow is not easily accomplished in the infant.

The formula for creatinine clearance is $C_{Cr} = U_{Cr} V/P_{Cr}$, where C_{Cr} = clearance of creatinine, mL/min; U_{Cr} = urine concentration of creatinine, mg/mL; V = urine volume, mL/min; and P_{Cr} = plasma concentration of creatinine, mg/dL.

1. Barratt, T. M., and Chantler, C., Clinical assessment of renal function. In *Pediatric Nephrology,* M. I. Rubin and T. M. Barratt, Eds. Williams and Wilkins, Baltimore, MD, 1975, p 55.

Commentary—Derek A. Applegarth

To express the output of many analytes, the output of a urinary solute is often determined in relation to the output of creatinine. This concept has been challenged for adults (1); moreover, although the adult output of creatinine probably correlates with lean body mass (2), the 24-h creatinine output is not sufficiently constant to justify its use as a reference standard for comparing the excretion of other substances (3).

Variation in creatinine output is even greater in children, who are growing more or less constantly throughout childhood. Creatinine excretion in children tends to increase more rapidly than the excretion of most other urinary analytes. Therefore, when the output of most analytes is expressed relative to creatinine concentration, the graph of output relative to creatinine concentration plotted vs age tends to show very high values for some analytes in the early years and tapers off to a rough nadir at approximately 12 to 14 years of age. Normal ranges for analytes *expressed relative to creatinine* are, therefore, strongly age-dependent (4). All laboratories attempting to use creatinine as a reference substance to express the output of various metabolites must be aware of this; as yet, however, no solution to the problem of expressing the output of urinary metabolites is forthcoming.

1. Peters, W. H., A study of the possible usefulness of the α-amino nitrogen/creatinine ratio in urine. *Clin. Chim. Acta* **45**, 387–390 (1973).
2. Forbes, G. B., and Bruining, G. J., Urinary creatinine excretion and lean body mass. *Am. J. Clin. Nutr.* **29**, 1359–1365 (1976).
3. Paterson, N., Relative constancy of 24-hour urine volume and 24-hour creatinine output. *Clin. Chim. Acta* **18**, 57–58 (1967).
4. Applegarth, D. A., and Ross, P. M., The unsuitability of creatinine excretion as a basis for assessing the excretion of other metabolites by infants and children. *Clin. Chim. Acta* **64**, 83–85 (1975).

Cyclic AMP (Adenosine 3′,5′-monophosphate)

Specimen Tested:

U.

Laboratory Reporting:

1.

Reference (Normal) Values:

		Daily excretion		
Age, yr	μmol	μmol/m^2 of body surface	μmol/g of creatinine	**Reference**
Child, 1–4			$8.00 \pm 0.70\,[a]$	1
16–18			$4.51 \pm 0.37\,[a]$	1
1–18	$9.09 \pm 0.05\,[a]$	$2.86 \pm 0.08\,[a]$		1
Child, 1–9.5		1.03–7.87		2
10–16		0.90–3.54		2
Adult	0.6–7.0			3

[a] Mean $\pm$ SEM.

Sources of Reference (Normal) Values:

1. Murad, F., Moss, W. W., Johanson, A. J., and Selden, R. F., Urinary excretion of adenosine 3′,5′-monophosphate and guanosine 3′5′-monophosphate in normal children and those with cystic fibrosis. *J. Clin. Endocrinol. Metab.* **40,** 552–559 (1975).
2. Vitek, V., and Lang, D. I., Urinary excretion of cyclic adenosine 3′,5′-monophosphate in children of different ages. *J. Clin. Endocrinol. Metab.* **42,** 781–784 (1976).
3. Consolidated Biomedical Labs.

Specimen Volume, Collection, and Preservation:

Collect 24-h U; store and ship frozen (−20 °C) without added preservative.

Analytical Method:

Gilman, A. G., A protein-binding assay for adenosine 3′,5′-cyclic monophosphate. *Proc. Natl. Acad. Sci. USA* **67,** 305–312 (1970).

Dehydroepiandrosterone (DHEA)

Specimen Tested:

P, S.

Laboratory Reporting:

1.

Reference (Normal) Values:

Age, yr	**DHEA, nmol/L**	
	M	**F**
7–8	0.6–4.9	0.4–5.2
9–10	1.7–5.4	0.6–6.3
11–12	0.7–18.3	2.1–20.3
13–14	1.4–18.8	—
Adult	6.7–31.3	2.4–32.2

Sources of Reference (Normal) Values:

Based on a survey made of normal school children and adults in Winnipeg, Manitoba, Canada.

Specimen Volume, Collection, and Preservation:

0.1 mL. Store S in FR.

Analytical Method:

RIA. Direct assay, charcoal separation, ^{3}H-labeled tracer from Amersham; antibody produced in Winnipeg; Carter, J. N., Tyson, S. E., Warne, G. L., McNeilly, A. S., Faiman, C., and Friesen, H. G., Adrenocorticol function in hyperprolactinemic women. *J. Clin. Endocrinol. Metab.* **45**, 973–980 (1977).

Instrumentation:

Packard 2425 liquid scintillation counter.

Note: See Commentary for **DHEA-S.**

Dehydroepiandrosterone Sulfate (DHEA-S)

Specimen Tested:

P, S.

Laboratories Reporting:

2.

Reference (Normal) Values:

Age	Range (not 2 SD)	
	µg/dL	µmol/L
Newborn		0.5–7.0
Premature	25–1000	
Full-term	25–200	
1–3 mo		<1.0
3 mo–8 yr		<1.4
1–6 yr	<50	
7 yr through puberty	gradual increase to adult value	
8–13 yr		1.6–5.6
Adult		1.9–9.4
M	130–550	
F	60–340	

Sources of Reference (Normal) Values:

Reiter, E. O., Fauldauer, V. G., and Root, A. W., Secretion of adrenal androgen, dehydroepiandrosterone sulfate during normal infancy, childhood, and adolescence, in sick infants, and in children with endocrinologic disorders. *J. Pediatr.* **90**, 766–770 (1977); Korth-Schutz, S., Levine, L. S., and New, M. I., Dehydroepiandrosterone sulfate (DS) levels, a rapid test for abnormal adrenal androgen secretion. *J. Clin. Endocrinol. Metab.* **42**, 1005–1013 (1976); dePeretti, E., and Forest, M. G., Pattern of plasma dehydroepiandrosterone sulfate levels in humans from birth to adulthood: Evidence for testicular production. *J. Clin. Endocrinol. Metab.* **47**, 572–577 (1978); Nichols Institute, San Pedro, CA.

Specimen Volume, Collection, and Preservation:

25 µL. Store P, S in FR. Prefer sample taken at 0800 hours.

Analytical Method:

RIA, ^{3}H; Endocrine Sciences Antibody DS-17-61. Buster, J. E., and Abraham, G. E., Radioimmunoassay of plasma dehydroepiandrosterone sulfate. *Anal. Lett.* **5**, 543–551 (1972).

Instrumentation:

Packard 3375 and 2425 liquid scintillation spectrometers.

Commentary—Elizabeth K. Smith

Dehydroepiandrosterone (DHEA) and its sulfate (DHEA-S) are produced primarily by the androgenic zone of the adrenal cortex; dexamethasone decreases plasma concentrations of DHEA and DHEA-S, and corticotropin (ACTH) increases them (1). The peripheral concentration of the two steroids differs markedly; DHEA is expressed in ng/dL or nmol/L, whereas the concentration of DHEA-S is much greater and is expressed in µg/dL or µmol/L.

Because of the increased activity of the fetal zone of the adrenal cortex, high concentrations of both hormones are found in cord blood and during the first few days of life. dePeretti and Forest (2) found that concentrations of DHEA were slightly higher in cord blood of male infants than in females, and that concentrations in peripheral blood on the first day of life were even higher than in cord blood. Serum concentrations of DHEA-S are higher in healthy premature infants than in full-term infants (3,4), and higher still in sick infants, both premature and full-term (3). Values decrease precipitously during the first week of life and then progressively for the first six months to very low concentrations, which are maintained to about six years of age, with no difference between sexes (2,5).

Serum concentrations begin to increase before the onset of puberty and continue through puberty. DHEA was significantly higher in pre-pubertal children older than seven years than in younger children (6). A rapid increase occurs in both boys and girls about the time of appearance of pubic hair. In boys significant increases of DHEA occur with the onset of pubic hair and voice change; DHEA-S increases with onset of genital and axillary hair growth. Adult values are reached by completion of puberty. In girls with precocious adrenarche, plasma DHEA values are significantly high for their age and correspond to reference values for the Tanner stage of puberty *(6,8)*.

Both the free steroid and its sulfate can be measured with specific RIA methods. The high concentration of DHEA-S makes the assay relatively easy, requiring only dilution of a small volume of serum without column-chromatographic purification. Secretion of both hormones is episodic; the significant circadian rhythm of DHEA, paralleling changes in cortisol *(9)*, is established by five years of age *(2)*. For DHEA-S the diural variation is much less than for DHEA, and values at 0900 hours are not significantly different from those at 1700 hours *(6)*. Day-to-day variations are small.

Plasma values for DHEA-S are positively correlated with urinary 17-ketosteroid excretion in boys and girls *(6)*, and measurement of DHEA-S is proposed as a rapid test for abnormal androgen secretion. Values are markedly increased in patients with congenital adrenal hyperplasia but can be suppressed with dexamethasone. Highest values are seen in patients with congenital adrenal hyperplasia related to deficiency of 3β-ol dehydrogenase. Values also are increased in adrenal carcinoma, but are not suppressible with dexamethasone. In Cushing's syndrome due to bilateral adrenal hyperplasia, DHEA-S concentrations in plasma were high, whereas in patients with Cushing's syndrome due to benign adrenal cortical adenoma, the plasma values were significantly lower *(10)*. In the differential diagnosis between hypogonadotropic hypogonadism and idiopathic delayed puberty, Copeland et al. *(11)* found that, with the former, plasma DHEA-S usually was normal for chronologic age and high for bone age, whereas with the latter, DHEA-S was low relative to chronologic age and normal relative to bone age.

1. Sizonenko, P. C., Endocrinology in preadolescents and adolescents. *Am. J. Dis. Child.* **132,** 704–712 (1978).
2. dePeretti, E., and Forest, M. G., Unconjugated dehydroepiandrosterone plasma levels in normal subjects from birth to adolescence in humans: The use of a sensitive radioimmunoassay. *J. Clin. Endocrinol. Metab.* **43,** 982–991 (1976).
3. Reiter, E. O., Fauldauer, V. G., and Root, A. W., Secretion of the adrenal androgen, dehydroepiandrosterone sulfate, during normal infancy, childhood and adolescence, in sick infants and in children with endocrinologic abnormalities. *J. Pediatr.* **90,** 766–770 (1977).
4. Korth-Schutz, S., Levine, L. S., and New, M. I., Dehydroepiandrosterone sulfate (DS) levels, a rapid test for abnormal adrenal androgen secretion. *J. Clin. Endocrinol. Metab.* **42,** 1005–1013 (1976).
5. dePeretti, E., and Forest, M. G., Pattern of plasma dehydroepiandrosterone sulfate levels in humans from birth to adulthood: Evidence for testicular production. *J. Clin. Endocrinol. Metab.* **47,** 572–577 (1978).

6. Korth-Schutz, S., Levine, L. S., and New, M. I., Serum androgens in normal prepubertal and pubertal children and in children with precocious adrenarche. *J. Clin. Endocrinol. Metab.* **42,** 117–124 (1976).
7. Lee, P. A., and Migeon, C. J., Puberty in boys: Correlation of plasma levels of gonadotropins (LH, FSH), androgens (testosterone, androstenedione, dehydroepiandrosterone and its sulfate), estrogens (estrone and estradiol) and progestins (progesterone and 17-hydroxyprogesterone). *J. Clin. Endocrinol. Metab.* **41,** 556–562 (1975).
8. Sizonenko, P. C., and Paunier, L., Hormonal changes in puberty III. Correlation of plasma dehydroepiandrosterone, testosterone, FSH and LH with stages of puberty and bone age in normal boys and girls and in patients with Addison's disease or hypogonadism or with premature or late adrenarche. *J. Clin. Endocrinol. Metab.* **41,** 894–905 (1975).
9. Rosenfeld, R. S., Rosenberg, B. J., and Fukushima, D. K., 24-Hour secretory pattern of dehydroisoandrosterone and dehydroisoandrosterone sulfate. *J. Clin. Endocrinol. Metab.* **40,** 850–855 (1975).
10. Yamaji, T., and Ibayashi, H., Plasma dehydroepiandrosterone sulfate in normal and pathological conditions. *J. Clin. Endocrinol. Metab.* **29,** 273–287 (1969).
11. Copeland, K. C., Paunier, L., and Sizonenko, P. C., The secretion of adrenal androgens and growth patterns of patients with hypogonadotropic hypogonadism and idiopathic delayed puberty. *J. Pediatr.* **91,** 985–990 (1977).

11-Deoxycortisol

Specimen Tested:

P, S.

Laboratories Reporting:

2.

Reference (Normal) Values:

Age	ng/dL (Lab. 1)	nmol/L (Lab. 2)
All ages, baseline	< 200[a]	< 50
Child	40–220 (range)[a]	
Adult	26–140 (range)[a]	

After midnight oral dose (30 mg/kg of body weight) of metyrapone; 0800 hour sample:

Child	> 7000	> 60
Adult		200–400

[a] Institutional study on 42 healthy children and 22 healthy adults.

Sources of Reference (Normal) Values:

Institutional; Endocrine Sciences Bulletin.

Specimen Volume, Collection, and Preservation:

200 to 300 μL. Heparin anticoagulant. Centrifuge specimen promptly after collection. Store in FR.

Analytical Method:

RIA. **Lab. 1:** Lee, L. M. Y., and Schiller, H. S., Nonchromatographic radioimmunoassay of plasma 11-deoxycortisol for use in the metyrapone test, with polyethylene glycol as the precipitant. *Clin. Chem.* **21**, 719–724 (1975). **Lab. 2:** Jubiz, W., Meikle, A. W., West, C. D., and Tyler, F. H., Single-dose metyrapone test. *Arch. Intern. Med.* **125**, 472–474 (1970); Murphy, B. E. P., Hood, A. B., and Pattee, C. J., Clinical studies utilizing a new method for the serial determination of plasma corticoids. *Can. Med. Assoc. J.* **90**, 775–780 (1964).

Instrumentation:

Packard 3375 and 2425 liquid scintillation spectrometers.

Commentary—Elizabeth K. Smith

11-Deoxycortisol, a steroid intermediate in the biosynthesis of cortisol from 17-hydroxyprogesterone, normally circulates in the blood at very low concentrations. It is metabolized to tetrahydro-11-deoxycortisol (THS) and excreted in the urine as a 17-hydroxycorticosteroid (17-OHCS), where it can be measured as a Porter–Silber 17-OHCS or a ketogenic steroid, 17-KGS.

Reference values for 11-deoxycortisol in serum, measured by a specific RIA method, are less than 200 μg/dL and appear to be independent of age or sex. Studies of 42 healthy children three to 15 years old showed no definite pattern of change with age; the mean for 22 boys was 126.8 $\pm$ 38.9 μg/dL (range), compared with 105.5 $\pm$ 54 μg/dL for 20 girls (E. K. Smith, unpublished data).

Measurement of 11-deoxycortisol as part of the metyrapone test has an important clinical application in evaluating pituitary–adrenal reserve. Metyrapone produces a chemical block of steroid 11β-hydroxylase (EC 1.14.15.4), inhibiting conversion of 11-deoxycortisol to cortisol. With less negative feedback from cortisol, release of corticotropin (ACTH) is increased, resulting in increased secretion of 11-deoxycortisol. With normal pituitary function, plasma 11-deoxycortisol concentration 8 h after a large oral dose of metyrapone will exceed 7000 ng/dL (7 μg/dL) *(1)*. Patients with panhypopituitarism and ACTH deficiency show very little increase in 11-deoxycortisol after metyrapone. In Cushing's snydrome, patients with adrenal hyperplasia respond vigorously to metyrapone, whereas those with adrenal tumors do not *(2)*.

In one form of congenital adrenal hyperplasia due to deficiency of the 11β-hydroxylase enzyme and consequent decreased biosynthesis of cortisol, plasma concentrations of 11-deoxycortisol and urinary excretion of THS are markedly above normal.

1. Jubiz, W., Meikle, A. W., West, C. D., and Tyler, F. H., Single dose metyrapone test. *Arch. Intern. Med.* **125,** 472–474 (1970).
2. Liddle, G. W., Estep, H. L., Kendall, J. W., Williams, C., and Townes, A. W., Clinical application of a new test of pituitary reserve. *J. Clin. Endocrinol. Metab.* **19,** 875–894 (1959).

Digoxin

Specimen Tested:

P, S.

Laboratories Reporting:

3.

Reference (Normal) Values:

Therapeutic values:

Lab. 1: Newborn, infant: 2–4 ng/mL (2.6–5.1 nmol/L)
Child–adult: 1–2 (1.3–2.6)
Time to reach equilibrium: 4–5 d; longer in presence of renal failure
Draw blood at least 6–8 h post dose.

Lab. 2: < 0.5 ng/mL (< 0.6 nmol/L) = under-digitalized
0.5–2.5 (0.6–3.2) = optimal
2.5–3.0 (3.2–3.8) = overlap
> 3.0 (> 3.8) = over-digitalized

Lab. 3: (1.0–2.5 nmol/L)

Toxicity (> 3 nmol/L)

Sources of Reference (Normal) Values:

Lab. 1: Smith, T. W., and Haber, E., Digitalis. *N. Engl. J. Med.* **289,** 945–952, 1010–1015, 1063–1072, 1125–1129 (1973). **Lab. 2:** institutional; Doherty, J. E., How and when to use the digitalis serum levels. *J. Am. Med. Assoc.* **239,** 2594–2596 (1978). **Lab. 3:** Goodman, L. S., and Gilman, A., *The Pharmacologic Basis of Therapeutics.* MacMillan, New York, NY, 1965.

Specimen Volume, Collection, and Preservation; Patient Preparation:

0.1 to 1.0 mL. For plasma use heparin as anticoagulant. Serum or plasma can be stored temporarily in FR. For storage > 48 h, use FR. Do not thaw and refreeze samples. Patient should not be receiving digitoxin.

Analytical Method:

Lab. 1: Smith, T. W., Butler, V. P., Jr., and Haber, E., Determination of therapeutic and toxic serum digoxin concentrations by radioimmunoassay. *N. Engl. J. Med.* **281,** 1212–1216 (1969); Becton-Dickinson digoxin solid-phase radioimmunoassay (^{125}I) single-lot component system. **Lab. 2:** unpublished institutional RIA method. **Lab. 3:** RIA; Diagnostic Products Corp.

Instrumentation:

Searle, LKB 80000 gamma counters.

Commentary—Joan H. and Peter J. Howanitz

Digoxin is a cardiac glycoside commonly used in treating congestive heart failure and supraventricular cardiac arrhythmias. Digoxin toxicity may be associated with a wide variety of symptoms related to the central nervous system and gastrointestinal tract. Cardiac manifestations of digoxin toxicity include increasing severity of congestive heart failure as well as alterations in cardiac rate and rhythm, which may be fatal.

In all age groups, only a small margin of error exists between the effective digitalizing dose and a dose that causes toxicity. In children, it has been particularly difficult to determine digoxin dosages that are both safe and effective. Recommendations for dosage schedules in neonates and infants have been based largely on clinical response and occurrence of cardiac toxicity. Compared on the basis of either surface area or weight, the digoxin doses usually used in pediatric patients are higher than those used in adults *(1–3)*. These doses are generally inversely proportional to age except in premature infants *(4)*.

The absorption of digoxin and its relative distribution to different tissues is similar in adults and infants. However, in infants the binding of digoxin to certain tissues may be more extensive *(5)*. Infants have an apparent volume of distribution about twice as great as adults *(2)*. During maintenance therapy, daily excretion of digoxin by the kidney is somewhat lower in children than in adults *(6)*. Data from a number of groups indicate that renal clearance of digoxin is low during the first few weeks of life but increases with age, reaching values similar to those of adults by three to four months *(5)*.

Although increased digoxin concentrations in serum are not diagnostic of toxicity, in conjunction with certain clinical manifestations they may indicate a high probability that toxicity is present *(7)*. In the clinical laboratory, digoxin concentrations in serum are usually determined by immunoassay. Although digoxin antibodies may cross react with certain steroids, no interference generally occurs with the antisera currently in use *(7)*. Because the cardiac glycosides are structurally similar, however, antibodies to one tend to cross react with other cardiac glycosides and their metabolites. Thus, immunoassays are meaningful only when the cardiac glycoside the patient is receiving is known. For example, another commonly used cardiac glycoside, digitoxin, has a relatively long half-life and thus a relatively high concentration in serum. This compound may interfere with digoxin assays for several weeks after having been discontinued.

To interpret digoxin values correctly, specimens for digoxin determinations must be obtained when tissue and serum concentrations are in equilibrium. After an oral dose of digoxin, equilibrium may not be complete for 4 to 6 h. Thus, specimens for digoxin analysis should be collected at least 6 h and preferably 8 h after the last oral dose *(7)*. Digoxin reaches equilibrium 12 h after intramuscular administration and 2 to 4 h after intravenous administration of the drug *(8)*. When these routes of administration are used, adjust the blood-collection times accordingly.

In adults, the usual therapeutic range for digoxin is 0.5 to 2.0 ng/mL, although some laboratories report somewhat higher values *(7)*. There is, however, significant overlap of toxic and nontoxic serum digoxin concentrations. Up to 10% of nontoxic adults have serum digoxin concentrations greater than 2 ng/mL but usually in the 2 to 3 ng/mL range *(7)*. Some patients who are treated with relatively large doses of digoxin to control supraventricular arrhythmias have serum digoxin concentrations in the range of 2 to 4 ng/mL without clinical evidence of toxicity *(9)*. In most adult patients with evidence of digoxin toxicity, serum concentrations of digoxin exceed 2.0 ng/mL. Some patients show toxicity, however, with digoxin in the range of 1.4 to 2.0 ng/mL *(7)*. Hypokalemia, hypomagnesemia, hypercalcemia, diffuse heart disease, and hypoxia may predispose patients to digoxin toxicity *(7,9)*.

Even when digoxin dosage schedules are comparable on the basis of body size, serum digoxin concentrations range widely among individuals, owing to a variety of factors, including intercurrent illness and drug interactions. For example, in patients with malabsorption or hyperthyroidism, serum concentrations for a given digoxin dose are less than in patients without these disorders. Because digoxin is excreted mainly by the kidneys, renal insufficiency prolongs digoxin half-life, and high concentrations are reached if the digoxin dose is not reduced. Several drugs such as cholestyramine and antacids may decrease gastrointestinal absorption of digoxin and thus possibly lead to lower serum digoxin values. Concomitant administration of quinidine increases serum digoxin, mainly by reducing renal clearance of the digoxin *(10)*.

Especially during the first few months of life, the dosage schedule used in infants may yield higher mean serum concentrations of digoxin than those usually attained in adults *(1,3,4,6,11)*. It is not known, however, whether such high concentrations are necessary to obtain adequate ionotropic effects *(5)*. There is evidence that in young infants higher serum digoxin concentrations are reached for a given dose of the drug than in older infants *(11,12)*. It has been suggested that the usual digoxin doses for infants younger than three months may be excessive *(13)*.

Infants have been found to tolerate high digoxin concentrations in serum without developing signs of toxicity *(9,13,14)*. Although the half-life of digoxin is significantly longer in premature than in mature infants, Lang et al. *(15)* found no significant differences in serum digoxin concentrations between these two groups. Hayes et al. *(14)* reported that the mean serum concentration in a group of nontoxic infants (age, one week to 11 months) was 2.8 ng/mL; in toxic infants it was 4.4 ng/mL.

Results of several studies have indicated that, in infants, digoxin concentrations between 2.0 and 3.5 ng/mL may or may not be associated with toxicity; values exceeding 3.5 ng/mL in infants usually are associated with signs of toxicity; and some nontoxic patients have serum digoxin values in the range of 5 ng/mL *(5)*. Recently it has been suggested that, to avoid toxicity, digoxin dosage schedules in neonates and infants should be adjusted to maintain serum digoxin steady-state concentrations of less than 2.0 ng/mL *(16)*.

In older children, therapeutic values for serum digoxin are similar to those found in adults. Krasula et al. *(13)* report that in spite of the relatively high doses used in children, serum digoxin concentrations in the age groups six months to two years, two to five years, and older than five years are comparable with each other and equivalent to adult values. In the study of Hayes et al. *(14)*, the mean serum digoxin concentration in children ages two to 14 years was 1.3 ng/mL, the same as in adults in their study; the mean serum digoxin concentration in toxic children, however, was 3.4 ng/mL, compared with 2.9 ng/mL in toxic adults *(14)*.

Digitoxin

Clinical use and toxic manifestations of digitoxin are similar to digoxin. Compared with digoxin, digitoxin has a longer half-life and a higher degree of binding to serum proteins; moreover, digitoxin is metabolized extensively in the liver. Concurrent administration of digitoxin and other drugs such as phenobarbital and phenytoin increases the digitoxin dosage requirement necessary to maintain constant digitoxin concentrations in serum, presumably because of increased hepatic metabolism of digitoxin *(7,17)*.

Digitoxin is usually measured by immunoassay. To interpret the results correctly, blood specimens for digitoxin assay must be obtained when serum and tissue concentrations are in equilibrium. Doherty and Kane suggest that specimens for digitoxin determinations should be collected at least 6 to 8 h after the last oral or parenteral dose *(8)*.

As with digoxin, there is an overlap between toxic and therapeutic ranges in patients treated with digitoxin. In adults with toxicity, serum digitoxin concentrations usually exceed 25 ng/mL. In patients without toxicity, values are in the range of 5 to 50 ng/mL, but most patients have concentrations less than 30 ng/mL *(7)*. Digitoxin concentrations greater than 35 to 40 ng/mL generally are considered to be associated with potential toxicity, while concentrations of 15 to 25 ng/mL are considered to be within the therapeutic range *(17)*.

There is some evidence that, as with digoxin, infants and children tolerate higher serum digitoxin concentrations than adults, without showing evidence of toxicity. Giardina et al. *(18)* found that in infants less than two years of age and in older children two to 13 years old, mean serum digitoxin concentrations were higher than in adults. However, their data showed no significant difference between the mean concentrations in nontoxic infants and children. These workers reported that digitoxin concentrations in four toxic infants ranged from 68 to 72 ng/mL; in four toxic children, digitoxin concentrations ranged from 53 to 84 ng/mL.

1. Rogers, M. C., Willerson, J. T., Goldblatt, A., and Smith, T. W., Serum digoxin concentrations in the human fetus, neonate, and infant. *N. Engl. J. Med.* **287,** 1010–1013 (1972).
2. Gorodischer, R., Jusko, W. J., and Yaffe, S. J., Tissue and erythrocyte distribution of digoxin in infants. *Clin. Pharmacol. Ther.* **19,** 256–263 (1976).
3. O'Malley, K., Coleman, E. N., Doig, W. B., and Stevenson, I. H., Plasma digoxin levels in infants. *Arch. Dis. Child.* **48,** 55–57 (1973).
4. Krasula, R. W., Pellegrino, P. A., Hastreiter, A. R., and Soyka, L. F., Serum levels of digoxin in infants and children. *J. Pediatr.* **81,** 566–569 (1972).
5. Wettrell, G., and Andersson, K. E., Clinical pharmacokinetics of digoxin in infants. *Clin. Pharmacokinet.* **2,** 17–31 (1977).
6. Iisalo, E., and Dahl, M., Serum levels and renal excretion of digoxin during maintenance therapy in children. *Acta Paediatr. Scand.* **63,** 699–704 (1974).
7. Butler, V. P., Assays of digitalis in the blood. *Prog. Cardiovas. Dis.* **14,** 571–600 (1972).
8. Doherty, J. E., and Kane, J. J., Clinical pharmacology of digitalis glycosides. *Ann. Rev. Med.* **26,** 159–171 (1975).
9. Butler, V. P., and Lindenbaum, J., Serum digitalis measurements in the assessment of digitalis resistance and sensitivity. *Am. J. Med.* **58,** 460–469 (1975).
10. Doering, W., Quinidine–digoxin interaction, pharmacokinetics, underlying mechanism and clinical implications. *N. Engl. J. Med.* **301,** 400–404 (1979).
11. Neutze, J. M., Rutherford, J. D., and Hurley, P. J., Serum digoxin levels in neonates, infants, and children with heart disease. *N. Z. Med. J.* **86,** 7–10 (1977).
12. Cree, J. E., Coltart, D. J., and Howard, M. R., Plasma digoxin concentration in children with heart failure. *Br. Med. J.* **i,** 443–444 (1973).
13. Krasula, R., Yanagi, R., Hastreiter, A. R., Levitsky, S., and Soyka, L. F., Digoxin intoxication in infants and children: Correlation with serum levels. *J. Pediatr.* **84,** 265–269 (1974).

14. Hayes, C. J., Butler, V. P., and Gersony, W. M., Serum digoxin studies in infants and children. *Pediatrics* **52,** 561–568 (1973).
15. Lang, D., and Von Bernuth, G., Serum concentration and serum half-life of digoxin in premature and mature newborns. *Pediatrics* **59,** 902–906 (1977).
16. Halkin, H., Radomsky, M., Blieden, L., Frand, M., Millman, P., and Boichis, H., Steady state serum digoxin concentration in relation to digitalis toxicity in neonates and infants. *Pediatrics* **61,** 184–188 (1978).
17. Perrier, D., Mayersohn, M., and Marcus, F. J., Clinical pharmacokinetics of digitoxin. *Clin. Pharmacokinet.* **2,** 292–311 (1977).
18. Giardina, A. C. V., Ehlers, K. H., Morrison, J. B., and Engel, M. A., Serum digitoxin concentrations in infants and children. *Circulation* **51,** 713–717 (1975).

1,25-Dihydroxyvitamin D

Specimen Tested

S.

Laboratory Reporting:

1.

Reference (Normal) Values:

Age	pg/mL
Newborn	21 ± 2 (SEM)
Child, 2–15 yr	43.6 ± 3 (SEM)
6–17 yr	13.3–60.9 (range, 16–64)
Adult	29 ± 2 (SEM)

Sources of Reference (Normal) Values:

Scriver, C. R., Reade, T. M., DeLuca, H. F., and Hamstra, A. J., Serum 1,25-dihydroxyvitamin D levels in normal subjects and in patients with hereditary rickets or bone disease. *N. Engl. J. Med.* **299,** 976–979 (1978); Chesney, R. W., Hamstra, A. J., and DeLuca, H. F., Serum 1,25-$(OH)_2$ vitamin D_3 levels in children and alteration with disorders of vitamin D metabolism. *Pediatr. Res.* **12,** 503 (1978), abstract.

Specimen Volume, Collection, and Preservation:

Collect blood in chilled tube; allow to clot at 4 °C. Centrifuge in refrigerated centrifuge. Store in FR.

Analytical Method:

Extraction; LH-20 Sephadex chromatography; HPLC; competitive binding assay with intestinal cytosol preparation from rachitic chicks; Eisman, J. A., Hamstra, A. J., and Kream, B. E., A sensitive, precise and convenient method for determination of 1,25-dihydroxyvitamin D in human plasma. *Arch. Biochem. Biophys.* **176,** 235–243 (1976).

Estradiol

Specimen Tested:

P, S.

Laboratories Reporting:

2.

Reference (Normal) Values:

Lab. 1: prepubertal children: < 20 pg/mL or < 2 ng/dL
Lab. 2: M: poorly defined; values decrease from about 10 ng/dL at birth to
< 2 ng/dL at 1 yr
1 yr–adrenarche[a]: < 2 ng/dL
F: Birth–adrenarche[a]: same as for M
Adrenarche through puberty: increases to adult values, correlating
with pubertal stage and phase of cycle
Adult, follicular phase: 4–15 ng/dL
luteal phase: 10–40 ng/dL
treated with synthetic estrogen: < 7 ng/dL

[a] At adrenarche, adrenal steroids start to increase in preparation for puberty. These changes occur as early as 7–8 yr in girls and 1–2 yr later in boys. In women, most of the estradiol is produced by the ovaries.

Sources of Reference (Normal) Values:

Lab. 1: *Radioimmunoassay Manual,* Nichols Institute, 4th ed., San Pedro, CA, 1977, p 219. **Lab. 2:** Sizonenko, P. C., Endocrinology in preadolescents and adolescents. I. Hormonal changes during normal puberty. *Am. J. Dis. Child.* **132,** 704–712 (1978); Thorner, M. O., Round, J., Jones, A., Fahmy, D., Groom, G. V., Butcher, S., and Thompson, K., Serum prolactin and oestradiol levels at different stages of puberty. *Clin. Endocrinol.* **7,** 463–468 (1977); Kletzky, O. A., Mishell, D. R., Davajan, V., Nicoloff, J., Mins, R., and Nakamura, R. M., Pituitary stimulation test in amenorrhoeic patients with normal or low serum oestradiol. *Acta Endocrinol.* **87,** 456–466 (1978).

Specimen Volume, Collection, and Preservation:

1 to 2 mL. Store in FR.

Analytical Method:

Lab. 1: RIA, double-antibody after LH-20 Sephadex chromatography with [³H]estradiol; Nichols Institute. **Lab. 2:** RIA; kit from Endocrine Sciences.

Instrumentation:

Liquid scintillation counter.

Note: SI conversion factor: pg/mL × 3.671 = pmol/L.

Commentary—Elizabeth K. Smith

Estradiol-17β is the major secretory product of the ovary and is physiologically the most potent estrogen. In women the measurement of estradiol is useful in evaluating the status of ovarian function. In children the concentration is extremely low and measurement has very limited application. However, the low peripheral concentration of estradiol can be measured satisfactorily with sensitive RIA methods. As with other hormones regulated by tropic hormones from the hypothalamic–pituitary axis, blood concentrations vary episodically, even in the prepubertal child, but the magnitude of episodic change is relatively small.

Both male and female infants have high concentrations of estradiol in cord blood, as much as 200 to 1000 ng/dL (> 2000 pg/mL) (1). Concentrations in both sexes during the first week of life are lower than in cord serum, but higher than in later childhood (up to 10 ng/dL or 100 pg/mL), corresponding to the increased amounts of follitropin (FSH) and lutropin (LH) in infants at this time (2). During the first three days of life the percentage of free estradiol is very high, more than twice that of sexually mature women (3). These concentrations peak at about two months in females, but are markedly variable, with many values above the childhood range during the first six months.

In normal prepubertal children estradiol is less than 10 pg/mL, and is slightly higher in girls than in boys (3).

During puberty estradiol increases progressively in girls, in parallel with increases in gonadotropins, and continues to increase until menarche (4). Increases may begin as early as seven to eight years of age, but correlations with stage of puberty (Tanner), breast development, and bone age are better than with chronological age. In boys estradiol increases gradually, reaching adult values (about 30 pg/mL) at about 13 years of age (5).

In premature thelarche (early breast development) plasma estradiol may not be significantly greater than control values, but Radfar et al. (3) reported an increased percentage of free estradiol in nine of 11 children with this condition. Girls with true precocious puberty have total estradiol values corresponding to the stage of puberty (3). Because estradiol is very labile and concentrations are extremely low, blood for assay must be handled carefully. After being drawn, the specimen should be placed on ice without delay and centrifuged in the cold, and the plasma or serum frozen if the assay cannot be performed promptly.

1. Winter, J. S. D., Hughes, I. A., Reyes, F. I., and Faiman, C., Pituitary–gonadal relations in infancy: 2. Patterns of serum gonadal steroid concentrations in man from birth to two years of age. *J. Clin. Endocrinol. Metab.* **42,** 679–686 (1976).

2. Sizonenko, P. C., Endocrinology in preadolescents and adolescents. I. Hormonal changes during normal puberty. *Am. J. Dis. Child.* **132**, 704–712 (1978).
3. Radfar, N., Ansusingha, K., and Kenny, F. M., Circulating bound and free estradiol and estrone during normal growth and development and in premature thelarche and isosexual precocity. *J. Pediatr.* **89**, 719–723 (1976).
4. Lee, P. A., Xenakis, T., Winer, J., and Matsenbauch, S., Puberty in girls: Correlation of serum levels of gonadotropins, prolactin, androgens, estrogens, and progestins with physical changes. *J. Clin. Endocrinol. Metab.* **43**, 775–784 (1976).
5. Lee, P. A., and Migeon, C. J., Puberty in boys: Correlation of plasma levels of gonadotropins (LH, FSH), androgens (testosterone, androstenedione, dehydroepiandrosterone and its sulfate), estrogens (estrone and estradiol) and progestins (progesterone and 17-hydroxyprogesterone). *J. Clin. Endocrinol. Metab.* **41**, 556–562 (1975).

Ethosuximide (Zarontin)

Specimen Tested:

P, S.

Laboratories Reporting:

3.

Reference (Normal) Values:

Therapeutic range: All labs: 40–100 μg/mL (mg/L)
Toxic range: 150 μg/mL

Sources of Reference (Normal) Values:

Institutional.

Specimen Volume, Collection, and Preservation:

5 to 100 μL. Heparin anticoagulant. Specimen should not be grossly icteric, lipemic, or hemolyzed if the EMIT system is used. Store in FR, or 2 d in RR.

Analytical Method and Instrumentation:

Syva EMIT; Abbott ABA-100 Bichromatic Analyzer; GLC; modified method of Dukhuis, I. C., and Vervolet, E., *Pharm. Weekbl.* **109**, 1–4 (1974); Hewlett-Packard 5710A gas chromatograph with HP 3380A recording integrator; Damon-IEC 6000 centrifuge; Applied Science Mini-Aktor tubes; HPLC; Soldin, S. J., and Hill, J. G., A rapid micromethod for measuring anticonvulsant drugs in serum by high performance liquid chromatography. *Clin. Chem.* **22**, 856–859 (1976); Waters HPLC ALC/GPC-204/6000A, with a Perkin-Elmer LC Variable Wavelength spectrophotometer.

Commentary—Peter J. and Joan H. Howanitz

Ethosuximide is currently the drug of choice for treating "absence seizures" (petit mal). It is well absorbed from the gastrointestinal tract, with peak serum concentrations occurring within 3 to 7 h. Although ethosuximide as a syrup is absorbed faster than the capsular form, peak serum values occur at the same time after dosing (1). Whether ethosuximide is given in a single dose or in divided doses, steady-state serum concentrations and urinary excretion are equivalent (2). Protein-binding is negligible, and concentrations in serum, cerebrospinal fluid, and saliva are comparable (3). Although the half-life varies over a wide range in all groups studied, the half-life in children (about 30 h) is considerably less than in adults (about 60 h). In a small group of children, the half-life did not vary significantly within the age range of five to 15 years. In this study, serum half-life did not vary with dose, or with serum concentration (4). Ethosuximide is extensively metabolized in the liver, but apparently none of the metabolites are active.

Control of seizure activity generally is attained when serum concentrations exceed 40 μg/mL; however, there is poor correlation between dose and serum concentration (4). A therapeutic range of 40–100 μg/mL is commonly accepted (5,6), although ranges of 40–60 (2) and 40–70 μg/mL (7) have been suggested. In some patients with refractory seizures, concentrations as great as 150 μg/mL may prove useful (6). There is some evidence that ethosuximide concentrations in serum are age-dependent, with values attained for a given dose being higher in adults than in children. There are apparently no sex-related differences (6). Ethosuximide is well tolerated, and adverse reactions such as nausea do not necessarily correlate with serum concentrations.

Serum ethosuximide concentrations were monitored in a patient in the last trimester of pregnancy. Ethosuximide concentrations in cord blood and breast milk approximated those in the mother's serum. After delivery, despite constant dosage, concentrations in the mother's serum increased about 50% (6).

1. Buchanan, R. A., Fernandez, L., and Kinkel, A. W., Absorption and elimination of ethosuximide in children. *J. Clin. Pharmacol.* **9**, 393–398 (1969).
2. Goulet, J. R., Kinkel, A. W., and Smith, T. C., Metabolism of ethosuximide. *Clin. Pharmacol. Ther.* **20**, 213–218 (1976).
3. McAuliffe, J. J., Sherwin, A. L., Leppik, I. E., Fayle, S. A., and Pippenger, C. E., Salivary levels of anticonvulsants: A practical approach to drug monitoring. *Neurology* **27**, 409–413 (1977).
4. Browne, T. R., Dreifuss, F. E., Dyken, P. R., Goode, D. J., Penry, J. K., Porter, R. J., White, B. G., and White, P. T., Ethosuximide in the treatment of absence (petit mal) seizures. *Neurology* **25**, 515–524 (1975).
5. Kutt, H., and Penry, J. K., Usefulness of blood levels of antiepileptic drugs. *Arch. Neurol.* **31**, 283–288 (1974).
6. Sherwin, A. L., Clinical pharmacology of ethosuximide in antiepileptic drugs: Quantitative analysis and interpretation. In *Antiepileptic Drugs:*

Quantitative Analysis and Interpretation, C. E. Pippenger, J. K. Penry, and H. Kutt, Eds. Raven Press, New York, NY, 1978, pp 283–295.
7. Buchanan, R. A., Kinkel, A. W., Turner, J. L., and Heffelfinger, J. C., Ethosuximide dosage regimens. *Clin. Pharmacol. Ther.* **19**, 143–147 (1976).
8. Koup, J. R., Rose, J. Q., and Cohen, M. E., Ethosuximide pharmacokinetics in a pregnant patient and her newborn. *Epilepsia* **19**, 535–539 (1978).

Factor VIII-Related Antigen

Specimen Tested:

P.

Laboratory Reporting:

1.

Reference (Normal) Values:

Subjects	Factor VIII antigen, antigenic units/mL (95% confidence limits)	Mean ratio, F-VIII activity/ F-VIII antigen
"Normal," F	0.60–1.65	1.07
Carriers of Hemophilia A	0.52–2.70	0.35
von Willebrand's disease	0.20–0.62	1.01
Hemophilia-A patients	0.50–1.50	

Sources of Reference (Normal) Values:

Institutional; Bennett, B., and Ratnoff, O. D., Changes in anti-hemophilic factor (AHF, factor 8) procoagulant activity and AHF-like antigen in normal pregnancy and following exercise and pneumoencephalography. *J. Lab. Clin. Med.* **80**, 256–263 (1972).

Specimen Volume, Collection, and Preservation:

10 μL. Citrate anticoagulant. Use fresh plasma, or store in FR.

Analytical Method:

Electroimmunoassay; Laurell, C. B., Quantitative estimation of proteins by electrophoresis in agarose gel containing antibodies. *Anal. Biochem.* **15**, 45–52 (1966); Behring Diagnostics rabbit anti-human Factor VIII antiserum; lab-prepared antibody-containing agar plates.

Fat

Specimen Tested:

Feces.

Laboratories Reporting:

4.

Reference (Normal) Values:

< 2 yr: < 15% of fat intake[a]
> 2 yr: < 8.5% of fat intake; < 10%
 Child: < 5 g/d

[a] Generally calculated by the dietary department.

Sources of Reference (Normal) Values:

Institutional; Anderson, C. M., Intestinal malabsorption in children. *Arch. Dis. Child.* **41,** 571–596 (1966).

Specimen Volume, Collection, and Preservation:

Collect 72-h specimen in preweighed container (paint can). Store in RR.

Analytical Method:

Van deKamer, J. H., Huinink, H. T., and Weijers, H. A., Rapid method for the determination of fat in feces. *J. Biol. Chem.* **177,** 347–355 (1949); Amenta, J. S., A rapid extraction and quantification of total lipids and lipid fractions in blood and feces. *Clin. Chem.* **16,** 339–346 (1970).

Instrumentation:

Titration equipment, burette, for method of Van deKamer et al.; spectrophotometer for Amenta method.

Commentary—John F. Connelly and G. L. Barnes

The percentage of ingested fat excreted in feces varies with age *(1)* as follows:

Age	% excreted
Premature	up to 40
Newborn	up to 20
3 mo–1 yr	up to 15
1 yr	up to 8.5

Excreted fat is believed to originate from two common sources. Part is endogenous and largely represents the fat derived from desquamated mucosal cells. The rest of the fat excreted is exogenous and represents unabsorbed dietary fat; this fat is altered somewhat by bacteria.

The differences observed in fat excretion for children younger than one year can be attributed to increased desquamation of mucosal cells, but a more likely explanation is a relative impairment of absorption of exogenous fats. Premature infants may have a bile salt concentration in the small bowel that is less than the cortical micellar concentration, resulting in "physiological" fat malabsorption. Other possibilities can account for the increased excretion, but the exact explanation is unknown *(2,3)*.

Because interpretation of results in children requires calculation of percentage absorption, a detailed knowledge of fat intake during the test is necessary. An oral marker should be used to identify the beginning and end of the stool collections.

1. Weijers, H. A., and Van deKamer, J. H., Coeliac disease. 1. Criticism of the various methods of investigation. *Acta Paediatr. Scand.* **42,** 24–33 (1953).
2. The origin of foecal fat. *Lancet* **ii,** 627–628 (1969). Editorial.
3. Grand, R. J., Watkins, J. B., and Tarti, F. M., Development of the human gastrointestinal tract. A review. *Gastroenterology* **70,** 790–810 (1976).

Fatty Acids, Free and Total Esterified

Specimen Tested:

P, erythrocytes.

Laboratories Reporting:

2.

Reference (Normal) Values:

	Plasma "free" fatty acids, μmol/L	
	Lab. 1	**Lab. 2**[a]
Newborn	435–1375	
Infant		1015–1225
4 mo–10 yr	500–900 (14-h fast)	
	730–1200 (19-h fast)	
Child		580–920
Adult	310–590 (14-h fast)	
	405–720 (19-h fast)	

[a] Average of triplicate determinations.

	Total esterified fatty acids (fasting; Lab. 1)			
Fatty acid[a]	**Plasma**		**Erythrocytes**	
	mg/dL	**% of total**	**mg/dL**	**% of total**
16:0	29.4–55.8	20.7–28.3	24.8–49.0	18.5–28.3
16:1	1.4–6.8	1.1–3.5	0.0–9.4	0.0–4.9
18:0	11.2–28.6	6.9–16.1	13.7–47.3	13.1–26.5
18:1	21.9–51.1	16.9–24.5	11.6–46.8	12.7–23.3
18:2	24.5–78.5	19.5–39.1	0.7–47.9	6.1–22.1
20:3	0.0–8.0	0.0–4.9	0.8–7.6	0.8–4.4
20:4	5.5–26.9	3.2–15.6	14.2–46.2	12.5–26.3
Total	125–235		123–205	

[a] No. of carbons:degree of unsaturation.

Sources of Reference (Normal) Values:

Institutional (both labs.); Persson, B., and Gentz, J., The pattern of blood lipids, glycerol and ketone bodies during the neonatal period, infancy and childhood. *Acta Paediatr. Scand.* **55,** 353–362 (1966); Ways, P., and Hanahan, D. J., Characterization and quantification of red blood cell lipids in normal man. *J. Lipid Res.* **5,** 318–328 (1964).

Specimen Volume, Collection, and Preservation; Patient Preparation:

200 to 300 μL. EDTA (**Lab. 1**); collect blood without stasis into chilled heparinized plastic tubes (**Lab. 2**). Separate plasma from cells by using a refrigerated centrifuge (4 °C). Store in FR. For erythrocytes, wash cells immediately before storage. Patients must fast 10, 14, or 19 h (see reference values above).

Analytical Method:

Lab. 1: GLC; Ways and Hanahan, *op. cit.* **Lab. 2:** colorimetric; Novak, M., Colorimetric ultramicro method for the determination of free fatty acids. *J. Lipid Res.* **6,** 431–433 (1975).

Instrumentation:

Lab. 1: Perkin-Elmer 900 gas chromatograph. **Lab. 2:** Zeiss spectrophotometer.

Alpha-Fetoprotein

Specimen Tested:

S.

Laboratory Reporting:

1.

Reference (Normal) Values:

During the first 20 h postpartum, concentrations decrease from 10 to 2 mg/dL. By 2 wk of age, the concentration has decreased to 0.6 mg/dL. The half-life of α-fetoprotein is 5 d; therefore, the persistence of a tumor-related increase in plasma concentration for more than 25 d after surgery suggests incomplete tumor removal.

Sources of Reference (Normal) Values:

Karlsson, B. W., Bergstrand, C. G., Ekelund, H., and Lindberg, T., Postnatal changes of alpha-fetoprotein, albumin and total protein in human serum. *Acta Paediatr. Scand.* **61,** 133–139 (1972).

Specimen Volume:

1 mL.

Analytical Method:

RIA; Abbott α-Fetoprotein Kit.

Commentary—Leonard K. Dunikoski, Jr.

α-Fetoprotein (AFP) is a glycoprotein synthesized in the fetus by embryonic liver, yolk sac, and gastrointestinal tissues. Highest concentrations in serum occur during the 10th to 14th weeks of fetal life, and decline thereafter. Adult serum concentrations ($<$ 200 ng/dL) are reached after two years of life.

Earlier methods (immunodiffusion, counter immunoelectrophoresis) have been replaced by RIA procedures with sensitivities of 2 to 10 ng/mL. Serum AFP values determined by this procedure have been used to help in the diagnosis, prognosis, and monitoring of malignancy in adult patients. High adult serum AFP concentrations occur in primary liver carcinoma and malignant gonadal teratoma, and less frequently in other carcinomas and some noncancerous diseases (hepatitis, cirrhosis). In pediatric patients, persistance of AFP may indicate active liver disease, but some apparently healthy patients less than two years old also have very high concentrations. Cord blood AFP values are being evaluated to differentiate transient tyrosine increases from tyrosinemia (1). Serum AFP values in infants less than four months old may be useful to distinguish neonatal hepatitis from biliary atresia (1).

1. Hamilton, R., Liver function tests. In text ref. *17*, 11th ed., pp 1144–1147.

Note: Also see Chapter 10, **Specific Proteins in Pediatrics.**

Fibrinogen

Specimen Tested:

P.

Laboratories Reporting:

2.

Reference (Normal) Values:

Child–Adult: **Lab. 1:** 200–400 mg/dL (2.0–4.0 g/L)
                     Lab. 2: 200–500 mg/dL (2.0–5.0 g/L)

Sources of Reference (Normal) Values:

Institutional; Hemker, H. C., Loeliger, E. A., and Veltkamp, J. J., *Human Blood Coagulation.* Springer-Verlag, New York, NY, 1969, p 187.

Specimen Volume, Collection, and Preservation:

Lab 1: 0.8 mL. Collect blood into 38 g/L sodium citrate. Keep on ice until assayed. **Lab. 2:** 200 µL. Heparin anticoagulant. Fibrinogen is claimed to have a stability of 7 d at RT, and 4 wk in RR.

Analytical Method:

Lab. 1: Clauss, A., Gerinnungsphysiologische Schnellmethode zur Bestimmung des Fibrinogens. *Acta Haematol.* **17,** 237–246 (1957), cited in L. A. Harker, *Hemostasis Manual,* 2nd ed. F. A. Davis Co., Philadelphia, PA, 1974, p 62. **Lab. 2:** Campbell, W. R., and Hanna, M. I., The albumin, globulins and fibrinogen of serum and plasma. *J. Biol. Chem.* **199,** 15 (1937); Goodwin, J. F., Estimation of plasma fibrinogen using sodium sulfite fractionation. *Am. J. Clin. Pathol.* **35,** 227–232 (1961).

Instrumentation:

Lab. 1: Bioquest Fibrometer. **Lab. 2:** Beckman 25 spectrophotometer.

Commentary—Leonard K. Dunikoski, Jr.

Fibrinogen (Factor I) is a plasma protein essential for hemostasis (coagulation). Synthesized in hepatic parenchymal cells, it has a relative molecular mass of 340 000 and a plasma half-life of three to five days. Fibrinogen is split by thrombin into a fibrin monomer, polypeptides A and B, and a carbohydrate moiety. The fibrin monomers then polymerize to form a fibrin gel clot, which is further strengthened by subsequent polymer cross-linking. Because fibrinogen is consumed in the formation of a clot, plasma is used for quantitation.

Although immunochemical procedures for quantitation of fibrinogen are available, they are generally too slow to be used in a hospital laboratory, where "stat" quantitation and qualitative evaluation are often requested. Newer automated nephelometers may make rapid immunoquantitation possible but may not detect functionally abnormal fibrinogens (dysfibrinogens). Alternatively, chromogenic and (or) fluorogenic substrates may soon offer new functional methods of measuring this important protein.

For most laboratories, fibrinogen evaluation will consist of a procedure based on the time required for thrombin to produce a clot from plasma containing fibrinogen (thrombin time determination). Specimens for such clotting procedures must be obtained cleanly to avoid hemolysis or contamination from tissue juices, which might activate the clotting process. Nine volumes of blood are added rapidly to one volume of sodium citrate (109 mmol/L) and mixed by gentle inversion, avoiding foaming or excessive turbulence. Because heparin affects the test results, blood samples should not be obtained from an intravenous line that contained heparin. For the assay procedure itself, use of an automatic electronic timer such as the Fibrometer (Baltimore Biological Labs.) improves the precision of the test procedure *(1).*

The minimum concentration of functional fibrinogen required to maintain hemostasis is 50–100 mg/dL. Lower values may be related to congenital deficiencies (afibrinogenemia, dysfibrinogenemia) or acquired deficiencies (liver disease, intravascular coagulation, fibrinolysis). In the newborn, disseminated intravascular coagulation (DIC) has been associated with hypoxia (respiratory distress syndrome), obstetrical conditions (eclampsia, abruptio placentae), infectious diseases (bacterial septicemia), and ischemic necrosis (cardiovascular collapse) *(2)*. Severe DIC in the newborn is frequently associated with a generalized bleeding tendency and a very high mortality rate; some authors feel that severe DIC in newborn infants is due primarily to cardiovascular collapse *(3)*.

1. Okuno, T., and Selenko, V., Plasma fibrinogen determination by automated thrombin time. *Am. J. Med. Technol.* **38,** 196–201 (1972).
2. Corrigan, J. J., Jr., Activation of coagulation and disseminated intravascular coagulation in the newborn. *Am. J. Pediatr. Hematol./Oncol.* **1,** 245–249 (1979).
3. Zipursky, A., Johnston, M., DeSa, D., Milner, R., and Hsu, E., Clinical and laboratory diagnosis of hemostatic disorders in newborn infants. *Am. J. Pediatr. Hematol./Oncol.* **1,** 217–226 (1979).

Note: Also see Chapter 10, **Specific Proteins in Pediatrics.**

Folic Acid, Folate

Specimen Tested:

S.

Laboratory Reporting:

1.

Reference (Normal) Values:

Child–adult: 1.9–14.0 ng/mL (4.3–23.6 nmol/L)

Sources of Reference (Normal) Values:

Institutional.

Specimen Volume, Collection, and Preservation:

100 μL. Serum should be removed from clot immediately, with refrigerated centrifuge. If the serum is analyzed within 3 to 4 h after collection of blood, it may be stored in RR; otherwise, store in FR.

Analytical Method:

Radioassay with ^{125}I-labeled folic acid; Bio-Rad kit.

Instrumentation:

Sorval RC-3 centrifuge; Packard liquid scintillation counter.

Galactokinase, Erythrocyte
(EC 2.7.1.6; ATP:D-galactose 1-phosphotransferase)

Specimen Tested:

B.

Laboratory Reporting:

1.

Reference (Normal) Values:

1–6 mo: 0.44–1.25 arbitrary units
6–12 mo: 0.26–0.94
> 12 mo: 0.18–0.47

Sources of Reference (Normal) Values:

Ng, W. G., Donnell, G. N., and Bergren, W. R., Galactokinase activity in human erythrocytes of individuals at different ages. *J. Lab. Clin. Med.* **66,** 115–121 (1965); Donnell, G. N., Ng, W. G., Hodgman, J. E., and Bergren, W. R., Galactose metabolism in the newborn infant. *Pediatrics* **39,** 829–837 (1967).

Specimen Volume, Collection, and Preservation:

3 mL. Heparin anticoagulant. Preferable to run enzyme assay on day of collection, though there is a claim that the enzyme is stable at RT for 2 to 3 d.

Analytical Method:

Radioisotope method of Ng et al., *op. cit.* This procedure has been modified by a number of investigators; one of the most recent is: Stocchi, V., Dacha, M., Bossu, M., and Fornaini, G., Modification of the radioactive method for erythrocyte galactokinase assay. *Clin. Chim. Acta* **89,** 371–374 (1978).

Enzyme Data:

1. Enzyme unit definition: 1 arbitrary unit = 1 μmol of substrate utilized per hour per milliliter of packed erythrocytes.
2. Buffer, pH: Tris·HCl, 7.0.
3. Substrate: [^{14}C]galactose, ATP.
4. Reaction temperature: 37 °C
5. Temperature reported: 37 °C.

Instrumentation:

Searle Analytical liquid scintillation counter; Whatman DE 81 (ion-exchange paper chromatography).

Note: A *Philadelphia* variant of galatokinase has been described: Tedesco, T. A., Miller, K. L., Rawnsley, B. E., Adams, M. C., Markus, H. B., Orkwiszewski, K. G., and Mellman, W. J., The Philadelphia variant of galactokinase. *Am. J. Hum. Genet.* **29,** 240–247 (1977).

Commentary—Michael A. Pesce

The enzyme galactokinase phosphorylates galactose to galactose 1-phosphate. Galactokinase deficiency is a rare inborn error of galactose metabolism, the only clinical symptom of which is cataracts. None of the severe symptoms (failure to thrive, jaundice, liver damage, and mental retardation) usually associated with hexose-1-phosphate uridylyltransferase (EC 2.7.7.12) deficiency are observed. In galactokinase deficiency, abnormal amounts of galactose and galactitol are found in urine, and concentrations of galactose are increased in serum. Erythrocytes contain normal amounts of galactose 1-phosphate and hexose-1-phosphate uridylyltransferase, but the enzyme galactokinase is absent. The diagnosis of galactokinase deficiency is based on the measurement of galactokinase in erythrocytes.

Galactokinase activity in erythrocytes is usually determined by a radioisotopic procedure involving [1-^{14}C]galactose and adenosine triphosphate. The [1-^{14}C]galactose 1-phosphate formed is separated from the [1-^{14}C]galactose and related to the galactokinase activity. Galactokinase activity is about three times higher in newborns than in adults *(1),* gradually decreasing to adult values by three to six years of age.

1. Ng, W. G., Donnell, G. N., and Bergren, W. R., Galactokinase activity in human erythrocytes in individuals at different ages. *J. Lab. Clin. Med.* **66,** 115–121 (1965).

Galactose

Specimen Tested:

P, S.

Laboratories Reporting:

2.

Reference (Normal) Values:

Lab. 1: 0–0.5 mg/dL (0–0.03 mmol/L)
Lab. 2: 1.1–2.1 (0.061–0.12)

Sources of Reference (Normal) Values:

Institutional.

Specimen Volume, Collection, and Preservation; Patient Preparation:

50 to 100 μL. Blood is collected into heparinized tubes. Galactose is stable in P for at least 4 d in FR. Galactose is usually not present in the plasma of normal individuals, but can be found in the plasma of transferase-deficient and galactokinase-deficient individuals if the blood is obtained soon after the individual has ingested milk.

Analytical Method:

Lab. 1: Enzymic, with galactose dehydrogenase and NAD^+: Grenier, A., and Luberge, C., Rapid method for screening for galactosemia and galactokinase deficiency by measuring galactose in whole blood spotted on paper. *Clin. Chem.* **9**, 463–465 (1973). **Lab. 2:** Enzymic: Roth, H., Segal, S., and Bertoli, D., The quantitative determination of galactose—an enzymic method using galactose oxidase with applications to blood and other biological fluids. *Anal. Biochem.* **10**, 32–52 (1965); Worthington Diagnostics Galactostat Reagent Set.

Instrumentation:

Lab 1: Union Carbide CentrifiChem. **Lab. 2:** Zeiss spectrophotometer.

Commentary—Michael A. Pesce

Galactose is usually absent, or present in trace amounts, in the serum of normal individuals. High concentrations are observed in galactokinase deficiency because galactose cannot be metabolized to galactose 1-phosphate. In children deficient in hexose-1-phosphate uridylyltransferase (HPU; EC 2.7.7.12), normal or high serum galactose values may be observed *(1)*. Children with this disorder may have normal values, either because galactose is rapidly metabolized to galactose 1-phosphate by the enzyme galactokinase (if the blood was drawn several hours after the child had consumed galactose-containing foods) or because the child is on intravenous feedings and not receiving galactose-containing foods. High serum galactose concentrations are found in HPU-deficient children if the blood is drawn soon after the ingestion of milk or other galactose-containing foods.

Galactose concentrations in serum should not be used to diagnose HPU-deficient galactosemia because the results depend on diet and rate of metabolism. However, if the concentration of galactose in serum is high, the possibility of galactokinase or HPU deficiency must be considered.

1. Pesce, M. A., Pitfalls in the diagnosis of transferase deficient galactosemia. *Lab. Manage.* **7**, 27–33 (1979).

Galactose 1-Phosphate

Specimen Tested:

Erythrocytes.

Laboratories Reporting.

3.

Reference (Normal) Values:

Non-galactosemic infant–adult: all three labs report < 1 mg/dL of erythrocytes (Lab. 1 reports a mean of 27 μg/g of hemoglobin with a range of 5–49 μg/g, corresponding to a range of 0.11–1.6 mg/dL of erythrocytes);[a] values slightly higher in cord blood

Galactosemic (transferase-deficient) individuals on galactose- (and lactose-) restricted diet:

Lab. 1: < 4.0 mg/dL of erythrocytes, or 80–125 μg/g of hemoglobin

Lab. 2: 1–5 mg/dL

Lab. 3: < 2 mg/dL

Galactosemic (transferase-deficient) individuals on unrestricted diet:

Lab. 1: > 4.0 mg/dL of erythrocytes, or > 125 μg/g of hemoglobin

Lab. 2: Up to 135 mg/dL[b]

Lab. 3: 9–20 mg/dL

Infants of Duarte-galactosemia-component heterozygotes: Up to 33 mg/dL[b]

Infants of low transferase activity variant: Up to 86 mg/dL[b]

[a] Based on a study of 25 children, fasting 8–12 h, at Babies' Hospital. See Pesce and Bodourian, cited below. [b] Ng, W. G., unpublished data.

Sources of Reference (Normal) Values:

Lab. 1: institutional; Pesce, M. A., and Bodourian, S. H., A new method for measuring galactose-1-phosphate in erythrocytes. *Clin. Chem.* **23**, 1166 (1977), abstract. **Lab. 2:** Donnell, G. N., Bergren, W. R., Perry, G., and Koch, R., *Pediatrics* **31**, 802–810 (1963); Donnell, G. N., Bergren, W. R., and Ng, W. G., Galactosemia. *Biochem. Med.* **1**, 29–53 (1967); Ng, W. R., unpublished data. **Lab. 3:** institutional.

Specimen Volume, Collection, and Preservation;
Patient Preparation:

1 to 4 mL of B. Heparin anticoagulant only. Cool B in an ice bath. Separate and wash erythrocytes immediately. Galactose 1-phosphate is stable in erythrocytes for 9 d in RR or FR. Patient should *not* be fasting to detect galactosemia.

Analytical Method:

Lab. 1: Pesce and Bodourian, *op. cit.;* a fluorometric micromethod to be published soon. **Lab. 2:** Gitzelman, R., Estimation of galactose-1-phosphate in erythrocytes: A rapid and simple enzymatic method. *Clin. Chim. Acta* **26**, 313–316 (1969). **Lab. 3:** Kirkman, H. N., and

Maxwell, E. S., Enzymatic estimation of erythrocyte galactose-1-phosphate. *J. Lab. Clin. Med.* **56,** 161–166 (1960).

Instrumentation:

Lab. 1: Farrand Mark 1 spectrofluorometer. **Lab. 2:** Gilford spectrophotometer. **Lab. 3:** Beckman 25 K spectrophotometer.

Commentary—Michael A. Pesce

Galactose 1-phosphate is formed by the phosphorylation of galactose, which is catalyzed by the enzyme galactokinase. High concentrations of galactose 1-phosphate in erythrocytes are found in cases of uridine diphosphate galactose 4-epimerase (EC 5.1.3.2) deficiency *(1)* and in hexose-1-phosphate uridylyltransferase (HPU; EC 2.7.7.12) deficiency. Uridine diphosphate galactose 4-epimerase converts uridine diphosphogalactose to uridine diphosphoglucose. Patients with erythrocyte uridine diphosphate galactose 4-epimerase deficiency are asymptomatic because epimerase activity is found in the liver, skin fibroblasts, and lymphocytes of these children. In HPU deficiency, galactose 1-phosphate cannot be metabolized and accumulates in the liver, brain, lens, and erythrocytes of affected individuals. Galactose 1-phosphate may be the toxic substance that causes many of the clinical complications associated with this disorder.

When a diagnosis of HPU deficiency is confirmed, a galactose-restricted diet is immediately initiated. After several days of this diet, the individual's concentration of erythrocyte galactose 1-phosphate decreases and must be monitored frequently, to determine whether the patient is following the diet. Galactose 1-phosphate concentrations in children with normal HPU activity are about 40 μg/g of hemoglobin *(2)*. In HPU-deficient children who are adhering to their galactose-restricted diet, galactose 1-phosphate is usually about 100 μg/g of hemoglobin. Galactose 1-phosphate exceeding 110 μg/g of hemoglobin indicates that the HPU-deficient patient is consuming galactose-containing foods.

Measurement of galactose 1-phosphate in erythrocytes is difficult because of the small amount present. Recently, a new fluorometric assay for measuring galactose 1-phosphate was introduced *(3)*, in which blood obtained from microhematocrit tubes is centrifuged, lysed with water, and immediately deproteinized by boiling. An aliquot of protein-free supernate is mixed with a reagent consisting of NADP$^+$, uridine diphosphoglucose, and the enzymes HPU (obtained from calf liver), glucose-6-phosphate dehydrogenase, phosphoglucomutase, and phosphogluconate dehydrogenase. The NADPH formed is measured fluorometrically and related to the amount of galactose 1-phosphate in the sample. The method is fairly sensitive, 2 mol of NADPH being formed per mole of galactose 1-phosphate.

With this assay, galactose 1-phosphate can be measured in blood obtained by skin puncture. Galactose 1-phosphate is stable in erythrocytes for nine days if stored at $-20\ °C$.

1. Gitzelman, R., Steinmann, B., Mitchell, B., and Haigos, E., Uridine diphosphate galactose 4-epimerase deficiency. *Helv. Paediatr. Acta* **31**, 441–452 (1976).
2. Pesce, M. A., Pitfalls in the diagnosis of transferase-deficient galactosemia. *Lab. Manage.* **7**, 27–33 (1979).
3. Pesce, M. A., and Bodourian, S. H., A new method for measuring galactose-1-phosphate in erythrocytes. *Clin. Chem.* **23**, 1166 (1977). Abstract.

Alpha-D-Galactosidase (EC 3.2.1.22;
α-D-galactoside galactohydrolase),
Beta-D-Galactosidase (EC 3.2.1.23;
β-D-galactoside galactohydrolase)

Specimen Tested:

Leukocytes.

Laboratory Reporting:

1.

Reference (Normal) Values:

	Arbitrary units	
	α-D-Galactosidase	β-D-Galactosidase
Range:	42–108.3	163.3–395.8
Mean ± 2SD:	33.0– 98.2	114.9–376.5

Sources of Reference (Normal) Values:

Institutional; D. A. Applegarth (see list of **Contributors**).

Specimen Volume, Collection, and Preservation:

10 mL of heparinized B. Keep B on ice and prepare leukocyte pellets without delay.

Note: See discussion on leukocyte preparation in **Appendix 4.**

Analytical Method:

Measure 4-methylumbelliferone (4-MU) released from 4-MU-α (or β)-D-galactopyranoside.

Enzyme Data:

1. Enzyme unit definition: 1 arbitrary unit = the amount of enzyme that cleaves 1 nmol of 4-MU-α-, or 4-MU-β-D-galactopyranoside per hour per milligram of protein at 37 °C.

2. Buffer, pH: α-D-galactosidase: 0.2 mol/L acetate, 4.5; β-D-galactosidase: citrate–phosphate, 4.3.
3. Substrate, pH: α-D-galactosidase: 4-MU-α-D-galactopyranoside, 4.5; β-D-galactosidase: 4-MU-β-D-galactopyranoside, 4.3.
4. Reaction temperature: 37 °C.
5. Temperature reported: 37 °C.

Gastric Analysis

Specimen Tested:

Gastric fluid.

Laboratory Reporting:

1.

Reference (Normal) Values:

Free HCl,	without stimulation:	0–40 mmol/L
	after alcohol:	10–90
	after histamine or Histalog (Lilly):	10–130
Total acid,	without stimulation:	10–60

Sources of Reference (Normal) Values:

Text ref. *5;* Cannon, D. C., Examination of gastric and duodenal contents. In text ref. *18,* 14th ed., 1969, pp 762–780.

Analytical Method:

See references above.

Commentary—K. W. Schmitt

The secreting activity of the fundic glands within the stomach can be assessed in several ways. One important measurement is gastric acid production of parietal cells. These cells first appear in the mucosal lining of the stomach in the fourth fetal month. A close relationship exists between the parietal cell mass and the mucosal volume. Mucosal volume is directly related to the size of the stomach and to body weight. The following figures for acid output indicate that this relationship does not hold true for infants younger than three months:

(a) Mean acid output at birth, 0.15 mEq/10 kg per hour (1 mEq = 1 mmol).

(b) Mean acid output at one month, 0.31 mEq/10 kg per hour.

(c) Mean acid output at three months, 1.22 mEq/10 kg per hour.

(d) Range of acid output in the adult, 1.02–2.71 mEq/10 kg per hour.

The secretory activity of the fundic glands at birth is low. There is a high acid output within the first 48 h, followed by a progressive increase in acid output during the first two to three weeks of postnatal life. A transient decrease occurs at one month of age, with a subsequent steady increase lasting to about three months of age:

Age	Mean vol, mL/h	Mean titratable acid, mEq/L	Mean HCl output, mEq/h
1 d	3.3	8.1	0.03
3–8 d	3.7	14.4	0.06
10–11 d	4.0	34.4	0.12
14–17 d	6.4	26.7	0.19
25–32 d	3.1	26.4	0.08
67–110 d	13.4	34.8	0.47
4–7 yr	42.5	114.8	4.88
Adult	143.2	91.2	13.06

The buffering capacity of amniotic fluid ingested by the fetus could account for the low acid values observed in the newborn. The increase in gastric acid shortly after birth and the continuing increase for two to three weeks thereafter could result from having had a stimulating hormone, such as gastrin, from the mother cross the placenta and stimulate acid output as well as growth and development of the fundic glands.

Acid output in the premature infant is much less than in the full-term newborn infant, and remains lower for the first few weeks after birth.

Because the total volume of secretory fluid produced by an infant is low, care must be taken to aspirate a *complete* sample. A few milliliters left in the stomach will represent a large percentage error *(1,2)*.

1. Avery, G. B., Randolph, J. G., and Weaver, T., Gastric response to specific disease in infants. *Pediatrics* **38,** 874–878 (1966).
2. Agunod, M., Yamaguchi, N., Lopez, R., Luhby, A., and Glass, G. B. J., Correlative study of hydrochloric acid, pepsin, and intrinsic factor secretion in newborns and infants. *Am. J. Dig. Dis.* **14,** 400–414 (1969).

Gastrin

Specimen Tested:

S.

Laboratory Reporting:

1.

Reference (Normal) Values:

Normal: < 300 pg/mL
Nondefinitive: 300–500 pg/mL
> 500 pg/mL is indicative of pernicious anemia or the Zollinger–Ellison syndrome.

Sources of Reference (Normal) Values:

Text ref. *1.*

Volume and Source of Specimen:

2 mL; venous.

Analytical Method:

Yalow, R. S., and Berson, S. A., Radioimmunoassay of gastrin. *Gastroenterology* **58,** 1–14 (1970); Hansky, J., and Cain, M. D., Radioimmunoassay of gastrin in human serum. *Lancet* **ii,** 1388–1390 (1969).

Instrumentation:

Nuclear Chicago Model 4216 liquid scintillation gamma counter.

Commentary—Claude C. Roy

The antral hormone, gastrin, is the most potent agent for the stimulation of gastric acid secretion. Secreted by G-cells of the antrum, gastrin plays a crucial role in the regulation of acid secretion in humans *(1).* Normally, there is a close interdependency of serum gastrin and gastric HCl. Variable degrees of escape from the negative-feedback inhibition of gastrin secretion by gastric acid is seen in various conditions. In the Zollinger–Ellison syndrome associated with gastrinomas, there is severe hypergastrinemia despite massive acid hypersecretion. A lesser degree of escape occurs in antral G-cell hyperplasia, in duodenal ulcers with a large parietal cell mass, in long-standing pyloric obstruction, in some patients with renal failure, and during the first few months after massive resection of the small intestine. Hypergastrinemia is reported in patients with endocrinopathies such as hyperparathyroidism and multiple endocrine neoplasia type I, as well as in rare cases of type II, pheochromocytoma, and neurofibromatosis. Because of a lack of a parietal cell mass capable of secreting HCl, hypergastrinemia is regularly seen in achlorhydric subjects who have primary pernicious anemia or atrophic gastritis with a spared antrum.

Acid is not the only inhibitor of gastrin secretion; gastrointestinal hormones such as secretin, gastric inhibitory peptide, vasoactive peptide, glucagon, and calcitonin also play a role. Besides vagal stimulation, other stimuli of gastrin release include peptides, amino acids, coffee grains, and ethanol. The most effective bloodborne stimulant is calcium; consequently, the calcium infusion test (calcium gluconate: 5 mg of Ca^{++}/kg per hour for 3 h) is widely used in subjects with the Zollinger–Ellison syndrome in whom gastrin concentrations may be equivocal.

There are still few studies in the pediatric age group. Hypergastrinemia is present in cord blood (2) and is of fetal origin, because gastrin concentrations are higher than in the mother's blood (3). Continuous basal acid secretory studies have demonstrated hyposecretion of gastric acid for the first 5 h of life (4), with normal gastric acid secretion subsequently. Fasting serum gastrin concentrations in normal infants and children are similar to those in adults (5). Values tend to be higher during the first three years of life than in older children. The prolonged postprandial increase of serum gastrin seen in adults also occurs in children (5). Both normal and high gastrin values have been reported in congenital hypertrophic pyloric stenosis. However, the possibility that high gastrin concentrations in cord serum is implicated as a pathogenic factor has been dismissed (6). Gastrin concentrations are usually normal in children with primary gastric ulcers, or in those with secondary ulcers associated with sepsis, trauma, and shock. The deeply penetrating ulcers seen after neurosurgical procedures or intracranial trauma may be accompanied by hypergastrinemia. Studies in children with duodenal ulcers show higher gastric acid secretion in response to Histalog (7), but gastrin concentrations have not been reported for many of these patients. The main indication for the measurement of gastrin in children with peptic disease is suspicion of a Zollinger–Ellison syndrome in cases with a strong family history of duodenal ulcers resistent to medical management, and whenever hypercalcemia is present. The calcium-infusion test has been successfully used to document gastrinomas in children (8).

RIA is sufficiently sensitive and precise to permit measurement of changes in gastrin under physiologic conditions. Although all assays are based on inhibition of the reaction between labeled gastrin and gastrin antibodies, gastrin values vary between laboratories. Consequently, it is important to know the values obtained in fasting normal subjects for any RIA before values in patients can be interpreted.

1. Walsh, J. H., and Grossman, M. I., Gastrin. *N. Engl. J. Med.* **292,** 1324–1334, 1377–1384 (1975).
2. Rogers, I. M., Davidson, D. C., Lawrence, J., Ardill, J., and Buchanan, K. D., Neonatal secretion of gastrin and glucagon. *Arch. Dis. Child.* **49,** 796–801 (1974).
3. von Berger, L., Henrichs, I., Raptis, S., Heinze, E., Jonatha, W., Teller, W. M., and Pfeiffer, E. F., Gastrin concentration in plasma of the neonate at birth and after the first feeding. *Pediatrics* **58,** 264–267 (1976).
4. Euler, A. R., Byrne, W. J., Cousins, L. M., Ament, M. E., Leake, R. D., and Walsh, J. H., Increased serum gastrin concentrations and gastric

hyposecretion in the immediate newborn period. *Gastroenterology* **72,** 1271–1273 (1977).
5. Janik, J. S., Akbar, A. M., Burrington, J. D., and Burke, G., Serum gastrin levels in infants and children. *Pediatrics* **60,** 60–64 (1976).
6. Werlin, S. L., Grand, R. J., and Drum, D. E., Congenital hypertrophic pyloric stenosis: The role of gastrin reevaluated. *Pediatrics* **61,** 883–885 (1977).
7. Christie, D. L., and Ament, M. E., Gastric acid hypersecretion in children with duodenal ulcer. *Gastroenterology* **71,** 242–244 (1976).
8. Garcia, J. C., Carney, J. A., Stickler, G. B., Telander, R. L., and Malagelada, J. R., Zollinger–Ellison syndrome and neurofibromatosis in a 13 year old boy. *J. Pediatr.* **93,** 982–984 (1978).

Gentamicin

Specimen Tested:

S.

Laboratory Reporting:

1.

Reference (Normal) Values:

Therapeutic values: Peak serum concentration should be maintained above 4 mg/L (μg/mL), to exceed minimal inhibitory concentration for most Gram-negative bacilli. Concentrations above 12 mg/L, however, are associated with irreversible ototoxicity. The trough value should be kept below 2 mg/L to avoid nephrotoxicity.

Sources of Reference (Normal) Values:

Noone, P., Parsons, T. M. C., Pattison, J. R., Slack, R. C. B., Garfield-Davies, D., and Hughes, K., Experience in monitoring gentamicin therapy during treatment of serious Gram-negative sepsis. *Br. Med. J.* **i,** 477–481 (1974); Dahlgren, J. G., Anderson, E. T., and Hewitt, W. L., Gentamicin blood levels: A guide to nephrotoxicity. *Antimicrob. Agents Chemother.* **8,** 58–62 (1972); Schentag, J. J., Jusko, W. J., Plaut, M. E., Cumbo, T. J., Vance, J. W., and Abrutyn, E., Tissue persistence of gentamicin in man. *J. Am. Med. Assoc.* **238,** 327–329 (1977).

Specimen Volume, Collection, and Preservation; Patient Preparation:

0.5 to 1 mL. Gentamicin is stable for 7 d when stored in RR. Do not use grossly lipemic or hemolyzed specimens. Samples for determining trough values should be drawn just before the next dose. Peak blood readings should be taken 8 h after initiating intravenous infusion, 1 h after intramuscular administration, and 1 h after a rapid intravenous bolus. Steady-state peak serum concentrations should be reached within one day. In renal failure a much longer time may be required to reach equilibrium, depending on the severity of disease. During chronic treatment, the drug accumulates gradually in the kidney, as reflected by a slow increase in the trough value over a period of many days. Because this may lead to nephrotoxicity, continuous monitoring of the trough value of gentamicin, and of renal function, is advisable.

Analytical Method and Instrumentation:

RIA; Lewis, J. E., Nelson, J. C., and Elder, H. A., Radioimmunoassay of an antibiotic: Gentamicin. *Nature (New Biol.)* **239,** 214–216 (1972); Science Corporation Monitor Science kit; Searle 1185 gamma counter.

Globin-Chain Electrophoresis

Specimen Tested:

B.

Laboratory Reporting:

1.

Reference (Normal) Values:

Alkaline globin-chain electrophoresis (pH 8.9): Beta-A and gamma-A chains migrate to the same position near the positive pole, while alpha-A chains migrate to the negative pole.

Acid globin-chain electrophoresis (pH 6.0): Beta-A and gamma-A chains migrate to the positive pole but to different positions, while alpha-A chains migrate to the negative pole.

Sources of Reference (Normal) Values:

International Committee for Standardization in Hematology, Simple electrophoretic system for presumptive identification of abnormal hemoglobins. *Blood* **52,** 1058–1064 (1978); *ibid.,* p 1065.

Specimen Volume, Collection, and Preservation:

2 mL. Heparin or EDTA anticoagulant. Store in RR.

Analytical Method:

As in reference cited above. Buffers: urea/2-mercaptoethanol, pH 8.9, and urea/2-mercaptoethanol, pH 6.0. This method separates normal alpha and beta chains as well as abnormal globin chains. Comparison with nonvariants applied to the same strip or plate permits presumptive identification of the mutant chain. For quality control, include with each assay a hemolysate containing hemoglobins J, A, F, S, and C.

Instrumentation:

Helena Labs. Zip-Zone electrophoresis apparatus.

Commentary—Schlomo Friedman

Globin Synthesis

The synthesis of polypeptide globin chains is measured in vitro in intact reticulocytes. A radioactive amino acid, such as [^{14}C]leucine, is gently mixed with freshly drawn heparinized whole blood and 8 mg of dextrose for 2 h at 37 °C. Heme is removed with acid acetone, and globin is separated into beta and alpha chains by chromatography on carboxymethyl cellulose (CM-52) at pH 6.5 and 8 mol/L urea with a sodium phosphate gradient. Absorption at 280 nm and beta scintillation are measured in aliquots from the eluted globin peaks. The radioactive beta/alpha ratio is calculated by summing the net counts per minute from the tubes containing the beta-chain peak and the alpha-chain peak and dividing the former by the latter. The specific activity beta/alpha ratio is calculated by dividing the radioactivity counts by the absorbance value for each of the most active three or four tubes from the beta peak and the alpha peak; the mean specific activity value for the beta chain is then divided by that of the alpha chain.

The mean beta/alpha specific activity ratio in the peripheral blood of normal adults is 0.99 (SD 0.05) (1). Caucasian heterozygotes with high hemoglobin A$_2$ beta-thalassemia trait have a mean beta/alpha ratio of 0.57 (SD 0.08) (2). Caucasian patients with beta-thalassemia major have radioactive beta/alpha ratios of 0.2 to 0.25. Globin synthesis studies are particularly helpful in confirming a diagnosis of various beta- and alpha-thalassemia syndromes.

Globin-Chain Electrophoresis

Globin-chain separation by electrophoresis may be performed on cellulose acetate strips with Tris–EDTA–borate buffer at pH 8.9 and 6.0 in the presence of 6 mol of urea and 50 mmol of 2-mercaptoethanol per liter (3). This method separates normal alpha, beta, and gamma chains as well as abnormal globin chains. By comparing specimens with known variants run on the same strip or gel, one can make a presumptive identification of the mutant chain (4).

1. Schwartz, E., Abnormal globin synthesis in thalassemic red cells. *Sem. Hematol.* **11**, 549–567 (1974).
2. Friedman, S., Schwartz, E., Ahern, V., and Ahern, E., Globin synthesis in the Jamaican Negro with beta-thalassemia. *Br. J. Haematol.* **28**, 505–513 (1974).
3. International Committee for Standardization in Hematology: Recommendations of a system for identifying abnormal hemoglobins. *Blood* **52**, 1065–1067 (1978).
4. Friedman, S., Kinney, T. R., and Atwater, J., Laboratory evaluation of hemoglobin disorders. In *Hemoglobinopathies in Children*, E. Schwartz, C. Pochedly, and D. R. Miller, Eds. PSG (Publishing Sciences Group) Publishing Co., Inc., Littleton, MA (in press).

Gamma-Globulins

Specimen Tested:

CSF.

Laboratory Reporting:

1.

Reference (Normal) Values:

Child: Up to 9% of total CSF protein
Adult: 14%

Sources of Reference (Normal) Values:

Nellhaus, G., Cerebrospinal fluid immunoglobulin G in childhood. Measurement by electroimmunodiffusion. *Arch. Neurol.* **24,** 441–448 (1971).

Specimen Volume:

3 μL.

Analytical Method:

Merrill, D., Hartley, T. F., and Claman, H. N., Electroimmunodiffusion (EID): A simple, rapid method for quantitation of immunoglobulins in dilute biological fluids. *J. Lab. Clin. Med.* **69,** 151–159 (1967).

Instrumentation:

Buchler Instruments Universal Electrophoresis Cell.

Glucagon

Specimen Tested:

P.

Laboratory Reporting:

1.

Reference (Normal) Values:

Child–adult: 20–210 pg/mL

Sources of Reference (Normal) Values:

Faloona, G. R., and Unger, R. H., Glucagon. In *Hormones in Blood,* C. H. Gray, and A. L. Bacharach, Eds. Academic Press, New York, NY, 1967, pp 317–330.

Specimen Volume, Collection, and Preservation:

Draw 5 mL of blood into specially prepared tubes containing 500 units of "Trasylol" (aprotinin; an inhibitor of proteolylic enzymes) and 1.2 mg of EDTA Na₂ per milliliter of blood. Sample must be kept on ice and separated immediately. Store in FR.

Analytical Method:

RIA; Unger, R. H., Eisentraut, A. M., McCall, M. S., Keller, S., Lanz, H. C., and Madison, L. L., Glucagon antibodies and their use for immunoassay of glucagon. *Proc. Soc. Exp. Biol. Med.* **102,** 621–623 (1959).

Instrumentation:

Nuclear-Chicago gamma counter.

Commentary—Richard A. Guthrie

Glucagon assay in pediatrics is primarily a research tool with little clinical application. It is used primarily for the study of insulin–glucose–glucagon interrelationships in diabetes mellitus. Clinically, assay of glucagon is useful only in the detection of glucagonoma, a tumor of the alpha cells of the pancreas. This tumor is rare in children.

Potential usefulness of glucagon assay may be as a marker of diabetic control. Glucagon concentrations are increased in juvenile diabetics and were once thought to be a part of the genetic diabetic syndrome. It is now known that these increased glucagon concentrations are suppressible by insulin; thus the high values reflect inadequate insulinization or poor diabetic control.

In the newborn, glucagon assay is useful in the study of the metabolic abnormalities of the infant of a diabetic mother but has little clinical application.

Before further clinical applications of glucagon measurements are found, there must be better standardization of the assay, especially improved specificity. Assay for glucagon is by standard RIA, as for other protein hormones. There are multiple sources of glucagon, including pancreatic and gut glucagons; pancreatic glucagon is the one to be assayed, but gut glucagon cross reacts in many assays. Normal values and specificity for pancreatic glucagon must be established for each laboratory. Preferably, antibody for the assay should be obtained from a standard source whose specificity has been proven. In any event, careful standardization is required to make the results interpretable.

Glucose

In Cerebrospinal Fluid

Laboratories Reporting:
4.

Reference (Normal) Values:

All ages: 40–80% of blood glucose; 40–60%
           37–64 mg/dL (2.1–3.6 mmol/L); 40–70 (2.2–3.9); 50–75 (2.8–4.2)

Note: Further information for CSF glucose is included in the next section.

In Blood

Specimen Tested:

B, P, S.

Laboratories Reporting:

8.

Reference (Normal) Values:

Age	P, S, mg/dL (mmol/L)		B, mg/dL (mmol/L)	
	Lower limits	Upper limits	Lower limits	Upper limits
Newborn				
Premature	20–30	80	20–30	65
	(1.11–1.67)[a]	(4.44)	(1.11–1.67)[a]	(3.61)
Full-term	20–50	75–90	20–30	90
	(1.11–2.78)[a]	(4.16–5.00)	(1.11–1.67)[a]	(5.00)
0–2 yr	60	105–110		
	(3.33)	(5.83–6.38)		
>1 mo			(3.6)	(5.4)
Child–adult	60–70	105–115	60	90
	(3.33–3.89)	(5.83–6.38)	(3.83)	(5.00)

[a] Although these lower limits are frequently noted, their interpretation as "normal" is debatable.

Sources of Reference (Normal) Values:

Institutional; a retrospective study of hospital data on 399 children ages up to 16 years, and selected to exclude infectious and inflammatory disease, malignancy, and anemia; Cheng, M. H., Lipsey, A. I., Blanco, V., Wong, H. T., and Spiro, S. H., Microchemical analysis for 13 constituents of plasma from healthy children. *Clin. Chem.* **25,** 692–698 (1979).

Specimen Volume, Collection, and Preservation:

5 to 25 μL, in general. Samples not analyzed immediately ($<$ 30 min) must be preserved. P or S should be separated rapidly. B must be collected into preservative such as fluoride–iodoacetate. [See Meites, S., and Saniel-Banrey, K., Preservation, distribution, and assay of glucose in blood, with special reference to the newborn. *Clin. Chem.* **25**, 531–534 (1979).] Refrigeration or ice definitely retards glycolysis.

Analytical Method:

Glucose oxidase–rate sensing: Beckman Glucose Analyzer with Reagent Kit; Astra-8; Kadish, A. H., Litle, R. L., and Sternberg, J. C., A new and rapid method for the determination of glucose by measurement of rate of oxygen consumption. *Clin. Chem.* **14**, 116–131 (1968); Kadish, A. H., and Sternberg, J. C., Determination of urine glucose by measurement of rate of oxygen consumption. *Diabetes* **78**, 467–470 (1969); Sternberg, J. C., A new glucose analyzer based on an enzymatic rate-sensing oxygen method. *Clin. Chem.* **15**, 801 (1969), abstract; Sterling, R. E., and Nagao, R. R., Evaluation of the glucose analyzer. *Clin. Chem.* **15**, 801–802 (1969), abstract. **Hexokinase method:** Richterich, R., and Dauwalder, H., Zur Bestimmung der Plasmaglucosekonzentration mit der Hexokinase–Glucose-6-phosphat-dehydrogenase-methode. *Schweiz. Med. Wochenschr.* **101**, 615–618 (1971). **Glucose oxidase–*p*-aminophenazone technique:** Trinder, P. J., Determination of blood glucose using 4-aminophenazone as oxygen acceptor. *J. Clin. Pathol.* **22**, 246 (1969).

Instrumentation:

Beckman Instruments, Inc., instrumentation (see *Analytical method*); Greiner Selective Analyzer II; Abbott ABA-100, VP Bichromatic Analyzer, with A-Gent Glucose; Electro-Nucleonics GEMSAEC; Union Carbide CentrifiChem; Yellow Springs Instrument Glucose Analyzer; Technicon Instruments Corp. SMAC.

In Urine

Laboratories Reporting:

3.

Reference (Normal) Values:

Child–adult: Up to 50 mg/L (2.78 mmol/L)

Sources of Reference (Normal) Values:

Institutional; see report for glucose in blood.

Commentary—Richard A. Guthrie

Glucose determinations in various body fluids are among the most frequent measurements of clinical medicine. Though less common in pediatrics than in adult medicine, they are nonetheless common. Glucose concentration can be determined in any body fluid, but is most often determined in blood, urine, and cerebrospinal fluid. Methods for determining glucose vary, but in modern chemistry they usually involve microquantities of fluid (as little as 10 μL), a true or nearly true glucose method, and automatic equipment. Glucose oxidase and hexokinase methods are most common.

Glucose values can be obtained from whole blood, plasma, or serum. Serum is most commonly used. Before normal values can be interpreted, the fluid used and the method must be known. True glucose values will be lower than methods that measure glucose plus other reducing substances. Plasma and serum values will be higher than whole-blood values (by about 15% because of the lower glucose content of erythrocytes). The clinician must, therefore, know what lab methods were used, to interpret correctly the values he receives.

Glucose is measured in CSF primarily in the diagnosis of bacterial meningitis. CSF glucose values are usually about 60% as much as the blood values and should be combined with blood values for interpretation. Urine glucose values are used in the diagnosis and treatment of diabetes mellitus. Patients and medical personnel check urine glucose semiquantitatively several times a day to adjust insulin dosages. Quantitative determination of urine glucose in 24-h samples is a useful guide to therapy in diabetics, and is frequently performed.

Blood glucose determinations are used most commonly in the diagnosis and treatment of diabetes mellitus, but are also useful in the diagnosis of the hypoglycemias (see **Glucose tolerance test**). In the newborn, blood glucose values are useful in the detection of hypoglycemia, a common condition, especially in the premature, and a potential cause of brain damage and even death in these infants. Normal fasting blood glucose values in newborns are lower than in adults. I believe from studies in our program and others that 40 mg/dL should be the lower limit called normal for blood glucose in newborns, whether full-term or premature. Maintaining glucose above this concentration will protect the brain and prevent serious sequelae.

In the diagnosis of diabetes mellitus, fasting, postprandial, or glucose tolerance values may be used. Debate continues as to which fasting values should be considered normal or diabetic. Values listed here vary with method, but values for serum glucose methods generally accepted are about 70–115 mg/dL. Using potassium ferricyanide, which measures slightly more than true glucose, I have found values as great as 111 mg/dL for capillary whole blood. A panel of experts (not including pediatricians, however) have recently agreed that a fasting glucose value exceeding 140 mg/dL should be considered diagnostic of diabetes mellitus. Values between the normal value of 115 mg/dL and the 140 mg/dL value should be considered suspect for diabetes, and further studies should be performed.

There is no standardization for postprandial blood glucose values because of the variations in the size and content of the meal; consequently, these values are not helpful in diagnosis. Postprandial blood glucose values are most helpful in guiding therapy with insulin in diabetic mellitus.

Glucose tolerance testing is discussed elsewhere. The use of blood glucose in the diagnosis of hypoglycemia is discussed with insulin values that are helpful in the diagnosis of that problem. In my experience children with low insulin values associated with high glucose values are more likely to decompensate than are children with more normal or high insulin values—thus the value of the insulin determination.

There is no place for mass glucose tolerance testing or screening in children. Glucose tolerance testing has only limited value in children and should be carefully standardized and interpreted when used.

Glucose-6-Phosphatase (EC 1.1.1.49; D-glucose-6-phosphate:NADP$^+$ 1-oxidoreductase)

Specimen Tested:

Liver.

Laboratories Reporting:

2.

Reference (Normal) Values:

Lab. 1:   2–10 units
(near zero activity in Type 1 glycogen storage disease)
Lab. 2:   > 5 units (as in Lab. 1)

Sources of Reference (Normal) Values:

Lab. 1: Hers, H. G., Glycogen storage disease. *Adv. Metab. Disord.* **1**, 1–44 (1964); Huijing, F., Glycogen and enzymes of glycogen metabolism. In *Clinical Biochemistry, Principles and Methods*, H. C. Curtius and M. Roth, Eds. de Gruyter, New York, NY, 1974, p 1225. **Lab. 2:** text ref. 2, pp 159–163.

Specimen Volume, Collection, and Preservation:

Lab. 1: 5 to 10 mg of liver biopsy material. **Lab. 2:** 0.1 mL of liver extract (1 g/dL). Inappropriate handling of sample destroys enzyme activity. Rapidly ("snap") freeze the specimen and store it at −70 °C in an airtight container with minimum air space.

Analytical Method:

Lab 1: Hers, *op. cit.;* Ricketts, T. R., An improved micromethod for the determination of glucose-6-phosphatase activity. *Clin. Chim. Acta* **8**, 160–162 (1963).

Enzyme Data:

Lab. 1:
1. Enzyme unit definition: 1 unit = 1 μmol of glucose 6-phosphate hydrolyzed/min per gram of wet tissue.
2. Buffer, pH: maleate–acetate buffer, 5.0.
3. Substrate, pH: glucose 6-phosphate, 6.5.
4. Reaction temperature: 37 °C.
5. Temperature reported: 37 °C.

Instrumentation:

Lab. 1: Varian 635 spectrophotometer, and thermostatically controlled shaking waterbath. **Lab. 2:** Beckman 25 spectrophotometer.

Glucose-6-Phosphate Dehydrogenase
(EC 3.1.3.9; D-glucose-6-phosphate phosphohydrolase)

Specimen Tested:

Erythrocytes.

Laboratories Reporting:

5.

Reference (Normal) Values, and Sources; Analytical Method:

Note: Because of the diversity in the analytical kinetic methods used, reference (normal) values are listed separately for each institution's report, as are sources and methods.

Lab. 1: 7.0–18.6 U/g of hemoglobin; Stamatoyannopoulos, G., Papayannopoulou, T., Bakopoulos, C., and Motulsky, H. G., Detection of glucose-6-phosphate dehydrogenase deficient heterozygotes. *Blood* **29**, 87–101 (1967); Glock, J. E., and McClean, P., Further studies on the properties and assay of glucose-6-phosphate dehydrogenase and 6-phospho-gluconate dehydrogenase of rat liver. *Biochem. J.* **55**, 400–408 (1953).

Lab. 2: 2.1–4.0 U/mL of erythrocytes; institutional; Princeton Biomedix reagent kit (UV assay).

Lab. 3: 5–12 U/g of hemoglobin; an institutional study on 100 subjects, 50 from blood bank samples (0–3 wk old) and 50 on surgical patients; Calbiochem-Behring Stat-Pack.

Lab. 4: Mean: 11 U/g of hemoglobin; range: 6.4–15.6 U/g of hemoglobin. The range is not ± 2 SD, so that heterozygous individuals are excluded and only individuals with normal enzyme activity are present; from an institutional study on 107 children; Nicholson, J. F., Bodourian, S. H., and Pesce, M. A., Measurement of glucose-6-phosphate dehydrogenase and 6-phosphogluconate dehydrogenase activities in erythrocytes by use of a centrifugal analyzer. *Clin. Chem.* **20,** 1349–1352 (1974).

Lab. 5: 150–215 units/dL; institutional; Zinkham, W. H., Lenhard, R. E., Jr., and Childs, B., A deficiency of glucose-6-phosphate dehydrogenase activity in erythrocytes from patients with favism. *Bull. Johns Hopkins Hosp.* **102,** 169–175 (1958).

Specimen Volume, Collection, and Preservation:

10 to 100 μL of hemolysate. Anticoagulant is usually heparin, but EDTA is satisfactory. The enzyme is quite stable: 11 d at 23 °C, and up to 3 wk in RR (4 °C). *Do not freeze* (−20 °C) because the enzyme activity will rapidly decrease.

Instrumentation:

Beckman 35 and 25K spectrophotometers; Gilford 2000 and 300-N spectrophotometer with Data Lister; Union Carbide CentrifiChem.

Note: Enzyme data are presented in the literature cited with each analytical method.

Commentary—Michael A. Pesce

The enzyme glucose-6-phosphate dehydrogenase (GPD) is the first enzyme in the hexose monophosphate shunt and converts glucose 6-phosphate to 6-phosphogluconate with the concurrent reduction of NADP⁺ to NADPH. GPD deficiency is the most common genetic abnormality of the human erythrocyte. Inheritance of GPD deficiency is sex-linked, the abnormal gene being carried on the X chromosome. Sons inherit the mutant gene from their mother, whereas daughters inherit it from both parents. When present in the male (hemizygous) or on both X chromosomes in the female (homozygous), the trait is fully expressed. The most common clinical manifestation of GPD deficiency is acute hemolysis, usually following infection or ingestion of certain drugs or other hemolytic agents. Hemolysis presumably results from a failure to maintain sufficiently high concentrations of NADPH and reduced glutathione, which protect cellular components from oxidation.

In the hexose monophosphate shunt NADPH is produced by the following reaction scheme:

Glucose 6-phosphate + NADP⁺ $\xrightarrow{\text{GPD}}$ 6-phosphogluconate + NADPH

6-Phosphogluconate + NADP⁺ $\xrightarrow{\text{PGD}}$ ribulose 5-phosphate + CO$_2$ + NADPH

[PGD = phosphogluconate dehydrogenase (decarboxylating); EC 1.1.1.44]

Any method that determines GPD activity by measuring the rate of increase in production of NADPH must also consider the second reaction. Methods that do not take this reaction into consideration and assume that 1 mol of NADPH is formed per mole of glucose 6-phosphate oxidized will overestimate the GPD activity. GPD activity can be measured in erythrocytes by adding excess PGD activity to a reaction mixture containing glucose 6-phosphate and NADP+ to convert all of the 6-phosphogluconate formed in the first reaction to NADPH (1). With this procedure, 2 mol of NADPH are produced per mole of glucose 6-phosphate oxidized. Other methods for measuring GPD inhibit the PGD reaction by adding either 2,3-diphosphoglycerate (2) or maleimide (3), and only the NADPH produced from the first reaction is measured. GPD activity is stable for 11 days in heparinized blood stored at RT or at 4 °C.

1. Nicholson, J. F., Bodourian, S. H., and Pesce, M. A., Measurement of glucose-6-phosphate dehydrogenase and 6-phosphogluconate dehydrogenase activities in erythrocytes by use of a centrifugal analyzer. *Clin. Chem.* **20,** 1349–1352 (1974).
2. Catalano, E. W., Johnson, G. F., and Solomon, H. M., Measurement of erythrocyte glucose-6-phosphate dehydrogenase activity with a centrifugal analyzer. *Clin. Chem.* **21,** 134–138 (1975).
3. Deutsch, J., Maleimide as an inhibitor in measurement of erythrocyte glucose-6-phosphate dehydrogenase activity. *Clin. Chem.* **24,** 885–889 (1978).

Glucose Tolerance and Insulin Test, Oral

Specimen Tested:

B, S.

Laboratory Reporting:

1.

Reference (Normal) Values:

See Figure 1 in Guthrie's Commentary on **Insulin** (p 290).

Sources of Reference (Normal) Values:

Based on 400 oral glucose tolerance tests on nondiabetic, ambulatory healthy children with no family history of diabetes, at the University of Missouri. Glucose dose was 1.75 g/kg of ideal body weight for height to a maximum dose of 100 g; Guthrie, R. A., Guthrie, D. W., Murthy, D. Y. N., Jackson, R. L., and Lang, J., Standardization of the oral glucose tolerance test and the criteria for diagnosis of chemical diabetes in children. *Metabolism* **22,** 275–282 (1973); Pickens, J. M., Burkeholder, J. N., and Womack, W. N., Oral glucose tolerance test in normal children. *Diabetes* **16,** 11–14 (1967).

Glucose

Specimen Volume, Collection, and Preservation:

0.1 mL; skin-puncture blood. Somogyi filtrate prepared immediately from the B diluted 1 + 9 (10-fold) with water. Analyze the supernate after centrifugation.

Analytical Method and Instrumentation:

Ferricyanide method; Technicon Instrument Corp. AutoAnalyzer.

Insulin

Specimen Volume, Collection, and Preservation:

0.3 mL; skin-puncture blood collected into two Caraway tubes. After clotting is complete, centrifuge the tubes, remove the serum, and store frozen in FR.

Analytical Method and Instrumentation:

RIA, double antibody; Nuclear Chicago liquid-scintillation counter.

Commentary—Richard A. Guthrie

Glucose tolerance testing has limited value in children. It is used basically for two purposes: to rule out diabetes mellitus in high-risk groups, and to diagnose hypoglycemia, particularly reactive hypoglycemia. This problem is discussed in the section on **Insulin.** Glucose tolerance testing is rarely necessary to diagnose diabetes mellitus; personally, I use this test mainly to reassure parents who are concerned about their children because of close relatives with diabetes.

If glucose tolerance testing is to be done, it should be performed properly. It is unfair to label people diabetic (borderline, chemical, or otherwise) unless they are. Such a label may affect insurability, employability, etc. Because the natural history of glucose intolerance in children is not known (only a small percentage seems to progress to frank diabetes), and because there is really no known treatment, the legitimate question then is—why find it? Above all, do not over-diagnose by faulty standardization of the test.

If glucose tolerance testing is to be performed, follow this procedure:

1. Do not test a sick or bedfast child; an erroneous (abnormal) test will result.

2. Perform the test with the child quiet, but ambulatory.

3. Give the child a high-carbohydrate diet (60–65% of calories) for three days before the test, to increase all sensitivity to the glucose stimulus.

4. Give a sandwich and a glass of milk at 2200 hours the evening before the test, and start the test no later than 0800 hours, to standardize the fasting period.

5. Administer a dose of glucose of 1.75 g/kg of ideal body weight for height to a maximum dose (for children) of 75 g.

6. Use a glucose solution no more dilute than 20% glucose (200 g/L) (if more dilute, the values will be too high) and no more concentrated than 30% (300 g/L) (to avoid gastric stasis or vomiting) in a flavored base.

7. Be sure the child drinks the glucose quickly.

8. Measure values for fasting, and at 30 min, 1 h, 2 h, and 3 h after glucose administration. Extend the test to 5 to 6 h for hypoglycemia.

9. Allow no drugs, food, or smoking during the test.

10. Use well-standardized norms for children for interpretation; the largest group of children tested for pediatric norms are those of Pickens et al. *(1),* although their norms are for capillary whole blood and correction must be made for serum or plasma values.

11. Obtain insulin values for each sample; this will increase the sensitivity of the test, especially for hypoglycemia.

Remember that most hospital labs use the normal values of Fajans and Conn for interpretation of oral glucose tolerance tests. These norms are for adults, and are lower than pediatric norms. Pediatric values should be compared only with pediatric norms (see graphs with **Insulin** discussion—p 290—for Pickens, Burkeholder, and Womack norms for children). Abnormal test results should not be called diabetes or chemical diabetes. The official terminology recently adopted by the National Diabetes Data Group, "impaired glucose tolerance (IGTT)," is appropriate because the significance of these abnormal values is not known *(2).* Children with such results should be carefully observed, but parents and physicians should not panic because only a low percentage of these children decompensate to frank diabetes.

1. Pickens, J. M., Burkeholder, J. N., and Womack, W. N., Oral glucose tolerance test in normal children. *Diabetes* **16,** 11–14 (1967).
2. National Diabetes Data Group, Classification and diagnosis of diabetes mellitus and other categories of glucose intolerance. *Diabetes* **28,** 1039–1057 (1979).

Note: See also **Insulin.**

Alpha-D-Glucosidase
(EC 3.1.1.20; α-D-glucoside glucohydrolase)

Specimen Tested:

Leukocytes.

Laboratory Reporting:

1.

Reference (Normal) Values:

Range: 12.5–36.2 arbitrary units
Mean ± 2 SD: 8.9–36.5 arbitrary units

Sources of Reference (Normal) Values:

Institutional.

Specimen Volume, Collection, and Preservation:

10 mL. Heparinized B. Keep B on ice and prepare leukocyte pellets without delay.

Note: See discussion on leukocyte preparation in **Appendix 4.**

Analytical Method:

Measure 4-methylumbelliferone (4-MU) released from 4-MU-α-D-glucopyranoside.

Enzyme Data:

1. Enzyme unit definition: 1 arbitrary unit = the amount of enzyme that cleaves 1 nmol of 4-MU-α-D-glucopyranoside per hour per milligram of protein at 37 °C.
2. Buffer, pH: citric acid–sodium phosphate, 4.0.
3. Substrate, pH: 4 MU-α-D-glucopyranoside, about 4.0.
4. Reaction temperature: 37 °C.
5. Temperature reported: 37 °C.

Commentary—Derek A. Applegarth

The α-glucosidase isoenzyme with an acid pH optimum (acid maltase) is deficient in Pompe's disease. Normal values do not vary with age. In an affected patient, residual enzyme activity at pH 4 may not be due to "true" acid enzyme but to an overlap of neutral enzyme (pH optimum = 6). This contribution can be evaluated by assaying the enzyme over the pH range 3 to 6 and plotting the data to give a pH profile.

Alpha-D-Glucosidase, Lysosomal

Specimen Tested:

Liver, muscle.

Laboratory Reporting:

1.

Reference (Normal) Values:

Liver: about 0.7 U/g of tissue, wet weight
Muscle: about 0.03 U/g of tissue, wet weight

Sources of Reference (Normal) Values:

Hers, H. G., Glycogen storage disease. *Adv. Metab. Dis.* **1**, 1–44 (1964).

Specimen Volume, Collection, and Preservation:

20 to 50 mg. Specimen must be immediately "snap" frozen. Store at −70 °C in an air-tight container with minimal air space.

Analytical Method:

Hers, *op. cit.* Rat liver or muscle used for quality control.

Enzyme Data:

1. Enzyme unit definition: 1 IUB unit (U) = 1 μmol of maltose hydrolyzed per minute.
2. Buffer, pH: acetate, 4.0.
3. Substrate, pH: maltose, 4.0.
4. Reaction temperature: 37 °C.
5. Temperature reported: 37 °C.

Instrumentation:

Varian 635 spectrophotometer; thermostatically controlled, shaking waterbath.

Glutamine

Specimen Tested:
CSF.

Laboratories Reporting:
2.

Reference (Normal) Values:

Lab. 1: 0–12 mo: 3.7–15.7 mg/dL (0.253–1.072 mmol/L)
12–24 mo: 3.6–9.6 (0.246–0.656)
Lab. 2: <25 mg/dL (<1.708 mmol/L)

Sources of Reference (Normal) Values:

Institutional.

Specimen Volume, Collection, and Preservation:

Lab. 1: 20 μL; **Lab. 2:** 100 μL. Store samples up to 7 d in FR.

Analytical Method:

Lab. 1: Glasgow, A. M., and Dhiensiri, K., Improved assay for spinal fluid glutamine, and values for children with Reye's syndrome. *Clin. Chem.* **20**, 642–644 (1974). **Lab. 2:** Hourani, B. T., Hamlin, E. M., and Reynolds, T. B., Cerebrospinal fluid glutamine as a measure of hepatic encephalopathy. *Arch. Intern. Med.* **127**, 1033–1036 (1971).

Instrumentation:

Perkin-Elmer Model 55 B, and Beckman Acta V spectrophotometers.

Commentary—Roger L. Boeckx

Ammonia is exceedingly toxic to mammalian systems, and several mechanisms exist for its rapid removal. One of these involves amidation of glutamic acid to produce glutamine. This detoxification system is active in the brain and may serve as a major mechanism for the removal of brain ammonia.

Because the concentration of glutamine in the CSF of patients with Reye's syndrome is increased, the measurement of CSF glutamine has been proposed as a rapid diagnostic procedure for detection of this syndrome *(1)*.

High concentrations of glutamine have also been reported in meningitis, in patients receiving total parenteral nutrition, and in patients suffering cerebral hemorrhage *(2)*. Glasgow and Dhiensiri *(1)* found that CSF glutamine exceeded 15 mg/dL in 20 of 27 patients with Reye's syndrome, while values for a control group ranged from 6 to 14 mg/dL. Boeckx et al. *(2)* found considerable age variation in infancy, with higher concentrations in younger infants.

1. Glasgow, A. M., and Dhiensiri, K., Improved assay for spinal fluid glutamine, and values for children with Reye's syndrome. *Clin. Chem.* **20**, 642–644 (1974).
2. Boeckx, R. L., Iosefsohn, M., and Hicks, J. M., Reference values for cerebrospinal fluid glutamine concentration in infants. *Clin. Chem.* **25**, 1081 (1979). Abstract.

Gamma-Glutamyltransferase, GGT [EC 2.3.2.2; (5-glutamyl)-peptide：amino-acid 5-glutamyltransferase]

Specimen Tested:

P, S.

Laboratories Reporting:

5.

Reference (Normal) Values:

Note: All labs reporting use a similar kinetic analytical method except for the modifications by Lab. 5 listed below.

Age	Labs. 1–4: 37 °C, same buffer and pH	Lab. 5: 30 °C, different buffer and pH	
		Mean	Range
Cord	19–270 U/L	105.5 U/L	0–224 U/L
Premature	56–233		
1–3 d	13–198		
0–3 wk	0–103; 0–130		
0–1 mo		74.3	0–206
3 wk–3 mo	4–111; 4–120		
1–2 mo		49.6	0–118
2–4 mo		32.6	0–71
>3 mo M	5–65		
F	5–35		
4–7 mo		18.2	0–37
7–12 mo		11.7	1–22
1–2 yr		10.6	3–19
1–5 yr	0–23		
2–5 yr		10.9	4–18
5–10 yr		12.9	6–20
6–15 yr	0–23		
10–15 yr		13.8	6–22
16 yr–adult	0–35		
Adult M	9–69	18.0	5–38
F	3–33	13.0	5–27

Sources of Reference (Normal) Values:

Institutional; lab. 5 data to be published; Sitzmann, F. C., Die Enzym-diagnostik bei Erkrankungen in Kindesalter. *Arch. Kinderheilkd. Beih.* **57,** 1–59 (1968); Lum, G., and Gambino, S. R., Serum gamma-glutamyl transpeptidase activity as an indicator of disease of liver, pancreas, or bone. *Clin. Chem.* **18,** 358–362 (1972); Rosalki, S. B., Gamma-glutamyl transpeptidase. *Adv. Clin. Chem.* **17,** 53–101 (1975).

Specimen Volume, Collection, and Preservation:

5 to 50 μL. Heparin anticoagulant preferred; EDTA also used. All labs. prefer to analyze the specimen within 4 h of collection. If not, the specimen is stored in FR (up to 2 mo), or up to 1 d in RR. There is evidence that the enzyme is stable for 1 mo in RR, and up to 1 yr in FR; also up to 2 d at RT, but unverified.

Analytical Method:

All labs cite as a basis for analysis: Szasz, G., A kinetic photometric method for serum γ-glutamyl transpeptidase. *Clin. Chem.* **15,** 124–136 (1969); and additional reference to Orlowski and coworkers, e.g.,

Orlowski, M., and Szewczuk, A., Determination of γ-glutamyl tran-speptidase activity in human serum and urine. *Clin. Chim. Acta* **7**, 755–760 (1962); Orlowski, M., and Szewczuk, A., *Acta Biochim. Pol.* **8**, 189 (1961); Abbott A-Gent; Bio-Dynamics/*bmc* γ-GT C-System; Sigma Chemical Co. no. 415.

Enzyme Data:

1. Enzyme unit definition: 1 IUB unit (U) = the activity liberating 1 μmol of *p*-nitroaniline per minute. **Lab. 2:** liberating 1 μmol of 5-amino-2-nitrobenzoate per minute (report on cord serum, only).
2. Buffer, pH: **Labs. 1–4:** Tris, 8.25; **Lab. 5:** 2-amino-2-methyl-1, 3-propanediol, 8.6.
3. Substrate, pH: **Labs. 1, 3, 4:** L-γ-glutamyl-*p*-nitroanilide, 8.25; **Lab. 2:** L-γ-glutamyl-3-carboxy-4-nitroanilide-glycyglycine, 8.25; **Lab. 5:** L-γ-glutamyl-*p*-nitroanilide, 8.6.
4. Reaction temperature: **Labs. 1–4:** 37 °C; **Lab. 5:** 30 °C.
5. Temperature reported: **Labs. 1–4:** 37 °C; **Lab. 5:** 30 °C.

Instrumentation:

Abbott ABA-100; Union Carbide CentrifiChem; American Instrument Co. Rotochem; Beckman TR Enzyme Analyzer.

Commentary—J. A. Knight

γ-Glutamyltransferase (GGT) is a membrane-bound glycoprotein that catalyzes the transfer of the γ-glutamyl moiety of the tripeptide glutathione and other γ-glutamyl donors to various acceptor sub-strates, including certain peptides and amino acids. Although its specific functions are not fully understood, it appears to be important in glutathione metabolism, transport of amino acids across cell mem-branes, and nitrogen balance.

In 1961 GGT activity was first shown to be increased above normal in patients with hepatic disease *(1)*. Although now well established as a more sensitive indicator than alkaline phosphatase in obstruc-tive, infiltrative, and other hepatic disorders *(2–4)*, it has usually been relegated to a secondary role, i.e., to be measured as an aid in explaining the origin of an above-normal activity of alkaline phos-phatase when the source of the latter is in doubt *(5,6)*.

This limited use of GGT in adults can be somewhat justified, but clearly cannot be in infants, children, and adolescents. A single, ran-dom serum specimen analyzed for alkaline phosphatase is essentially uninterpretable in children, the normal range for the analyte being extremely wide and varying markedly with age as well as the stage of an individual child's growth *(7)*; in adolescents, sex difference is of considerable significance. GGT, on the other hand, is highest at birth and decreases rapidly *and predictably* with age *(8–10)*. There are slight, statistically significant differences with age from seven months to adulthood, but these are of little clinical importance. In addition, the activity of GGT in serum is unaffected by bone diseases or pregnancy. After puberty, GGT varies slightly with sex.

GGT is clearly more sensitive than alkaline phosphatase in childhood liver diseases (10). The only real drawback to measuring this enzyme instead of alkaline phosphatase is that GGT response is drug-inducible; that is, a variety of drugs, particularly the antiepileptic drugs but also the antirheumatic drug aminopyrine, cause increases of GGT, apparently without causing overt liver disease. Ethanol also induces GGT activity (11); however, this can be an asset to the clinician because it may bring to light otherwise unsuspected excessive use of alcohol in adolescents and adults (2,12). In patients on antiepileptic drugs, a high GGT value in the absence of liver disease suggests drug compliance, a well-known problem in medicine.

Men have slightly higher GGT activities than women (2). This sex differentiation begins with the onset of puberty (10), and is apparently related to estrogen production, because pregnant women and those taking birth-control pills have lower GGT values than nonpregnant women or those not taking this type of medication (13).

GGT is readily measured, the most common method used being that of Szasz (14). All normal values reported here were determined by that general method. Serum of plasma (heparin- or EDTA-treated) are equally suitable. Hemolysis is usually of no consequence because the reaction is generally measured kinetically. Rosalki et al. have reported the enzyme to be stable in serum for at least one week at 4 °C and for two months at −18 °C (11). Enzyme estimation is precise and accurate on microsamples, as measured with various instruments. Isoenzymes of GGT are known, but are generally difficult to measure routinely; they currently have little clinical usefulness.

1. Szczeklik, E., Orlowski, M., and Szewczuk, A., Serum G. G. T. P. activity in liver disease. *Gastroenterology* **41**, 353–359 (1961).
2. Lum, G., and Gambino, S. R., Serum gamma-glutamyl transpeptidase activity as an indicator of disease of liver, pancreas, or bone. *Clin. Chem.* **18**, 358–362 (1972).
3. Whitfield, J. B., Pounder, R. S., Neale, G., and Moss, D. W., Serum γ-glutamyl transpeptidase activity in liver disease. *Gut* **13**, 702–708 (1972).
4. Lum, G., Gamma-glutamyl transpeptidase in cancer diagnosis. *Ann. Clin. Lab. Sci.* **4**, 13–18 (1974).
5. Kampa, T. S., Jarzabek, J., and Clain, J., The use of gamma-glutamyl transpeptidase in differentiating liver from bone isoenzymes of alkaline phosphatase. *Clin. Biochem.* **9**, 234–236 (1976).
6. Betro, M. G., Oon, R. C. S., and Edwards, J. B., Gamma-glutamyl transpeptidase in diseases of the liver and bone. *Am. J. Clin. Pathol.* **60**, 672–678 (1973).
7. Fleisher, G. A., Eickelberg, E. S., and Elveback, L. R., Alkaline phosphatase activity in the plasma of children and adolescents. *Clin. Chem.* **23**, 469–472 (1977).

8. Shore, G. M., Haberman, L., Dowdey, A. B., and Combes, B., Serum gamma-glutamyl transpeptidase activity in normal children. *Am. J. Clin. Pathol.* **63**, 245–250 (1975).
9. Richterich, R., and Cantz, B., Normal values of plasma γ-glutamyl transpeptidase in children. *Enzyme* **13**, 257–260 (1972).
10. Knight, J. A., and Haymond, R. E., Reference values for γ-glutamyltransferase and its clinical usefulness compared to alkaline phosphatase in childhood liver diseases. Manuscript in preparation (1979).
11. Rosalki, S. B., Lehmann, D., and Prentice, M., Determination of γ-glutamyl transpeptidase activity and its clinical applications. *Ann. Clin. Biochem.* **7**, 143–147 (1970).
12. Westwood, M., Cohen, M. I., and McNamara, H., Serum γ-glutamyl transpeptidase activity: A chemical determinant of alcohol consumption during adolescence. *Pediatrics* **62**, 560–562 (1978).
13. Combes, B., Shore, G. M., Cunningham, F. G., Walker, F. B., Shorey, J. W., and Ware, A., Serum γ-glutamyl transpeptidase activity in viral hepatitis: Suppression in pregnancy and by birth control pills. *Gastroenterology* **72**, 271–274 (1977).
14. Szasz, G., A kinetic photometric method for serum γ-glutamyl transpeptidase. *Clin. Chem.* **15**, 124–136 (1969).

Commentary—Paul L. Wolf

Serum GGT activity is greater in neonates than in adults. Freer et al. analyzed the sera in 78 neonates and found a normal range of 19–407 U/L, compared with 5–37 U/L in adults *(1)*. This increase lasts for approximately three months. GGT is a very sensitive indicator of liver disease, but recently has been shown to be not specific. It is more sensitive than alkaline phosphatase because, although increased in the neonate, it is not increased in growing children as alkaline phosphatase is. Drugs such as phenobarbital and phenytoin (Dilantin) stimulate the cytochrome P_{450} microsomal system, resulting in an increase in GGT *(2)*.

The increased GGT in newborns may be caused by the increase in bilirubin, which stimulates the P_{450} system. Other conditions besides liver disease that will increase GGT activity include: renal disease, cardiac disease, prostatic cancer metastatic to bone, and postoperative condition *(3,4)*.

1. Freer, D. E., Statland, B. E., Johnson, M., and Felton, H., Reference values for selected enzyme activities and protein concentrations in serum and plasma derived from cord-blood specimens. *Clin. Chem.* **25**, 565–569 (1979).
2. Rosalki, S. B., Tarlow, D., and Rau, D., Plasma gammaglutamyl transpeptidase elevation in patients receiving enzyme-inducing drugs. *Lancet* **ii**, 376–377 (1971).
3. Rosalki, S. B., Rau, D., and Lehmann, D., Determination of serum gamma-glutamyl transpeptidase activity and its clinical applications. *Ann. Clin. Biochem.* **7**, 143–151 (1970).
4. Cohen, M. I., and McNamara, H., The diagnostic value of gamma-glutamyl transpeptidase in children and adolescents with liver disease. *J. Pediatr.* **75**, 838–842 (1969).

Glycerol

Specimen Tested:

P.

Laboratories Reporting:

1.

Reference (Normal) Values:

Child–adult: 30–100 μmol/L

Sources of Reference (Normal) Values:

Laurell, S., and Tibbling, G., The use of blood glycerol determination in the diagnosis of hypothyroidism. *Clin. Chim. Acta* **21,** 127–132 (1968).

Specimen Volume, Collection, and Preservation:

200 μL. Heparin anticoagulant. Collect blood into chilled tubes; separate plasma in refrigerated centrifuge (4 °C) and store in FR.

Analytical Method:

Fluorometric assay of NADH; Laurell and Tibbling, *op. cit.*

Instrumentation:

Aminco-Bowman fluorometer.

Glycogen

In Blood

Specimen Tested:

Erythrocytes.

Laboratory Reporting:

1.

Reference (Normal) Values:

Cord:	10–338 μg/g of hemoglobin
4.5–19 h:	48–361
2–12 mo:	32–134
1–12 yr:	22–109
Adult:	20–105

Sources of Reference (Normal) Values:

Sidbury, J. B., Cornblath, M., Fisher, J., and House, E., Glycogen in erythrocytes of patients with glycogen storage disease. *Pediatrics* **27**, 103–111 (1961).

Specimen Volume, Collection, and Preservation:

2 mL. Heparin anticoagulant. Separate and wash the cells without delay after collection.

Analytical Method:

Sidbury et al., *op. cit.;* text ref. 2, p 165.

Instrumentation:

Zeiss spectrophotometer.

In Tissue

Specimen Tested:

Liver, muscle.

Laboratory Reporting:

1.

Reference (Normal) Values:

Liver: 1–6% (10–60 mg/g of tissue) (based on "fasting" wet weight)
Muscle: 0.25–2.0% ("fasting" wet weight)
Up to 1.5% ("fasting" wet weight), with variation according to muscle type and development

Sources of Reference (Normal) Values:

Hers, H. G., private communication (1974); Morgan, T. E., Short, F. A., and Cobb, L. A., Muscle adaptation to exercise in man. Effects on glycogen and lipid. *J. Clin. Invest.* **47**, 71a (1968), abstract.

Specimen Volume, Collection, and Preservation:

5 to 10 mg. Inappropriate handling of the sample will destroy the enzyme and glycogen content. The tissue should be frozen immediately on foil on solid CO_2 (snap-freeze), and stored at $-70\ °C$.

Analytical Method:

Hers, H. G., Glycogen storage disease. *Adv. Metab. Disord.* **1**, 1–44 (1964); Seifter, S., Dayton, S., Novic, B., and Muntwyler, E., The estimation of glycogen with the anthrone reagent. *Arch. Biochem.* **25**, 191–200 (1950).

Instrumentation:

Varian 635 spectrophotometer.

Commentary—David J. Harris

Many clinicians wish to avoid liver and muscle biopsy in the diagnosis of glycogen storage disease, now classified into eight or 12 varieties *(1,2)*. Abnormally high erythrocyte glycogen should be found in most cases of glycogen storage disease III, the defect due to deficiency of the debrancher enzyme *(3)*. According to Williams and Field, type III accounted for 50% of the patients with glycogen storage disease *(3)*. Because the test can be performed on a readily obtained sample, and with generally available equipment and reagents, it should aid in evaluating a child whose symptoms suggest one of these disorders.

1. Howell, R. R., The glycogen storage diseases. In text ref. *11*, 4th ed., pp 137–159.
2. Hug, G., Glycogen storage diseases. *Birth Defects* **12**, 145–175 (1976).
3. Williams, C., and Field, J. B., Studies in glycogen storage disease. III. Limit dextrinosis: A genetic study. *J. Pediatr.* **72**, 214–221 (1968).

Glycohemoglobins, Hemoglobin A$_{1c}$

Specimen Tested:

B.

Laboratories Reporting:

3.

Reference (Normal) Values:

Lab.1: 3.1–6.3% HbA$_{1c}$[a]
4.7–8.8% HbA$_{1(a+b+c)}$[b]

Lab. 2:	**Controls (n = 28)**[c]		**Juvenile diabetes (n = 48)**[c]
	HbA$_{1c}$	3.5–6.3%	6.2–13.8
	HbA$_{1(a+b)}$	1.3–2.9	1.8–4.6
	HbA$_{1(a+b+c)}$	5.2–8.8	8.6–17.8
	Controls (n = 12)[d]		**Juvenile diabetes (n = 57)**[d]
	HbA$_{1c}$	2.3–6.3	4.2–14.6
	HbA$_{1(a+b)}$	1.2–3.2	1.5–5.1
	HbA$_{1(a+b+c)}$	3.5–9.5	6.4–19.2

Lab. 3: 5.3–8.2% HbA$_{1(a+b+c)}$

[a] Tze, W. J., Thompson, K. H., and Leichter, J., HbA$_{1c}$—an indicator of diabetic control. *J. Pediatr.* **93**, 13–16 (1978).

[b] Chou, J., Robinson, C. A., and Siegel, A. L., Simple method for estimating glycosylated hemoglobins and its application to evaluation of diabetic patients. *Clin. Chem.* **24**, 1708–1710 (1978).

[c] Gabbay, K. H., Hasty, K., Breslow, J. L., Ellison, R. C., Bunn, H. F., and Gallop, P. M., Glycosylated hemoglobins and long-term blood glucose control in diabetes mellitus. *J. Clin. Endocrinol. Metab.* **44**, 859–864 (1977).

[d] Abraham, E. C., Huff, T. A., Cope, N. D., Wilson, J. B., Jr., Bransome, E. D., Jr., and Huisman, T. H. J., Determination of glycosylated hemoglobins (hemoglobin A$_1$) with a new microcolumn procedure. *Diabetes* **27**, 931–937 (1978).

Sources of Reference (Normal) Values:

Lab. 1: Tze et al. and Chou et al., cited above. **Lab. 2:** Gabbay et al. and Abraham et al., cited above. **Lab. 3:** institutional.

Specimen Volume, Collection, and Preservation:

100 μL to 2 mL. Heparin or EDTA anticoagulant. Refrigerate the sample, if not soon analyzed.

Analytical Method:

Lab. 1: Tze et al., *op. cit.;* Chou et al., *op. cit.* **Lab. 2:** Bio Rex 70 microcolumn, or prepacked columns from Helena Labs. **Lab. 3:** Ion-exchange; Allen, D. W., Schroeder, W. A., and Balog, J., Observations on the chromatographic heterogeneity of normal adult and fetal human hemoglobin: A study of the effects of crystallization and chromatography on the heterogeneity and isoleucine content. *J. Am. Chem. Soc.* **80,** 1628–1634 (1958); Isolab Quick-Sep Fast Hemoglobin Test.

Instrumentation:

Lab. 1: Beckman DB spectrophotometer. **Lab. 2:** spectrophotometer. **Lab. 3:** Beckman spectrophotometer.

Commentary—J. A. Knight

Whereas early electrophoretic studies of normal adult hemoglobin by zone electrophoresis revealed only two fractions, designated HbA$_1$ (HbA) and HbA$_2$, the introduction of starch gel revealed an additional component, HbA$_3$. By the latter technique, these fractions constituted approximately 96%, 3–4%, and less than 1% of the total hemoglobin, respectively. Subjected to cation-exchange chromatography, adult hemoglobin separated into eight different components *(1–3)*, designated (on the basis of the rate at which they flowed through the column) as hemoglobin A$_{Ia}$, A$_{Ib}$, A$_{Ic}$, A$_{Id}$, A$_{Ie}$, A$_{II}$ (the major component), A$_{IIIa}$, and A$_{IIIb}$. The fractions separated by starch gel electrophoresis were shown to be related to those separated by column chromatography as follows:

$$HbA_1 = A_{Ic} + A_{Id} + A_{Ie} + A_{II}$$
$$HbA_2 = A_{IIIb} + \text{non-heme protein}$$
$$HbA_3 = A_{Ia} + A_{Ib} + \text{non-heme protein}$$

At first, most hematologists thought these minor components were artifacts. However, in 1968 Rahbar noted an unusual hemoglobin in the blood of certain diabetics *(4);* the following year, he noted that the abnormal hemoglobin had the same chromatographic properties as HbA$_{Ic}$ *(5).* By then, this component had been shown to be a glycosylated hemoglobin, produced by the nonenzymic reaction of glucose 6-phosphate and (or) glucose with the amino group of the terminal valine on the β-chains of hemoglobin A_1. This reaction forms a Schiff base, which then undergoes a stable rearrangement. HbA_{Ia} and A_{Ib} are also glycosylated hemoglobins, but are less well understood (6).

Beginning with Trivelli et al., numerous clinical reports have shown that the measurement of HbA_{Ic} is very helpful in evaluating long-term diabetic control (7–10). The modified method of Trivelli et al. (7), used in most of the early studies, involves overnight dialysis of the hemolysate and collection of both glycosylated hemoglobin and hemoglobin A fractions. Most clinical laboratories now measure $HbA_{Ia} + A_{Ib} + A_{Ic}$ together, this technique being easier, less expensive, and apparently of equivalent significance. Because diabetics have higher mean blood glucose concentrations than nondiabetics, they also have higher glycohemoglobin concentrations. The formation of glycohemoglobins is a slow, essentially irreversible process, so that glycohemoglobin in erythrocytes represents a blood glucose concentration averaged over the previous several weeks. This provides the physician an excellent tool to evaluate long-term therapy and (or) patient compliance.

Some have questioned the usefulness of this test in children, not because it does not measure this time-averaged glucose concentration, but because of the many other difficulties encountered in managing brittle childhood diabetes; however, it still should be quite helpful when one considers the alternatives (11). The technique may also be helpful in diagnosing borderline cases of adult-onset diabetes mellitus.

Normal concentrations of HbA_{Ic} in children appear to correlate well with those in adults, although adequate numbers of normal children have yet to be studied. In a recent report HbA_{Ic} concentrations are 3.1–6.3% of total hemoglobin (10). Normal values for total glycosylated hemoglobins (HbA_{Ia}, HbA_{Ib}, and HbA_{Ic}) are about 3 to 4% higher (12). Diabetics usually average about twice the mean of normal controls.

1. Allen, D. W., Schroeder, W. A., and Balog, J., Observations on the chromatographic heterogeneity of normal adult and fetal human hemoglobin: A study of the effects of crystallization and chromatography on the heterogeneity and isoleucine content. *J. Am. Chem. Soc.* **80**, 1628–1634 (1958).
2. Clegg, M. D., and Schroeder, W. A., A chromatographic study of the minor components of normal adult hemoglobin including a comparison of hemoglobin from normal and phenylketonuric individuals. *J. Am. Chem. Soc.* **81**, 6065–6069 (1959).
3. Schnek, A. G., and Schroeder, W. A., The relation between the minor components of whole normal human adult hemoglobin as isolated by chromatography and starch block electrophoresis. *J. Am. Chem. Soc.* **83**, 1472–1478 (1961).
4. Rahbar, S., An abnormal hemoglobin in red cells of diabetics. *Clin. Chim. Acta* **22**, 296–298 (1968).

5. Rahbar, S., Blumenfeld, O., and Ranney, H. M., Studies of an unusual hemoglobin in patients with diabetes mellitus. *Biochem. Biophys. Res. Commun.* **36,** 838–843 (1969).
6. Bunn, H. F., Gabbay, K. H., and Gallop, P. M., The glycosylation of hemoglobin: Relevance to diabetes mellitus. *Science* **200,** 21–27 (1978).
7. Trivelli, L. A., Ranney, H. M., and Lai, H.-T., Hemoglobin components in patients with diabetes mellitus. *N. Engl. J. Med.* **284,** 353–357 (1971).
8. Koenig, R. J., Peterson, C. M., Jones, R. L., Saudek, C., Lehrman, M., and Cerami, A., Correlation of glucose regulation and hemoglobin A_{Ic} in diabetes mellitus. *N. Engl. J. Med.* **295,** 417–420 (1976).
9. Gonen, B., Rochman, H., Rubenstein, A., Tanega, S. P., and Horowitz, D. L., Haemoglobin A_1: An indicator of the metabolic control of diabetic patients. *Lancet* **ii,** 734–736 (1977).
10. Tze, W. J., Thompson, K. H., and Leichter, J., HbA$_{Ic}$—an indicator of diabetic control. *J. Pediatr.* **93,** 13–16 (1978).
11. Malone, J. I., Hellrung, J. M., Malphus, E. W., Rosenbloom, A. L., Grgic, A., and Weber, F. T., Good diabetic control—study in mass delusion. *J. Pediatr.* **88,** 943–947 (1976).
12. Chou, J., Robinson, C. A., and Siegel, A. L., Simple method for estimating glycosylated hemoglobins, and its application to evaluation of diabetic patients. *Clin. Chem.* **24,** 1708–1710 (1978).

Gonadotropins (FSH, LH)[1]

Specimen Tested:

P, S.

Laboratories Reporting:

3 (reports from each lab. follow).

* * *

Reference (Normal) Values:

Age	FSH, int. units/L		LH, int. units/L	
	M	F	M	F
Prepubertal	<1–12		<1–12	
1–10 yr	1–8	1–10	1–6	1–8
11–16 yr	3–13	5–19	3–12	6–22
Adult	6–21	6–24[a]	6–24	6–22[a]

[a] Higher in midcycle.

Sources of Reference (Normal) Values:

Radioimmunoassay Manual, 4th ed., Nichols Institute, San Pedro, CA, 1977, p 264; Lee, P. A., Midgley, A. R., Jr., and Jaffe, R. B., Regulation of human gonadotropins. VI. Serum follicle stimulating and luteinizing hormone determinations in children. *J. Clin. Endocrinol. Metab.* **31,** 248–253 (1970).

---

[1] The internationally recommended names for these are follitropin (rather than follicle-stimulating hormone) and lutropin (rather than luteinizing hormone).

Specimen Volume, Collection, and Preservation:

600 μL each. Heparin anticoagulant. Store in FR.

Analytical Method:

RIA, double antibody; Nichols Institute, *op cit.;* Midgley, A. R., Jr., Radioimmunoassay for human follicle-stimulating hormone. *J. Clin. Endocrinol. Metab.* **27,** 295–299 (1967); Midgley, A. R., Jr., Radioimmunoassay: A method for human chorionic gonadotropin and human luteinizing hormone. *Endocrinology* **79,** 10–18 (1966).

*   *   *

Reference (Normal) Values:

Age	FSH, int. units/L		LH, int. units/L	
	M	**F**	**M**	**F**
0–3 mo			<45	
0–4 mo	<30 (most <12)			
0–6 mo		<75		
1–6 mo				<40
4 mo–2 yr	<5		<13	
6 mo–2 yr		<15 (most <1)		<14
2–6 yr			<10	
2–8 yr				<12
2–10 yr		<7		
2–11 yr	<7			
6–10 yr			<14	
8–12 yr				3–25
11 yr–adult	<14			
Puberty		increasing to adult values		
Adult		<18[a]	<30	<90[b]

[a] Includes follicular and luteal values, but ovulatory values that reach 25 are excluded. FSH is secreted episodically in pre- and postpubertal subjects. Values obtained on the same normal individual on the same or different days may vary widely within the normal range.

[b] Includes follicular and luteal values, but ovulatory values that reach 200 are excluded.

Sources of Reference (Normal) Values:

Institutional; Winter, J. S. D., Faiman, C., Hobson, W. C., Prasad, A. V., and Reyes, F. I., Pituitary–gonadal relations in infancy. I. Patterns of serum gonadotropin concentrations from birth to four years of age in man and chimpanzee. *J. Clin. Endocrinol. Metab.* **40,** 545–551 (1975); Apter, D., Pakarinen, A., and Vihko, R., Serum prolactin, FSH and LH during puberty in girls and boys. *Acta Pediatr. Scand.* **67,** 417–423 (1978); Job, J. C., Chaussain, J. L., and Garnier, P. E., The use of luteinizing hormone-releasing hormone in pediatric patients. *Horm. Res.* **8,** 171–187 (1977).

Specimen Volume:

1 mL each.

Analytical Method:

RIA (I^{125} tracer, NIH antibody, second-antibody separation).

*   *   *

Reference (Normal) Values:

Age	FSH	LH
Child, 1–11 yr	<1.3 int. unit/L	<0.7 int. unit/L
12–16 yr	<2.2	<1.2

Sources of Reference (Normal) Values:

Institutional.

Specimen Volume:

100 µL each.

Analytical Method:

RIA, double antibody, polyethylene glycol separation; standard reference is LER 907 containing both LH + FSH; the first antibody is rabbit anti-human LH + FSH, prepared locally; the second antibody is goat anti-rabbit (Burroughs-Wellcome); ^{125}I-labeled LH + FSH is from Serono (Switzerland); Greenwood, F. C., Hunter, W. M., and Glover, J. S., The preparation of I-131 labelled human growth hormone of high specific radioactivity. *Biochem. J.* **89,** 114–123 (1963); Feldman, H., and Rodbard, D., Mathematical theory of radioimmunoassay. In *Principles of Competitive Protein-Binding Assays*, W. D. Odell and W. H. Daughaday, Eds. J. B. Lippincott Co., Philadelphia, PA, 1971, pp 158–203.

Instrumentation:

LKB 80 000 gamma counter and dilutor; Oxford Microdoser.

Commentary—Ann Johanson

Gonadotropins, both LH and FSH, are measurable by RIA in children of all ages *(1–4)*. Concentrations vary with sex and age. In both males and females, LH and FSH are high for the first several months of life, after which they decrease to rather constant prepubertal values. At birth, FSH concentration may be as much as 30 int. units/ L in males and 80 int. units/L in females; LH may be 50 to 60 int. units/L in both sexes at birth, decreasing more slowly in females. FSH in females may be, to four years of age, twice those concentrations found in later prepubertal years *(3,5)*. LH and FSH after four years and until puberty are each less than 6 int. units/L in both sexes.

At puberty, from age nine to 10 years, there is a gradual increase in both LH and FSH, to reach mean adult values at ages 14 to 15. Gonadotropins are secreted in pulses, and therefore may vary within a several-hour period through the entire normal range—a difference of 300 to 400% (6,7). Pubertal girls, within two to three years of earliest sexual development, exhibit the cyclic pattern characteristic of the adult woman, with higher follicular-phase values than luteal-phase values, and strikingly higher midcycle values of LH (>100 int. units/d) and FSH (>40 int. units/d) for one to two days.

Agonadal individuals (e.g., with Turner's syndrome or anorchia) have modestly high FSH concentrations but normal LH concentrations, prepubertally. At adolescence LH and FSH greatly increase (4,5). Hypogonadotropic values are the same as prepubertal or low normal adult values, making diagnosis difficult (4).

Human choriogonadotropin concentrations are higher in mothers giving birth to girls than in mothers delivering boys, but cord blood values do not differ with sex (8). Values at later times have not been reported.

LH and FSH can also be measured by RIA in urine after acetone precipitation (9). Concentrations closely parallel serum values but are more discriminatory in distinguishing prepubertal, mid-pubertal, and adult values, as well as hypogonadotropic values, probably because urinary values reflect total daily secretion, or an integrated mean daily concentration in blood.

1. Kulin, H. E., and Reiter, E. O., Gonadotropins during childhood and adolescence: A review. *Pediatrics* **51**, 260–271 (1973).
2. Lee, P. A., Jaffe, R. B., and Midgley, A. R., Serum gonadotropin, testosterone and prolactin concentrations throughout puberty in boys: A longitudinal study. *J. Clin. Endocrinol. Metab.* **39**, 664–672 (1974).
3. Winter, J. S. D., Faiman, C., Hobson, W. C., Prasad, A. V., and Reyes, F. I., Pituitary–gonadal relations in infancy. I. Patterns of serum gonadotropin concentrations from birth to 4 years of age in man and chimpanzee. *J. Clin. Endocrinol. Metab.* **40**, 545–551 (1975).
4. Johanson, A. J., *Recent Advances in Endocrinology. Excerpta Med. Int. Congr. Ser.* **238**, 182–192 (1970).
5. Conte, F. A., Grumbach, M. M., and Kaplan, S. L., A diphasic pattern of gonadotropin secretion in patients with syndrome of gonadal dysgenesis. *J. Clin. Endocrinol. Metab.* **40**, 670–674 (1975).
6. Johanson, A., Fluctuations of gonadotropin levels in children. *J. Clin. Endocrinol. Metab.* **39**, 154–159 (1974).
7. Faiman, C., and Winter, J. S. D., Diurnal cycles in plasma FSH, testosterone and cortisol in men. *J. Clin. Endocrinol. Metab.* **33**, 186–192 (1971).
8. Penny, R., Olambiwonnu, N. A., and Frasier, S. E., A difference in maternal and chorionic gonadotropin (HCG) concentrations, but not in cord serum HCG concentrations, as related to the sex of the fetus. *Pediatr. Res.* **9**, 293 (1975).
9. Raiti, S., Light, C., and Blizzard, R. M., Urinary follicle stimulating hormone excretion in boys and adult males as measured by radioimmunoassay. *J. Clin. Endocrinol. Metab.* **29**, 884–890 (1969).

Growth Hormone, Human (Somatotropin)

Specimen Tested:

P, S.

Laboratories Reporting:

3 (reports from each lab. follow).

* * *

Reference (Normal) Values:

Note: Measurement of somatotropin in a single "fasting" blood sample is not an appropriate method for testing deficiency; provocative stimulation is required.

Child   Baseline, resting: 0–10 ng/mL
        After stimulation (exercise, hypoglycemia, L-dopa): >5 ng/mL

Sources of Reference (Normal) Values:

Keenan, B. S., Killmer, L. B., Jr., and Sode, J., Growth hormone response to exercise. *Pediatrics* **50,** 760–764 (1972); Frasier, S. D., A review of growth hormone stimulation tests in children. *Pediatrics* **53,** 929–937 (1974).

Specimen Volume, Collection, and Preservation;
Patient Preparation:

100 μL. Heparin or EDTA anticoagulant. Preserve specimen in a FR. Have patient fast overnight.

Analytical Method:

RIA, double antibody, with paper discs as solid phase, I^{125}; Phadebas hGH PRIST.

Instrumentation:

Liquid scintillation gamma counter.

* * *

Reference (Normal) Values

Child, prepubertal, and adult M: <5 ng/mL (fasting)
Adult F: <8 ng/mL

Sources of Reference (Normal) Values:

Alsever, R. N., and Gotlin, R. W., *Handbook of Endocrine Tests in Adults and Children.* Year Book Medical Publishers, Chicago, IL, 1975, p 14; institutional.

Specimen Volume:

200 μL.

Analytical Method:

RIA; Shalch, D. S., and Parker, M. L., A sensitive double antibody immunoassay for human growth hormone in plasma. *Nature* **203,** 1141–1142 (1964); Kallestad Lab., Inc., Quantitope ¹²⁵I Growth Hormone Radioimmunoassay kit.

Instrumentation:

Nuclear Chicago gamma counter; Clay-Adams adjustable volume dispenser.

*   *   *

Reference (Normal) Values:

As noted above, random samples have little diagnostic value.

After stimulation (exercise, arginine, insulin), peak value >5 ng/mL.

Sources of Reference (Normal) Values:

Institutional.

Specimen Volume:

100 μL.

Analytical Method:

Institutional; RIA; unpublished.

Commentary—Eleanor Colle

Growth hormone is secreted episodically throughout the day with a sleep-associated, major secretory burst *(1)*. Spontaneous peaks are more frequent in adolescent males than in prepubertal or adult males *(2)*. Females tend to have more frequent secretory bursts of greater amplitude *(2)*. Fasting values are low in both children and adults, unless sampling happens to occur during a spontaneous secretory burst. Infants have high concentrations that remain high for the first six to eight weeks of life *(3)*.

To rule out growth-hormone deficiency, one of several stimuli to growth-hormone secretion must be used, including the production of hypoglycemia by insulin injection, intravenous infusion of arginine (0.5 mg/kg of body wt), intramuscular glucagon with oral administration of propanolol, oral administration of L-dopa, or exercise *(4)*. The latter, the least invasive stimulatory test, is positive in 80% of children and adolescents, although adults may fail to respond with growth hormone unless exercise is strenuous *(5)*.

Children who are hypothyroid may fail to have normal growth-hormone release. Therefore, growth-hormone testing should be done only after a euthyroid state is induced by appropriate treatment *(6)*. Some boys with severe adolescent delay fail to release growth hormone until after three to five days of treatment with estrogens or testosterone *(7)*. Children with social deprivation may release growth hormone when stimulated with propanolol and L-dopa, when other stimulatory tests may have given negative results *(8)*. In general, results of two stimulatory tests should be negative before a diagnosis of growth-hormone deficiency is secure *(5)*.

1. Goldsmith, S. J., and Glick, S. M., Rhythmicity of growth hormone secretion. *Mt. Sinai J. Med. N.Y.* **37**, 501–509 (1970).
2. Finklestein, J. W., Rottwarg, H. P., Boyar, R. M., Kream, J., and Hellman, L., Age-related change in the 24 hour spontaneous secretion of growth hormone. *J. Clin. Endocrinol. Metab.* **35**, 665–670 (1972).
3. Cornblath, M., Parker, M. L., Reisner, S. H., Forbes, A. E., and Daughaday, W. H., Secretion and metabolism of growth hormone in premature and full-term infants. *J. Clin. Endocrinol. Metab.* **25**, 209–218 (1965).
4. Frasier, S. D., A review of growth hormone stimulation tests in children. *Pediatrics* **53**, 929–937 (1974).
5. Johanson, A. J., and Morris, G. L., A single determination to rule out growth hormone deficiency. *Pediatrics* **56**, 467–468 (1971).
6. Iawatsubo, H., Omori, K., Okado, Y., Fukuchi, M., Kiyoshi, M., Abe, H., and Kumahara, Y., Human growth hormone secretion in primary hypothyroidism before and after treatment. *J. Clin. Endocrinol. Metab.* **27**, 1751–1754 (1967).
7. Frantz, A. G., and Rapkin, M. T., Effects of estrogen and sex difference on secretion of human growth hormone. *J. Clin. Endocrinol. Metab.* **25**, 1470–1480 (1965).
8. Collu, R., Brun, G., Milsant, F., Leboeuf, G., Letarte, J., and Ducharme, J., Reevaluation of levodopa–propanolol as a test of growth hormone reserve in children. *Pediatrics* **61**, 242–244 (1978).

Haptoglobins (Serum Hemoglobin-Binding Capacity)

Specimen Tested:

S.

Laboratories Reporting:

2.

Reference (Normal) Values:

Newborn: detectable haptoglobin in only 10–20% of infants

1 yr and older (Lab. 1):　400–1800 mg of Hb bound/L (748–1118 μmol/L)
　　　　　　　　(Lab. 2):　500–1500

Sources of Reference (Normal) Values:

Institutional; Giblett, E. R., *Genetic Markers in Human Blood.* Davis, Philadelphia, PA, 1969, p 66.

Specimen Volume, Collection, and Preservation:

1 mL. Reportedly stable for 3 d at RT, 7 d in RR, 1 yr in FR.

Analytical Method:

Electrophoresis; Valeri, C. R., Bond, J. C., Fowler, K., and Sobucki, J., Quantitation of serum hemoglobin-binding capacity using cellulose acetate membrane electrophoresis. *Clin. Chem.* **11,** 581–588 (1965).

Instrumentation:

Beckman R-101 Microzone electrophoretic cell and Analytrol densitometer.

Commentary—T. A. Blumenfeld

Haptoglobins are a group of α_2-glycoproteins in plasma that possess several common properties, principally the capacity to bind free hemoglobin. Haptoglobins occur in normal plasma, lymph, and urine, and in pleural, synovial, ascitic, and spinal fluids. Three phenotypes of haptoglobin have been described, Hp 1–1, Hp 2–1, and Hp 2–2 *(1).* The amount in urine partly depends on the phenotype, because the smaller molecule Hp 1–1 is more rapidly released through the diseased kidney. One milligram of hemoglobin combines with 1.3 mg of Hp 1 or Hp 2, and the hemoglobin/haptoglobin complex is removed by the reticuloendothelial system. When all of the haptoglobin is saturated, excess hemoglobin appears in the free state, first in the plasma and then in the urine.

Normally, the binding capacity of haptoglobins for free hemoglobin in the total circulating blood of an adult totals 1–4 g. Under normal physiological conditions, breakdown of erythrocytes releases 0.7 g of hemoglobin per day. Thus, 1 g of haptoglobin per day is involved with normal hemoglobin catabolism, and is therefore subtracted from values calculated to be circulating in blood. After intravenous injection of enough hemoglobin to saturate the hemoglobin-combining capacity of plasma, the injected hemoglobin is complexed with haptoglobin within 10 min and the hemoglobin/haptoglobin complex is catabolized at the rate of about 13 mg/dL per hour. Therefore, the hemoglobin-binding capacity of the serum decreases perceptibly within 10 min and the total serum haptoglobin, including that complexed in vivo with hemoglobin, will reach its lowest value after 8 h. Haptoglobin synthesis, probably in the liver, causes serum haptoglobins to return to their previous concentration in four to seven days.

Low values for serum haptoglobins may be attributed to the presence of free hemoglobin in the plasma, to severe hepatic disease, or, rarely, to congenital ahaptoglobinemia. Values increase after steroid administration or in the presence of malignancy or inflammation. Intravascular hemolysis in patients with an average blood volume of 5 L will decrease the haptoglobin value about 100 mg/dL for every 20 mL of whole blood (or 10 mL of erythrocytes) lysed. Because the average normal serum haptoglobin is 100 mg/dL, this small amount of lysis results in a decrease of serum haptoglobin to very low values *(2)*.

Before 1966 it was thought that haptoglobins might be present in the serum of newborns in very small amounts, even though hemoglobinuria is extremely rare *(3)*. In 1971, Philip *(4)*, using the method described by Owen *(5)*, measured haptoglobin in 50 newborns and found that all had detectable haptoglobin. Owen's method is based on peroxidase activity of the haptoglobin/methemoglobin complex and expresses values for haptoglobin in terms of hemoglobin-binding capacity. In Philip's study, mean haptoglobin increased from 24.4 mg/dL in cord-blood samples to 49 mg/dL of circulating whole blood on the fifth day. Infants with low birth weight and (or) gestation periods of less than 32 to 38 weeks have lower haptoglobin values at birth and after 28 days than do full-term infants at these times *(6)*.

There are two possible explanations for the lower haptoglobin concentrations in the serum of newborns. Maybe the values are in fact quantitatively less than in adults and gradually increase to adult values in the first weeks or months; this would be similar to the gradual increase in immunoglobulins and total proteins, principally albumin, both produced almost exclusively in the liver. It is also possible that the amount of antigenically competent haptoglobin is the same as in the adult, but that because of certain differences in structure, the normal change in peroxidase activity of hemoglobin is not seen when this "immature" haptoglobin is added.

In a study of serum haptoglobin in 305 children, 20 days to 14 years of age, mean haptoglobin concentrations ranged from 89 to 110 mg/dL. The mean for adults in the same study was 97 mg/dL *(7)*.

1. Jayle, M. F., and Moretti, J., Haptoglobin. Biochemical, genetic and physiopathologic aspects. *Progr. Hematol.* **3**, 342–359 (1962).
2. Fink, D. J., Petz, L. D., and Black, M. B., Serum haptoglobin. *J. Am. Med. Assoc.* **199**, 615–618 (1967).
3. Drakowa, D., The relation of serum haptoglobin levels to age and sex in healthy children. *Arch. Immunol. Ther. Exp.* **14**, 47–55 (1966).
4. Philip, A. G. S., Haptoglobins in the newborn. 1. Full-term infants. *Biol. Neonate* **19**, 185–193 (1971).
5. Owen, J. A., Better, F. C., and Hoban, J., A simple method for the determination of serum haptoglobins. *J. Clin. Pathol.* **13**, 163–164 (1960).
6. Philip, A. G. S., Haptoglobins in the newborn. II. Low birth weight babies. *Biol. Neonate* **19**, 322–328 (1971).

7. Sklavunu-Zurukzoglu, S., and Malaka, K., Serum-haptoglobins in childhood. *Lancet* **ii,** 722 (1961).

Note: See also Chapter 10, **Specific Proteins in Pediatrics.**

Hematocrit

Specimen Tested:

B.

Laboratories Reporting:

3.

Reference (Normal) Values:

Age	%
Birth	44–64
14–90 d	35–49
6 mo–1 yr	30–40
4–10 yr	31–43

Sources of Reference (Normal) Values:

Institutional.

Specimen Volume, Collection, and Preservation:

50 μL. Heparin or EDTA anticoagulant.

Analytical Method:

Text ref. 2, p 187.

Instrumentation:

IEC Hematocrit Microcentrifuge; International Clinical or Micro Capillary Reader; Coulter Electronics, Inc., Model S.

Hemoglobin

In Blood

Specimen Tested:

B.

Laboratories Reporting:

3.

Reference (Normal) Values:

Age	Hemoglobin, g/L	Age	Hemoglobin, g/L
Birth	150–240; 180–265	3–5 mo	100–145
1 d	140–240	6 mo	105–145; 106–154
2 d	150–230	1 yr	110–150
4–8 d	140–220	2 yr	120–150
6 d	130–230	3 yr	102–148
9–13 d	130–200	4–5 yr	103–149
2 wk	134–192; 150–200	6–10 yr	106–152
2 wk–2 mo	107–173	6–12 yr	100–143
1 mo	110–170; 121–173	11–15 yr	111–157
2 mo	110–140	Adult, M	140–160
3 mo	100–130; 98–162	F	120–160

Sources of Reference (Normal) Values:

Wintrobe, M. M., *Clinical Hematology,* 5th ed. Lea and Febiger, Philadelphia, PA, 1961, p 105; institutional.

Specimen Volume, Collection, and Preservation:

20 to 50 μL. Heparin or EDTA anticoagulant. Stable up to 1 wk in RR.

Analytical Method:

Cyanmethemoglobin; Miale, J. B., *Laboratory Medicine Hematology,* 4th ed. C. V. Mosby Co., St. Louis, MO, 1972, p 1216; Harboe, M., Studies on the conversion of oxyhemoglobin to alkaline hematin in dilute alkaline solution. *Scand. J. Lab. Clin. Invest.* **11,** 138–142 (1959).

Instrumentation:

Coulter-S; Zeiss spectrophotometer.

Commentary—T. A. Blumenfeld

The mean concentration of hemoglobin in cord blood at birth is 170 g/L and the mean hematocrit is 55% (range, 43–73%). These values may be modified by several factors that must be considered when interpreting hematological data on the newborn.

Gestational age may affect the hemoglobin and hematocrit values: during the final weeks of intrauterine life, the hemoglobin concentration of whole blood rapidly increases, with average increments of 10–30 g/L between the 39th and 40th weeks. This magnitude of change is reflected in the lower hemoglobin concentration at birth in prematures.

The length of time elapsing before the umbilical cord is clamped at delivery can considerably affect the newborn's blood volume and total circulating erythrocyte mass. Placental vessels contain about 100 mL of blood at term. A major fraction of the placental blood can be transfused into the infant if the clinician attempts to empty the placental vessels at delivery—i.e., by placing the infant lower than the placenta and delaying clamping the cord for several minutes after birth, the blood volume of the infant can be increased by as much as 40–60%. Newborn infants with delayed clamping of the cord have mean blood volumes of 126 mL/kg of body weight, compared with 78 mL/kg in infants whose cords are clamped immediately at delivery. In both groups of infants the average hematocrit is the same at birth, but after 48 h the mean hematocrit is 65% in those with delayed cord clamping and 48% in those in whom placental transfusion is prevented (2). Increased hemoglobin and hematocrit values can be demonstrated for at least three to four days in infants for whom cord clamping was delayed.

Transfusion of placental blood into the infant at birth may result in even greater increases in the blood volume in the case of premature infants. The quantity of blood in the placenta undergoes little change in the last two to three months of gestation, during which time the blood volume of the infant increases greatly. The premature infant can thereby receive a proportionately larger fraction of blood volume by the addition of placental blood.

In the newborn, hemoglobin values in samples obtained by puncture of the infant's heel or finger are usually increased by 20–30 g/L over values for simultaneously obtained venous blood, a difference attributable to the sluggish peripheral circulation of the newborn. Values obtained for venous blood are generally more reliable and reproducible, and are preferable for very accurate assessment of hemoglobin concentration during the first few days of life.

Additionally, during the first few hours after delivery there is a shift in the distribution of fluid, which may modify the hemoglobin and hematocrit value; this shift results in a decreased circulating plasma volume and a proportionately increased erythrocyte concentration. Consequently, hemoglobin is typically increased about 20 g/L above cord blood values within the first 24 h of life.

Within hours after birth of a normal infant, the low oxygen saturation of the blood increases, reaching about 93% saturation. The striking changes in erythropoiesis in the first weeks of life are largely due to the improved oxygenation of the blood and tissues. Erythropoietin concentrations, which are relatively high at birth, rapidly decline to undetectable values, and the erythropoietic activity of the bone marrow is decreased.

The postnatal suppression of erythropoiesis and the expansion of the infant's blood volume due to rapid growth result in a progressive decrease in the infant's hemoglobin concentration, beginning near the end of the first week and reaching a low point after two to three months. This "physiological anemia" may result in a hemoglobin concentration as low as 90 (110 ± 20) g/L in a normal full-term infant. These changes do not represent any abnormality or nutritional deficiency, and hematological events at this stage are not affected by administration of iron or other hematinic agents. Active erythropoiesis resumes after the second to third month if iron supplies are adequate, and the mean concentration of hemoglobin gradually increases to 125 g/L, which persists throughout early childhood.

Premature infants, particularly those with birth weights of less than 1500 g, undergo a physiological decrease in hemoglobin concentration earlier than full-term infants, and ultimately reach a lower concentration. Minimum values are achieved by four to seven weeks, and hemoglobin concentrations may be 70–80 g/L at this time in apparently healthy premature infants. They resume active erythropoiesis earlier in postnatal life than do full-term infants.

1. Honig, G. R., Disorders of the blood and vascular system. In *Neonatology, Diseases of the Fetus and Infant*, R. E. Behrman, Ed. C. V. Mosby Co., St. Louis, MO, 1973, pp 171–217.
2. Usher, R., Shephard, M., and Lind, J., The blood volume of the newborn infant and placental transfusion. *Acta Paediatr. Scand.* **52**, 497–512 (1963).

In Plasma

Specimen Tested:

P.

Laboratories Reporting:

4.

Reference (Normal) Values:

Lab. 1 (data for plasma obtained solely by skin puncture):

Age	No.	mg/L (mean)
0–13 d	176	390; 73% <500; <3% above 1000; highest value: 1470
14 d–3 mo	47	220
>3 mo–2 yr	49	160
>2 yr	145	100
All ages	417	260
Adults	(literature)	190

Labs. 2–4: up to 500 mg/L

Sources of Reference (Normal) Values:

Institutional study; Meites, S., and Lin, S. S., Hemolysis in plasma samples from skin puncture of children. *Clin. Chem.* **26**, 987 (1980), abstract; Dacie, J. V., and Lewis, S. M., *Practical Haematology*, 3rd ed. Grune and Stratton, New York, NY, 1963, pp 380–382.

Specimen Volume, Collection, and Preservation:

10 µL to 5 mL. Heparin anticoagulant. Store P in FR.

Analytical Method:

Lab. 1: Elson, E. C., Ivor, L., and Gochman, N., Substitution of a nonhazardous chromogen for benzidine in the measurement of plasma hemoglobin. *Am. J. Clin. Pathol.* **69,** 354–355 (1978). **Lab. 2:** Cripps, C. P., Rapid method for the estimation of plasma hemoglobin levels. *J. Clin. Pathol.* **21,** 110–111 (1968). **Lab. 3:** Hunter, F. T., Grove-Rasmussen, M., and Soutter, L., A spectrophotometric method for quantitating hemoglobin in plasma or serum. *Am. J. Clin. Pathol.* **20,** 429–433 (1950). **Lab. 4:** Shinowara, G. Y., Spectrophotometric studies on blood serum and plasma. *Am. J. Clin. Pathol.* **24,** 696–710 (1954).

Commentary—T. A. Blumenfeld

		Values from the literature, mg/L	Ref.
Infant:	Umbilical vein plasma	80	*1*
Adult:	Circulating plasma	1.6–5.8	*2*
	Venous plasma	20–30	*3*
	Venous serum	90 (10–220)	*4*
	Capillary plasma	190 (100–320)	*1*
	Capillary plasma (warmed hand)	110 (20–210)	*4*
	Capillary plasma (unwarmed hand)	160 (30–230)	*4*
	Capillary serum (warmed hand)	130 (50–230)	*4*
	Capillary serum (unwarmed hand)	130 (40–260)	*4*

The normal range for free hemoglobin in plasma is 1.6–5.8 mg/L. Unless the patient has intravascular hemolysis, the serum or plasma hemoglobin measured in the laboratory is most affected by the method of obtaining the specimen, the hematocrit, and the fragility of the erythrocytes. Because abnormal amounts of hemoglobin in serum or plasma can interfere with laboratory determination of potassium, bilirubin, hemoglobin, haptoglobin, iron, and enzymes, it is important to know the range of hemoglobin values to be expected when different methods of specimen collection are used, and the values for different sorts of populations.

Venous serum contains more hemoglobin than does venous plasma. The values for hemoglobin in serum and plasma stated in the literature are from different studies, and it is not possible to know whether the mean difference (60 mg/L) is statistically significant; however, this difference probably would interfere with no clinical laboratory tests. Capillary (skin-puncture) blood specimens from adults contain more hemoglobin in the serum and plasma than do venous samples from adults (mean difference, 40 mg/L in serum) *(4);* however, this small difference also will not interfere with clinical laboratory tests.

If no special precautions are taken before obtaining a sample by skin puncture in an adult, the capillary plasma hemoglobin value is higher than the capillary serum hemoglobin value, but the difference is neither statistically nor clinically significant. Heating increases blood flow about sevenfold, makes specimen collection easier, increases the volume of the specimen obtained, and speeds collection, but it does not significantly decrease the serum or plasma hemoglobin in adults *(4)*.

Plasma hemoglobin is much higher in capillary (skin-puncture) specimens from infants than from adults, probably because of the infant's higher hematocrit and more fragile erythrocytes. In a study comparing different methods of specimen collection from skin-puncture sites in infants under the best conditions, with use of thin-wall capillary tubes with siliconized puncture site, the plasma hemoglobin concentration was 1000 mg/L (range 250–2700) *(1)*. The highest values for free hemoglobin were reported when the blood was collected drop by drop into test tubes.

To the unaided eye, plasma appears faintly pink when the free hemoglobin concentration is 200 mg/L, red when 1000 mg/L *(3)*. However, to the unaided eye, a free hemoglobin concentration of 2000 mg/L will be undetectable if the bilirubin is 200 mg/L and will appear faintly pink if the bilirubin is 100 mg/L *(5)*.

1. Michaëlsson, M., and Sjölin, S., Haemolysis in blood samples from newborn infants. *Acta Paediatr. Scand.* **54,** 325–330 (1965).
2. Hanks, G. E., Cassell, M., Ray, R. N., and Chaplin, H., Jr., Further modification of the benzidine method for measurement of hemoglobin in plasma; definition of a new range of normal values. *J. Lab. Clin. Med.* **56,** 486–498 (1960).
3. Mollison, P. L., *Blood Transfusion in Clinical Medicine,* 3rd ed. Blackwell, Oxford, England, 1961.
4. Blumenfeld, T. A., Hertelendy, W. G., and Ford, S. H., Simultaneously obtained skin-puncture serum, skin-puncture plasma, and venous serum compared, and effects of warming the skin before puncture. *Clin. Chem.* **23,** 1705–1710 (1977).
5. Watson, D., A note on the haemoglobin error in some non-precipitation diazo-methods for bilirubin determinations. *Clin. Chim. Acta* **5,** 613–615 (1960).

Hemoglobin, Electrophoresis of

Specimen Tested:

B.

Laboratories Reporting:

2.

Reference (Normal) Values:

Lab. 1: $HbA_1 + HbA_3$: 96.0–98.5% of total hemoglobin
HbA_2:   1.5–4.0%
Lab. 2: HbA migrates to the postive pole. HbF is cathodal to HbA (behind HbA). HbS migrates half-way between HbA_2 and HbA. HbC migrates to the position of HbA_2.

Note: See also Commentary for **Glycohemoglobins.**

Sources of Reference (Normal) Values:

Lab. 1: Institutional; Helena Labs., Procedure No. 15, March, 1978.
Lab. 2: Atwater, J., and Schwartz, E., Separation of hemoglobin. In *Hematology,* 2nd ed., W. J. Williams, E. Beutler, A. J. Erslev, and R. W. Rundles, Eds. McGraw-Hill, New York, NY, 1977, pp 1597–1601.

Specimen Volume, Collection, and Preservation:

5 μL. Heparin or EDTA anticoagulant. Store in RR. Samples in Alsever's solution (20.5 g of glucose, 8 g of sodium citrate, 0.5 g of citric acid, and 4.2 g of NaCl per liter) are stable for mailing; stability of Hb variants is not established, however, so specimens for this determination should not be mailed.

Analytical Method:

Lab. 1: Schmidt, R. M., and Holland, S., Standardization in abnormal hemoglobin detection. An evaluation of hemoglobin electrophoresis kits. *Clin. Chem.* **20,** 591–594 (1974); Helena Hb Electrophoresis kit.
Lab. 2: vertical starch gel hemoglobin electrophoresis in Tris–EDTA–borate buffer, pH 8.6, 4 °C, 15–20 h, at 25 mA, 200 V, with electrostarch; control: hemolysate containing J, A, F, S, and C hemoglobins with each run. For further details, see **Hemoglobin Variants.**

Instrumentation:

Lab. 1: Helena Labs. Electrophoresis System.

Commentary—Jeanne M. Lusher

Hemoglobin electrophoresis is a very useful tool for identification of specific hemoglobin types. By electrophoresis proteins can be separated and classified on the basis of their surface charge and their migration in an electric field. When hemoglobin (or other protein) molecules are in solution, they are partially ionized and acquire a net electrical charge. The latter depends not only on the number of uncombined ionizable groups in the molecule, but also on the pH of the solution.

Amino acid substitutions in the various abnormal hemoglobins result in different net charges in solution, which can be used to separate the abnormal hemoglobins on the basis of their movement in an electrical field. The hemoglobin will migrate at a rate determined by the net charge of the molecule, the pH, the ionic strength of the buffer, and the type of supporting medium.

Electrophoresis is not definitive as a test to identify specific hemoglobin types because many hemoglobins move to the same position under specific conditions of the test. For example, hemoglobins D, Flatbush, Zurich, Lepore, and others migrate to the same position as hemoglobin S at pH 8.0–8.9 *(1)*. Thus a combination of tests must be used to identify hemoglobin types with certainty. To identify hemoglobin S, either a sickling or solubility test should be used in conjunction with electrophoresis.

Most electrophoresis techniques involve the use of stabilizing media such as agar, starch gel, cellulose acetate, or acrylamide gel. Cellulose acetate has gained increasing popularity over the last decade as a support medium for hemoglobin electrophoresis, allowing rapid (1–1.5 h) separation of hemoglobins. In addition, a micromethod for cellulose-acetate electrophoresis of capillary blood samples is quite reliable. Distinct bands clearly separate hemoglobins A, C, and S, as well as A_2, allowing detection of some cases of β-thalassemia trait. Samples containing abnormal hemoglobins should be subjected to additional testing, such as agar gel electrophoresis at an acid pH if hemoglobin D is suspected, a sickling or solubility test if S is suspected, or quantitation of hemoglobins A_2 and F if β-thalassemia trait is suspected.

Hemoglobin types in cord blood or neonatal samples can be accurately determined as long as certain technical difficulties are understood. In the newborn the detection of abnormal hemoglobins is dependent on the identification of small quantities of hemoglobin A, S, C, etc. in the presence of large quantities of hemoglobin F, which can be done by using agar gel electrophoresis at pH 6.2 *(2)*. Other forms of electrophoresis are unsuitable because of their inability to separate A from F.

Starch gel electrophoresis at pH 6.8–7.0 can clearly separate hemoglobins H and Barts from all other hemoglobins. Hemoglobin H is a tetramer of β chains (β_4), while Barts is a tetramer of γ chains (γ_4). Trace amounts of hemoglobin H may be found in normal cord blood, but values greater than 1% (usually 5–15%) indicate a relative deficiency of α-chain synthesis (α-thalassemia). In α-thalassemia trait the concentration of hemoglobin Barts decreases after birth, in parallel with the decline of hemoglobin F ($\alpha_2\gamma_2$). Thus, by three or four months of age hemoglobin Barts is no longer detectable in infants with α-thalassemia trait. Persistence of high amounts of hemoglobin H (hemoglobin-H disease) indicates interaction of two different α-thalassemia genes (α-thal$_1$, α-thal$_2$).

Hemoglobins Barts and H are unique in their anodal migration at pH 6.5–7.0, making them easy to identify. Starch gel electrophoresis at a more alkaline pH of 8.8 can distinguish many other hemoglobins from hemoglobin A. It is also the method of choice for detecting hemoglobin constant spring, an α-chain variant *(3)*.

1. Barnhart, M. I., Henry, R. L., and Lusher, J. M., *Sickle Cell.* The Upjohn Co., Kalamazoo, MI, 1976, pp 72–85.
2. Pearson, H. A., and O'Brien, R. T., Sickle cell testing programs. *J. Pediatr.* **81,** 1201–1204 (1972).
3. Weatherall, D. J., The thalassemias. In *Hematology,* 2nd ed., W. J. Williams, E. Beutler, A. J. Erslev, and R. W. Rundles, Eds. McGraw-Hill, New York, NY, 1977, pp 391–413.

Hemoglobin Variants

Hemoglobin Variant A$_2$

Specimen Tested:

B.

Laboratories Reporting:

2.

Reference (Normal) Values:

Lab. 1: Newborn: not detectable (by chromatography)
Child: reaches adult values at about 6 mo
Adult: 1.9–3.2% of total Hb

		% of total hemoglobin (and no. tested)	
	Analytical technique	Controls	Beta-thalassemia trait
Lab. 2:	Chromatography	1.6 –2.9% (99)	4.1 –5.4% (24)
	Cellulose acetate electrophoresis	1.94–3.18% (3)	3.38–5.82% (28)

Sources of Reference (Normal) Values:

Lab. 1: Huisman, T. H. J., Chromatographic determination of Hb-A$_2$. *CRC Crit. Rev. Clin. Lab. Sci.* **5,** 57–61 (1974). **Lab. 2:** *chromatography:* Schleider, C. T. H., Mayson, S. M., and Huisman, T. H. J., Further modifications of the microchromatographic determination of hemoglobin A$_2$. *Hemoglobin* **1,** 503–504 (1977); *electrophoresis:* Schmidt, R. M., Rucknagel, D. L., and Necheles, T. F., Comparison of methodologies for thalassemia screening by hemoglobin A$_2$ quantitation. *J. Lab. Clin. Med.* **86,** 873–882 (1975).

Specimen Volume, Collection, and Preservation:

Lab. 1: 100 μL. **Lab. 2:** 2 to 3 mL. Heparin or EDTA anticoagulant. Store in RR.

Analytical Method:

Lab. 1: Efremov, C. D., Huisman, T. H. J., Bowman, K., Wrightstone, R. N., and Schroeder, W. A., Microchromatography of hemoglobins. II. A rapid method for the determination of hemoglobin A_2. *J. Lab. Clin. Med.* **83**, 657–664 (1974). **Lab. 2:** Huisman, *op. cit;* Weatherall, D. J., and Clegg, J. B., *The Thalassemia Syndromes*, 2nd ed. Blackwell Scientific Publications, Oxford, 1972, pp 311–312.

Instrumentation:

Lab. 1: Gilford 2400 S spectrophotometer; Pasteur pipette chromatography columns. **Lab. 2:** Spectrophotometer (chromatography); Helena Labs. Zip-Zone electrophoresis apparatus. Do *not* scan the cellulose acetate plates by densitometry.

Commentary—Jeanne M. Lusher

HbA_2 ($\alpha_2\delta_2$) is 2–3% of hemoglobin in the adult. The amounts of HbA_2 in cord blood are quite low, however, because δ-chain synthesis does not begin until late in fetal life. Cord-blood values range from 0 to 1.8% *(1)*. After birth, A_2 values increase steadily, reaching the normal adult range at approximately five months of age *(2)*.

Many methods are available for quantitating HbA_2, the most rapid and reliable of which is diethylaminoethyl (DEAE)–cellulose chromatography *(3,4)*. The microchromatographic methods mentioned above are ideally suited for the small sample size from pediatric patients. By use of a special buffer, A_2 may be quantitated in the presence of hemoglobin S or other hemoglobins of similar electrophoretic mobility. The method is equally applicable to hemolysate, whole blood, or blood collected on filter paper *(4)*.

Another reliable method involves separation of hemoglobin A_2 by starch block electrophoresis, followed by elution and quantitation. This method, however, is much more time-consuming than DEAE–cellulose chromatography.

Some quantitate A_2 by scanning cellulose acetate strips, but this method is not always reliable and thus is not recommended. However, one can reliably quantitate A_2 after elution from the strip.

Clinical application is in the diagnosis of the most common form of β-thalassemia trait, where the A_2 fraction is increased. However, quantitation of HbA_2 is not useful during the first few months of life. In addition, some forms of β-thalassemia trait are characterized by increased HbF only, with normal values for A_2.

1. Minnich, V., Cordonnier, J. K., Williams, W. J., and Moore, C. V., Alpha, beta and gamma polypeptide chains during the neonatal period with description of a fetal form of hemoglobin Dα-St. Louis. *Blood* **19**, 137–167 (1962).
2. Erdem, S., and Aksoy, M., The increase of hemoglobin A$_2$ to adult level. *Isr. J. Med. Sci.* **5**, 427–428 (1969).
3. Bernini, L. S., Rapid estimation of HbA$_2$ by DEAE chromatography. *Biochem. Genet.* **2**, 305–310 (1969).
4. Efremov, C. D., Huisman, T. H. J., Bowman, K., Wrightstone, R. N., and Schroeder, W. A., Microchromatography of hemoglobins. II. A rapid method for the determination of hemoglobin A$_2$. *J. Lab. Clin. Med.* **83**, 657–664 (1974).

Hemoglobin Variant F

Specimen Tested:

B.

Laboratories Reporting:

3.

Reference (Normal) Values:

Lab. 1: Birth: 50–85% of total Hb; gradual decline, reaching adult values by about 1 yr
>2 yr: 0.25–0.75%
Lab. 2: >5 yr: 0–1%
Lab. 3: Birth: 50–85%
1 yr: <15%
Up to 2 yr: Up to 5%
>2 yr–adult: <2%

Sources of Reference (Normal) Values:

Lab. 1: Garby, L., Sjolin, S., and Vuille, J. C., Studies on erythrokinetics in infancy. II. The relative rate of synthesis of haemoglobin F and haemoglobin A during the first months of life. *Acta Paediatr.* **51**, 245–254 (1965); private communication: Detter, J. C., Dept. Lab. Med., Univ. of Washington, Seattle, WA. **Lab. 2:** Betke, K., Marti, H. R., and Schlicht, I., Estimation of small percentages of foetal hemoglobin. *Nature* **184**, 1877–1878 (1959); Weatherall, D. G., and Clegg, J. B., *The Thalassemia Syndromes*, 2nd ed. Blackwell Scientific Publications, Oxford, 1972. **Lab. 3:** institutional; Chernoff, A. I., and Singer, K., Studies on abnormal hemoglobins. IV. Persistence of fetal hemoglobin in the erythrocytes of normal children. *Pediatrics* **9**, 469–474 (1952).

Specimen Volume, Collection, and Preservation:

1.6 to 2 mL. Heparin or EDTA anticoagulant. Store in RR.

Analytical Method:

All labs use alkali-denaturation technique. **Lab. 1:** Betke et al., *op. cit.* **Lab. 2:** Betke et al., *op. cit.;* Weatherall and Clegg, *op. cit.;* the alkali-denaturation test used gives reliable results only when the HbF concentration is <20% of the total. For values >20%, an alternative method is used. **Lab. 3:** Beaven, G. H., Ellis, M. J., and White, J. C., Studies on human foetal hemoglobin. I. Detection and estimation. *Br. J. Haematol.* **6,** 1–22 (1960).

Instrumentation:

Gilford 2400 S, Zeiss, other spectrophotometers; shaking-waterbath.

Commentary—Jeanne M. Lusher

Fetal hemoglobin ($\alpha_2\gamma_2$) is the major hemoglobin in cord blood. Several properties distinguish HbF from adult hemoglobin and serve as the basis for quantitative tests for HbF.

That HbF is resistant to alkali denaturation is utilized in most of the chemical methods for determining its concentration in blood samples. With the 1-min alkali denaturation test of Singer *(1)* cord-blood proportions of HbF range from 50 to 85% of total hemoglobin, steadily decrease to <10% by four months of age, and reach adult values of <2% by two years of age. Although easy to perform, the alkali denaturation test is less sensitive at higher proportions of HbF. If more precise values are desired, column chromatography is recommended.

HbF is oxidized to methemoglobin more readily than is HbA. Because fetal methemoglobin is denatured by alkali, the sample for determining HbF should be free of methemoglobin. Therefore, use freshly prepared rather than stored hemolysates *(2)*.

In addition to its alkali resistance, HbF has a different absorption spectrum in the ultraviolet region than does HbA. This characteristic is the basis for another sensitive method for estimating HbF concentration.

The rate of decline of HbF is delayed in certain hematologic disorders such as thalassemia, sickle-cell disease, congenital and acquired hypoplastic anemias, certain forms of childhood leukemia, and the condition called "hereditary persistence of fetal hemoglobin."

Because HbF is also resistant to acid elution, an acid-elution staining technique has proved useful in several clinical situations. If anemia in the newborn is suspected to be related to fetomaternal hemorrhage, one can detect even a very small number of fetal cells in the mother's circulation by use of the acid-elution staining technique *(3)*. This method has also been used to study the distribution of HbF among erythrocytes in various hematologic disorders.

1. Singer, K., Chernoff, A. I., and Singer, L., Studies on abnormal hemoglobins. I. Their demonstration in sickle-cell anemia and other hematologic disorders by means of alkali denaturation. *Blood* **6**, 413–428 (1951).
2. Atwater, J., and Erslev, A. J., Fetal hemoglobin–alkali denaturation test. In *Hematology*, 2nd ed., W. J. Williams, E. Beutler, A. J. Erslev, and R. W. Rundles, Eds. McGraw-Hill, New York, NY, 1977, pp 1602–1603.
3. Kleihauer, E. F., Tang, T. E., and Betke, K., Die intrazelluläre Verteilung von embryonalem Hämoglobin in roten Blutzellen menschlicher Embryonen. *Acta Haematol.* **38**, 264–272 (1967).

Other Variants (Qualitative)

Specimen Tested:

B.

Laboratory Reporting:

1.

Reference (Normal) Values:

Solubility test to confirm presence of HbS: Deoxy-HbS is less soluble in concentrated salt solutions than HbS and most other Hb mutants, except HbC Harlem. This distinguishes HbS from hemoglobins G, D, and Lepore, which have similar mobilities on cellulose acetate electrophoresis.

Shaking test to confirm presence of HbS and unstable hemoglobins: Oxy-HbS and other unstable hemoglobins denature and precipitate rapidly upon mechanical shaking.

Isopropanol precipitation test to detect unstable hemoglobins: Unstable Hb becomes cloudy in 5 min; precipitate forms in 20 min. Control remains cloudy for 40 min.

Sources of Reference (Normal) Values:

Solubility test: Schmidt, R. M., and Wilson, S. M., Standardization in detection of abnormal hemoglobins. Solubility tests for hemoglobin S. *J. Am. Med. Assoc.* **225**, 1225–1230 (1973).

Shaking test: Asakura, T., Segal, M. E., Friedman, S., and Schwartz, E., A rapid test for sickle hemoglobin. *J. Am. Med. Assoc.* **233**, 156–157 (1975).

Isopropanol precipitation test: Carrell, R. W., and Kay, R. A., A simple method for detection of unstable hemoglobins. *Br. J. Haematol.* **23**, 615–619 (1972).

Specimen Volume, Collection, and Preservation:

Solubility test: 1 mL. Heparin or EDTA anticoagulant. Test fresh specimen.

Shaking and isopropanol precipitation tests: 100 µL. EDTA anticoagulant, microhematocrit tube. Store in RR.

Analytical Method:

Solubility test: Schmidt and Wilson, *op. cit.*
Shaking test: Asakura et al., *op. cit.*
Isopropanol precipitation test: Carrell and Kay, *op. cit.*

Instrumentation:

Shaking test: Technical Consulting Services Shaker.
Isopropanol precipitation kit: Centrifuges.

Notes:

1. *Solubility test:* Use positive and negative controls with each test: positive control = known HbS; negative control = known negative. This test often gives false results. High concentrations of plasma proteins or lipids cause false-positive results. False negatives may be obtained in anemic individuals with HbS, and in newborns or infants with low concentrations of HbS.

2. *Shaking test:* Use positive and negative controls with each test: positive control = known HbS; negative control = blood without HbS and unstable Hb. The shaking test is recommended in the study of unstable hemoglobins as an adjunct to tests for heat and isopropanol stability and to the brilliant cresyl blue test. This technique is good for screening HbS before using electrophoresis; it is preferable to the dithionide solubility test as a fast screening test because false-negative results have not been observed with it, and because abnormal Hb can also be detected.

3. *Isopropanol precipitation test:* Use a negative control (normal HbA) with each test. A positive test should be confirmed with a heat-stability test.

Commentary—Jeanne M. Lusher

Solubility tests, electrophoresis, chromatographic techniques, and determinations of amino acid sequences have lead to the identification of more than 160 hemoglobin variants. The existence of these variants has demanded the development of rapid and specific diagnostic tests. Most tests proposed are nonspecific and unreliable when used alone; in general, a combination of tests is necessary for the specific identification of a given hemoglobinopathy.

For example, available diagnostic tests for hemoglobin S include erythrocyte sickling tests, low-solubility tests, and electrophoresis with various supporting media and pHs. None of these methods used alone can identify HbS with certainty. Although rare, several other hemoglobins sickle, and several give a positive solubility test, e.g., HbC Georgetown, Hb Barts, HbI. In addition, the finding of a positive solubility test does not distinguish between sickle trait (AS), sickle-cell anemia (SS), or S in combination with another abnormal Hb, such as C. Thus, a positive solubility test result should always be followed by electrophoresis. Because several other hemoglobin variants are electrophoretically identical to HbS under specified conditions *(1)*, electrophoresis alone also cannot be considered definitive as a test to identify a specific hemoglobin. A combination of solubility test and electrophoresis is most desirable. If hemoglobin D is suspected, electrophoresis on agar gel at pH 6.25 should be used to distinguish between S and D.

In addition to their lack of specificity, common reasons for the unreliability of these tests include collecting blood samples within 100 days after blood transfusion; using sodium metabisulfite at >2% (>20 g/L); not using freshly prepared reagent, in the case of erythrocyte sickling tests; and testing blood too early in infancy, in the case of solubility tests.

Unstable Hemoglobins

The unstable hemoglobins, structural variants of hemoglobin A, undergo denaturation within the erythrocyte, resulting in precipitation of insoluble inclusions called Heinz bodies. The disorders formerly referred to as "congenital Heinz body anemia" are more accurately termed "unstable hemoglobin hemolytic anemia." More than 65 unstable hemoglobins have been described *(2)*.

The heat-stability and isopropanol-precipitation tests are relatively specific for unstable hemoglobin. Normal hemoglobin is somewhat unstable at 37 °C in a 17% (170 mL/L) isopropanol solution, but unstable hemoglobins precipitate much more rapidly. Isopropanol weakens the internal bonding of hemoglobin, decreasing the stability of the molecule. The isopropanol precipitation test is simple and rapid to perform; however, hemoglobin F may be largely precipitated as well. Thus, a hemolysate from an infant, or from an older child with a high proportion of hemoglobin F, may give a false-positive precipitation test result. Equivocal clouding of the solution may result from small amounts of methemoglobin, particularly if the blood sample is old. The use of fresh hemolysates is important. An advantage of the isopropanol method over the heat method is that the flocculent precipitate of unstable hemoglobin is suitable for further analysis *(3)*. Note that the proportion of hemoglobin A_2 is increased with most β-chain (but not α-chain) unstable hemoglobins.

The shaking test provides an alternative method for detecting heat-unstable hemoglobins or hemoglobin S; the presence of turbidity after shaking indicates the presence of hemoglobin S or a heat-unstable hemoglobin.

1. Barnhart, M. I., Henry, R. L., and Lusher, J. M., *Sickle Cell.* The Upjohn Co., Kalamazoo, MI, 1976, 1979.
2. Lehmann, H., Huntsman, R. G., Casey, R., Lang, A., and Lorkin, P. A., Hemoglobinopathies associated with unstable hemoglobin. In *Hematology,*

2nd ed., W. J. Williams, E. Beutler, A. J. Erslev, and R. W. Rundles, Eds. McGraw-Hill, New York, NY, 1977, pp 531–544.

3. Carrell, R. W. and Kay, R. A., A simple method for the detection of unstable haemoglobins. *Br. J. Haematol.* **23**, 615–619 (1972).

Hexose-1-Phosphate Uridylyltransferase
(EC 2.7.7.12; UDP glucose:α-D-galactose-1-phosphate uridylyltransferase)[1]

Specimen Tested:

Erythrocytes.

Laboratories Reporting:

4.

Reference (Normal) Values:

Zygosity	Arbitrary enzyme units		
	Labs. 1, 2	Lab. 3	Lab. 4
"Normal"	17–30; 15–47	18–26	16.7–37.4
Heterozygote	3–12; 5–12	5–17	
Homozygote	<3	0–2	

Sources of Reference (Normal) Values:

Labs. 1, 2: institutional. **Lab. 3:** institutional; normal values obtained on 205 children; Pesce, M. A., Bodourian, S. H., Harris, R. C., and Nicholson, J. F., Enzymatic micromethod for measuring galactose-1-phosphate uridylyltransferase activity in human erythrocytes. *Clin. Chem.* **23**, 1711–1717 (1977). **Lab. 4:** Ng, W. G., Bergren, W. R., and Donnell, G. N., A new variant of galactose-1-phosphate uridyltransferase in man: The Los Angeles variant. *Ann. Hum. Genet.* **37**, 1–8 (1973); Ng, W. G., Bergren, W. R., Donnell, G. N., and Hodgman, J. E., Galactose-1-phosphate uridyltransferase activity in hemolysates of newborn infants. *Pediatrics* **39**, 293–294 (1967).

Specimen Volume, Collection, and Preservation:

100 μL to 3 mL. Heparin anticoagulant. Washed cells or hemolysates stored in FR. Obtain sample before blood transfusion.

Analytical Method:

Lab. 1, 2: Beutler, E., and Baluda, M. C., Improved method for measuring galactose-1-phosphate uridyltransferase activity of erythrocytes. *Clin. Chim. Acta* **13**, 369–379 (1966); Kalckar, H. M., Anderson, E. P., and Isselbacher, K. J., Galactosemia, a congenital defect in a

---

[1] Not to be confused with galactose-1-phosphate uridylyltransferase (EC 2.7.7.10), which catalyzes another reaction.

nucleotide transferase. *Biochim. Biophys. Acta* **20,** 262–268 (1956); Anderson, E. P., Kalckar, H. M., Kurahasi, K., and Isselbacher, K. J., A specific assay for the diagnosis of galactosemia. *J. Lab. Clin. Med.* **50,** 464–476 (1958); Sigma Tech. Bull. 600-UV; Bretthauer, R. K., Hansen, R. G., Donnell, G. N., and Bergren, W. R., A procedure for detecting carriers of galactosemia. *Proc. Natl. Acad. Sci. USA* **45,** 328 (1959); *Galactosemia,* D. Y.-Y. Hsia, Ed. Charles C Thomas, Springfield, IL, 1969. **Lab. 3:** Pesce et al., *op. cit.* **Lab. 4:** Ng, W. G., Bergren, W. R., and Donnell, G. N., An improved procedure for the assay of hemolysate galactose-1-phosphate uridyl transferase activity by the use of ^{14}C-labeled galactose-1-phosphate. *Clin. Chim. Acta* **15,** 489–492 (1967).

Enzyme Data:

Labs. 1, 2:
1. Enzyme unit definition: 1 arbitrary unit is the amount of enzyme activity that will transform 1 μmol of UDP glucose to UDP galactose in 1 h per gram of hemoglobin at 37 °C. 1 IUB unit (U) = this unit/60.
2. Buffer, pH: glycine, 1 mol/L, 8.7.
3. Substrate, pH: UDP glucose + galactose 1-phosphate, 8.7.
4. Reaction temperature: 37 °C.
5. Temperature reported: 37 °C.

Lab. 3:
1. Enzyme unit definition: 1 arbitrary unit is the amount of enzyme activity that will transform 1 μmol of UDP galactose to UDP glucose in 1 h per gram of hemoglobin at 37 °C.
2. Buffer, pH: glycine, 50 mmol/L, with EDTA, 8.6.
3. Substrate, pH: UDP glucose + galactose 1-phosphate, 7.8.
4. Reaction temperature: 37 °C.
5. Temperature reported: 37 °C.

Lab. 4:
1. Enzyme unit definition: Same as Labs. 1, 2.
2. Buffer, pH: glycine, 200 mmol/L, 8.7.
3. Substrate, pH: [U-^{14}C]galactose 1-phosphate and UDP glucose, 8.7.
4. Reaction temperature: 37 °C.
5. Temperature reported: 37 °C.

Instrumentation:

Labs. 1–3: Zeiss PMQ II, Varian 635, Rohm and Haas Micromedic spectrophotometers. **Lab. 4:** Searle analytical liquid scintillation counter, with ion-exchange paper chromatography, DE-81 Whatman.

Notes: **Lab. 4:** The erythrocyte transferase is polymorphic. The Duarte and Los Angeles variants have quite variable enzyme activities, but can be distinguished by gel electrophoresis. The affected patients who are galactosemia homozygotes have no transferase activity. The presence of low transferase-activity variants in the population complicates the diagnosis of galactosemia.

Commentary—Michael A. Pesce

Hexose-1-phosphate uridylyltransferase converts galactose 1-phosphate to glucose 1-phosphate, and uridine diphosphoglucose to uridine diphosphogalactose. In transferase-deficient galactosemia, this enzyme is absent. Transferase-deficient galactosemia is an autosomal recessive disorder, occurring in about 1 in 70 000 children born in the United States (1). Affected infants usually appear normal at birth. Vomiting, diarrhea, jaundice, and failure to thrive are the earliest and most common symptoms, and usually appear after milk is given to the infant. If milk feedings are continued, hepatic failure, cataracts, and mental retardation may occur; death can result.

Because the hexose-1-phosphate uridylyltransferase is absent, the galactose 1-phosphate formed from the phosphorylation of galactose by the enzyme galactokinase cannot be metabolized. As a result, galactose 1-phosphate accumulates in erythrocytes, liver, lens, and brain of affected individuals, and may contribute to many of the clinical problems (except cataracts) associated with this disorder. (This is supported by the fact that cataracts are the only clinical symptom in galactokinase deficiency.)

Treatment for transferase-deficient galactosemia is a galactose-restricted diet. Once patients are on this diet, many of their clinical problems regress. Mental retardation, however, is irreversible and is not affected by the galactose-restricted diet, but can be prevented if the diet is initiated early in life.

In transferase-deficient galactosemia, galactose concentrations in serum and urine may increase. However, the amount of galactose present depends on diet and the rate of metabolism to galactose 1-phosphate. Because the galactose concentration depends on many variables, it should be used only to aid in the diagnosis of transferase-deficient galactosemia (2). The diagnosis of transferase-deficient galactosemia must be based on the activity of hexose-1-phosphate uridylyltransferase in erythrocytes, which is usually measured by the uridine diphosphoglucose consumption test (3) or a radioisotopic procedure (4). Recently, a kinetic enzymic procedure has been developed for measuring this activity in blood collected in microhematocrit tubes (5). Hexose-1-phosphate uridylyltransferase is stable in erythrocytes stored at −20 °C for at least two days.

1. Levy, H. L., and Hammersen, G., Newborn screening for galactosemia and other galactose metabolic defects. *J. Pediatr.* **92,** 871–877 (1978).
2. Pesce, M. A., Pitfalls in the diagnosis of transferase deficient galactosemia. *Lab. Manage.* **17,** 27–33 (1979).

3. Anderson, E. P., Kalckar, H. M., Kurahashi, K., and Isselbacher, K. J., A specific enzymatic assay for the diagnosis of congenital galactosemia. *J. Lab. Clin. Med.* **50,** 469–477 (1957).
4. Ng, W. G., Bergren, W. R., and Donnell, G. N., An improved procedure for the assay of hemolysate galactose-1-phosphate uridyl transferase activity by the use of ^{14}C-labeled galactose-1-phosphate. *Clin. Chim. Acta* **15,** 489–492 (1967).
5. Pesce, M. A., Bodourian, S. H., Harris, R. C., and Nicholson, J. F., Enzymatic micromethod for measuring galactose-1-phosphate uridylyltransferase activity in human erythrocytes. *Clin. Chem.* **23,** 1711–1717 (1977).

High-Density Lipoprotein (HDL) Cholesterol
(Alpha Cholesterol)

Specimen Tested:

P.

Laboratory Reporting:

1.

Reference (Normal) Values:

HDL cholesterol, mg/L (mmol/L)

	M		F	
Age, yr	**White**	**Black**	**White**	**Black**
6–7	240–780 (0.62–2.02)	300–900 (0.78–2.33)	310–670 (0.80–1.73)	350–790 (0.91–2.04)
8–9	360–760 (0.93–1.97)	360–880 (0.93–2.28)	310–750 (0.80–1.94)	460–780 (1.19–2.02)
10–11	360–760 (0.93–1.97)	450–810 (1.16–2.09)	310–710 (0.80–1.94)	350–730 (0.85–1.89)
12–13	250–850 (0.65–2.20)	290–810 (0.75–2.09)	380–780 (0.98–2.09)	300–820 (0.78–2.12)
14–15	280–680 (0.72–1.76)	330–730 (0.85–1.89)	300–700 (0.78–1.81)	340–780 (0.88–2.02)
16–17	280–680 (0.72–1.76)	260–740 (0.67–1.91)	310–790 (0.80–2.04)	340–780 (0.88–2.02)

Sources of Reference (Normal) Values:

Morrison, J. A., deGroot, I., Edwards, B. K., Kelly, K. A., Mellies, M. J., Khoury, P., and Glueck, C. J., Lipids and lipoproteins in 927 school children, ages 6 to 17 years. *Pediatrics* **62,** 990–995 (1978).

Specimen Volume, Collection, and Preservation;
Patient Preparation:

2 mL. EDTA·Na$_2$ anticoagulant. Place specimen in wet ice or RR after collection. Separate P within 8 h. Store 1 wk in RR, or several months in FR. Patient must fast 12–16 h before blood collection.

Analytical Method:

Isolation of HDL by precipitation of low-density and very-low density lipoprotein, as described by Burstein, M., and Samaille, J., Sur un dosage rapide du cholesterol lié aux α- et aux β-lipoprotéines du sérum. *Clin. Chim. Acta* **5,** 609 (1960); measurement of cholesterol by the Lieberman–Burchard reaction, modified: Abell, L. L., Levy, B. B., Brodie, B. B., and Kendall, F. E., Simplified method for estimation of total cholesterol in serum and demonstration of its specificity. *J. Biol. Chem.* **195,** 357 (1952); *Manual of Laboratory Operations,* Lipid Research Clinic Program, I. Lipid and Lipoprotein Analysis, DHEW Publication No. (NIH) 75–628.

Instrumentation:

Technicon Corp. AutoAnalyzer II; Micromedic automatic dilutor; SMI pipettes.

Note: Serum calibrator standards and quality-control materials were obtained from the Center for Disease Control, Atlanta, GA. Zeolite prefilled in disposable tubes was obtained from Standard Scientific.

Commentary—John E. Sherwin

HDL-cholesterol is most frequently measured by selective precipitation with manganese salts *(1).* This requires approximately 1 mL of serum or plasma collected in EDTA. Recently, an electrophoretic procedure has been reported *(2,3)* that requires only 2 μL of sample; however, results are 5 to 10% lower than by the precipitation method.

HDL-cholesterol measurement provides a more specific assessment than total cholesterol of risk for coronary heart disease in adults *(4),* but has been used for less than five years to assess potential risk in adolescents for development of coronary heart disease. Because longitudinal studies have not yet been completed, the validity of studying adolescent HDL-cholesterol to predict coronary heart disease risk has not been established. HDL-cholesterol values are frequently used in diagnosing and managing hereditary hyperlipoproteinemia in infants and children *(5).*

1. Warnick, G. R., and Albers, J. J., A comprehensive evaluation of the heparin–manganese precipitation procedure for estimating high-density lipoprotein cholesterol. *J. Lipid Res.* **19,** 65–71 (1978).
2. Stein, E. A., McNeely, S., and Steiner, P., Electrophoretic separation of high-density lipoprotein cholesterol evaluated and compared with the modified Lipid Research Clinic procedure. *Clin. Chem.* **25,** 1934–1938 (1979).
3. Conlon, D. R., Blankstein, L. A., Pasakarnis, P. A., Steinberg, C. A., and D'Amelio, J. E., Quantitative determination of high-density lipoprotein cholesterol by agarose gel electrophoresis. *Clin. Chem.* **25,** 1965–1970 (1979).

4. Miller, N. E., Thelle, D. S., Førte, O. H., and Mjøs, O. D., The Trømsø heart study. High-density lipoprotein and coronary heart disease. A prospective case control study. *Lancet* **i,** 965–967 (1977).
5. Levy, R. I., and Rifkind, B. M., Diagnosis and management of hyperlipoproteinemia in infants and children. *Am. J. Cardiol.* **31,** 547–551 (1973).

Homovanillic Acid (HVA; 3-methoxy-4-hydroxyphenylacetic acid)

Specimen Tested:

U.

Laboratories Reporting:

6.

Reference (Normal) Values:

	μg/mg of creatinine				
Age	**Labs. 1, 2**	**Lab. 3**[a]	**Lab. 4**	**Lab. 5**	**Lab. 6**
0–12 mo	6–30				
1–6 mo		<56 (15)			
1–12 mo			to 35		3.3–44.1
1–24 mo		<37 (32)	to 23		
1–2 yr					4.7–41.5
1–5 yr	8.5–23.5				
2–5 yr		<27 (33)	to 14		3.1–28.7
5–10 yr	3.5–18		to 9		0.6–19.4
Child				3–16	
5–18 yr		<17 (27)			
10–15 yr			to 12		0.0–18.1
10 yr	2.5–11.0				
15 yr			to 9		
Adult				2–4	

[a] Study on 107 random (untimed) urine specimens obtained from 107 children, ages 1 mo–18 yr. Subjects were ambulatory patients and those admitted for elective surgery. Values reported are at upper limit of 95% confidence limit. The number of individuals studied is in parentheses.

Sources of Reference (Normal) Values:

Labs. 1, 2: Addanki, S., Hinnenkamp, E. R., and Sotos, J. F., Simultaneous quantitation of 4-hydroxy-3-methoxymandelic (vanilmandelic) and 4-hydroxy-3-methoxy phenylacetic (homovanillic) acids in human urine. *Clin. Chem.* **22,** 310–314 (1976). **Lab. 3:** institutional. **Lab. 4:** institutional; Gitlow, S. E., Mendlowitz, M., Wilk, E. K., Wilk, S., Wolf, R. L., and Bertani, L. M., Excretion of catecholamine catabolites by normal children. *J. Lab. Clin. Med.* **72,** 612–620 (1968). **Lab. 5:** institutional.

Specimen Volume, Collection, and Preservation:

Aliquot of 24-h urine preferred. Preservatives used: dark bottle containing 10–20 mL of 50% (6 mol/L) HCl; 6 mol/L HCl to pH 2–3; 5 g of boric acid.

Analytical Method:

Lab. 1: Addanki et al., *op. cit.* **Lab. 2:** Goldenberg, H., and Friedland, M., Specificity of the nitrosophenol reaction. Detection of metanephrine and other guaiacol derivatives. *Clin. Chem.* **13**, 698 (1967), abstract. **Labs. 3, 5:** Sarkoff, I., and Sourkes, T. L., Determination by thin-layer chromatography of urinary homovanillic acid in normal and disease states. *Can. J. Biochem.* **4**, 1381–1388 (1963). **Lab. 4:** modification of the method of Huck, H., and Dworzak, E., Quantitative Analyse von Katecholamin- und Serotonin Metaboliten auf der Dünnschichtplatte 2. mitt. Remissions Messung nach einer specifischen photochemischen Reaktion. *J. Chromatog.* **74**, 303–310 (1972). **Lab. 6:** Knight, J. A., and Haymond, R. E., Improved colorimetry of urinary 3-methoxy-4-hydroxyphenylacetic acid. *Clin. Chem.* **23**, 2007–2010 (1977).

Instrumentation:

Lab. 1: Varian GLC, with 600-cm (20 ft.) glass coil column. **Labs. 3,5:** Coleman Jr., Zeiss spectrophotometers; Shandon Universal Chromatography tank. **Lab. 6:** Beckman DB spectrophotometer; Eberbach 6000 variable speed mechanical shaker.

Note: **Lab. 2:** For young children, from whom a 24-h urine is difficult to obtain, results are reliable on fresh, random urine, acidified upon arrival in the lab (see Knight and Haymond, *op. cit.*). In neuroblastoma, HVA may be increased alone or with vanillylmandelic acid *(q.v.)*. If increased, the value will usually be at least double or triple the upper limit of the reference range.

Commentary—J. A. Knight

Homovanillic acid (HVA) is the major metabolite of dopamine, one of three compounds known collectively as catecholamines. For the other two, epinephrine and norepinephrine, vanillylmandelic acid (VMA; 4-hydroxy-3-methoxymandelic acid) is the major end-metabolite. The excretion of HVA exceeds that of VMA in children of all ages and in adults *(1–4)*. Urinary HVA excretion is reportedly increased in 74% of patients with neuroblastoma, essentially the same as for VMA. When both substances are simultaneously measured, approximately 95% of all tumors are detected *(5)*.

Having fewer reactive functional groups than VMA, HVA is more difficult to measure by classic chemical analysis; hence, there are no "spot tests," as are so well known for VMA. HVA can, however, be measured simultaneously with VMA by paper chromatography, to obtain semiquantitative results *(6–8)*. This technique is widely used and will detect most cases of neuroblastoma (9). In the only reliable colorimetric quantitative method published, HVA is reacted with 2-nitroso-1-naphthol-4-sulfuric acid (2). The method is rapid, simple, and highly reliable, and the reported normal values obtained from random urine samples allow measurement of HVA in micrograms per milligram of creatinine (2).

| Age | n | Normal values for urinary HVA in children,[a] μg/mg of creatinine | | |
		Range	Mean (SD)	Mean ± 2 SD
1–12 mo	42	2.9–46.8	23.7 (10.2)	3.3–44.1
1–2 yr	42	7.0–45.6	23.1 (9.2)	4.7–41.5
2–5 yr	55	1.7–34.3	15.9 (6.4)	3.1–28.7
5–10 yr	48	0.6–21.8	10.0 (4.7)	0.6–19.4
10–15 yr	42	1.6–26.8	8.3 (4.9)	0–18.1

[a] Data from ref. 2.

Although not available in most laboratories, GLC methods are well developed, accurate, and highly reliable (10,11). In addition to HVA, they simultaneously measure VMA and various other metabolic products from these tumors.

Whatever the method used, the measurement of both HVA and VMA is highly recommended when neuroblastoma is suspected. Not only is the accuracy of the diagnosis increased thereby, but also the VMA/HVA ratio reportedly has prognostic importance (12).

Although HVA is quite stable, either preservation with boric acid or acid fixation with HCl to pH 2–3 is recommended. The effect of diet and drugs on HVA excretion has not been studied to the same extent as for VMA, but one would expect similar problems, and should exercise appropriate precautions. (See also Commentary on **Vanillylmandelic Acid.**)

1. Gitlow, S. E., Mendlowitz, M., Wilk, E. K., Wilk, S., Wolf, R. L., and Bertani, L. M., Excretion of catecholamine catabolites by normal children. *J. Lab. Clin. Med.* **72,** 612–620 (1968).
2. Knight, J. A., and Haymond, R. E., Improved colorimetry of urinary HVA. *Clin. Chem.* **23,** 2007–2010 (1977).
3. Haymond, R. E., Knight, J. A., and Bills, A. C., Normal values for urinary 3-methoxy-4-hydroxymandelic acid (VMA) in children. *Clin. Chem.* **24,** 1853–1854 (1978).
4. *The Bio-Science Handbook,* 11th ed. Bio-Science Laboratories, Van Nuys, CA, 1975, pp 82–83.
5. Williams, C. M., and Greer, M., Homovanillic acid and vanilmandelic acid in diagnosis of neuroblastoma. *J. Am. Med. Assoc.* **183,** 134–138 (1963).
6. Armstrong, M. D., Shaw, K. N. F., and Wall, P. E., The phenolic acids of human urine: Paper chromatography of phenolic acids. *J. Biol. Chem.* **218,** 293–303 (1956).
7. Duke, P. S., and Demopoulos, H. B., One-dimensional paper chromatographic method for determination of urinary homovanillic acid. *Clin. Chem.* **14,** 212–221 (1968).

8. Eichorn, E., and Rutenberg, A., A simple and rapid method for estimating 3,4-dihydroxyphenethylamine (dopamine), 3,4-dihydroxyphenylalanine (dopa), and homovanillic acid (HVA) with "two-solutions paper electrophoresis." *Clin. Chem.* **11,** 563–569 (1965).
9. Bray, P. F., Wu, J. T., and Myers, G. G., Reliable chemical diagnosis of neuroblastoma better than screening. *N. Engl. J. Med.* **295,** 230–231 (1976).
10. Addanki, S., Hinnenkamp, E. R., and Sotos, J. F., Simultaneous quantitation of 4-hydroxy-3-methoxymandelic (vanilmandelic) and 4-hydroxy-3-methoxyphenylacetic (homovanillic) acids in human urine. *Clin. Chem.* **22,** 310–314 (1976).
11. Brewster, M. A., Berry, D. H., and Moriarty, M., Urinary 3-methoxy-4-hydroxyphenylacetic (homovanillic) and 3-methoxy-4-hydroxymandelic (vanillylmandelic) acids: Gas–liquid chromatographic methods and experience with 13 cases of neuroblastoma. *Clin. Chem.* **23,** 2247–2249 (1977).
12. Laug, W. E., Siegel, S. E., Shaw, K. N. F., Landing, B., Baptista, J., and Gutenstein, M., Initial urinary catecholamine metabolite concentrations and prognosis in neuroblastoma. *Pediatrics* **62,** 77–83 (1978).

17-Hydroxycorticosteroids

Specimen Tested:

U.

Laboratories Reporting:

2.

Reference (Normal) Values:

Age		mg/d (μmol/d)	
		Lab. 1	**Lab. 2**
Newborn–2 wk		0.05–0.3 (0.14–0.8)	
0–1 yr			0.2–2.0 (0.6–5.5)
2 wk–1 yr		0.10–0.5 (0.3–1.4)	
1–2 yr			0.5–2.5 (1.4–6.9)
1–3 yr		0.5–1.0 (1.4–2.8)	
2–4 yr			1.0–4.0 (2.8–11.0)
3–6 yr		0.6–1.8 (1.7–5.0)	
5–6 yr			1.0–4.8 (2.8–13.2)
6–8 yr			1.0–5.6 (2.8–15.4)
6–9 yr		0.9–3.3 (2.5–9.1)	
8–10 yr			1.0–7.0 (2.8–19.3)
9–12 yr		1.2–5.2 (3.3–14.3)	
10–12 yr			1.5–8.0 (4.1–22.1)
12 yr			2.0–10.0 (5.5–28.0)
12–16 yr,	M	2.0–6.0 (5.5–16.0)	
	F	2.8–6.8 (7.7–18.8)	
16–20 yr,	M	3.0–10 (8.3–28.0)	
	F	2–7 (5.5–19.3)	
Adult,	M	5–10 (13.8–28.0)	
	F	3–7 (8.3–19.3)	

Sources of Reference (Normal) Values:

Lab. 1: institutional study of 119 healthy children, ages 3–17 yr, and 24 adults, ages 21–40 yr. **Lab. 2:** institutional.

Specimen Volume, Collection, and Preservation:

5–10 mL. Collect over 5 g of boric acid crystals. Acidified urine is claimed to be stable for this assay for up to 45 d at RT.

Analytical Method:

Silber, R. H., and Porter, C. C., The determination of 17,21-dihydroxy-20-ketosteroids in urine and plasma. *J. Biol. Chem.* **210**, 923–932 (1954); Peterson, R. E., Karrer, A., and Guerra, S. L., Evaluation of the Silber–Porter procedure for determination of plasma hydrocortisone. *Anal. Chem.* **29**, 144–149 (1957); Silber, R. H., Free and conjugated 17-hydroxycorticosteroids in urine. *Stand. Methods Clin. Chem.* **4,** 113–120 (1963).

Instrumentation:

Gilford 200 and Zeiss PMQ II spectrophotometers.

Commentary—Elizabeth K. Smith

Urinary 17-hydroxycorticosteroids (17-OHCS) measured by the Porter–Silber reaction represent specifically the urinary metabolites of cortisol, including cortisol, tetrahydrocortisol, and tetrahydrocortisone; their measurement is a valuable indirect indicator of the rate of secretion of cortisol and hence of the functional activity of the adrenal cortex.

Children show wide individual variation in excretion of 17-OHCS. Normal values increase with age to adult values at ages 16–20 years in males and 12–16 years in females. Values for adults are higher in men than in women. Excretion is positively correlated with body weight; therefore, if results are expressed as mg/kg of body weight per day, changes with age are minimized, with mean values of about 90 mg/kg per day after nine years of age (E. K. Smith, unpublished data).

Excretion values for newborn infants are very low, and mean values in the healthy premature infant (62 μg/24 h) are lower than in the healthy full-term infant (207 μg/24 h), even when related to body weight (33.7 and 62.6 μg/kg per 24 h, respectively) *(1)*. However, the Porter–Silber assay method is relatively unreliable in the first week of life, owing to interference from the increased excretion of metabolites of unusual steroids produced by the neonate. This problem is enhanced in newborns with congenital adrenal hyperplasia, whose urinary steroids produce unusual colors with the Porter–Silber reagent.

Diurnal variation in adrenocortical activity and plasma cortisol is reflected in the excretion of 17-OHCS; hence, an accurate 24-h urine collection is essential to assess normal functioning and pathological changes. Corticosteroid excretion values may also reflect transient increases in plasma cortisol that are caused by various stresses. A mild preservative such as boric acid (*not* HCl) should be included in the urine-collection bottles.

Values for 17-OHCS are decreased in adrenal insufficiency (Addison's disease), and values may be normal or low in pituitary hypofunction with secondary adrenal insufficiency. Values are increased in adrenocortical hyperfunction, Cushing's syndrome (either primary or secondary to pituitary hyperfunction), and adrenal carcinoma. In simple obesity, excretion values expressed in mg/24 h may appear to be increased; if expressed in mg/kg per 24 h, however, these values are not significantly above the mean for age. More definitive diagnostic information is obtained by observing responses of 17-OHCS excretion to dynamic testing procedures involving suppression (with dexamethasone, metyrapone) and stimulation (with corticotropin).

Many drugs interfere with the assay of Porter–Sibler chromogens, including reserpine, chlorpromazine, meprobamate, spironolactone, and others; e.g., carbamazepine produces a purple color (2). In addition, many drugs cause physiological changes in pituitary–adrenal activity, resulting in changes in urinary 17-OHCS excretion.

1. Smith, E. K., and Tippitt, D. F., Evaluation of steroid hormone metabolism. In text ref. 7, vol. 1, p 319.
2. Young, D. L., Pestaner, L. C., and Gibberman, V., Effects of drugs on clinical laboratory tests. *Clin. Chem.* **21,** 1D–432D (1975).

5-Hydroxyindoleacetic Acid (5-HIAA)

Specimen Tested:

U.

Laboratories Reporting:

1.

Reference (Normal) Values:

0.11–0.61 μmol/kg of body weight per 7 h

Sources of Reference (Normal) Values:

Institutional; text ref. *1.*

Specimen Volume, Collection, and Preservation; Patient Preparation:

6 mL. Collect U into 25 mL of glacial acetic acid. Certain foods must be withheld. Stable for several days at RT for screening test.

Analytical Method:

Udenfriend, S., Titus, E., and Weissbach, H., The identification of 5-hydroxy-3-indoleacetic acid in normal urine and a method for its assay. *J. Biol. Chem.* **216**, 499–505 (1955).

Instrumentation:

Zeiss spectrophotometer.

Commentary—Elizabeth K. Smith

Serotonin (5-hydroxytryptamine) is a derivative of tryptophan, formed primarily in the argentaffine cells of the gastrointestinal tract. Normal adults convert about 2% (10 mg) of their average daily intake of tryptophan to serotonin. Patients with carcinoid tumors convert as much as 60%.

Virtually all of the serotonin in blood is in the platelets. The primary metabolite of serotonin is 5-hydroxyindoleacetic acid (5-HIAA), which is excreted in the urine in amounts of 2–9 mg/d in normal adults. Greatly increased amounts are excreted in the carcinoid syndrome, and constitute a valuable diagnostic test for this condition *(1)*.

Foods containing serotonin (avocados, bananas, tomatoes, and walnuts) and various drugs increase 5-HIAA output, and should be restricted for one to two days before urine collection. Drugs such as phenothiazines, methyldopa, and ethanol decrease output. Malabsorptive diseases may cause modest increases in 5-HIAA output (to 10–25 mg/d). Presumptive indications of a serotonin-producing tumor are, in the absence of malabsorption disease, excretion of 15 mg of 5-HIAA per day, and in the presence of malabsorption, >30 mg/d.

1. Chattoraj, S. C., Endocrine function. In text ref. *5*, 2nd ed., pp 818–821.

17-Hydroxyprogesterone

Specimen Tested:

P, S.

Laboratories Reporting:

2.

Reference (Normal) Values:

Lab. 1:

Age	ng/dL (nmol/L)
Cord blood	Up to 5000 (151); ref. *1, 2, 3*[a]
Newborn, <4 d	Up to 1000 (up to 30); ref. *3, 4*
>4 d	<300 (<9); ref. *3, 4*
1–4 mo	<200 (<6.1); slightly higher in M; ref. *1, 2*
4–24 mo	<100 (<3.0); ref. *1, 2*
Child, prepubertal	<100 (<3.0); ref. *1, 4*
3–10 yr (F)	range, 11–54 (0.33–1.33); mean, 25 (0.76)
3–15 yr (M)	range, 17–86 (0.52–2.61); mean, 44 (1.33)
11–14 yr (F)	range, 33–163 (1.0–4.9); mean, 96 (2.9)
Adult	<200 (<6.1); range, 34–141 (1.0–4.3); mean 82 (2.5)

Note: Congenital hyperplasia (untreated 21-hydroxylase deficiency)
>5000 (>151) up to 100 000 (3030)

Lab. 2:

Child: <10 nmol/L (most children, 1–8 yr old, will have <4 nmol/L)

[a] Reference numbers refer to sources, below.

Sources of Reference (Normal) Values:

Lab. 1: *(1)* Hughes, I. A., and Winter, J. S. D., The application of a serum 17OH-progesterone radioimmunoassay to the diagnosis and management of congenital hyperplasia. *J. Pediatr.* **88,** 766–773 (1976); *(2)* Forest, M. G., and Cathiard, A. M., Ontogenic study of plasma 17α-hydroxyprogesterone in the human. I. Postnatal period: Evidence for a transient ovarian activity in infancy. *Pediatr. Res.* **12,** 6–11 (1978); *(3)* Sippell, W. G., Becker, H., Versmold, H. T., Bidlingmaier, F., and Knorr, D., Longitudinal studies of aldosterone, 17-hydroxyprogesterone, cortisol and cortisone determined simultaneously in mother and child at birth and during the early neonatal period. I. Spontaneous delivery. *J. Clin. Endocrinol. Metab.* **46,** 971–984 (1978); *(4)* institutional. **Lab. 2:** institutional.

Specimen Volume, Collection, and Preservation; Patient Preparation:

200 to 500 µL. Heparin anticoagulant. Separate serum promptly. Store in FR. Obtain (fasting) specimen at 0800 hours. If monitoring therapy, note time of last corticosteroid dose.

Analytical Method:

Lab. 1: RIA, after LH-20 Sephadex chromatography, ^{3}H; precipitation of bound hormone with polyethylene glycol; Plasma 17-hydroxyprogesterone RIA procedure, Technical Bulletin, Endocrine Sciences; Anderson, P. H., Fukishima, K., and Schiller, H. S., Radioimmunoassay of plasma testosterone with use of polyethylene glycol to separate antibody-bound and free hormone. *Clin. Chem.* **21,** 708–714 (1975). **Lab. 2:** unpublished institutional RIA method.

Instrumentation:

Packard 3375 scintillation counter; fraction collector.

Commentary—Elizabeth K. Smith

The steroid 17-hydroxyprogesterone (17-OHP) is a key intermediate in the biosynthesis of cortisol in the adrenal cortex, and in the synthesis of testosterone and estradiol in the testis and ovary.

Methods utilizing both competitive protein binding and RIA have been reported and are currently in use. Both procedures are sensitive enough to be used with the small amounts of blood (50–200 μL) obtained by skin puncture in infants. RIA with a specific antibody gives lower values than competitive protein binding and is more sensitive at low concentrations, but either method provides clinically useful data.

The concentration of 17-OHP in blood varies widely with age and clinical condition. In the newborn infant the concentration is increased during the first week, reflecting the increased secretory activity of the fetal adrenal and the very high concentration in cord blood (1). Forest and Cathiard (2) found that pre-term infants had cord blood values higher than full-term infants, with somewhat higher values in female infants than in males. The concentration decreases rapidly during the first week of life. With an RIA method, 17-OHP concentrations in plasma during the first few days may be as much as 600–1000 ng/dL, but by seven days mean values are approximately 100 ng/dL (3,4). Values obtained with the less-specific method of Barnes and Atherden (5) are: younger than four days, up to 1500 ng/dL; older than four days <500 ng/dL. During the first few months plasma concentrations of 17-OHP may range as high as 300 ng/dL, especially in boys (4), but after nine months and throughout childhood the concentrations are less than 100 ng/dL. At about eight years of age, blood concentrations of 17-OHP increase, in a prepubertal and pubertal surge. In adults the values usually are less than 200 ng/dL, with greater values in women during the luteal phase of the menstrual cycle.

Blood concentration varies episodically throughout the day (6), and also exhibits a circadian rhythm, with peak values in early morning and low values in the late afternoon; this is similar to the pattern for cortisol, but with less dramatic changes.

The primary clinical application of 17-OHP is in the diagnosis of congenital adrenal hyperplasia (CAH) caused by a deficiency of the 21-hydroxylase enzyme for conversion of 17-OHP to 11-deoxycortisol. In this most common form of CAH, the deficiency of 21-hydroxylase results in decreased or no synthesis of cortisol, little or no negative feedback control of corticotropin (ACTH), increased ACTH, and increased synthesis of androgens with virilization. A marked deficiency of 21-hydroxylase, also affecting the aldosterone biosynthetic pathway, results in less aldosterone and, consequently, salt-losing symptoms in some patients.

In untreated CAH the concentration of 17-OHP is markedly increased *(1)*, with highest values in the severe salt-losing form. In a recent study of 17-OHP in differential diagnosis of CAH, the highest value in 17 infants with electrolyte imbalance of ambiguous genitalia not due to CAH was 630 ng/dL, whereas in 14 infants with similar presenting symptoms due to CAH the 17-OHP values ranged from 8700 to 106 000 ng/dL (E. K. Smith, unpublished observations). Age at time of blood sampling is important: one infant at 3 h of age had a serum concentration of 1400 ng/dL, but after one week without treatment the value was 22 700 ng/dL.

Measurement of 17-OHP also may be useful in distinguishing precocious pubarche (pubic or axillary hair), in which serum concentrations of 17-OHP are normal, from virilizing CAH, with high serum concentrations of 17-OHP *(7)*. Although potentially useful as a replacement for cumbersome assays for urinary 17-ketosteroid and pregnanetriol (used to monitor effectiveness of glucocorticoid therapy in CAH), reports are conflicting as to the critical concentration of 17-OHP that represents suppression of the pituitary but will still allow adequate growth. The diurnal variation in serum 17-OHP concentration is retained during corticoid therapy, making critical the time of sampling. If plasma values are low to normal for age, the patient may be overtreated.

The response of plasma 17-OHP to intravenous ACTH is significantly higher in heterozygous carriers for 21-hydroxylase deficiency CAH than in normal individuals *(8)*. Such a challenge test with ACTH is valuable for detecting carriers in families of CAH patients for genetic counselling.

Walker et al. *(9)* reported an RIA method for 17-OHP in saliva. Values obtained with 200 µL of parotid fluid gave a good correlation for matched samples of saliva and plasma, and showed marked increases to 26 000 pmol/L in patients with CAH compared with a mean of 527 pmol/L for healthy children. A screening test for CAH involving a micro filter-paper method for RIA of 17-OHP also has been reported *(10)*.

1. Hughes, I. A., and Winter, J. S. D., The application of a serum 17OH-progesterone radioimmunoassay to the diagnosis and management of congenital adrenal hyperplasia. *J. Pediatr.* **88,** 766–773 (1976).
2. Forest, M. G., and Cathiard, A. M., Ontogenic study of plasma 17α-hydroxyprogesterone in the human. I. Postnatal period: Evidence for a transient ovarian activity in infancy. *Pediatr. Res.* **12,** 6–11 (1978).

3. Sippell, W. G., Becker, H., Versmold, H. T., Bidlingmaier, F., and Knorr, D., Longitudinal studies of plasma aldosterone, corticosterone, deoxycorticosterone, progesterone, 17-hydroxyprogesterone, cortisol and cortisone determined simultaneously in mother and child at birth and during the early neonatal period. I. Spontaneous delivery. *J. Clin. Endocrinol. Metab.* **46,** 971–984 (1978).

4. Winter, J. S. D., Hughes, I. A., Reyes, F. I., and Faiman, C., Pituitary-gonadal relations in infancy: 2. Patterns of serum gonadal steroid concentrations in man from birth to two years of age. *J. Clin. Endocrinol. Metab.* **42,** 679–686 (1976).

5. Barnes, N. D., and Atherden, S. M., Diagnosis of congenital adrenal hyperplasia by measurement of plasma 17-hydroxyprogesterone. *Arch. Dis. Child.* **47,** 62–65 (1972).

6. West, C. D., Mahajan, D. K., Chavre, V. S., Nabors, C. J., and Tyler, F. H., Simultaneous measurement of multiple plasma steroids demonstrating episodic secretion. *J. Clin. Endocrinol. Metab.* **36,** 1230–1236 (1973).

7. August, G. P., Hung, W., and Tnayas, D. M., Plasma androgens in premature pubarche: Value of 17-hydroxyprogesterone in differentiation from congenital adrenal hyperplasia. *J. Pediatr.* **87,** 246–248 (1975).

8. Krensky, A. M., Bongiovanni, A. M., Marina, J., Parks, J., and Tenore, A., Identification of heterozygote carriers of congenital adrenal hyperplasia by radioimmunoassay of serum 17-OH progesterone. *J. Pediatr.* **90,** 930–933 (1977).

9. Walker, R. F., Read, G. F., Hughes, I. A., and Riad-Fahmy, D., Radioimmunoassay of 17α-hydroxyprogesterone in saliva, parotid fluid, and plasma of congenital adrenal hyperplasia patients. *Clin. Chem.* **25,** 542–545 (1979).

10. Pang, S., Hotchkiss, J., Drash, A., Levine, L., and New, M. I., Microfilter paper method for 17α-hydroxyprogesterone radioimmunoassay: Its application for rapid screening for congenital adrenal hyperplasia. *J. Clin. Endocrinol. Metab.* **45,** 1003–1008 (1977).

Hydroxyproline

Specimen Tested:

U.

Laboratory Reporting:

1.

Reference (Normal) Values:

Age	Total, mmol/m^2 of body surface	Free
1 wk–12 mo	0.42–1.68	>33% of total, decreasing to 3–5% of total by 12 mo
1–13 yr	0.19–0.61	
14–21 yr	wide fluctuations	
22–65 yr	0.05–0.17	
>66 yr	0.04–1.13	

Sources of Reference (Normal) Values:

Turek, J., and Goverde, B. C., The significance of hydroxyproline assay in the urine. Organon Diagnostics (manufacturers of "Hypronosticon kit" for determination of hydroxyproline); Lenzi, F., Ravenni, G., Rubegni, M., and Del Giovane, L., The significance of urinary hydroxyproline in osteoporosis. *Panminerva Med.* **5**, 155–158 (1963).

Specimen Volume, Collection, and Preservation:

Collect 24-h U; keep U in RR during collection. Store aliquot in FR. Stability to 5 d at RT is claimed if U is adjusted to pH 1–2.

Analytical Method:

Bergman, I., and Loxley, R., The determination of hydroxyproline in urine hydrolysates. *Clin. Chim. Acta* **27**, 347–349 (1970).

Instrumentation:

LKB 7400 calculating absorptiometer.

25-Hydroxyvitamin D, 25-Hydroxycalciferol[1]

Specimen Tested:

S.

Laboratories Reporting:

2.

Reference (Normal) Values:

Age	ng/mL (nmol/L)	
	Lab. 1	**Lab. 2**[a]
Newborn, premature		44
full-term		5.5–17.7[b]
Child, 8–36 mo	11.6–28.8 (29.0–72.0)[c]	
extreme range	13.9–38.1 (34.8–95.2)	
1–18 yr		38.4–70.4
		2.1–54.8[b]
Adult		15–60

[a] These data are highly tentative. [b] Data obtained with a specific method after LH-20 chromatography. [c] Based on a study of 40 out-patients having no liver abnormality or overt bone disease. Diets were normal, but not supplemented with vitamin D, except that found in milk (360 USP units/L). Blood collected in morning.

---

[1] Also 25-hydroxycholecalciferol, 25-hydroxy D_3. Calciferol and its hydroxylated derivative refer to both endogenous (vitamin D_3 or cholecalciferol) and exogenous (vitamin D_2 or ergocalciferol) sources of vitamin D.

Sources of Reference (Normal) Values:

Lab. 1: institutional. **Lab. 2:** Chan, G. M., Tsang, R. C., Chen, I. W., DeLuca, H. F., and Steichen, J. J., The effect of 1,25-$(OH)_2$ vitamin D_3 supplementation in premature infants. *J. Pediatr.* **93**, 91–96 (1978); Weisman, Y., Reiter, E., and Root, A., Measurement of 24,25-dihydroxyvitamin D in sera of neonates and children. *J. Pediatr.* **91**, 904–908 (1977); Consolidated Biomedical Labs., Columbus, OH.

Specimen Volume, Collection, and Preservation:

100 μL to 1 mL. Collect blood into chilled tube. Allow to clot at 4 °C. Centrifuge in a refrigerated centrifuge. Store in FR.

Analytical Method:

Lab. 1: Haddad, J. G., and Chyu, K. J., Competitive protein binding radioassay for 25-hydroxycholecalciferol. *J. Clin. Endocrinol.* **33**, 992–995 (1971). **Lab. 2:** competitive binding radioassay with protein from rachitic rat serum, [^{3}H]25-hydroxy D_3; Belsey, R. E., DeLuca, H. F., and Potts, J. T., A rapid assay for 25-OH vitamin D_3 without preparative chromatography. *J. Clin. Endocrinol. Metab.* **38**, 1046–1051 (1974).

Instrumentation:

Packard Tri-Carb scintillation counter.

Hypoxanthine Phosphoribosyltransferase, HPRT
(EC 2.4.2.8; IMP:pyrophosphate phosphoribosyltransferase)

Specimen Tested:

B.

Laboratory Reporting:

1.

Reference (Normal) Values:

640–2884 arbitrary units; with saturating substrates.
318–1490 arbitrary units; with subsaturating substrates.

Sources of Reference (Normal) Values:

Institutional (experimental).

Specimen Volume, Collection, and Preservation:

10 μL of 1:9 (10-fold diluted) hemolysate. Heparin anticoagulant. HPRT is usually stable for about 2 wk. Blood should be shipped at RT as soon as possible after collection. A "control" blood should also be sent for comparison. Ship at RT. Do not freeze.

Analytical Method:

Bakay, B., Telfer, M. A., and Nyhan, W. L., Assay of hypoxanthine–guanine and adenine phosphoribosyl transferases. A simple screening test for the Lesch–Nyhan syndrome and related disorders of purine metabolism. *Biochem. Med.* **3**, 230–243 (1969); Sweetman, L., Hoch, M. A., Bakay, B., Borden, M., Lesch, P., and Nyhan, W. L., A distinct human variant of hypoxanthine–guanine phosphoribosyl transferase. *J. Pediatr.* **92**, 385–389 (1978).

Enzyme Data:

1. Enzyme unit definition: 1 arbitrary unit = 1 nmol of IMP (inosinic acid) per minute per milliliter of packed erythrocytes.
2. Buffer, pH: Tris/HCl/phosphate, 7.4.
3. Substrate, pH: [8-^{14}C]hypoxanthine-5-phosphoribosyl-1-pyrophosphate, 7.4.
4. Reaction temperature: 60 °C.
5. Temperature reported: 60 °C.

Instrumentation:

Beckman LS-250 liquid scintillation system.

Note: See Commentary with **Adenine phosphoribosyltransferase.**

Immunoglobulins

Immunoglobulin E (IgE)

Specimen Tested:

P, S.

Laboratories Reporting:

2.

Reference (Normal) Values:

	IgE, units/mL[a]	
Age, yr	**Lab. 1**	**Lab. 2**[b]
0–3	<10	
1		58
2		61
3		40
3–4	<25	
4		70
4–7	<50	
7		221
7–14	<100	
10		337
14		187
14–adult:	<150	150

[a] 1 unit = 2 ng of IgE.   [b] Upper limit.

Sources of Reference (Normal) Values:

Lab. 1: institutional; *Phadebas IgE PRIST by RIA, Directions for Use*, Pharmacia Diagnostics; Kjellman, N. I., Johannson, S. G. O., and Roth, A., Serum IgE levels in healthy children quantified by a sandwich technique (PRIST). *Clin. Allergy* **6**, 51–59 (1976). **Lab. 2:** Kjellman et al., *op. cit.*

Specimen Volume, Collection, and Preservation:

10 to 50 μL. Heparin as anticoagulant. Store specimens in FR. **Lab. 1** ultracentrifuges lipemic specimen for 5 min in Beckman Airfuge at 85 000 rpm, before storage or use.

Analytical Method:

Pharmacia Diagnostics Phadebas IgE PRIST; Ceska, M., and Lundkvist, U., A new and simple radioimmunoassay method for the determination of IgE. *Immunochemistry* **9**, 1021–1030 (1972).

Instrumentation:

Lab. 1: Searle 1185 Automatic Gamma System; Sorvall RC-3 refrigerated centrifuge. **Lab. 2:** Packard 5110 Auto-Gamma scintillation spectrometer; Micromedic automatic pipette and diluter; Eberbach 5900 reciprocating centrifuge and shaker.

Commentary—Leonard K. Dunikoski, Jr.

IgE is an immunoglobulin with a relative molecular mass of 197 000 and a half-life of two to three days; it may be formed in response to antigenic stimulation. The IgE effects release of pharmacologically active agents from the mast cell, causing asthma, hay fever, and signs of anaphylaxis. Above-normal concentrations of serum IgE are found in children in response to particular allergens (such as ascaris). Atopic individuals form IgE antibodies on exposure to pollens, dust, and other common environmental substances, suggesting the possibility of a different mechanism of disposition of antigens coming in contact with mucosal surfaces. Serum IgE may be used as a screening test for atopy, although a significant number of allergic individuals have normal total IgE concentrations. Determination of IgE concentrations in response to specific antigens may be performed with the radioallergosorbent test (RAST).

Although anaphylaxis is uncommon in children, almost any foreign substance is capable of developing an IgE-mediated anaphylactic sensitivity. Penicillin administration and Hymenoptera sting are the most common examples in pediatrics.

Immunoglobulin G (IgG)

Specimen Tested:

CSF.

Laboratories Reporting:

2.

Reference (Normal) Values:

Lab. 1: Child: range: u[a]–5.6 mg/dL; mean = 2.63
Lab. 2: Child: <10% of total CSF protein.

[a] Undetectable by the RID method used. Values based on 68 subjects.

Sources of Reference (Normal) Values:

Lab. 1: institutional. **Lab. 2:** Berner, J. J., Ciemins, V. A., and Schroeder, E. F., Jr., Radial immunodiffusion of spinal fluid: Diagnostic value in multiple sclerosis. *Am. J. Clin. Pathol.* **58,** 145–152 (1972).

Specimen Volume, Collection, and Preservation:

10 to 20 μL. Use fresh specimen on day of collection, without freezing.

Analytical Method and Instrumentation:

RID: Mancini, G., Carbonara, A. O., and Heremans, J. F., Immunochemical quantitation of antigens by single radial immunodiffusion. *Int. J. Immunochem.* **2,** 235–254 (1965); Calbiochem-Behring Diagnostics low-level immunodiffusion plates and LC-Partigen RID Plates, working range 1.0–13 mg/dL.

Commentary—Leonard K. Dunikoski, Jr.

Quantitation of CSF immunoglobulins usually means IgG analysis, which may be performed by RID or electroimmunodiffusion. Most often these determinations are used in the diagnosis of multiple sclerosis, and CSF-protein electrophoresis may be performed concurrently. Increased IgG in CSF is found in 75% of patients with multiple sclerosis; the percentage is even higher if the ratio of IgG/albumin is measured in both CSF and plasma *(1)*:

(CSF IgG/plasma IgG)/(CSF albumin/plasma albumin)

1. Tibbling, G., Link, H., and Ohman, S., Principles of albumin and IgG analyses in neurological disorders. I. Establishment of reference values. *Scand. J. Clin. Lab. Invest.* **37**, 385–390 (1977).

Immunoglobulins in Duodenal Fluid

Specimen Tested:

Duodenal fluid.

Laboratory Reporting:

1.

Reference (Normal) Values:

	mg/g of protein (mean; upper limit)		
Age	**IgA**	**IgM**	**IgG**
2–4 wk	8.7; up to 20.1	11.7; up to 16.7	20.7; up to 55.5
1–2 mo	8.8; up to 20.6	14.2; up to 27.2	28.0; up to 61.6
3–4 mo	11.3; 21.7	16.1; 28.1	26.6; 55.2
5–7 mo	13.3; 27.9	15.4; 31.8	23.6; 53.6
8–10 mo	11.3; 21.5	15.7; 32.5	24.4; 43.6
11–12 mo	10.1; 20.5	14.1; 36.3	23.4; 50.2
13–24 mo	11.7; 22.7	10.1; 17.7	32.2; 54.6
25 mo–5 yr	11.5; 25.5	10.0; 14.4	35.5; 68.9
6–8 yr	11.8; 20.8	8.8; 11.0	
9–12 yr	14.8; 25.8	14.3; 31.5	28.4; 67.2
13–19 yr	12.3; 21.7		27.4; 59.6

Sources of Reference (Normal) Values:

Institutional.

Specimen Volume, Collection, and Preservation:

5 μL. Collect fluid from duodenum through nasogastric tube. Store in FR.

Analytical Method and Instrumentation:

Single RID; Mancini, G., Carbonara, A. O., and Heremans, J. F., Immunochemical quantitation of antigens by single radial immunodiffusion. *Int. J. Immunochem.* **2**, 235–254 (1965); Kallestad Quantiplate, low-level plates.

Commentary—Emanuel Lebenthal

The effects of proteolytic enzymes are among the major problems in the determination of duodenal fluid immunoglobulins. IgA is susceptible to pepsin digestion, and IgG and IgM are digested by trypsin *(1)*. Several techniques, including heating, cooling, and the addition of antitryptic agents, have been tried to overcome this problem *(2)*, but none has met with complete success, as evidenced by the presence of immunoglobulin fragments in duodenal secretions *(1)*. Thus underestimation of immunoglobulin concentrations is probable, and sometimes only semiquantitative results are obtained.

In the quantitation of IgA in duodenal fluid the IgA reference (standard) used is usually a 7S monomer *(3)*, whereas the IgA in the specimen normally contains both 11S and 7S components *(4)*.

As yet unpublished data from this laboratory indicate no statistical difference in duodenal fluid immunoglobulin concentrations in children from two weeks through 19 years of age.

Immunoglobulin concentrations can be used to determine isolated, selective-immunoglobulin deficiencies, as well as the general immunoglobulin deficiency.

1. Samson, R. R., McClelland, D. B. L., and Shearman, J. C., Studies on the quantitation of immunoglobulin in human intestinal secretions. *Gut* **14**, 616–626 (1973).
2. Plaut, A. G., and Keonil, B., Immunoglobulins in human small intestinal fluid. *Gastroenterology* **56**, 522–530 (1969).
3. Tomsai, T. B., Tan, E. M., Soloman, A., and Pendergast, R. A., Characteristics of an immune system common to certain external secretions. *J. Exp. Med.* **121**, 101–124 (1965).
4. Clancy, R., and Bienenstock, J., Secretion of immunoglobulins. *Clin. Endocrinol.* **5**, 229–249 (1976).

Immunoglobulins in Blood

Specimen Tested:

S.

Laboratories Reporting:

3.

Reference (Normal) Values:
See page 284.

Sources of Reference (Normal) Values:

Lab. 1: Cejka, J., Mood, D. W., and Kim, C. S., Immunoglobulin concentrations in sera of normal children: Quantitation against an international reference preparation. *Clin. Chem.* **20**, 656–659 (1974). **Lab.**

Immunoglobulins, mg/dL

Age	IgG			IgA			IgM		
	Labs. 1, 2		Lab. 3	Labs. 1, 2		Lab. 3	Labs. 1, 2		Lab. 3
	Lower limits	Upper limits		Lower limits	Upper limits		Lower limits	Upper limits	
Cord S	766–788	1633–1693		0.04–0.05	8–9		4	24–26	
0.5–3 mo	299–310	821–852		3–3.5	60–66		15–16	101–149	
3–6 mo	142–147	952–988		4–5	82–90		18–20	109–118	
6 mo			150–470			20–130			30–60
6–12 mo	418–434	1102–1142		14–15	86–95		43–47	207–223	
1 yr			140–1030			20–130			30–160
1–2 yr	356–359	1162–1204		13–14.5	108–118		37–39	224–239	
2 yr			280–960			20–110			30–150
2–3 yr	492–510	1224–1269		23–25	124–137		49–53	190–204	
5 yr			370–1500			30–200			20–220
3–6 yr	564–585	1332–1381		35–38	190–209		51–55	199–214	
6–9 yr	658–682	1480–1535		29–32	258–384		50–54	211–228	
9–12 yr	625–648	1541–1598		60–66.5	270–294		64–69	258–278	
10 yr			440–1550			50–230			30–170
>10 yr			450–1440			40–240			40–200
12–16 yr	680–706	1493–1548		81–89	232–252		45–48	237–256	

2: Allansmith, M., McClellan, B. H., Butterworth, M., and Maloney, J. R., The development of immunoglobulin levels in man. *J. Pediatr.* **72,** 279–290 (1968). **Lab. 3:** institutional.

Specimen Volume, Collection, and Preservation:

5 to 20 μL. Serum is stable for several days (2–3) in RR.

Analytical Method:

Lab. 1: RID; Mancini et al., cited in previous section; Meloy Labs. RID plates; for low levels of IgG, Calbiochem-Behring Diagnostics low-level plates (CSF). **Lab. 3:** nephelometry.

Instrumentation:

Lab. 3: Technicon Instruments Corp. Automated Immunoprecipitin System.

Commentary—Leonard K. Dunikoski, Jr.

Immunoglobulins may be quantitated by RID or immunonephelometric techniques. Some data suggest that automated nephelometry may provide better precision than manual procedures, especially those involving manual dilution of serum or antiserum. Intralaboratory comparisons of results should include normal ranges by age and sex, because of the large changes involved. This may present a problem in large, computerized laboratories, where "normal ranges" are limited to a small number of age/sex combinations; in such laboratories, reference values should be entered on the patient's chart.

A comprehensive discussion of the immunoglobulins is beyond the scope of this book. In pediatrics, quantitation of immunoglobulins is requested most often in the diagnosis of immunodeficiency states and diagnosis of intrauterine immunization or infections. Most states of true immunodeficiency in children are associated with IgG concentrations less than 200 mg/dL, and undetectable IgA or IgM [1]. Normal or high values may be found, however, in dysgammaglobulinemia, unusual forms of combined T- and B-cell deficiency, and IgG subgroup deficiency (where total IgG may be normal but specific subgroups are absent). To detect selective IgA deficiency, use of rabbit antiserum to human IgA has been advocated instead of goat antiserum, to minimize cross reaction with dietary antigens. The reader is referred to the comprehensive discussion in a recent pediatric text for a full discussion of implications of immunoglobulin concentrations [1].

1. Hong, R., The immunologic system. In text ref. *17*, 11th ed., pp 582–598.

Note: Also see Chapter 10, **Specific Proteins in Pediatrics.**

Insulin

Specimen Tested:

P, S.

Laboratories Reporting:

3.

Reference (Normal) Values:

Fasting concentration: 6–18; 20 or less; <25 micro-USP units/mL

Sources of Reference (Normal) Values:

Labs. 1, 3: institutional. **Lab. 2:** *Radioimmunoassay Manual,* 4th ed. Nichols Institute, San Pedro, CA, 1977, pp 255–259.

Specimen Volume, Collection, and Preservation:

100 to 300 µL. Heparin as anticoagulant. Specimen is chilled at all stages of preparation and transport. Store in FR.

Analytical Method:

Lab. 1: Herbert, V., Lau, K. S., Gottlieb, C. W., and Bleicher, S. J., Coated charcoal immunoassay of insulin. *J. Clin. Endocrinol. Metab.* **25,** 1375–1384 (1965). **Lab. 2:** RIA, double antibody, ^{125}I-labeled insulin. **Lab. 3:** RIA, modified Corning Medical IMMO PHASE RIA test system Insulin.

Instrumentation:

All use gamma counters.

* * *

Laboratories reporting:

1.

Reference (Normal) Values:

	Oral glucose tolerance test values[a]		
Time	Glucose, mg/dL (mmol/L)	Insulin, micro-USP units/mL	Phosphorus, mg/dL (mmol/L)
Fasting	56–96 (3.11–5.33)	5–40	3.2–4.9 (1.2–1.58)
30 min	91–185 (5.05–10.32)	36–110	2.0–4.4 (0.65–1.42)
60 min	66–164 (3.66–9.10)	22–124	1.8–3.6 (0.58–1.16)
90 min	68–148 (3.77–8.21)	17–105	1.6–3.6 (0.52–1.16)
2 h	66–122 (3.66–6.77)	6–84	1.8–4.2 (0.58–1.36)
3 h	47–99 (2.61–5.50)	2–46	2.0–4.6 (0.65–1.49)
4 h	61–93 (3.39–5.16)	3–32	2.7–4.3 (0.87–1.39)
5 h	63–86 (3.50–4.77)	5–37	2.9–4.4 (0.94–1.42)

[a]Based on 13 healthy children given an oral dose of glucose, 1.75 g/kg of body weight, after two weeks on a high-carbohydrate diet.

Sources of Reference (Normal) Values:

Institutional.

Specimen Volume:

200 μL. See precautions in preceding report.

Analytical Method:

RIA; Wide, L., Radioimmunoassays employing immunosorbents. *Acta Endocrinol.*, Suppl. 142, 207–221 (1969); Wide, L., Axen, R., and Porath, J., Radioimmunosorbent assay for proteins. Chemical couplings of antibodies to insoluble dextran. *Immunochemistry* **4**, 381–386 (1967); Pharmacia Diagnostics Phadebas Insulin Test.

Instrumentation:

Nuclear Chicago gamma counter.

Commentary—Eleanor Colle

Fasting insulin values are lower in infants and children than in adults. Obesity leads to increased fasting values for insulin in both children and adults *(1)*.

Insulin values increase after ingestion of glucose or mixed meals. The insulin response to glucose loading also increases with age *(2)*. There is wide variation in the amount of insulin released in response to glucose loading, and the long-term significance of low and high responders is not yet clear. Obese children will usually release more insulin after glucose loading than normal children will *(1)*.

Newborn infants generally have a sluggish response to glucose loading for the first few days of extrauterine life, except for infants of hyperglycemic diabetic mothers *(3)*.

Intravenous infusion of tolbutamide, arginine, or glucagon will cause an immediate increase in plasma insulin concentrations *(4)*. Although these tests may be of diagnostic value for the delineation of hyperinsulinemic states (insulinomas, nesidioblastosis, or Beckwith's syndrome), the most useful test is the demonstration of failure of insulin concentrations to decrease in the face of hypoglycemia. In young infants, nesidioblastosis may be present with insulin values that are not very high except when interpreted in view of the blood glucose value *(5)*. In the majority of the fasting hypoglycemias due to defects in glycogen formation or release, or due to defects in new glucose formation, plasma insulin values are at the limits of detection for most assay systems.

1. Paulsen, E. P., Richenderfer, L., and Ginsberg-Fellner, F., Plasma glucose, free fatty acids and immunoreactive insulin in sixty-six obese children. *Diabetes* **17**, 261–269 (1968).
2. Lestradet, H., Deschamps, I., and Giron, B., Insulin and free fatty acid levels during oral glucose tolerance tests and their relations to age in the healthy children. *Diabetes* **25**, 505–508 (1976).

3. Falorni, A., Fracassini, F., Massi-Beneditti, F., and Mattei, S., Glucose metabolism and insulin secretion in the newborn infant. *Diabetes* **23,** 172–178 (1974).
4. Parker, M. D., Pildes, R. S., Chao, K. L., Cornblath, M., and Kipnis, D. M., Juvenile diabetes mellitus, a deficiency in insulin. *Diabetes* **17,** 27–32 (1968).
5. Stanley, C. A., and Baker, L., Hyperinsulinism in infancy: Diagnosis by demonstration of an abnormal response to fasting hypoglycemia. *Pediatrics* **57,** 702–711 (1976).

Commentary—Richard A. Guthrie

The measurement of serum insulin in children and newborns has limited usefulness. In the newborn, measurement of insulin may be useful for research on infants of diabetic mothers, for research on carbohydrate metabolism, and, clinically, for studying various hypoglycemic states. In older children, the primary clinical use of serum insulin values is in the study of hypoglycemic states and research on carbohydrate metabolism, especially the study of early states of carbohydrate intolerance.

In the insulin-dependent diabetic, insulin-binding antibodies are formed after about three months of exogenous insulin therapy. These antibodies can react in the insulin immunoassay procedure and give falsely high insulin values. Whenever insulin is to be measured in persons who have received exogenous insulin therapy, procedures that can separate the insulin from the antibody (e.g., acid–alcohol extraction) must be followed. Insulin-binding antibodies are transmitted transplacentally, and are present in the infant of the insulin-dependent diabetic mother. They must be removed before true insulin values can be measured.

Hypoglycemia of the newborn is fairly common. Most causes of this are related to lack of glucose substrate and are unrelated to insulin. Insulin-producing tumors that occur in the newborn period must be found and removed. A more common cause of hypoglycemia of the newborn is nesidioblastosis, a congenital defect of B-cell formation. This produces a hyperinsulinemic state and can cause a profound, refractory hypoglycemia. The usefulness of serum insulin determinations in the newborn period, then, is to differentiate hyperinsulinemic from normoinsulinemic causes of hypoglycemia, the treatment of the two being vastly different (diazoxide or surgery in the hyperinsulinemic state; glucose etc. in the nonhyperinsulinemic state).

In infants and older children, hypoglycemia also occurs and requires differentiation of the hyperinsulinemic from the nonhyperinsulinemic state. Insulin adenomas, insulin-producing adenocarcinoma of the pancreas, and leucine-induced hypoglycemia are the most important hyperinsulinemic states in children. Ketotic hypoglycemia and glycogen-storage disease are the primary nonhyperinsulinemic hypoglycemic states in infants and children. Serum insulin measurements are valuable in differentiating these various problems.

In older children, a common problem is reactive hypoglycemia (probably an early diabetic state). Reactive hypoglycemia is thought to involve an altered carbohydrate metabolism, in which hypoglycemia occurs after meals, especially after the ingestion of concentrated sweets. There is a delayed secretion of insulin, with a late secretion and overshoot, resulting in the hypoglycemic state. The condition is usually diagnosed when an oral glucose tolerance test shows a decrease in blood glucose to 50 mg/dL or less.

I believe serum insulin concentrations are useful in the diagnosis of reactive hypoglycemia, and have established four criteria for the diagnosis: (a) occurrence of symptoms of hypoglycemia between meals or 30–120 min after ingestion of concentrated sweets, (b) relief of symptoms quickly by food, (c) a characteristic oral glucose tolerance test with high glucose values early in the test and a rapid decrease to low values late in the test (I believe the shape of the curve is more important than absolute values), and (d) a late peak in insulin values, corresponding to the decrease in glucose values late in the test. Testing for reactive hypoglycemia is the most important use for serum insulin measurements in children.

Another potential use of serum insulin measurements in children is in differentiating the various kinds of diabetes. In our early studies, some children with early or mild carbohydrate intolerate had high serum insulin values and some had low values during carbohydrate tolerance tests. I and others now believe that the children with low serum insulin values will progress to insulin-dependent (Type I) diabetes mellitus, whereas the children with high serum insulin values may eventually develop non-insulin-dependent (adult onset or Type II) diabetes mellitus. I believe glucose tolerance testing has limited value in children but, when performed, should include insulin measurements to differentiate the type of diabetes found (if any), because prognosis, clinical course, and perhaps treatment will be different for each type.

Serum insulin is measured by RIA, but the procedures vary considerably between laboratories. Some differences in normal values occur with the various procedures, especially those used for separation of bound from non-antibody-bound insulin, so each laboratory must establish its own norms.

Normal values in children differ from adult values and vary somewhat with age. Insulin secretion in the newborn period is low. Prematures have much less insulin responsiveness than full-term infants. Insulin secretion increases with age into adulthood, decreasing again in old age. The largest group of normal children (200) studied are those studied by Jackson and Guthrie (1). The limitation of these norms is that they were performed only in children between three and 17 years old, and thus do not represent younger infants or newborns.

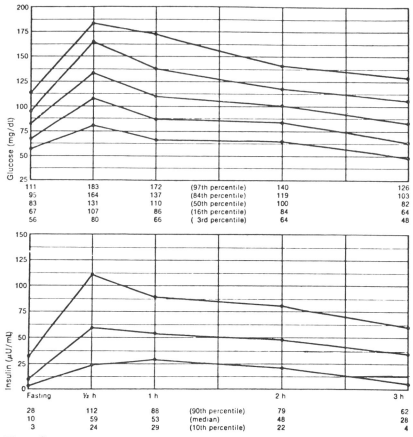

Fig. 1. Serum insulin values (*lower graph,* micro-USP units/mL) in 40 normal children during a standard oral glucose tolerance test *(upper graph)*

Based on data in ref. 2

Because insulin can be determined in samples as small as 100 μL of serum (200–500 μL of blood), newborns can be tested with heel-stick samples. Blood should be chilled when drawn and the clotted blood separated; the serum can then be frozen for later assay, and is stable for many months.

1. Jackson, R. L., and Guthrie, R. A. *The Child with Diabetes Mellitus.* Monograph published by The Upjohn Co., Kalamazoo, MI, 1975.
2. Guthrie, R. A., Guthrie, D. W., Murthy, D. Y. N., Jackson, R. L., and Lang, J., Standardization of the oral glucose tolerance test and the criteria for diagnosis of chemical diabetes in children. *Metabolism* **22,** 275–282 (1973).

Inulin Clearance

Specimen Tested:

P, U.

Laboratory Reporting:

1.

Reference (Normal) Values:

Age	mL/min per 1.73 m^2 of body surface
<1 mo	29–88
1–6 mo	40–112
6–12 mo	62–121
>1 yr	78–164

Sources of Reference (Normal) Values:

Institutional.

Specimen Volume:

0.2 mL of P; 1.0 mL of U.

Analytical Method:

Heyrovsky, A., A new method for the determination of inulin in plasma and urine. *Clin. Chim. Acta* **1**, 470–474 (1956).

Instrumentation:

Beckman 25 or Zeiss spectrophotometer.

Commentary—Garry M. Lum

Inulin is a fructose polymer. It can be used as a standard for the determination of glomerular filtration rate because it is a physiologically inert substance not bound to protein and is freely filtered by the glomerulus; furthermore, it is neither secreted nor reabsorbed by the tubules. Plasma and urine concentrations are easily measured, but the test is not routinely used clinically because it requires constant intravenous infusion and timed simultaneous urine collection. Ingestion of fruits and fruit drinks that contain fructose should be avoided when the test is performed.

When equilibrium of arterial to venous plasma is reached, venous sampling can be used for determination. Inulin clearance is then calculated by the standard formula:

$$C_{IN} = U_{IN}V/P_{IN}$$

where C_{IN} = inulin clearance, mL/min; U_{IN} = urine concentration of inulin, mg/mL; V = urine flow rate, mL/min; P_{IN} = plasma concentration, mg/mL.

The test is rather cumbersome in most clinical settings: disturbances in arterial and venous concentrations can introduce error; the flow of urine must be constant; large areas of urinary dead space (e.g., in a child with obstructive uropathy) alter the volume and concentration of urine. In children there is the further difficulty of obtaining accurate timed collections of urine unless catherization is used. Thus, unless such exacting calculation of clearance is mandatory, estimates by techniques such as creatinine clearance rather than the complexities of inulin clearance are usually more suitable in children.

1. Leake, R. D., Trygstad, C. W., and Oh, W., Inulin clearance in the newborn infant: Relationship to gestational and postnatal age. *Pediatr. Res.* **10,** 759–762 (1976).

Iron and Iron-Binding Capacity

Specimen Tested:

P, S.

Laboratories Reporting:

4.

Reference (Normal) Values:

Age	µg/dL (µmol/L)	
	Total iron	**Iron-binding capacity**
Birth	110–270 (19.7–48.3), then decreases for 4–6 mo	
Newborn	20–157 (3.6–28.1) (n = 26)[a]	59–175 (10.6–31.3)
6 wk–3 yr	20–115 (3.6–20.6) (n = 70)[a]	
4–10 mo	30–70 (5.4–12.5)	
6 mo–3 yr	Increases gradually to 59–175 (10.6–31.3)	
3–9 yr	20–141 (3.6–25.2) (n = 137)[a]	
3–10 yr	53–151 (9.5–27.0)	250–400 (45–72)
9–14 yr	21–151 (3.8–27.0) (n = 132)[a]	
Child	50–150 (9.0–26.9)	250–400 (45–72)
14–16 yr	20–181 (3.6–32.4) (n = 85)[a]	
Adult	72–186 (12.9–33.3); 40–175 (7.2–31.3) (n = 150)[a]	250–400 (45–72)

[a] Number tested in an institutional study of this age group. A retrospective study was made of patients' charts, and those used showed no evidence of active infectious or inflammatory disease, malignancy, or anemia.

Sources of Reference (Normal) Values:

Institutional; text ref. *2*, pp 5, 195; Fischer, D. S., and Price, D. C., A simple serum iron method using the new sensitive chromogen tripyridyl-s-triazine. *Clin. Chem.* **10**, 21–31 (1964).

Specimen Volume, Collection, and Preservation:

0.1 to 1.0 mL. Stability is claimed for up to 4 d at RT, and 1 wk in RR.

Analytical Method:

Ferrozine-based method: Carter, P., Spectrophotometric determination of serum iron at the submicrogram level with a new reagent (Ferrozine). *Anal. Biochem.* **40**, 450–458 (1971); Stookey, L. L., Ferrozine—a new spectrophotometric reagent for iron. *Anal. Chem.* **42**, 779–781 (1970); Giovaniello, T. J., DiBenedetto, G., Palmer, D. N., and Peters, T., Jr., Fully automated method for the determination of serum iron and total iron-binding capacity. In *Automation in Analytical Chemistry, Technicon Symposia 1967,* **1.** Mediad, Inc., White Plains, NY, 1968, pp 185–188; Sigma Chemical Co. iron and total iron-binding capacity kit; Hyland-Travenol Labs. Ferro-Chek II; O'Malley, J. A., Hassan, A., Shiley, J., and Traynor, H., Simplified determination of serum iron and total iron-binding capacity. *Clin. Chem.* **16**, 92–96 (1970); Goodwin, J. F., Direct estimation of serum iron and unsaturated iron-binding capacity in a single aliquot. *Clin. Biochem.* **3**, 307–314 (1970).

Instrumentation:

Zeiss spectrophotometer; Abbott ABA-100 Bichromatic Analyzer; Technicon smac; Greiner Selective Analyzer II.

17-Ketogenic Steroids

Specimen Tested:

U.

Laboratory Reporting:

1.

Reference (Normal) Values:

0–1 yr: <1 mg/d
1–10 yr: 1 mg/d per year of age

Sources of Reference (Normal) Values:

Institutional.

Specimen Volume

5 mL.

Analytical Method:

Birke, G., Diczfalusy, E., and Plantin, L. O., Assessment of the functional capacity of the adrenal cortex. *J. Clin. Endocrinol. Metab.* **18,** 736–754 (1958).

Instrumentation:

Zeiss spectrophotometer.

Commentary—Elizabeth K. Smith

Urinary 17-hydroxycorticosteroids (17-OHCS) oxygenated at C-20 may be oxidized by sodium bismuthate or sodium periodate to 17-ketosteroids and measured by the Zimmerman reaction. These 17-ketogenic steroids include the cortisol metabolites, tetrahydrocortisol and tetrahydrocortisone, plus cortol, cortolone, pregnanetriol, etc., and may be considered "total" 17-OHCS.

Normal values for 17-ketogenic steroids increase with age to adulthood and are approximately 50% higher than Porter–Silber 17-OHCS values in the same child *(1)*.

Changes in the excretion of 17-ketogenic steroids with hypo- and hyperfunction of the pituitary–adrenal axis generally parallel changes in Porter–Silber values for 17-OHCS. However, a marked discrepancy occurs in congenital adrenal hyperplasia from 21-hydroxylase deficiency, where Porter–Silber 17-OHCS values are very low but 17-ketogenic steroids values are markedly increased, because of the inclusion of high concentrations of pregnanetriol.

Precautions regarding urine collection are similar to those for Porter–Silber 17-OHCS (see **17-Hydroxycorticosteroids**). Interferences include any drugs that interfere with the physiological activity of the adrenal cortex or with the Zimmerman color reaction.

1. Smith, E. K., and Tippit, D. F., Evaluation of steroid hormone metabolism. In text ref. 7, vol. **1,** p 318.

17-Ketosteroids

Specimen Tested:

U.

Laboratories Reporting:

3.

Reference (Normal) Values:

Age	M	mg/d (μmol/d) M & F	F
0–14 d		up to 1.0 (3.5); (5–9); 0.5 to 2.5 (1.73–8.7)	
2 wk–1 yr		(0–0.7)	
2 wk–2 yr		0.0–0.5 (0.0–1.73)	
1–3 yr		<2.0 (<6.9)	
2–6 yr		0.0–2.0 (0.0–6.9); (0–7)	
3–6 yr		0.5–3.0 (1.73–10.4)	
6–8 yr		0.0–2.5 (0.0–8.7); (0.7–7)	
6–9 yr		0.8–4.0 (2.77–13.9)	
8–10 yr		0.7–4.0 (2.43–13.9); (2–10)	
9–12 yr		2.0–6.0 (6.9–20.8)	
10–12 yr	0.7–6.0 (2.43–20.8)	(4–26)	0.7–5.0 (2.43–17.3)
12–13 yr		(6–45)	
12–14 yr	1.3–10.0 (4.5–35)		1.3–8.5 (4.5–29.5)
12–16 yr	3.0–12.0 (10.4–41.6)		3.0–14 (10.4–48.2)
13–15 yr	(9–45)		(9–38)
14–16 yr	2.5–13.0 (8.7–45)		2.5–11.0 (8.7–38)
16–20 yr	5–21 (17.3–69)		4–18 (13.9–62)
Adult	7–23 (24.3–80); (35–85)		5–15 (17.3–52); (17–50)

Sources of Reference (Normal) Values:

Institutional; study on 119 healthy children and 24 normal adults.

Specimen Volume, Collection, and Preservation:

10 mL. Collect 24-h U over 5 g of boric acid crystals. Keep U in RF during collection and storage.

Analytical Method:

Zimmerman reaction; Kraushaar, L. A., Epstein, E., and Zak, B., Characteristics of a 17-ketosteroid reaction. *Clin. Chem.* **12**, 282–288 (1966); Sobel, C., Golub, O. J., Henry, R. J., Jacobs, S. L., and Basu, G. K., Study of the Norymberski method for determination of 17-ketogenic steroids (17-hydroxycorticosteroids) in urine. *J. Clin. Endocrinol. Metab.* **18**, 208–221 (1958); B. M. Hudson (private communication); modification of the method of Callow, N. H., Callow, R. K., and Emmens, C. W., Colorimetric determination of substances containing the grouping $-CH_2 \cdot CO-$ in urine extracts as an indication of androgen content. *Biochem. J.* **32**, 1312–1331 (1938).

Instrumentation:

Gilford 300 N, Zeiss spectrophotometers; LKB 7400 calculating absorptiometer; Eberbach 5900 reciprocating shaker; Oxford sampler, pipettor; rotating mixer; 40 °C waterbath with overhead air or nitrogen lines to evaporate solvent.

Commentary—Elizabeth K. Smith

The 17-ketosteroids (17-KS) are compounds having a ketone group on C-17. The "total neutral 17-ketosteroids" excreted in the urine, and measured by the Zimmerman reaction with alkaline *m*-dinitrobenzene, represent a mixture of metabolites of testosterone and adrenal androgens, plus small amounts of cortisol metabolites. Urinary 17-KS is often measured as an index of androgen secretion. In the normal man approximately one-fourth to one-third of the 17-KS is derived from the testes, the remainder from the adrenal cortex. In the normal woman most of the 17-KS is derived from the adrenal cortex, with perhaps a trace from the ovary. In prepubertal children of either sex, the primary source of 17-KS is the adrenal cortex.

The daily excretion of 17-KS increases throughout childhood, increasing abruptly with the onset of puberty in either sex. The earlier maturation of girls is reflected in the attainment of adult values at age 12–16 years, with mean values often higher than those for boys of the same age (1). Boys show a rapid increase at age 16–20 years as the testes mature, reaching final adult values that exceed those for women. Excretion seems to correlate best with stage of skeletal maturation (2).

In the newborn, urinary excretion of 17-KS is high (up to 2.5 mg/d) during the first two to three days of postnatal life. The excretion decreases rapidly, seeming to parallel closely the neonatal involution of the fetal zone of the adrenal cortex, to reach the very low concentrations that persist throughout infancy (3).

Many medications produce colors with the Zimmerman reagent, resulting in unpredictable interference, usually as falsely high results. Recognized offenders are meprobamate, reserpine, chlorpromazine, ethinamate, and spironolactone (1). Avoid administration of drugs when urine is being collected for steroid assays.

In children, determination of 17-KS is useful as a screening test for adrenal dysfunction. Values are increased in congenital adrenal hyperplasia and can be reduced to normal with adequate glucocorticoid-replacement therapy. Values also are increased in virilizing adrenal tumors. Precocious puberty with advanced bone age from whatever cause usually is accompanied by an increase in 17-KS above the normal range for chronologic age. Low values for age are found in Addison's disease, hypothyroidism, hypopituitarism, and generally in growth retardation with retarded bone age from any cause.

1. Smith, E. K., and Tippit, D. F., Evaluation of steroid hormone metabolism. In text ref. 7, vol. 1, p 312.
2. Tanner, J. M., Growth and endocrinology of the adolescent. In text ref. 6, pp 46–48.
3. Seely, J. R., The fetal and neonatal adrenal cortex. In text ref. 7, vol. 1, p 239.

Lactate

Specimen Tested:

B, CSF, P.

Laboratories Reporting:

5.

Reference (Normal) Values:

Source	Lactate, mg/dL (mmol/L)
Capillary B (newborn)	(up to 3.0)
Capillary P (child)	5–20 mg/dL (0.56–2.25)
Venous B	5–18 (0.5–2.0); (1.0–1.8)
Arterial B	3–7 (0.3–0.8)
CSF	8.0–25.0 (0.9–2.8)

Sources of Reference (Normal) Values:

Institutional; Calbiochem-Behring Rapid Lactate package insert; Bio-Dynamics/ bmc Lactate package insert; *Documenta Geigy Scientific Tables*, 6th ed., Geigy Pharmaceuticals, Ardsley, NY, 1962, p 563; CSF values are institutional.

Specimen Volume, Collection, and Preservation;
Patient Preparation:

10 to 500 μL. Heparin as anticoagulant. Collect blood without stasis. Preservation is critical. **B:** collect into protein-precipitating agent directly (trichloroacetic acid; perchloric acid). **P:** centrifuge heparinized blood without delay. If blood is kept in an ice bath for 15 min before centrifuging, no significant change is observed, but if kept there for 1 h, the change is significant. Lactate is stable in P for 2 h in RR, and 4 h in FR; protein-free filtrate may be stable longer. Patient should preferably fast for 8 to 12 h before blood is drawn. Reference values are based on fasting subjects.

Analytical Method:

All methods used are enzymic. **B:** Calbiochem-Behring Rapid Lactate kit; Olson, G. F., Optimal conditions for the enzymatic determination of L-lactic acid. *Clin. Chem.* **8,** 1–10 (1962); Bio-Dynamics/ bmc Lactate kit; Bergmeyer, H. U., Ed., *Methods of Enzymatic Analysis,* **2,** 2nd English ed. Academic Press, Inc., New York, NY, 1974, p 1464. **P:** Pesce, M. A., Bodourian, S. H., and Nicholson, J. F., Rapid kinetic measurement of lactate in plasma with a centrifugal analyzer. *Clin. Chem.* **21,** 1932–1934 (1975). **CSF:** Marbach, E. P., and Weil, M. H., Rapid enzymatic measurement of blood lactate and pyruvate. *Clin. Chem.* **13,** 314–325 (1967); text ref. *4,* 1st ed., pp 664–666.

Instrumentation:

Abbott ABA-100 and ABA-50 Bichromatic Analyzers; Zeiss and Varian 635 spectrophotometers; Union Carbide CentrifiChem System 400.

Commentary—Michael A. Pesce

Lactate, the end product of the anaerobic metabolism of glucose, is formed from the reduction of pyruvate by the enzyme lactate dehydrogenase (EC 1.1.1.27). The concentration of lactate in blood is determined by the production of lactate, primarily by the muscles and erythrocytes, and by its removal by the liver. Lactic acidosis may be the most frequent cause of metabolic acidosis and results usually from an overproduction or underutilization of lactate. Increased lactate concentrations are usually observed in tissue hypoxia, diabetes mellitus, malignancies such as leukemia, and after ingestion of drugs such as ethanol, methanol, and salicylate (1). High concentrations of lactate and pyruvate are usually seen in congenital disorders such as Type I glycogen storage disease (glucose-6-phosphatase deficiency), and deficiencies of fructose-1,6-diphosphatase, pyruvate dehydrogenase, or pyruvate carboxylase. The lactate-to-pyruvate ratio, which is usually less than 10, is increased when there is an excess production of lactate, as in tissue hypoxia, but is normal in glucose-6-phosphatase deficiency, in which both lactate and pyruvate concentrations increase.

Lactate is measured through its oxidation to pyruvate and the accompanying reduction of NAD^+ to NADH by lactate dehydrogenase at a pH greater than 9.0. The equilibrium of the reaction favors lactate production but is shifted by the removal of the pyruvate formed. The NADH produced is measured at 340 nm and is related to the concentration of lactate. Pyruvate is determined by reversing the reaction used for measuring lactate: at pH 7.5 pyruvate is converted to lactate and NADH to NAD^+. The change in absorbance of NADH is measured at 340 nm and related to the concentration of pyruvate.

Lactate is unstable in whole blood and increases in concentration because of glycolysis; therefore, as soon as the blood is collected, it should be either deproteinized or centrifuged at 4 °C. Lactate is stable in the protein-free filtrate for several days at 4 °C. Because lactate values determined in blood and plasma are not significantly different, lactate can be measured in plasma. Lactate is stable in plasma for at least 4 h at 4 °C (2). Using plasma instead of blood simplifies the assay, and results are rapidly obtainable.

1. Olvia, P. B., Lactic acidosis. *Am. J. Med.* **48**, 209–225 (1970).

2. Pesce, M. A., Bodourian, S. H., and Nicholson, J. F., Rapid kinetic measurement of lactate in plasma with a centrifugal analyzer. *Clin. Chem.* 21, 1932–1934 (1975).

Commentary—J. A. Knight

Increased concentrations of lactate in CSF in cases of bacterial meningitis were first noted in 1924 *(1)*. However, the general recognition of the clinical value of this fact, as well as an appreciation of its worth in distinguishing bacterial from viral meningitis, has only recently been realized *(2–4)*.

CSF lactate is readily measured by either enzymic *(5)* or GLC techniques *(4);* the latter authors show that these two methods give essentially identical results. A reliable normal range, determined by enzymic analysis, is 100–253 mg/L (1.11–2.81 mmol/L) *(6)*. Values in the 250–300 mg/L range are considered equivocal, because an occasional normal spinal fluid will have values in this range. In essentially all bacterial infections, the value will exceed 300 mg/L *(3,4,6);* in very early or mild cases, values in the 250–300 mg/L range may rarely be seen. In viral meningitis, however, the concentration is invariably less than 250 mg/L, although rare cases may be in the borderline range *(3)*.

Occasionally, xanthochromic fluid will be sent to the laboratory for lactate determination. These fluids usually yield high values, but have no diagnostic significance and should probably not be recommended for analysis. High values may also be seen in a wide variety of other central nervous system conditions *(2)*. Increased lactate concentrations are apparently caused by tissue hypoxia, owing to increased intracranial pressure with subsequent impairment of the central blood supply *(7,8);* they are apparently unrelated to phagocytic destruction of bacteria by neutrophilic leukocytes. This explains why lactate concentrations are high in tuberculous meningitis, where mononuclear cells usually predominate and microorganisms are few. Appropriate serological tests must be carried out to identify infections from *Mycoplasma;* cultures here are negative, but lactate values are high *(4)*. If serological tests are not performed, one may mistake these for cases of viral meningitis with high lactate values.

1. Nishimura, K., The lactic acid content of blood and spinal fluid. *Proc. Soc. Exp. Biol. Med.* 22, 322–324 (1924).
2. Pryce, J. D., Gant, P. W., and Saul, K. J., Normal concentrations of lactate, glucose, and protein in cerebrospinal fluid, and the diagnostic implications of abnormal concentrations. *Clin. Chem.* 16, 562–565 (1970).
3. Bland, R. D., Lister, R. C., and Ries, J. P., CSF lactic acid levels and pH in meningitis. *Am. J. Dis. Child.* 128, 151–156 (1974).
4. Controni, G., Rodriguez, W. J., Hicks, J. M., Ficke, M., Ross, S., Friedman, G., and Khan, W., Cerebrospinal fluid lactic acid levels in meningitis. *J. Pediatr.* 91, 379–384 (1977).

5. Marbach, E. P., and Weil, M. H., Rapid enzymatic measurement of blood lactate and pyruvate. *Clin. Chem.* **13**, 314–325 (1967).
6. Knight, J. A., Dudek, S. M., and Haymond, R. E., Increased cerebrospinal fluid lactate and early diagnosis of bacterial meningitis. *Clin. Chem.* **25**, 809–810 (1979).
7. Kopetsky, S. J., and Fishberg, E. H., Changes in distribution ratio of constituents of blood and spinal fluid in meningitis. *J. Lab. Clin. Med.* **18**, 796–801 (1933).
8. Poulson, O. B., Hansen, E. L., Christensen, H. S., and Brodersen, P., Cerebral blood flow, cerebral metabolic rate of oxygen and CSF acid–base parameters in patients with acute pyrogenic meningitis and with acute encephalitis. *Acta Neurol. Scand.* **48**, Suppl. 51, 407–408 (1972).

Lactate Dehydrogenase (LD; EC 1.1.1.27; L-lactate:NAD⁺ oxidoreductase)

Specimen Tested:

S.

Laboratories Reporting:

3.

Reference (Normal) Values:

	U/L	
Age	**37 °C**	**30 °C**
2.5 h–10 d		308–1780
At birth	upper limit: 3–9 × adult values	
1 d–1 mo	upper limit: 2–5 × adult values	
1 mo–2 yr	2–3 × adult values	
Up to 2 yr	150–360	
Up to 4 yr		60–170
2–5 yr	150–350	
3–17 yr	1–2 × adult values	
5–8 yr	150–300	
5 yr–adult		40–110
8–12 yr	130–300	
12–14 yr	130–280	
14–16 yr	130–230	
16 yr–adult	110–200	
Adult	109–193	

Sources of Reference (Normal) Values:

Lab. 1: Cheng, M. H., Lipsey, A. I., Blanco, V., Wong, H. T., and Spiro, S. H., Microchemical analysis for 13 constituents of plasma from healthy children. *Clin. Chem.* **25,** 692–698 (1979). **Lab. 2:** institutional; text ref. *2*, p. 202. **Lab. 3:** institutional.

Specimen Volume, Collection, and Preservation:

5 µL. Heparin *only* as anticoagulant. Separate S *without delay* after clotting. Remarkable stability (1 wk) is claimed at RT, but this is not true of all S specimens. Do not refrigerate or freeze. Reject hemolyzed samples.

Analytical Method:

All three labs. use Abbott ABA-100 with a modified method of Wacker. **Lab. 1:** Amador, E., Dorfman, L. E., and Wacker, W. E. C., Serum lactic dehydrogenase activity: An analytical assessment of current assays. *Clin. Chem.* **9,** 391–399 (1963); Mallinckrodt Gran-U-Chem LDH-L; Harleco Ultrazyme-PLUS LDH. **Labs. 2, 3:** Abbott A-Gent; Wacker, W. E. C., Ulmer, D. D., and Vallee, B. L., Metalloenzymes and myocardial infarction. Malic and lactic dehydrogenase activities and zinc concentrations in serum. *N. Engl. J. Med.* **55,** 449–456 (1956).

Enzyme Data:

1. Enzyme unit definition: 1 IUB unit (U) = that activity yielding 1 µmol of NADH per minute, under the conditions specified.
2. Buffer, pH: **Lab. 1:** Tris, 8.8; **Lab. 2, 3:** glycine–Na_2CO_3, 8.6 ± 0.20 at 25 °C.
3. Substrate, pH: L-lactate, 8.6–8.8.
4. Reaction temperature: **Lab. 1, 3:** 37 °C; **Lab. 2:** 30 °C.
5. Temperature reported: **Lab. 1, 3:** 37 °C; **Lab. 2:** 30 °C.

Instrumentation:

Abbott ABA-100 Bichromatic Analyzer.

*   *   *

Laboratory Reporting:

1.

Reference (Normal) Values:

Age	No.	U/L
Newborn	24	>500
6 wk–18 mo	36	208–473
18 mo–3 yr	32	249–403
3–8 yr	117	191–381
8–11 yr	59	187–325
11–14 yr	81	144–316
14–16 yr	81	129–279
Adult	150	99–207

Sources of Reference (Normal) Values:

An institutional, retrospective study of patients' charts. Patients included were free of active infectious, inflammatory disease, malignancy, and anemia.

Analytical Method and Instrumentation:

Technicon Instruments Corp. SMAC; Wacker et al., *op. cit.;* Morganstern, S., Flor, R., Kessler, G., and Klein, B., Automated determination of NAD-coupled enzymes, determination of lactic dehydrogenase. *Anal. Biochem.* **13,** 149–161 (1965); Morganstern, S., Rush, R., and Lehmann, D., SMAC: Chemical methods for increased specificity. In *Advances in Automated Analysis 1972, International Congress,* **1.** Mediad Inc., Tarrytown, NY, 1973, pp 27–31; Technicon Instruments Corp. SMAC/SDM.

Enzyme Data:

Same as in previous report except:
Substrate, pH: lactate, 9.0.
Reaction temperature: 37 °C.
Temperature reported: 37 °C.

*   *   *

Specimen Tested:

CSF, P, S.

Laboratory Reporting:

1.

Reference (Normal) Values:

P, S: Newborn, 1–3 d: 40–348 U/L
         Adult, M: 70–178; F: 42–166
CSF: Child: 17–59

Analytical Method and Instrumentation:

Amador et al., *op. cit.;* Bio-Dynamics/*bmc* LDH L kit; Beckman TR Enzyme Analyzer.

Enzyme Data:

1. Enzyme unit: same as in preceding reports.
2. Buffer, pH: pyrophosphate, 8.6.
3. Substrate, pH: L-lactate, 8.6.
4. Reaction temperature: 37 °C.
5. Temperature reported: 37 °C.

*   *   *

Laboratories Reporting:

2.

Reference (Normal) Values:

	Lab. 1	Lab. 2
Cord blood S	337–871 U/L	24–436 U/L

Sources of Reference (Normal) Values:

Lab. 1: institutional study made on 69 cord specimens. **Lab. 2:** institutional.

Analytical Method:

Lab. 1: Bio-Dynamics/*bmc* UV System-LDH; Wroblewski, F., and LaDue, J. S., Lactate dehydrogenase activity in blood. *Proc. Soc. Exp. Biol. Med.* **90,** 210–213 (1955). **Lab. 2:** Technicon SMA II method; Fisher Diagnostics reagents.

Enzyme Data:

Lab. 1:
1. Enzyme unit definition: 1 IUB unit (U) = activity utilizing 1 μmol of NADH per minute.
2. Buffer, pH; phosphate, 7.5.
3. Substrate, pH: pyruvate, 7.5.
4. Reaction temperature: 30 °C.
5. Temperature reported: 30 °C.

Lab. 2: Same conditions as reported previously for Technicon SMAC.

Instrumentation:

Lab. 1: American Instrument Corp. Rotochem. **Lab. 2:** Technicon SMA II system.

LD Isoenzymes

Specimen Tested:

S.

Laboratory Reporting:

1.

Reference (Normal) Values:

Isoenzyme	% of total LD activity
LD$_1$ (heart)	24–34
LD$_2$ (heart, erythrocytes)	35–45
LD$_3$ (muscle)	15–25
LD$_4$ (liver, trace; muscle)	4–10
LD$_5$ (liver, muscle)	1–9

Sources of Reference (Normal) Values:

Institutional.

Specimen Volume, Collection, and Preservation:

5 μL. Heparin *only* as anticoagulant. Separate S *without delay* after clotting. Remarkable stability (1 wk) is claimed at RT, but this is not true of all S specimens. Do not refrigerate or freeze. Reject hemolyzed samples.

Analytical Method:

Electrophoresis; Galen, R. S., The enzyme diagnosis of myocardial infarction. *Hum. Pathol.* **6,** 141–155 (1975); Helena Labs. LDH Isoenzyme kit.

Instrumentation:

Helena Labs. electrophoresis system.

Commentary—Paul J. Wolf

Howell *(1)* and Matsuoka *(2)* demonstrated that serum and plasma LD values are increased in the newborn. King and Morris *(3)* found that cord blood and serum LD had a mean activity of 330 (150–590) U/L. Adult values are reached gradually. Freer et al. recently studied 69 newborns and determined that the LD range was 327–874 U/L *(4);* the LD isoenzyme pattern in their study indicated that LD_5 was especially increased. This is confirmed by King and Morris, who found that the more slowly moving isoenzymes of LD predominate in the newborn *(3)*. This pattern indicates that the increased LD in newborns results from the neonate's skeletal muscle and liver. The immature hepatocyte may, because of defective membranes, release LD into the serum or may synthesize excess enzyme. LD_5 also may be released from renal tubular medullary cells. Another source of the LD_5 may be the mother's skeletal muscle activity during labor. A minor part is probably derived from the fetal erythrocytes that undergo physiological hemolysis, and is LD_1.

When LD is increased above the normal range in children, owing to pathologic lesions, the pediatrician should consider a number of conditions, primarily skeletal muscle lesions such as dystrophy, myositis, or rhabdomyolysis. Other causes would include viral hepatitis, toxic hepatitis, and malignant infiltrative hepatic disease. Other conditions causing a high LD activity are well-advanced malignancies such as neuroblastoma and Wilms' tumor. Lymphomas and leukemia cause a prominent increase in LD_2 and LD_3. Finally, rare causes of increased LD in children include hemolytic anemia, megaloblastic anemia, myocardial damage, pulmonary or renal infarction, and acute pancreatitis.

1. Howell, R. R., The diagnostic value of serum enzyme measurements. *J. Pediatr.* **68,** 121–134 (1966).
2. Matsuoka, S., Studies on lactic dehydrogenase (LDH) during development. Part 1: Changes of LDH activity and isoenzyme patterns in healthy human serum during development. *Acta Paediatr. Jpn.* **10,** 13–21 (1968).
3. King, J., and Morris, M. B., Serum enzyme activity in the normal newborn infant. *Arch. Dis. Child.* **36,** 604–609 (1961).
4. Freer, D. E., Statland, B. E., Johnson, M., and Felton, H., Reference values for selected enzyme activities and protein concentrations in serum and plasma derived from cord-blood specimens. *Clin. Chem.* **25,** 565–569 (1979).

Commentary—Michael A. Pesce

Lactate dehydrogenase (LD) catalyzes the reversible reaction of lactate to pyruvate. In normal serum, LD is separated by electrophoresis into five isoenzymes. Each isoenzyme is a tetramer composed of two subunits, designated H for heart muscle and M for skeletal muscle. These subunits are combined into five possible tetramers, H_4, H_3M, H_2M_2, HM_3, and M_4, corresponding to LD_1, LD_2, LD_3, LD_4, and LD_5, respectively. Those isoenzymes with more H units have an increasingly negative charge and migrate closest to the anode, whereas the M_4 isoenzyme (LD_5) has a slightly positive net charge and is located closest to the cathode. The migration of LD isoenzymes can be related to the serum proteins. LD_1 is the fastest moving fraction and migrates in the α_1-globulin region; LD_2 and LD_3 migrate in the α_2- and β-globulin region; LD_4 in the fast gamma-globulin region; and LD_5, the slowest moving fraction, migrates in the slow gamma-globulin region.

LD_1 is found primarily in heart muscle, erythrocytes, and kidneys; LD_5 is found mainly in the skeletal muscle and liver. The other isoenzymes are distributed in all tissues. The relative concentration of the isoenzymes in normal serum, in descending order, are LD_2, LD_1, LD_3, LD_4, and LD_5. In myocardial infarcts the total serum LD begins to increase 12 to 24 h after the infarction, and at about 48 h the LD_1 fraction exceeds the LD_2 fraction. This "flipped" LD isoenzyme ratio (LD 1 > 2), in combination with an increased serum creatine kinase MB isoenzyme fraction in the appropriate clinical setting, is diagnostic of myocardial infarction. A "flipped" LD isoenzyme ratio is also observed in hemolytic disease and in renal infarction, but the creatine kinase MB fraction is absent in these cases. An increase in LD_5 indicates hepatic or skeletal muscle injury. The midzone fractions LD_2, LD_3, and LD_4 can be increased in pulmonary infarctions and in certain neoplasms.

The isoenzymes of LD are separated by electrophoresis on either cellulose acetate membranes or agarose gels and then incubated with a buffered solution of lactate and NAD^+. The NADH formed is quantitated either fluorometrically by measurement of NADH or colorimetrically by reduction of a tetrazolium salt to produce a formazan.

The LD isoenzymes are stable for at least one day in serum stored at room temperature. LD_5 is unstable in serum stored at 4 °C or above 45 °C, whereas LD_1 is stable at temperatures up to 65 °C. A hemolyzed specimen will show increased LD_1 and LD_2 fractions because of the substantial amounts of these isoenzymes in erythrocytes. The percentage of LD_1 in neonates is less than in normal adults, but LD_5 is increased in neonates (1); LD isoenzymes 2, 3, and 4 are at the same percentage in neonates as in adults.

1. Freer, D. E., Statland, B. E., Johnson, M., and Felton, H., Reference values for selected enzyme activities and protein concentrations in serum and plasma derived from cord-blood specimens. *Clin. Chem.* **25,** 565–569 (1979).

Lactose Tolerance

Specimen Tested:

P, S.

Laboratory Reporting:

1.

Reference (Normal) Values:

Increase of 20 mg/dL (as glucose) from fasting value

Note: mg/dL × 0.055 = mmol/L, as glucose.

Sources of Reference (Normal) Values:

Text ref. *2*, p 312.

Volume and Source of Specimen:

5 µL; capillary.

Analytical Method:

Text ref. *2*, p 312.

Instrumentation:

Beckman Glucose Analyzer.

Commentary—S. Meites

The disaccharidase lactase (EC 3.2.1.25) is present in human intestinal mucosa at birth. Lactase deficiency is very rare in infants and young children. It may be caused by temporary injury, delayed production, disease, or surgery at the intestinal site of enzyme production. In adolescence and young adulthood, idiopathic lactase deficiency develops in surprisingly vast segments of the human population, with a wide variation of incidence in different racial groups.

The deficiency develops in almost 100% of Orientals, 70–75% of American Negroes, and 3–19% of Caucasians. In a few instances, lactose per se may be toxic, despite the presence of adequate concentration of lactase.

Diagnosis of lactase deficiency may be helped with the oral lactose tolerance test, by analysis of capillary (*not* venous) blood sugar at intervals (30, 60, 90, 120, and 150 min) after ingestion of 2 g of aqueous lactose (100 g/L) solution per kilogram of body weight by the fasting subject. Because the hydrolysis and absorption of lactose is a comparatively slow process, results of the test are often inconclusive. Assay of peroral biopsy is preferable, except for small children on whom the biopsy is too risky to perform. Because lactose is hydrolyzed to glucose and galactose and the monosaccharides are actively absorbed, any of the specific ultramicro methods for quantitative blood glucose determination may be used in the tolerance test as a measure of lactose digestion.

1. Gray, G. M., Intestinal disaccharidase deficiencies and glucose–galactose malabsorption. In text ref. *11*, pp 1453–1464.
2. Hsia, D. Y.-Y., In text ref. *13*, pp 199–203.
3. Hsia, D. Y.-Y., and Inouye, T., In text ref. *14*, pp 132–134, 223.

Commentary—G. L. Barnes and John F. Connelly

Methods of assessing disaccharide intolerance include:
1. Measurement of reducing sugars in feces *(1)*.
2. Disaccharide tolerance tests.
3. Disaccharidase assays on small-bowel biopsy specimens *(2)*.
4. Breath-hydrogen measurement after disaccharide challenge *(3)*.

The first has proved very useful in children with lactose intolerance secondary to gastroenteritis; it is not invasive and does not require laboratory facilities. In contrast, disaccharide tolerance tests are often difficult to interpret and can be dangerous by provoking severe osmotic diarrhea in an intolerant infant. Disaccharidase measurements are more reliable but require small-bowel biopsy facilities; moreover, there is sometimes lack of correlation between results and symptoms.

The breath-hydrogen test after disaccharide challenge, although still in the development stage, may prove to be the most useful and reliable test of disaccharide tolerance. It has the advantage of measuring function of the whole small bowel.

1. Kerry, K. R., and Anderson, C. M., A ward test for sugar in the faeces. *Lancet* **i**, 981–982 (1964).
2. Dahlqvist, A., Method for assay of intestinal disaccharidases. *Anal. Biochem.* **7**, 18–25 (1964).
3. Maffei, H. V. L., Metz, G. L., and Jenkins, D. J. A., Hydrogen breath test: Adaptation of a simple technique to infants and children. *Lancet* **i**, 1110–1111 (1976).

Lead

Specimen Tested:

B, U.

Laboratories Reporting:

4

Reference (Normal) Values:

	Lead in blood, μg/dL (μmol/L)		
Age	**Lab. 1**	**Labs. 2, 3**	**Lab. 4**
0–6 yr	29 or less (1.40 or less)		
Child		up to 40 (1.93)	
4–12 yr			1.0–39.0 (0.05–1.88)
Adult	59 or less (2.85 or less)		

U (Lab. 1): <500 μg/L, post-chelation (<2.42 μmol/L)

Sources of Reference (Normal) Values:

Preventing Lead Poisoning in Young Children, Center for Disease Control, USDHEW 00–2629, April, 1978; *Occupational Exposure to Lead, Federal Register* 43 (2), 54353, Nov. 21, 1978; U.S. Public Health Service, Department of Health, Education and Welfare: The Surgeon General's policy statement on medical aspects of childhood lead poisoning (Bureau of Community Environmental Management PHS, 5600 Fisher's Lane, Rockville, MD 20852) Nov. 1970; institutional. **Lab. 4:** based on analysis of specimens from 415 elementary school children, ages 4–12 yr.

Specimen Volume, Collection, and Preservation:

B: 20 to 100 μL. Heparin or EDTA as anticoagulant. Use only pre-tested Pb-free containers. Careful cleaning of the patient's puncture site and the phlebotomist's hands is important. **U:** 8-h collection, after chelation challenge.

Analytical Method:

Labs. 1, 2, 4: anodic stripping voltammetry; Therell, B. L., Drosche, J. M., and Dziuk, T. W., Analysis for lead in undiluted whole blood by tantalum ribbon atomic absorption spectrophotometry. *Clin. Chem.* **24,** 1182–1185 (1978); Morrell, G., and Giridhar, G., Rapid micromethod for blood lead analysis by anodic stripping voltammetry. *Clin. Chem.* **22,** 221–223 (1976). **Lab. 3:** Fernandez, F. J., Progress report—preliminary results on the determination of lead in blood with the HGA 2100 graphite furnace. Atomic Absorption Application Study No. 562, Perkin-Elmer Corp., Norwalk, CT, May, 1974.

Instrumentation:

Urine: Instrumentation Laboratory Inc. 251 atomic absorption spectrophotometer and 355 flameless atomizer; Micromedic diluter.

Blood: **Labs. 1, 2, 4:** Enviromental Sciences Associates 2014 Anodic Stripping Voltameter. **Lab. 3:** Perkin-Elmer Corp. 360 atomic absorption spectrophotometer.

Commentary—Roger L. Boeckx

After absorption from the lung or gastrointestinal tract, lead concentration in blood increases, then decreases rapidly as lead is deposited in the calcified matrix of bone (1). The total body burden of lead increases throughout life, but this is not necessarily reflected in an increasing blood lead (PbB) concentration. Metabolic tests such as erythrocyte protoporphyrin and urinary δ-aminolaevulinate correlate best with the total lead burden, whereas PbB reflects the extent of recent or current absorption of lead. Intake in children may fluctuate widely, which would be reflected in varying PbB concentrations; consequently, PbB concentrations could, under certain circumstances, correlate poorly with the clinical effects of plumbism, as observed in the nervous system and the hematopoietic system.

In studies where PbB was monitored in men continually exposed to high concentrations of airborne lead, PbB attained an equilibrium after 100 days of exposure, with a return to pre-exposure values in 20 weeks (1). Other studies have reported increased PbB in children as long as 10 years after exposure (2). The short-term clearance of lead apparently involves deposition of lead in bone, i.e., redistribution, whereas long-term clearance involves actual elimination of the metal. In dogs, the biological half-life of lead has been estimated to exceed five years, reflecting the long-term storage of lead in bone.

Because of the complex nature of lead redistribution and excretion, it is doubtful that the lead concentration in urine (PbU), even in a timed collection, can be relied upon to provide accurate information on lead exposure. Some investigators have used chelating agents such as calcium disodium EDTA (3–5) or penicillamine (6) to mobilize lead from bone, thereby causing a lead diuresis. Although PbB and PbU concentrations do not correlate well, PbB and post-chelation PbU do show good agreement (6). This so-called "EDTA mobilization test" is particularly useful in children who show some evidence of lead absorption but for whom it is not certain whether the lead burden is sufficient to warrant chelation therapy (7).

Although spectrophotometric and colorimetric methods were the first to be developed, they are tedious, imprecise, and subject to contamination and interference. PbB concentration is most commonly determined by atomic absorption spectrophotometry or anodic stripping voltammetry. Atomic absorption techniques can be divided into two categories, based on the method used to atomize the sample: *(a)* flame atomization and *(b)* electrothermal atomization.

Flame atomization techniques are of two types: *(a)* direct aspiration and *(b)* indirect flame atomization. For direct-aspiration techniques, the sensitivity of lead analysis, expressed as the concentration required to produce an absorbance of 0.2, is approximately 25 µg/mL. In other words, to get reasonable absorption, the solution aspirated into the flame must contain lead concentrations of at least 1000 µg/dL. The lead in blood must be extracted and concentrated for direct-aspiration techniques to be applicable to biological samples. The relatively large sample sizes required make this approach unsuitable for pediatric work.

In an attempt to overcome the problems caused by the low sensitivity of the direct-aspiration methods, Delves *(8)* developed an indirect flame atomization technique. In this method, the sample is placed in a nickel crucible, and the crucible is heated in the flame. The atomized metal is collected in a nickel or ceramic absorption tube to concentrate the vapor. This system provides a 100-fold increase in sensitivity over direct atomization methods.

Hicks et al. *(9)* found that correlation between the Delves method and a direct-aspiration method was excellent; furthermore, the use of capillary blood obtained by fingerstick provided PbB results as reliable as those involving blood obtained by venipuncture. The development of screening techniques that allowed the use of 50–100 µL of fingerstick blood was one of the major factors in the establishment of routine community screening programs in high-risk areas in the early 1970s.

Electrothermal atomization systems offer another approach for the microanalysis of trace metals. In these "flameless" atomic absorption systems electrical current is used to produce the high temperatures (2200–2500 °C) necessary to atomize lead. Various designs have been developed, including carbon cups, graphite tubes, and tantalum ribbons.

Polarography has been of great interest to clinical chemists recently. Beginning with the earliest mercury-drop electrode systems, polarography has progressed to anodic stripping voltammetry. Modern anodic stripping voltammetry systems can accurately measure 10 µg/dL or less PbB in 100-µL aliquots of blood. Several authors have reported good correlation between anodic stripping voltammetry and atomic absorption techniques *(10,11)*.

Boone et al. *(12)* of the Center for Disease Control compared various methodologies for PbB; the precision of the assays ranged from an average CV of 12% for anodic stripping voltammetry to 32% for carbon rod atomic absorption spectrophotometry. When compared with a definitive method (mass spectroscopy–isotopic dilution), all analytical approaches showed significant positive bias. The lowest bias (8%) was observed with extraction atomic absorption, while the highest bias (13%) was observed with carbon rod atomic absorption spectrophotometry.

Proper diagnosis and treatment of childhood lead poisoning can be a complex issue. The proper interpretation of results for PbB and erythrocyte protoporphyrin is discussed elsewhere (7) and the reader is strongly urged to follow the guidelines for risk classification and interpretation of data described there.

1. Hammond, P. B., Exposure of humans to lead. *Ann. Rev. Pharmacol. Toxicol.* **17,** 197–214 (1977).
2. Chisolm, J. J., The use of chelating agents in the treatment of acute and chronic lead intoxication in childhood. *J. Pediatr.* **73,** 1–38 (1968).
3. Teisinger, J., and Srbova, J., The value of mobilization of lead by calcium ethylenediaminetetraacetate in the diagnosis of lead poisoning. *Br. J. Ind. Med.* **16,** 148–152 (1959).
4. Hammond, P. B., and Aaronson, A. L., The mobilization and excretion of lead in cattle: A comparative study of various chelating agents. *Ann. N.Y. Acad. Sci.* **88,** 498–511 (1960).
5. Lahaye, D., Roosels, D., and Verwilghen, R., Diagnostic sodium calcium edetate mobilization test in ambulant patients. *Br. J. Ind. Med.* **25,** 148–149 (1968).
6. Selander, S., Cramer, K., and Hallberg, L., Studies in lead poisoning. Oral therapy with penicillamine: Relationship between lead in blood and other laboratory tests. *Br. J. Ind. Med.* **23,** 282–291 (1966).
7. *Preventing Lead Poisoning in Young Children.* Center for Disease Control, Atlanta, GA, 1978.
8. Delves, M. T., A micro-sampling method for the rapid determination of lead in blood by atomic absorption spectrophotometry. *Analyst* **95,** 431–438 (1970).
9. Hicks, J. M., Gutierrez, A. M., and Worthy, B. E., Evaluation of the Delves micro system for blood lead analysis. *Clin. Chem.* **19,** 322–325 (1973).
10. Searle, B., Chan, W., and Davidow, B., Determination of lead in blood and urine by anodic stripping voltammetry. *Clin. Chem.* **19,** 76–80 (1973).
11. Morrell, G., and Giridhar, G., Rapid micromethod for blood lead analysis by anodic stripping voltammetry. *Clin. Chem.* **22,** 221–223 (1976).
12. Boone, J., Hearn, T., and Lewis, S., Comparison of interlaboratory results for blood lead with results from a definitive method. *Clin. Chem.* **25,** 389–393 (1979).

Leucine Aminopeptidase [EC 3.4.11.1; α-aminoacyl-peptide hydrolase (cytosol)]

Specimen Tested:

S.

Laboratory Reporting:

1.

Reference (Normal) Values:

Newborn: 29–59 arbitrary units/L
1 mo–adult: 15–50

Source of Reference (Normal) Values:

Text ref. *1*.

Volume and Source of Specimen:

40 μL; venous.

Analytical Method:

Sigma Tech. Bull. 251; text ref. *2*.

Enzyme Data:

1. Enzyme unit definition: 1 arbitrary unit is that activity that will cause release of 1 μmol of β-naphthylamine from L-leucyl-β-naphthylamide per hour at 37 °C.
2. Buffer: *N*-(1-naphthyl)ethylenediamine.
3. Substrate, pH: L-leucyl-β-naphthylamide, 7.1.
4. Reaction temperature: ambient.

Instrumentation:

Beckman Model DU spectrophotometer.

Commentary—T. A. Blumenfeld

Leucine aminopeptidase is a peptidolytic enzyme catalyzing the hydrolysis of *N*-terminal residues from certain peptides and amides containing a free amino group. Activity is especially favored when the *N*-terminal residue is leucine. The enzyme is widely distributed in human tissues and is found (in order of decreasing activity) in pancreas, gastric mucosa, liver, spleen, large intestine, brain, small intestine, and kidney. Significant activity has also been demonstrated in plasma, urine, and bile. The enzyme is excreted by the liver into the bile.

Leucine aminopeptidase activity is probably the composite of the activity of a group of closely related enzymes. Either magnesium or manganese ions can serve as activators. EDTA inhibits the enzyme, but citrate, fluoride, and oxalate do not.

Most investigators now believe that leucine aminopeptidase activity cannot be used to differentiate hepatocellular from obstructive jaundice, nor does it provide any useful information that cannot be obtained by other tests. Serum leucine aminopeptidase activity in cord blood, in the blood of newborns, and in the mother's blood during pregnancy, especially during the third trimester, is greater than in the blood of normal, nonpregnant adults. The enzyme is present in urine but, owing to the presence of other chromogens, the urine must be dialyzed before determining the enzyme's activity. When serum activity is increased, urinary leucine aminopeptidase is also increased in 98% of the cases.

In the newborn, leucine aminopeptidase activity is normal in hemolytic disease (Rh and ABO incompatabilities) and in physiological jaundice. In a study of the activity in normal infants, infants with biliary atresia, and infants with other diseases, marked increases were suggestive of biliary obstruction, but normal values did not rule out the possibility of biliary obstruction.

1. Text ref. 5.
2. Rutenburg, A. M., Pineda, E. T., Goldbarg, J. A., Levitan, R., Gellis, S. S., and Silverberg, M., Serum leucine aminopeptidase. *Am. J. Dis. Child.* **103,** 47–54 (1962).

Lipase (EC 3.1.1.3; triacylglycerol lipase)

Specimen Tested:

Duodenal fluid, S.

Laboratories Reporting:

2.

Reference (Normal) Values:

	Lab. 1, arbitrary units	Lab. 2, U/L
S: Newborn, full-term, 0–5 d	0.1–0.7	
Child		20–136
Adult	0.0–1.5	
Duodenal fluid:		8 000–35 000

Sources of Reference (Normal) Values:

Lab. 1: institutional study on 50 infants; adult values based on manufacturer's insert (below). **Lab. 2:** institutional; P, S values based on 4-h incubation.

Specimen Volume, Collection, and Preservation:

Lab. 1: 50 µL; **Lab. 2:** 1.0 mL. Lipase is claimed to be stable for 1 wk at RT or in RR.

Analytical Method:

Lab. 1: Perkin-Elmer 91 Amylase-Lipase Analyzer; Zinterhofer, L., Wardlaw, S., Jatlow, P., and Seligson, D., Nephelometric determination of pancreatic enzymes. I. Amylase. *Clin. Chim. Acta* **43,** 5–12 (1973); Vogel, W. C., and Zieve, L., A rapid and sensitive turbidimetric method for serum lipase based upon differences between the lipases of normal and pancreatitis serum. *Clin. Chem.* **9,** 168–181 (1963). **Lab. 2:** titrimetric determination; Tietz, N. W., and Fiereck, E. A., A specific method for serum lipase determination. *Clin. Chim. Acta* **13,** 352–358 (1966); Sigma Chemical Co. Lipase kit.

Enzyme Data:

Lab. 1:

1. Enzyme unit definition: the rate of change of turbidity in the method was adjusted so that the arbitrary unit values numerically approximate Cherry–Crandall units.
2. Buffer, pH: Tris, 9.0 ± 0.2.
3. Substrate, pH: olive oil, 8.8 ± 0.2.
4. Reaction temperature: 37 °C.
5. Temperature reported: 37 °C.

Lab. 2:

1. Enzyme unit definition: Sigma–Tietz units of lipase are exactly equal to the milliliters of NaOH (50 mmol/L) required to neutralize the fatty acids liberated during the incubation period of the test. These units × 280 = IUB units (U)/L; 1 U is the enzyme activity catalyzing the liberation from the substrate of 1 μmol of fatty acid per minute at 37 °C.
2. Buffer, pH: Tris, 8.0.
3. Substrate, pH: olive oil, 50% (500 mL/L), 8.0.
4. Reaction temperature: 37 °C.
5. Temperature reported: 37 °C.

Instrumentation:

Lab. 1: Perkin-Elmer 91 Amylase-Lipase Analyzer. **Lab. 2:** Corning burette.

Commentary—Paul L. Wolf

The most common disease state associated with an increase in serum lipase is acute pancreatitis. Acute pancreatitis is an unusual condition in children but may occur as a result of viral infections, especially secondary to mumps or coxsackie. The increase in serum lipase may lag behind the increase in amylase by 12 to 24 h and may persist for 10 to 14 days. Chronic renal failure will also cause increased serum lipase because of decreased excretion *(1)*.

Fat embolism from bone marrow to the pulmonary circulation as a result of bone fractures in children will cause an increased serum lipase. The lipase is liberated from pulmonary alveolar cells *(2)*.

1. Berk, J. E., Serum amylase and lipase. *J. Am. Med. Assoc.* **199,** 98–102 (1967).
2. Adler, F., and Peltier, L. F., The laboratory diagnosis of fat embolism. *Clin. Orthop.* **21,** 226–231 (1961).

Low-Density Lipoprotein (LDL) Cholesterol

Specimen Tested:

P.

Laboratory Reporting:

1.

Reference (Normal) Values:

	mg/L (mmol/L)			
	M		**F**	
Age, yr	**White**	**Black**	**White**	**Black**
6–7	520–1360	410–1450	630–1390	680–1400
	(1.34–3.52)	(1.06–3.75)	(1.63–3.58)	(1.76–3.60)
8–9	560–1280	570–1490	600–1360	810–1270
	(1.45–3.34)	(1.47–3.87)	(1.55–3.52)	(2.09–3.31)
10–11	400–1560	410–1570	560–1400	590–1390
	(1.03–4.02)	(1.06–4.04)	(1.45–3.60)	(1.53–3.58)
12–13	520–1400	240–1800	580–1480	540–1500
	(1.34–3.60)	(0.62–4.66)	(1.50–3.84)	(1.40–3.90)
14–15	420–1500	610–1290	530–1290	640–1400
	(1.09–3.90)	(1.58–3.37)	(1.37–3.37)	(1.66–3.60)
16–17	500–1380	500–1220	490–1370	390–1490
	(1.29–3.56)	(1.29–3.16)	(1.27–3.54)	(1.01–3.87)

Sources of Reference (Normal) Values:

Morrison, J. A., deGroot, I., Edwards, B. K., Kelly, K. A., Mellies, M. J., Khoury, P., and Glueck, C. J., Lipids and lipoproteins in 927 school children, ages 6 to 17 years. *Pediatrics* **62,** 990–995 (1978).

Specimen Volume, Collection, and Preservation; Patient Preparation:

7 mL. EDTA-Na$_2$ as anticoagulant. Place specimen in wet ice or RR after collection. Separate P within 8 h. Store 1 wk in RR, or several months in FR. Patient must fast 12–16 h before blood collection.

Analytical Method:

Calculated as difference between $d > 1.006$ cholesterol fraction (separated by ultracentrifugation) and high-density lipoprotein (HDL) cholesterol. Measurement of cholesterol by modified Lieberman–Burchard reaction: Abell, L. L., Levy, B. B., Brodie, B. B., and Kendall, F. E., Simplified method for estimation of total cholesterol in serum and demonstration of its specificity. *J. Biol. Chem.* **195,** 357 (1952); *Manual of Laboratory Operations,* Lipid Research Clinic Program, I. Lipid and Lipoprotein Analysis, DHEW Publication No. (NIH) 75–268. Low-density lipoproteins may also be calculated from the Friedewald formula [LDL cholesterol = total cholesterol − HDL cholesterol − (triglyceride/5)]: Friedewald, W. T., Levy, R. I., and Frederickson, D. S., Estimation of the concentration of low-density lipoprotein cholesterol in plasma, without use of the preparative ultracentrifuge. *Clin. Chem.* **18**, 499–502 (1972); see also **High-Density Lipoprotein.**

Instrumentation:

Beckman Instruments preparative ultracentrifuge; Technicon Instruments Corp. AutoAnalyzer II; Micromedic dilutor.

Note: Also see Frederickson, D. S., Levy, R. I., and Lindgren, F. T., A comparison of heritable abnormal lipoprotein patterns in serum as defined by two different techniques. *J. Clin. Invest.* **47**, 2446–2457 (1968).

Commentary—John E. Sherwin

Measurement of HDL and LDL cholesterol has been reported to provide a specific assessment of risk for coronary heart disease *(1)*. Increases of LDL cholesterol are associated with higher risk. The relationship between high values of LDL cholesterol in adolescence and subsequent risk for heart disease has not been satisfactorily studied at this time.

Measurement of LDL cholesterol requires 7 mL of blood and a preparative ultracentrifuge, thus preventing routine measurement in the younger pediatric age group. The principal use of LDL cholesterol measurement is in the diagnosis and management of hereditary hyperlipoproteinemias *(2)*.

1. Morrison, J. A., deGroot, I., Edwards, B. K., Kelly, K. A., Mellies, M. J., Khoury, P., and Glueck, C. J., Lipids and lipoproteins in 927 school children, ages 6 to 17 years. *Pediatrics* **62**, 990–995 (1978).
2. Levy, R. I., and Rifkind, B. M., Diagnosis and management of hyperlipoproteinemia in infants and children. *Am. J. Cardiol.* **31**, 547–551 (1973).

Magnesium

Specimen Tested:

P, S, erythrocytes.

Laboratories Reporting:

4.

Reference (Normal) Values:

	mEq/L (mmol/L)	
Age	**Labs. 1, 2**	**Labs. 3, 4**
P, S:		
Newborn	1.5–2.3 (0.75–1.15)	
Child		1.4–1.9 (0.7–0.95)
Adult	1.4–1.8; 2.0 (0.70–0.90; 1.00)	1.3–2.5 (0.65–1.25)
Erythrocytes:	3.92–5.28 (1.96–2.64)[a]	

[a] Lab. 1 only.

Sources of Reference (Normal) Values:

Lab. 1, 2, 4: institutional. **Lab. 3:** text ref. *2,* p 6; Pruden, E. L., Meier, R., and Plaut, D., Comparison of serum magnesium values by photometric, fluorometric, atomic absorption, and flame emission methods. *Clin. Chem.* **12,** 613–619 (1966).

Specimen Volume, Collection, and Preservation:

10 to 100 μL. Heparin only as anticoagulant. Stable at RT or in RR for 1 wk.

Analytical Method:

Atomic absorption: **Labs. 1, 2:** Zettner, H., and Seligson, D., Determination of serum magnesium by atomic absorption spectrophotometry. *Clin. Res.* **11,** 406 (1963); Paschen, K., and Fuchs, C., A new micromethod for Na, K, Ca, and Mg determinations in a single serum dilution by atomic-absorption spectrophotometry. *Clin. Chim. Acta* **35,** 401–408 (1971); Pybus, J., Determination of calcium and magnesium in serum and urine by atomic absorption spectrophotometry. *Clin. Chim. Acta* **23,** 309–317 (1969); Fleming, L. W., and Stewart, W. K., The effect of the atomiser on the estimation of magnesium by atomic absorption spectrophotometry. *Clin. Chim. Acta* **14,** 131–134 (1966).
Dye-chelation: **Lab. 3:** Gindler, E. M., and Heth, D. A., Colorimetric determination with bound "Calmagite" of magnesium in human blood serum. *Clin. Chem.* **17,** 662 (1971), abstract; Pierce Chemical Co. Magnesium Rapid Stat kit. **Lab. 4:** Magon dye; Baginski, E. S., Marie, S. S., Karcher, R., and Zak, B., Magnesium in serum. In *Selected Methods for the Small Clinical Chemistry Laboratory,* W. R. Faulkner and S. Meites, Eds. American Association for Clinical Chemistry, Washington, DC, 1981 (in press).

Instrumentation:

Lab. 1, 2: Perkin-Elmer 290, Varian 1200 atomic absorption spectrophotometers; Micromedic diluter. **Labs. 3, 4:** Gilford Stasar II and III spectrophotometers.

Commentary—M. J. Levitt

Concentrations of magnesium in serum or plasma at birth are lower than in older children or adults, averaging 1.35–1.45 mEq/L (0.675–0.725 mmol/L) *(1)*. They are, however, higher than magnesium concentrations in the mother's blood at the time of birth *(2,3)*. There are different mechanisms controlling magnesium and calcium homeostasis during the first week of postnatal life: the magnesium concentration remains relatively constant during this period while calcium varies *(1,2,4)*. Serum magnesium is lower in the infant with respiratory distress or with above-normal birth weight, but is not correlated with sex or race *(2,4)*.

Parathyrin (parathyroid hormone) may unequally control serum magnesium and calcium ion concentration. While it is true that familial hypoparathyroidism can result in subnormal serum magnesium concentrations of 0.4–0.5 mEq/L (0.20–0.50 mmol/L) and calcium concentrations of 2.2 mEq/L (1.1 mmol/L), the postulated hypoparathyroidism during the first week of neonatal life does not result in hypomagnesemia *(5)*.

Similarly, malabsorption of magnesium can exist without corresponding defects in the absorption of calcium. This condition can result in serum magnesium concentrations as low as 0.5 mEq/L (0.25 mmol/L) with nearly normal calcium values of 3.8 mEq/L (1.9 mmol/L). Malabsorption of magnesium alone can also accompany abnormally low circulating concentrations of both magnesium and calcium *(7)*. Both ions may also be decreased in children with prolonged diarrhea.

Hypomagnesemia of < 1 mEq/L (0.50 mmol/L) is associated with convulsions, but this may be due to the correlation between low serum concentrations of total magnesium and ionized calcium. Symptoms of neuromuscular irritability in infants can be observed with serum magnesium concentrations up to 1.6 mEq/L (0.80 mmol/L), but only if serum ionized calcium values are < 1.8 mEq/L (0.9 mmol/L) *(1)*.

Hypermagnesemia > 2.5 mEq/L (1.25 mmol/L) may be asymptomatic, although concentrations exceeding 6 mEq/L (3.0 mmol/L) cause drowsiness. Serum magnesium values > 10 mEq/L (5.0 mmol/L) can result in respiratory failure and heart block *(8)*. Hypermagnesemia at birth occurs as a result of treatment of the mother with magnesium salts before delivery.

Atomic absorption spectrometry is the preferred method for measuring magnesium, but is not well suited to around-the-clock operation. Manual precipitation methods for measuring magnesium may come into prominence in pediatric laboratories because they apparently can be performed on small volumes of samples without interference from bilirubin or lipids *(9)*.

1. Raade, I. C., Parkinson, D. K., Höffken, B., Appiah, K. E., and Hanley, W. B., Calcium ion activity in the sick neonate: Effect of bicarbonate administration and exchange transfusion. *Pediatr. Res.* **6**, 43–49 (1972).

2. Tsang, R. C., Kleinman, L. I., Sutherland, J. M., and Light, I. J., Hypocalcemia in infants of diabetic mothers. *J. Pediatr.* **80,** 384–395 (1972).

3. Tsang, R. C., Chen, I. W., Friedman, M. A., and Chen, I., Neonatal parathyroid function: Role of gestational age and postnatal age. *J. Pediatr.* **83,** 728–738 (1973).

4. de Baare, L., Lewis, J., and Sing, H., Ultramicroscale determination of clinical chemical values for blood during the first four days of postnatal life. *Clin. Chem.* **21,** 746–750 (1975).

5. Niklasson, E., Familial early hypoparathyroidism associated with hypomagnesemia. *Acta Pediatr. Scand.* **59,** 715–719 (1970).

6. Strömme, J. H., Nesbakken, R., Norman, T., Skjorten, F., Skyberg, D., and Johannessen, B., Familial hypomagnesemia. *Acta Pediatr. Scand.* **58,** 433–444 (1969).

7. Friedman, M., Hatcher, G., and Watson, L., Primary hypomagnesemia with secondary hypocalcemia in an infant. *Lancet* **i,** 703–705 (1967).

8. Text ref. *16,* pp 931, 974, 991.

9. Pragay, D. A., Casey, S. J., and Cross, L. C., Evaluation of a new magnesium kit. *Clin. Chem.* **19,** 671 (1973).

Manganese

Specimen Tested:

B.

Laboratory Reporting:

1.

Reference (Normal) Values:

Newborn: 2.4–9.6 μg/dL (2.44–1.75 μmol/L)
2–18 yr: 0.8–2.1 (0.15–0.38)

Sources of Reference (Normal) Values:

Institutional study of 457 full-term newborns, 4 d old, and 29 healthy children, 2–18 yr old.

Specimen Volume, Collection, and Preservation:

50 μL. Heparin or EDTA as anticoagulant. Refrigerate sample until assayed, although there is a claim of stability at RT for 45 d. See *Notes* below.

Analytical Method:

Atomic absorption spectrophotometry: Muzzarelli, R.A.A., and Rocchetti, R., Atomic absorption determination of manganese, cobalt, and copper in whole blood and serum with a graphite atomizer. *Talanta* **22,** 683 (1975). The validity of this procedure was confirmed by analyses of dry-ashed blood samples, and by the method of standard additions.

Instrumentation:

Perkin-Elmer 306 atomic absorption spectrophotometer; deuterium background corrector and HGA-2000 graphite furnace.

Notes:
1. No sex differences were observed. The range in children is the same as that found in adults. The high value seen in the newborn appears to decrease gradually during the first two years of life, to a plateau at the child–adult concentration.
2. Skin-puncture (capillary) blood gives slightly higher values than venous blood.

Alpha-D-Mannosidase
(EC 3.2.1.24; α-D-mannoside mannohydrolase)

Specimen Tested:

Leukocytes.

Laboratory Reporting:

1.

Reference (Normal) Values:

Range: 108.8–433.3 arbitrary units
Mean ± 2 SD: 7.15–382.8 arbitrary units

Sources of Reference (Normal) Values:

Institutional; D. A. Applegarth (see list of **Contributors**).

Specimen Volume, Collection, and Preservation:

10 mL of heparinized B. Keep B on ice and prepare leukocyte pellets without delay.
  Note: See discussion on leukocyte preparation in **Appendix 4.**

Analytical Method:

Measure release of 4-methylumbelliferone (4-MU) from 4-MU-α-D-mannopyranoside.

Enzyme Data:

1. Enzyme unit definition: 1 arbitrary unit = the amount of enzyme that cleaves 1 nmol of 4-MU-α-D-mannopyranoside per hour per milligram of protein, at 37 °C.
2. Buffer system, pH: acetate, 4.0
3. Substrate, pH: 4-MU-α-D-mannopyranoside.
4. Reaction temperature: 37 °C.
5. Temperature reported: 37 °C.

Mercury

Specimen Tested:

U.

Laboratory Reporting:

1.

Reference (Normal) Values:

Child: < 50 μg/d (< 250 nmol/d)

Sources of Reference (Normal) Values:

Institutional.

Specimen Volume, Collection, and Preservation:

50 mL. Collect timed urine specimen in an acid-washed container.

Analytical Method:

Atomic absorption spectrophotometry: Hatch, W. R., and Ott, W. L., Determination of submicrogram quantities of mercury by absorption spectrophotometry. *Anal. Chem.* **40,** 2085 (1968).

Instrumentation:

Perkin-Elmer 360 atomic absorption spectrophotometer.

Metanephrine, Normetanephrine

Specimen Tested:

U.

Laboratories Reporting:

2.

Reference (Normal) Values:

Age, yr	Lab. 1, mg/g of creatinine (μmol)	Lab. 2, mg/d (μmol/d)
<2	up to 4.6 (23.3)	
2–10	up to 3 (15.2)	
10–15	up to 2 (10.3)	
>15	up to 1 (5.1)	
Adult		<1 (<5.1)

Sources of Reference (Normal) Values:

Lab. 1: institutional; Bio-Rad Labs. instruction manual. **Lab. 2:** institutional; Gitlow, S. E., Mendlowitz, M., Wilk, E. K., Wilk, S., Wolf,

R. L., and Bertani, L. M., Excretion of catecholamine metabolites by normal children. *J. Lab. Clin. Med.* **72,** 612–620 (1968).

Specimen Volume, Collection, and Preservation; Patient Preparation:

Aliquot of 24-h U. For children, collect U in a bottle containing 15 mL of 6 mol/L HCl; for adults, use 30 mL. U may be stored in RR for 3 d, although some claim that acidified U may be stored at RT for several days. The patient should not take drugs for 72 h before U collection. Diet has no effect: Weetman, R. M., Rider, P. S., Oei, T. O., Hempel, J. S., and Baehner, R. L., Effect of diet in urinary excretion of VMA, HVA, metanephrine and total catecholamine in normal preschool children. *J. Pediatr.* **88,** 46–50 (1976).

Analytical Method:

Bio-Rad Labs. Metanephrine Assay; Pisano, J. J., A simple analysis for normetanephrine and metanephrine in urine. *Clin. Chim. Acta* **5,** 406–414 (1960).

Instrumentation:

Lab. 1: Micromedic MS2 spectrophotometer.

Note:
1. Absorbance should also be measured at 350 nm to determine whether interfering substances are present. If the absorbance at 360 nm is less than one-half of the absorbance at 350 nm, then interfering substances are in the urine and invalidate the assay.
2. See also **Catecholamines.**

Commentary—Michael A. Pesce

The metanephrines (normetanephrine and metanephrine) are 3-methoxy metabolites of norepinephrine and epinephrine, and are formed mainly in the liver and kidneys by the enzyme catechol methyltransferase (EC 2.1.1.6). Normetanephrine and metanephrine can be excreted in the urine, either as the free form or as the conjugated sulfate or glucuronide, or can be metabolized to vanillylmandelic acid by the enzyme monoamine oxidase (EC 1.4.3.4). Metanephrines are usually determined by the procedure of Pisano *(1).* Urine is hydrolyzed and passed through an ion-exchange column. The metanephrines are eluted from the column and oxidized to vanillin, which is measured spectrophotometrically at 360 nm. Absorbance should also be measured at 350 nm to determine whether chromogens are present that would interfere with the assay. If the absorbance at 360 nm is less than one-half the absorbance at 350 nm, then interfering substances are present.

A 24-h urine should be collected in a bottle containing 15 mL of HCl (6 mol/L) and the urine kept refrigerated during the collection. Metanephrines are stable in acidified urine for one week at 4 °C.

There is a diurnal variation in excretion of metanephrines (2). Urine collected from 0800 to 2000 hours shows a greater excretion of metanephrines than that collected from 2000 to 0800 hours. Diet does not affect metanephrine excretion (2)—children ingesting vanilla ice cream, vanillin, or bananas did not show any increase in their urinary metanephrines. Drugs, however, can significantly alter the excretion of metanephrines (3), so that urine should be collected from a patient who is not receiving medication. The normal concentrations of urinary metanephrines, expressed as milligrams per 24 h, are lower in children than in adults (4) but increase with age and reach adult values between the ages of 10 and 16. Increased concentrations of urinary metanephrines are usually observed in patients with neuroblastoma and pheochromocytoma.

1. Pisano, J. J., A simple analysis for normetanephrine and metanephrine in urine. *Clin. Chim. Acta* **5**, 406–414 (1960).
2. Weetman, R. M., Rider, P. S., Oei, T. O., Hempel, J. S., and Baehner, R. L., Effect of diet on urinary excretion of VMA, HVA, metanephrine and total free catecholamine in normal preschool children. *J. Pediatr.* **88**, 46–50 (1976).
3. Young, D. S., Pestaner, L. C., and Gibberman, V., Effects of drugs on clinical laboratory tests. *Clin. Chem.* **21**, 328D (1975).
4. De Schaepdryver, A. F., Hooft, C., Delbeke, M. J., and Van den Noortgaete, M., Urinary catecholamines and metabolites in children. *J. Pediatr.* **93**, 266–268 (1978).

Methemoglobin

Specimen Tested:

B.

Laboratories Reporting:

4.

Reference (Normal) Values:

3 Labs.: Up to 3 g/L; 5; 10
2 Labs.: Up to 2% of total Hb; 3%

Sources of Reference (Normal) Values:

Institutional.

Specimen Volume, Collection, and Preservation:

50 to 200 μL. Heparin or EDTA (K_3) anticoagulant. Store in RR, but perform analysis within 2 h of collection.

Analytical Method:

Evelyn, K. A., and Malloy, H. T., Microdetermination of oxyhemoglobin, methemoglobin and sulfhemoglobin in a single sample of blood. *J. Biol. Chem.* **126**, 655–662 (1938); also see Miale, J. B., *Laboratory Medicine and Hematology*, 4th ed., C. V. Mosby Co., St. Louis, MO, 1972, pp 1223–1224.

Instrumentation:

Varian 635, Coleman Jr. II, Zeiss, Gilford 200 spectrophotometers.

Commentary—T. A. Blumenfeld

Methemoglobin is an oxidized form of hemoglobin, i.e., the heme iron is in the ferric rather than in the normal ferrous state. Methemoglobin is totally nonfunctional as an oxygen carrier and normally constitutes no móre than 2% of the circulating hemoglobin. If more than 10% of the hemoglobin is in this oxidized state, the skin color is dusky and the blood has a brown discoloration that persists after oxygenation.

Normally, methemoglobin forms slowly and the oxidized hemoglobin iron is reduced by enzymes in the erythrocyte. The most important of the reductive enzymes is the NADH-dependent diaphorase, NADH-methemoglobin reductase (no EC no. assigned). The activity of this enzyme is substantially less in the erythrocytes of newborns, particularly if the newborns are premature. As a result of this deficiency, there is during infancy a higher concentration of methemoglobin in blood and an increased susceptibility to formation of methemoglobin.

Various drugs and chemicals such a nitrites, aniline, phenacetin, certain sulfonamides, and benzene derivatives produce acute episodes of methemoglobin in newborns. Acute methemoglobinemia may develop after exposure to the offending agent; the interval varies. Although marked cyanosis may be present, symptoms are usually mild. Occasionally, however, methemoglobinemia may exceed 30 to 50% of total hemoglobin and the infant may develop respiratory distress and tachycardia.

In addition to acute drug- or chemical-induced methemoglobinemia, congenital forms of this disorder may occur, due to enzyme deficiency and structural abnormalities of the hemoglobin molecule, resulting in lifelong cyanosis. Congenital deficiency of NADH-dependent methemoglobin reductase activity is associated with various abnormalities that affect this enzyme; they are inherited as an autosomal recessive trait. In various affected individuals, 20 to 50% of the hemoglobin exists as methemoglobin, resulting in cyanosis, which often is apparent at birth. The diagnosis is established by demonstrating subnormal activity of the enzyme in the erythrocytes. Studies of kinetic properties and electrophoretic mobility of the abnormal enzymes are the basis for more definitive identification of the abnormality.

Congenital methemoglobinemia (also recessive form only; the homozygous form would be lethal) due to structural abnormalities of the hemoglobin molecule occurs because of amino acid substitutions in the region of the globin chain at which the heme groups are attached. Because of the altered protein/heme interactions, the affected heme groups remained oxidized and are unable to bind oxygen. Several such mutant forms of hemoglobin have been identified and are collectively classified as hemoglobin M disease. These patients exhibit lifelong cyanosis but are asymptomatic. Amino acid substitutions in the alpha chain may produce cyanosis from birth; substitutions in the beta chain produce cyanosis that becomes apparent at two to six months of age.

Acute methemoglobinemia, resulting from drugs or chemical exposure, will subside spontaneously when the explosure is discontinued. The condition may be treated with methylene blue or ascorbic acid, both reducing agents. Prolonged administration of either of these agents will reduce methemoglobin concentrations in patients with the enzyme deficiency but not in patients with hemoglobin M disease.

1. Jaffé, E. R., and Heller, P., Methemoglobinemia in man. *Prog. Hematol.* **4**, 48–71 (1964).
2. Jaffé, E. R., and Neumann, G., Hereditary methemoglobinemia, toxic methemoglobinemia, and the reduction of methemoglobin. *Ann. N.Y. Acad. Sci.* **151**, 795–806 (1968).

Methotrexate

Specimen Tested:

S.

Laboratory Reporting:

1.

Reference (Normal) Values:

Toxic concentrations are greater than 1 μmol/L at 48 h after infusion of high doses of methotrexate.

Sources of Reference (Normal) Values:

Institutional.

Specimen Volume, Collection, and Preservation:

10 μL. Do not expose the sample to light. Stable 3 d in FR.

Analytical Method and Instrumentation:

Modification of the method of: Finley, P. R., and Williams, R. J., Methotrexate assay by enzymatic inhibition with use of the centrifugal analyzer. *Clin. Chem.* **23**, 2139–2141 (1977); Union Carbide Centrifichem 400 centrifugal analyzer system. *Note:* With this procedure, there is no interference from bilirubin at 10 mg/dL or from hemoglobin at 100 mg/dL. When bilirubin concentration is 15 mg/dL, there is a 20% positive interference; and when hemoglobin concentration is 200 mg/dL, there is a 15% positive interference. Lipemic samples decrease the methotrexate values by about 15%.

Commentary—Michael A. Pesce

Therapy with high doses of methotrexate has been used to treat osteogenic sarcoma, acute lymphatic leukemia, cancer of the head and neck, and other malignancies. Methotrexate acts as an antitumor agent because it is tightly bound to the enzyme dihydrofolate reductase (EC 1.5.1.3), and blocks the metabolism of folic acid. Prolonged high doses of methotrexate have been associated with myelosuppression, renal failure, vomiting, dermatitis, alopecia, and hepatotoxicity. High-dose methotrexate therapy has also been suspected of contributing to death.

The major route of elimination of methotrexate is by the kidneys. Recently, a metabolite of methotrexate, 7-hydroxymethotrexate, has been detected in serum *(1)* and urine *(2)* of patients receiving high-dose therapy. 7-Hydroxymethotrexate neither significantly inhibits the enzyme dihydrofolate reductase nor has any other antifolate activity. Methotrexate and 7-hydroxymethotrexate will precipitate in renal tubules at acid pH, causing renal failure and delayed excretion of methotrexate, the situation responsible for the resulting toxicity. Because high-dose methotrexate therapy can be dangerous, routine monitoring in serum will identify patients at high risk of impending toxicity.

Methotrexate in serum can be measured by enzyme-multiplied immunoassay (EMIT) (Pesce, M. A., and Bodourian, S. H., unpublished observations) or enzymic inhibition techniques *(3)*. With the EMIT assay, serum is mixed with a reagent consisting of antibodies to methotrexate, NAD^+, and glucose 6-phosphate. The methotrexate in serum binds the antibody; this solution is then added to a reagent containing methotrexate bound to glucose-6-phosphate dehydrogenase (EC 1.1.1.49), and the enzyme-labeled drug combines with any remaining unfilled antibody sites. The residual enzyme activity is determined by measuring the increase in absorbance of NADH at 340 nm and is related to the concentration of methotrexate in the sample. With the enzyme-inhibition system, dihydrofolic acid is reduced to tetrahydrofolic acid and NADPH is oxidized to $NADP^+$ by the dihydrofolate reductase; methotrexate in the sample binds the active sites on the dihydrofolate reductase molecule and inhibits the oxidation of NADPH. The change in absorbance of NADPH at 340 nm is related to the concentration of methotrexate in the sample. With this procedure, there is no interference from bilirubin (up to 10 mg/dL) or hemoglobin (up to 100 mg/dL). Lipemic samples will lower the methotrexate values by about 15%. Methotrexate is stable in serum stored at 4 °C in the dark for at least seven days.

1. Watson, T., Cohen, J. L., and Chan, K. K., High pressure liquid chromatographic determination of methotrexate and its major metabolite, 7-hydroxymethotrexate, in human plasma. *Cancer Treat. Rep.* **62**, 381–387 (1978).
2. Jacobs, S. A., Stoller, R. G., Chabner, B. A., and Johns, D. G., 7-Hydroxymethotrexate as a urinary metabolite in human subjects and rhesus monkeys receiving high dose methotrexate. *J. Clin. Invest.* **57**, 534–538 (1976).
3. Falk, L. C., Clark, D. R., Kalman, S. M., and Long, T. F., Enzymatic assay for methotrexate in serum and cerebrospinal fluid. *Clin. Chem.* **22**, 785–788 (1976).

Mucopolysaccharides; Ratio of High/Low M_r Mucopolysaccharides; Oligosaccharides

Specimen Tested:

U.

Reference (Normal) Values:

Lab. 1			
Age, yr	μg of uronic acid/mg of creatinine	Age, yr	μg of uronic acid/mg of creatinine
2–16	<20	10	1–13
2	6–20	12	0–11
4	5–18	14	0–10
6	4–16	16	0–9
8	3–14		

Lab. 2: Child: < 20 mg/d (expressed as hexuronic acid)
Lab. 3: Child: 0–2.5 mg/dL

Sources of Reference (Normal) Values:

Lab. 1: Institutional verification of private communication from Dr. W. Van B. Robertson, Dept. of Pediatrics, Stanford University. **Lab. 2:** Institutional. **Lab. 3:** institutional study on 674 urines, for which metabolic screens were requested. Urines with values greater than 2.5 mg/dL are reassayed. A blood smear study for Alder–Reilly inclusions was made, and those with values exceeding 4.0 mg/dL were subjected to thin-layer chromatography, as well as reassay of urine and another blood smear.

Specimen Volume, Collection, and Preservation:

Four of the five labs. use random urine collection, the volumes analyzed varying with the analytical method. At least 50 mL of urine should be collected and stored in FR, though it is best analyzed when fresh. **Lab. 2:** 40-μL aliquot of 24-h collection.

Analytical Method:

Lab. 1: Galambos, J. T., The reaction of carbazole with carbohydrates. I. Effect of borate and sulfamate on the carbazole color of sugars. *Anal. Biochem.* **19,** 119–132 (1967). **Lab. 2:** Whiteman, P., The quantitative measurement of Alcian Blue–glycosaminoglycan complexes. *Biochem. J.* **131,** 343–350 (1973); Whiteman, P., The quantitative determination of glycosaminoglycans in urine with Alcian Blue 8GX. *Biochem. J.* **131,** 351–357 (1973). **Lab. 3:** Carter, C. H., Wan, A. T., and Carpenter, D. G., Commonly used tests in the detection of Hurler's syndrome. *J. Pediatr.* **73,** 217–221 (1968); Dorfman, A., and Ott, M. L., A turbidimetric method for the assay of hyaluronidase. *J. Biol. Chem.* **172,** 367 (1948).

Instrumentation:

Lab. 2: Coleman Jr. II spectrophotometer.

Ratio of High/Low M_r Mucopolysaccharides[1]

Laboratories Reporting:

1.

Reference (Normal) Values:

Child: ratio 0.2–0.4

Sources of Reference (Normal) Values:

Institutional; DiFerrante, N., Nichols, B. L., Donnelly, P. V., Neri, G., Hrgovcic, R., and Berglund, R. K., Induced degradation of glycosaminoglycans in Hurler's and Hunter's syndromes by plasma infusion. *Proc. Natl. Acad. Sci. USA* **68,** 303–307 (1971).

Analytical Method:

DiFerrante et al., *op. cit.*

Oligosaccharides

Laboratories Reporting:

1.

---

[1] M_r, relative molecular mass.

Reference (Normal) Values:

Slowly migrating fractions are absent.

Sources of Reference (Normal) Values:

For detecting mannosidosis, mucolipidosis I, myoclonus syndrome, GM_1 gangliosidosis, fucosidosis, aspartylglucosaminuria: Humbel, R., and Collart, M., Oligosacchardes in urine of patients with glycoprotein storage diseases. I. Rapid detection by thin-layer chromatography. *Clin. Chim. Acta* **60,** 143–145 (1975).

Analytical Method:

Humbel and Collart, *op. cit.* Use MN silica gel N-HR (Brinkmann), 0.2-mm thick layer.

Instrumentation:

Eastman 13259 chromatogram-developing apparatus. *Note:* Apply sample 2-cm from edge in a 1.5-cm streak. Develop 5 h in butanol/acetic acid/water (100/50/50 by vol). After drying, spray with orcinol, 0.2 g/dL of 20% (200 mL/L) sulfuric acid. Heat at 100 °C for 10 min.

Commentary—J. A. Knight

The genetic mucopolysaccharidoses represent a group of disorders characterized by the accumulation of complex polyanionic macromolecules known as glycosaminoglycans (mucopolysaccharides). These conditions were reclassified in 1972 by McKusick *(1)*. All are inherited as autosomal recessives, except Hunter's syndrome, which is sex-linked. They are all characterized by the urinary excretion of excessive quantities of acid mucopolysaccharides. Except for Morquio's syndrome, in which large quantities of keratan sulfate are excreted, all others show increased, but varying, amounts of both dermatan and heparan sulfate.

There are several screening tests for acid mucopolysaccharides. Some are simple metachromatic "spot" tests *(2–4)*, while others are quantitative *(5–7)*. Of the latter, the Dische carboxazole reaction *(8)*, as modified *(6)*, is commonly used. The major limitation of this technique is that it measures uronic acid, a substance not present in keratan sulfate, the excretion product in Morquio's syndrome.

The modified turbidometric method involving acid albumin has been recommended by some as the procedure of choice in screening *(8)*. Using this method, Dr. Haymond and I measured mucopolysaccharides in 674 random urine specimens from hospital and ambulatory patients who showed no evidence of a mucopolysaccharidosis (Figure 1). The curve is skewed to the high side and best fits a log-

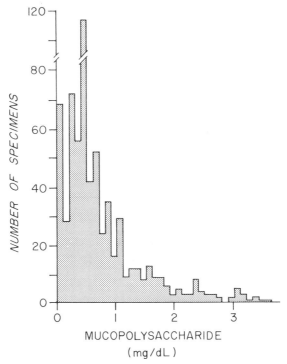

Fig. 1. Frequency distribution of acid mucopolysaccharide in 674 normal random urine specimens, determined by the acid albumin method (R. E. Haymond and J. A. Knight, unpublished observations, 1978)

normal distribution. The upper limit of normal is considered to be 2.5 mg/dL. Specimens that exceeded this concentration were dialyzed and requantitated. If they were still in excess of the upper limit of normal, they were subjected to thin-layer chromatography, which often gives a reliable preliminary diagnosis (S. Goodman, personal communication).

An alternative approach of apparent value is to measure the ratio of high M_r mucopolysaccharides to those with relatively low M_r (9). Normal individuals invariably have ratios less than 1.0, and usually less than 0.5. Patients with mucopolysaccharidoses have ratios greater than 1.0.

An accurate diagnosis, however, requires the demonstration of a specific enzyme deficiency. This technique usually requires cultured fibroblasts from an appropriate skin biopsy.

Oligosaccharides

Many lysosomal storage diseases share similarities, in that part of the complex stored material represents carbohydrate. The partial degradation of this material results in the urinary excretion of various oligosaccharides, among other products. Although there are more than 25 known genetic disorders in this category, these conditions are relatively rare *(10)*. Nevertheless, there is considerable interest in this fascinating area.

Definitive diagnosis of these conditions—mucopolysaccharidoses, sphingolipidoses, mucolipidoses, and others—depends on demonstrating specific enzyme deficiencies, usually in leukocytes or cultured fibroblasts, depending on the specific disorder. In recent years, thin-layer chromatography has been used to demonstrate the urinary excretion of neutral oligosaccharides *(11–13)*. The patterns produced have been quite specific for the presumptive diagnosis of mannosidosis, fucosidosis, aspartylglucosaminuria, Type I GM_1 gangliosidosis, and others. Related disorders need to be carefully studied and compared, to evaluate fully the usefulness of this technique in the preliminary diagnosis of these inherited biochemical disorders.

1. McKusick, V., *Heritable Disorders of Connective Tissue*, 4th ed. C. V. Mosby Co., St. Louis, MO, 1972, p 525.
2. Heremans, J. F., Vaerman, V. P., and Heremans, M. T., Acid mucopolysaccharides of normal urine. *Nature* **183,** 1606 (1959).
3. Berry, H. K., and Spinager, J. J., A paper spot test useful in the study of Hurler's syndrome. *J. Lab. Clin. Med.* **55,** 136–138 (1960).
4. Berman, E. R., Vered, J., and Bach, G., A reliable spot test for mucopolysaccharidoses. *Clin. Chem.* **17,** 886–890 (1971).
5. Dorfman, A., and Ott, M. L., A turbidimetric method for the assay of hyaluronidase. *J. Biol. Chem.* **172,** 367–375 (1948).
6. Galambos, J. T., The reaction of carbazole with carbohydrates. I. Effect of borate and sulfamate on the carbazole color of sugars. *Anal. Biochem.* **19,** 119–132 (1967).
7. Whiteman, P., The quantitative determination of glycosaminoglycans in urine with Alcian Blue 8GX. *Biochem. J.* **131,** 351–357 (1973).
8. Lorincz, A. E., Screening measurements of urinary acid mucopolysaccharides for detection of the Hurler syndrome. In *The Clinical Pathology of Infancy*, F. W. Sunderman and F. W. Sunderman, Jr., Eds. Charles C Thomas, Springfield, IL, 1967, pp 68–71.
9. DiFerrante, N., Giovanni, N., Neri, M. E., and Hogsett, W. E., Measurement of urinary glycosaminoglycans with quaternary ammonium salts: An extension of the method. *Connect. Tissue Res.* **1,** 93–101 (1972).
10. Kolodny, E. H., Lysosomal storage diseases. *N. Engl. J. Med.* **294,** 1217–1220 (1976).
11. Humbel, R., and Collart, M., Oligosaccharides in urine of patients with glycoprotein storage disease. I. Rapid detection by thin-layer chromatography. *Clin. Chim. Acta* **60,** 143–145 (1975).
12. Friedman, R. B., Williams, M. A., Moser, H. W., and Kolodny, E. H., Improved thin-layer chromatographic method in the diagnosis of mannosidosis. *Clin. Chem.* **24,** 1576–1577 (1978).

13. McLaren, J., and Ng, W. G., Radial and linear thin-layer chromatographic procedures compared for screening urines to detect oligosaccharidoses. *Clin. Chem.* **25,** 1289–1292 (1979).

Commentary—Derek A. Applegarth

Mucopolysaccharides in Urine

Screening techniques used to detect the presence of increased mucopolysaccharide excretion can be subject to error because of the possibility of examining a dilute urine sample and missing a slightly increased excretion of mucopolysaccharide. It is preferable, therefore, to check all suspected cases of mucopolysaccharide storage disease by measuring quantitative mucopolysaccharides by a technique such as precipitation with cetylpyridium chloride. The normal values for this technique are expressed in terms of creatinine coefficients and are related to age. We have found that, in the age group of two- to three-year olds, the upper limit of normal excretion is 20 μg of uronic acid per milligram of creatinine. The upper limit of normal for children aged 14 years and older is 10 μg of uronic acid per milligram of creatinine. The uronic acid output appears to decrease in an approximately linear fashion for children between three and 14 years of age. In the cases of mucopolysaccharide storage disease in children we have studied, we have found values exceeding 45 μg of uronic acid per milligram of creatinine. If any doubt remains about whether the result is abnormal, we assess the ratio of high M_r to low M_r mucopolysaccharides *(1)*. All of our patients have given a clearcut result with this assay. Details of column techniques available to assess mucopolysaccharide output are given in reference 2.

The problem of assessing urinary mucopolysaccharide output in terms of creatinine is also discussed in the Commentary for **Creatinine Clearance Coefficients.** A complete work-up of a mucopolysaccharide storage disease will necessarily involve the assay of the specific enzymes involved in these diseases. These enzymes are best measured in cultured skin fibroblasts or leukocytes *(3–5)*.

1. DiFerrante, N., Nichols, B. L., Donnelly, P. V., Neri, G., Hrgovcic, R., and Berglund, R. K., Induced degradation of glycosaminoglycans in Hurler's and Hunter's syndromes by plasma infusion. *Proc. Natl. Acad. Sci. USA* **68,** 303–307 (1971).
2. Applegarth, D. A., Bozoian, G., and Lowry, R. B., Analysis of urinary mucopolysaccharides using small ion exchange columns. *Clin. Biochem.* **8,** 151–160 (1975).
3. Pennock, C. A., and Barnes, I. C., The mucopolysaccharidoses. *J. Med. Genet.* **13,** 169–181 (1976).
4. Dorfman, A., and Matalon, R., The mucopolysaccharidoses (a review). *Proc. Natl. Acad. Sci. USA* **73,** 630–637 (1976).
5. Gantz, M., and Gehler, J., The mucopolysaccharidoses: Inborn errors of glycosaminoglycan catabolism. *Hum. Genet.* **32,** 233–255 (1976).

Mucoprotein Tyrosine

Specimen Tested:

P, S.

Laboratory Reporting:

1.

Reference (Normal) Values:

25–35 mg/L

Sources of Reference (Normal) Values:

Walker, C. H. M., O'Brien, D., Gibson, M. L., Ibbott, F. A., and Swanziger, J. L., Indices of activity in rheumatic fever treated with corticosteroids. *J. Pediatr.* **60,** 815–822 (1962).

Specimen Volume:

0.25 mL.

Analytical Method:

Modified procedure of Winzler, R. J., Devor, A. N., Mehl, J. W., and Smyth, I. M., Studies on the mucoproteins of human plasma. I. Determination and isolation. *J. Clin. Invest.* **27,** 609–615 (1948), according to Walker et al., *op. cit.*

Instrumentation:

Gilford Stasar II spectrophotometer.

Commentary—J. A. Knight

Protein–carbohydrate complexes (mucoproteins, glycoproteins) are now known to be widely distributed and to participate in many metabolic processes. In fact, the majority of known proteins contain various amounts of carbohydrate. Although there is some disagreement in the classification of these substances, the following designation is useful: those containing less than 4% hexosamines and up to 15% carbohydrate are glycoproteins, and those with more than 4% hexosamines and from 10 to 75% carbohydrate are mucoproteins *(1)*.

Concentrations of mucoprotein in serum have long been known to be increased in a wide variety of pathological states, including cancer, various infectious processes, and certain collagen disorders, especially rheumatoid arthritis and rheumatic fever. The measurement of the mucoprotein tyrosyl groups with Folin–Ciocalteu reagent *(2)* is not only the most commonly used technique, but also the clinically most useful, at least in certain conditions *(3)*.

The increase of serum mucoprotein concentrations is highly non-specific, and normal concentrations often overlap pathologic ones. Inasmuch as these substances represent acute-phase reactants, they can be estimated by protein electrophoresis, mainly the α_2-globulins, or by specific determinations for haptoglobin, α_1-antitrypsin, and others. Because requests for the estimation of total serum mucoproteins are now infrequent and measurements of other substances are generally more specific, one might consider total mucoprotein determinations to be outdated.

1. Kent, P. W., Structure and function of glycoproteins. In *Essays in Biochemistry*, P. N. Campbell and G. A. Greville, Eds. Academic Press, Inc., New York, NY, 1967, p 105.
2. Winzler, R. J., Devor, A. W., Mehl, J. W., and Smyth, I. M., Studies on the mucoproteins of human plasma. I. Determination and isolation. *J. Clin. Invest.* **27,** 609–615 (1948).
3. Walker, C. H. M., O'Brien, D., Gibson, M. L., Ibbott, F. A., and Swanziger, J. L., Indices of activity in rheumatic fever treated with corticosteroids. *J. Pediatr.* **60,** 815–822 (1962).

NADH–Methemoglobin Reductase
(Ferrihemoglobin reductase)

Specimen Tested:

B.

Laboratory Reporting:

1.

Reference (Normal) Values:

2.0–4.0 arbitrary units

Sources of Reference (Normal) Values:

Institutional; Hegesh, E., Calmanovici, N., and Avron, M., New method for determining ferrihemoglobin reductase (NADH–methemoglobin reductase) in erythrocytes. *J. Lab. Clin. Med.* **72,** 339–344 (1968); Agar, N. S., Irvine, S., Davis, J. R., and Harley, J. D., Enzymopenic methaemoglobinemia and spastic diplegia in an Italian–Yugoslavian child. *Med. J. Aust.* **2,** 429–430 (1972).

Specimen Volume, Collection, and Preservation:

40 µL. Heparin or citrate anticoagulant. Store B in RR.

Analytical Method:

Hegesh et al., *op. cit.*

Enzyme Data:

1. Enzyme unit definition: 1 arbitrary unit = 1 nmol of methemoglobin reduced per minute per milligram of Hb.
2. Buffer, pH: citrate, 4.7.
3. Substrate: hemoglobin.
4. Reaction temperature: 25 °C.
5. Temperature reported: 25 °C.

Instrumentation:

Varian 635 recording spectrophotometer.

Orotic Acid

Specimen Tested:

U.

Laboratory Reporting:

1.

Reference (Normal) Values:

2.2–12.8 µg/mg of creatinine (14.1–82.0 nmol/mg)

Sources of Reference (Normal) Values:

Institutional.

Specimen Volume, and Collection:

2 mL of random (untimed) U.

Analytical Method:

Colorimetric; Adachi, T., Tanimura, A., and Asahina, M., A colorimetric determination of orotic acid. *J. Vitaminol.* **9,** 217–226 (1963); Goldstein, A. S., Hoogenraad, N. J., Johnson, J. D., Fukanoga, K., Swierczewski, E., Cann, H. M., and Sunshine, P., Metabolic and genetic studies of a family with ornithine transcarbamylase deficiency. *Pediatr. Res.* **8,** 5–12 (1974).

Instrumentation:

Beckman DB spectrophotometer.

Commentary—Roger L. Boeckx

The colorimetric methods of Adachi et al. *(1)* and Goldstein et al. *(2)* have severe limitations. The methods are nonspecific, with poor recovery *(3;* and A. M. Glasgow, unpublished results). Compounds such as ornithine, lysine, citrulline, proline, hydroxyproline, and gly-cine inhibit color formation, whereas histidine, tryptophan, and hista-mine cause extensive production of interfering color *(3)*.

Kesner et al. *(3)* report a modification of the original method *(1)*, as well as a chromatographic method, that may eliminate some of these difficulties. Extraction of the final chromophore and the use of enzymic conversion of orotic acid have also been proposed by Glas-gow as improvements on the available colorimetric procedures.

Orotic acid, an intermediate in the pathway of pyrimidine synthe-sis, is excreted in increased amounts in the urine in orotic aciduria and pregnancy, during total parenteral nutrition, after allopurinol and azathioprine therapy, in purine nucleoside phosphorylase defi-ciency, and in some urea-cycle disorders (ornithine transcarbamylase deficiency, citrullinemia, argininosuccinic aciduria, and argininemia). Urinary orotic acid excretion may be useful in screening for urea-cycle disorders, and urinary orotic acid excretion combined with serum and urine amino acid quantitation can be helpful in localizing defects in patients with urea-cycle disorders.

Urinary orotic acid concentration tends to be greater in urines with low creatinine concentrations and in urines from young chil-dren. Glasgow (unpublished results) has studied several children with ornithine transcarbamylase deficiency and has found urinary orotic acid concentrations ranging from 56 to 1010 μg/mg of creatinine; he also found that 46 normal children had urinary orotic acid concen-trations of less than 4 μg/mg of creatinine.

1. Adachi, T., Tanimura, A., and Asahina, M., A colorimetric determination of orotic acid. *J. Vitaminol.* **9,** 217–226 (1963).
2. Goldstein, A. S., Hoogenraad, N. J., Johnson, J. D., Fukanoga, K., Swier-czewski, E., Cann, H. M., and Sunshine, P., Metabolic and genetic studies of a family with ornithine transcarbamylase deficiency. *Pediatr. Res.* **8,** 5–12 (1974).
3. Kesner, L., Aronson, F. L., Silverman, M., and Chan, P. C., Determination of orotic and dihydroorotic acids in biological fluids and tissues. *Clin. Chem.* **21,** 353–355 (1975).

Osmolality

Specimen Tested:

P, S, U.

Laboratories Reporting:

5.

Reference (Normal) Values:

P, S:[a]
Minimum range: 275–296 mmol/kg of P, S, or water
Maximum range: 295–317

U (random specimens):
Infant: 50–645
Child–adult, maximum (dehydration):   800–1500
                    minimum (water diuresis)   50–80

   [a] mmol/kg water = (100/93) × mmol/L water

Sources of Reference (Normal) Values:

Institutional; text ref. *2*, p 7; text ref. *5*, p 949; Faulkner, W. R., and King, J. W., Renal function. In text ref. *5*, 2nd ed., p 1012; Johnson, R. B., and Hoch, H., Osmolality of serum and urine. *Stand. Methods Clin. Chem.* **5**, 159–168 (1965).

Specimen Volume, Collection, and Preservation:

7 to 300 µL. Heparin only as anticoagulant. Random U. Store 1 to 3 d in RR, 1 wk in FR. There is a claim that specimens may be stored 1 to 3 d at RT.

Analytical Methods and Instrumentation:

Freezing point depression: Fiske Osmometer 130; Precision Systems Osmette A automatic osmometer; Knaver Halemikro osmometer. **Relative vapor pressure:** Barlow, W., Vapor pressure osmometry. *Med. Electron. Data,* July, 1975; Wescor Inc. 5100, 5100 B vapor pressure osmometer.

Commentary—Garry M. Lum

The osmolality of serum or urine is determined by comparing the specimen's freezing point or vapor pressure with that of a solution (e.g., NaCl) of known osmotic pressure. Body water moves freely between cell membranes, but its distribution is governed by the law of osmosis. It thus must follow an osmotic gradient and must redistribute relative to changes in the gradient until iso-osmolality is reached. Outside the cells the primary osmotically active particles are sodium and accompanying anions, chloride and bicarbonate. Glucose can be considered to contribute to overall serum osmolality as well, but once it moves inside the cells, it quickly enters metabolic pathways. Urea is osmotically active but diffuses freely across cell membranes and so becomes equally distributed among the body's fluid compartments. Inside the cells the primary osmotically active ions are potassium, magnesium, sulfate, and phosphate. Thus, analysis of readily accessible serum osmolality enables an evaluation of the status of the body's fluid/solute, intra- and extra-cellular balance, thereby drawing attention to threats to osmotic homeostasis.

Urine osmolality may also be determined, to assess renal participation in body fluid regulation. In various clinical settings the ability of the kidneys to concentrate or dilute urine can be a helpful guide to renal function or response to appropriate or inappropriate stimuli (e.g., antidiuretic hormone). Because renal function is designed to defend serum osmolality, one would expect an appropriate concentration or dilution of urine relative to serum osmolality; however, the movement of excess osmotically active solutes into the urine can increase urine osmolality, regardless of total body-water status.

Oxalate

Specimen Tested:

U.

Laboratories Reporting:

2.

Reference (Normal) Values:

1–3 mo:	<0.2 mmol/d
1–10 yr:	<0.7 mmol/d
>10 yr:	<1.1 mmol/d

Sources of Reference (Normal) Values:

Institutional.

Specimen Volume, Collection, and Preservation:

2 to 10 mL. Refrigerate U during 24-h collection. Store in FR. There is a claim that oxalate is stable for 7 d at RT.

Analytical Method:

Lab. 1: Zarembski, R. M., and Hodgkinson, A., The fluorimetric determination of oxalic acid in blood and other biological materials. *Biochem. J.* **96,** 717–721 (1965); Hodgkinson, A., and Zarembski, R. M., The determination of oxalic acid in urine. *Analyst* **86,** 16 (1961). **Lab. 2:** Mayer, G. G., Markow, D., and Karp, F., Enzymatic oxalate determination in urine. *Clin. Chem.* **9,** 334–339 (1963).

Instrumentation:

LKB 7400 calculating absorptiometer.

Commentary—John F. Connelly and H. E. Davies

The urine excretion of oxalate is affected by several factors, including age, sex, time of day, diet, and certain pathological conditions. Although children excrete less oxalate than adults, and women excrete less than men, values for each group become comparable when correction is made for body surface area (1,2). Diurnal variation has been demonstrated in adults by Hargreave et al. (3), with highest amounts in the late morning and evening and lowest in the early morning. The authors considered that these changes were probably of dietary origin. No diurnal variation was shown by Hatch et al. (4), investigating concentrations in plasma. No similar studies appear to have been reported for children.

Dietary factors such as ingestion of oxalate or one of its precursors increases oxalate excretion. Whether ascorbic acid ingestion significantly affects oxalate concentrations is still a matter of contention (5–8). Increased oxalate excretion has been reported in pyridoxine deficiency and malabsorption; and in primary hyperoxaluria, by definition, there is increased oxalate excretion with no demonstrable increase in plasma concentrations. Primary hyperoxaluria may be further subdivided into two types: type I, with increased glycolic acid excretion, and type II, with increased glyceric acid excretion. These two types may be differentiated by quantitative analysis for glycolic or glyceric acid or by separative techniques such as GLC or GLC/mass spectrometry.

Analysis of specimens as soon as possible after collection is most desirable. A bacteriostatic agent should be added during collection. If storage is necessary, colder than 4 °C is best; even at this temperature, however, an increase in oxalate concentration has been reported (9,10). According to Harris (6), ascorbate is rapidly oxidized to oxalate in voided urine on contact with air. Smith (7) reported that alkalinization of urine may yield spuriously high results by allowing in vitro oxidation of ascorbate to oxalate.

Many methods have been published for measurement of oxalate, including precipitation, titration, extraction, isotope dilution, atomic absorption, colorimetry, GLC, and enzymic techniques. Each has been criticized for various reasons such as specificity and interference. Laboratorians should be aware of the limitations of and the precautions for the method chosen.

1. Hockaday, T. D. R., Frederick, E. W., Clayton, J. E., and Smith, L. H., Jr., Studies on primary hyperoxaluria II. Urinary oxalate, glycolate and glyoxylate measurement by isotope dilution methods. *J. Lab. Clin. Med.* **65**, 677–687 (1965).
2. Gibbs, D. A., and Watts, R. W. E., The variation of urinary oxalate excretion with age. *J. Lab. Clin. Med.* **73**, 901–908 (1969).
3. Hargreave, T. B., Sali, A., MacKay, C., and Sullivan, M., Diurnal variation in urinary oxalate. *Br. J. Urol.* **49**, 597–600 (1977).

4. Hatch, M., Bourke, E., and Costello, J., New enzymatic method for oxalate determination. *Clin. Chem.* **23,** 76–78 (1977).
5. Briggs, M. H., Vitamin-C-induced hyperoxaluria. *Lancet* **i,** 154 (1976). Letter.
6. Harris, A. B., Vitamin-C-induced hyperoxaluria. *Lancet* **i,** 366 (1976). Letter.
7. Smith, L. H., Risk of oxalate stones from large doses of vitamin C. *N. Engl. J. Med.* **298,** 856 (1978). Letter.
8. Costello, J., Hatch, M., and Keogh, B., Urinary oxalate excretion during ascorbic acid loading. *N. Engl. J. Med.* **299,** 1469 (1978). Letter.
9. Mayer, G. G., Markow, D., and Karp, F., Enzymatic oxalate determination in urine. *Clin. Chem.* **9,** 334–339 (1963).
10. Hodgkinson, A., Determination of oxalic acid in biological material. *Clin. Chem.* **16,** 547–557 (1970).

Oxygen Capacity of Blood

Specimen Tested:

B.

Laboratory Reporting:

1.

Reference (Normal) Values:

1.34 mL/g of hemoglobin

Sources of Reference (Normal) Values:

Text ref. *1.*

Oxygen Saturation/Tension

Specimen Tested:

B.

Laboratory Reporting:

1.

Reference (Normal) Values:

Newborn: 30–80% of complete saturation
Thereafter: 65–85%

Sources of Reference (Normal) Values:

Text ref. *1.*

Volume and Source of Specimen:

30 μL; venous.

Analytical Method:

Text ref. *2*.

Instrumentation:

Beckman DU spectrophotometer.

*　　　*　　　*

Laboratory Reporting:

1.

Reference (Normal) Values:

Vigorous, full-term infants, vaginal delivery:	mm Hg[a]	
	Arterial	**Venous**
Birth	19.8	47.6
1 h	93.8	
3 h	94.7	
24 h	93.2	

[a] 1 mm Hg $\approx$ 133 N/m² $\approx$ 133 Pa.

Sources of Reference (Normal) Values:

Weisbrot, I. M., James, L. S., Prince, C. E., Holaday, D. A., and Apgar, V., Acid–base homeostasis of the newborn infant during the first 24 hours of life. *J. Pediatr.* **52,** 395–403 (1958).

Volume of Specimen:

40 μL of hemolyzed erythrocytes.

Analytical Method:

Spectrophotometric.

Instrumentation:

Radiometer Hemolyzer type Hem 1; Oxygen Saturation Meter Type OSM 1.

Parathyrin (Parathyroid hormone, PTH; Parathormone)

Specimen Tested:

S.

Laboratory Reporting:

1.

Reference (Normal) Values:

With adult control subjects' serum calcium at 8.8–10.4 mg/dL (2.11–2.62 mmol/L), PTH (C-terminal) = 40–100 μL Eq/mL.

Sources of Reference (Normal) Values:

Radioimmunoassay Manual, 4th ed., Nichols Institute, San Pedro, CA, 1977, pp 108, 286.

Specimen Volume, Collection, and Preservation:

150 μL. Collect blood in chilled tube. Allow blood to clot in an icebath (1 to 4 h). Centrifuge in refrigerated centrifuge. Store S in FR.

Analytical Method and Instrumentation:

RIA, double antibody, with ^{125}I-labeled bPTH (b = bovine); gamma counter.

Note: According to the *Radioimmunoassay Manual (op. cit.),* p 277: "A pool of serum or plasma samples from patients with hyperparathyroidisms is chosen as the reference standard. One then determines, for each patient sample or unknown, the concentration of immunoreactive PTH present relative to the concentration in the hyperparathyroid pool. Results are expressed as microliter equivalents per milliliter of blood. For example, if a patient has a high concentration of hormone, the response given by 1000 μL of patient's serum may equal that of 300 μL of the standard hyperparathyroid serum (300 μL Eq/mL)."

Commentary—Peter J. and Joan H. Howanitz

Measurement of PTH in serum potentially provides important information useful in the assessment of parathyroid function. However, several problems limit the availability and reliability of this laboratory determination. The interpretation of PTH measurements is complicated by the heterologous nature of RIA for PTH. Until recently, only non-human PTH was available for the production of anti-PTH antibodies, which led to wide variability in antibody crossreactivity with human PTH [1]. In addition, these assays usually involve bovine PTH for preparation of assay standards and tracers.

More importantly, PTH exists in many immunoreactive forms: pre-pro-PTH, pro-PTH, and native PTH have been identified in parathyroid glands. Forms larger than native PTH also have been identified in serum from patients with primary hyperparathyroidism or ectopic production of PTH [2]. Native PTH, containing 84 amino acids and having a serum half-life of about 20 min, is cleaved into a biologically inactive carboxy(C)-terminal fraction and a biologically active amino(N)-terminal fraction. The C-terminal fraction, which is about two-thirds the size of the native molecule, has a half-life of 1 to 2 h, whereas the N-terminal fragment has a half-life of only a few minutes. Because the intact hormone and the C-terminal fraction are cleared by the kidney, their half-life is extended in renal failure.

Antibodies have been developed to each of the three circulating PTH moieties: intact PTH, the C-terminal fraction, and the N-terminal fraction. Generally, antibodies that react with the C-terminal fraction and those that react with the N-terminal fraction also react to a lesser degree with the intact hormone. Several laboratories report that PTH assays with the C-terminal antiserum better identify patients with primary hyperparathyroidism, and assays with antibody to the N-terminal fragment better reflect acute changes in glandular secretion of PTH *(3,4)*. The N-terminal PTH assay is also useful in localizing parathyroid adenomas: PTH is measured in venous effluents from the parathyroid gland, obtained by catheterization *(5)*. Certain antisera with specificity directed against N-terminal PTH also have been utilized successfully in the differentiation of disorders of calcium metabolism *(6)*.

Antisera that show other kinds of specificity have also been developed. One appears to be highly specific and sensitive for intact PTH, and has little reactivity with the C- or N-terminal fragment *(7)*; another recognizes the C- and N-terminal ends of PTH equally well *(8)*. Both types of antisera are useful in catheterization studies and in discriminating among normals, patients with hyperparathyroidism, and patients with tumor-associated hypercalcemia.

In normal subjects, serum PTH is inversely correlated to serum calcium. PTH values are controlled tightly, secretion being suppressed by slight increases in serum calcium and stimulated by slight decreases in serum calcium. In contrast, patients with primary hyperparathyroidism have increased concentrations of PTH, while those with secondary hyperparathyroidism have, as a rule, even greater PTH increases *(4,6–8)*. In most patients with hypercalcemia of malignancy, the parathyroid glands are suppressed by the above-normal serum calcium and PTH values are not increased. However, there is a large overlap of PTH values in these groups of patients, as well as in patients with other disorders of calcium metabolism.

Expressing PTH values as a function of ionized or total calcium in serum has led to better discrimination among groups of patients with disorders of calcium metabolism. Five distinct groups of patients may be delineated: *(a)* normals, *(b)* those with primary hyperparathyroidism and ectopic PTH production (increased calcium and PTH), *(c)* secondary hyperparathyroidism (decreased calcium and increased PTH), *(d)* tumors associated with hypercalcemia (increased calcium and decreased PTH), *(e)* primary hypoparathyroidism (decreased calcium and PTH). An overlap of PTH values in these conditions still occurs and possibly is dependent on the immunological characteristics of the PTH antibody used in the assay.

The ectopic production of PTH is associated with a number of tumors. The frequency and quantity of immunoactive PTH detected in sera from patients with hypercalcemia of malignancy are apparently assay-dependent. For example, in patients with similar types of tumors, some immunoassays detect PTH in a large percentage of the patients, whereas other assays detect no PTH *(9)*. In addition, serum samples from patients with malignancy show high PTH values with some assays but low values with others.

PTH values in pregnant women increase in the second half of pregnancy, probably secondary to a decrease in ionized calcium *(11)*, and exceed the values in cord blood *(12)*. After birth, PTH values in full-term infants peak and surpass adult values in the first few days of life, while in premature infants this surge occurs in the first hours of life *(13)*. During middle childhood PTH values decrease, and by adolescence approximate adult values *(14)*. In a reference population of adults, PTH values gradually increase with age so that elderly individuals have values roughly double those of young adults *(5)*.

Although PTH has not been studied extensively in children, it is reportedly increased in a few children with vitamin-D-resistant rickets or pseudohypoparathyroidism, and in some children receiving anticonvulsant drugs *(16)*. In children with renal insufficiency, immunoreactive PTH concentrations are increased; progression of renal failure progressively increases PTH. These increases are reversed by renal transplantation or treatment with calcitriol (1,25-hydroxyvitamin D_3) *(17)*.

1. Di Bella, F. P., Gilkinson, J. B., Flueck, J., and Arnaud, C. D., Carboxyl-terminal fragments of human parathyroid tumors: Unique new source of immunogens for the production of antisera potentially useful in the radioimmunoassay of parathyroid hormone in human serum. *J. Clin. Endocrinol. Metab.* **46,** 604–612 (1978).
2. Benson, R. C., Riggs, B. L., Pickard, B. M., and Arnaud, C. D., Immunoreactive forms of circulating parathyroid hormone in primary and ectopic hyperparathyroidism. *J. Clin. Invest.* **54,** 175–181 (1974).
3. Arnaud, C. D., Goldsmith, R. S., Bordier, P. J., Sizemore, G. W., Larsen, J. A., and Gilkinson, J. B., Influence of immunoheterogeneity of circulating parathyroid hormone on results of radioimmunoassay of serum in man. *Am. J. Med.* **56,** 785–793 (1974).
4. Parthemore, J. G., Roos, B. A., Parker, D. C., Kripke, D. F., Avioli, L. A., and Deftos, L. J., Assessment of acute and chronic changes in parathyroid hormone secretion by a radioimmunoassay with predominant specificity for the carboxy-terminal region of the molecule. *J. Clin. Endocrinol. Metab.* **47,** 284–289 (1978).
5. Arnaud, C. D., Parathyroid hormone: Coming of age in clinical medicine. *Am. J. Med.* **55,** 577–581 (1973).
6. Woo, J., and Singer, R. F., Radioimmunoassay for human parathyroid hormone. *Clin. Chim. Acta* **54,** 161–168 (1974).
7. Hawker, C. D., and Di Bella, F. P., Human parathyroid hormone: A review of the radioimmunoassay procedures and clinical interpretation. In *Clinical Immunochemistry,* S. Natelson, A. J. Pesce, and A. A. Dietz, Eds. Washington, DC, 1978, pp 329–343.
8. Krutzik, S., Segre, G., and Potts, J., PTH RIA, methodologic and clinical aspects. *Clin. Chem.* **24,** 993 (1978). Abstract.
9. Raisz, L. G., Mundy, G. R., and Eilon, G., Hypercalcemia of neoplastic diseases. In *Endocrinology of Calcium Metabolism; Proceedings of the*

Sixth Parathyroid Conference, Amsterdam, D. H. Copp and V. Talmage, Eds., Excerpta Medica, 1978, no. 421, 1978.

10. Raisz, L. G., Yajnik, C. H., Bockman, R. S., and Bower, B. F., Comparison of commercially available parathyroid hormone immunoassays in the differential diagnosis of hypercalcemia due to primary hyperparathyroidism or malignancy. *Ann. Intern. Med.* **91**, 740–741 (1979).

11. Drake, T. S., Kaplan, R. A., and Lewis, T. A., The physiologic hyperparathyroidism of pregnancy. *Obstet. Gynecol.* **53**, 746–749 (1979).

12. Fairney, A., Jackson, D., and Clayton, B. E., Measurement of serum parathyroid hormone, with particular reference to some infants with hypercalcemia. *Arch. Dis. Child.* **48**, 419–424 (1973).

13. Mallet, E., Basuyau, J., Brunelle, P., Devaux, A., and Fessard, C., Neonatal parathyroid secretion and renal receptor maturation in premature infants. *Biol. Neonate* **33**, 304–308 (1978).

14. Arnaud, S. B., Goldsmith, R. S., Stickler, G. B., McCall, J. T., and Arnaud, C. D., Serum parathyroid hormone and blood minerals: Interrelationships in normal children. *Pediatr. Res.* **7**, 485–493 (1973).

15. Wiske, P. S., Epstein, S., Bell, N. H., Queener, S. F., Edmondson, J., and Johnston, C. C., Increase in immunoreactive parathyroid hormone with age. *N. Engl. J. Med.* **300**, 1419–1421 (1979).

16. Root, A., Gruskin, A., Reber, R. M., Stopa, A., and Duckett, G., Serum concentrations of parathyroid hormone in infants, children, and adolescents. *J. Pediatr.* **85**, 329–336 (1974).

17. Chan, J. C. M., and DeLuca, H. F., Calcium and parathyroid disorders in children. *J. Am. Med. Assoc.* **241**, 1242–1244 (1979).

Phenobarbital (Luminal, Phenobarb)

Specimen Tested:

P, S.

Laboratories Reporting:

5.

Reference (Normal) Values:

Therapeutic range: 3 labs.: 15–40 mg/L; 1 lab.: 14–37 (60–160 μmol/L); 1 lab.: 10–30
Toxic concentration: 50 mg/L

Note: mg/L × 4.306 = μmol/L

Sources of Reference (Normal) Values:

Institutional; Kutt, H., Pharmacodynamic and pharmacokinetic measurements of antiepileptic drugs. *Clin. Pharmacol. Ther.* **16**, 243–250 (1974); Kutt, H., and Penry, J. K., Usefulness of blood levels of antiepileptic drugs. *Arch. Neurol.* **31**, 283–288 (1974); Kutt, H., and McDowell, F., Management of epilepsy with diphenylhydantoin sodium. *J. Am. Med. Assoc.* **203**, 969–972 (1968).

Specimen Volume, Collection, and Preservation:

5 to 200 μL. Heparin anticoagulant. Store in FR for prolonged period, or 2 d in RR.

Analytical Method and Instrumentation:

Labs. 1, 2: Syva EMIT (homogenous enzyme immunoassay); Kananen, G., Osiewicz, J. R., and Sunshine, I., Barbiturate analysis—a current assessment. *J. Chromatogr. Sci.* **10,** 283–287 (1972); Bausch and Lomb Spectronic 710 spectrophotometer with thermally regulated flow cell, timer-printer, semi-automatic pipetter-dilutor, conical bottom disposable beakers. **Labs. 3, 4:** GLC modified from Joern, W. A., Gas chromatography of anticonvulsant drugs, with no solvent incorporation. *Clin. Chem.* **21,** 1548–1549 (1975); Beckman GC-4 or Hewlett-Packard 5710A gas chromatograph, H-P 3380A recording integrator, Damon-IEC 6000 centrifuge, Applied Science Labs Mini-Aktor tubes; modification of the method by Magee, J., Rapid determination of diphenylhydantoin in blood plasma by gas–liquid chromatography. *Anal. Chem.* **42,** 421 (1970); L'Etrange Orme, M., Borga, O., Cook, C. E., and Sjoqvist, F., Measurement of diphenylhydantoin in 0.1-mL plasma samples: Gas chromatography and radioimmunoassay compared. *Clin. Chem.* **22,** 246–249 (1976); Perkin-Elmer GLC, with Spectra Physics Autolab System electronic integrator. **Lab. 5:** HPLC; Soldin, S. J., and Hill, J. G., A rapid micromethod for measuring anticonvulsant drugs in serum by high performance liquid chromatography. *Clin. Chem.* **22,** 856–859 (1976); Waters HPLC ALC/GPC 6000 A, with a Perkin-Elmer LC 55 Variable Wavelength spectrophotometer.

Commentary—Peter J. and Joan H. Howanitz

Phenobarbital has been used effectively for the treatment of generalized clonic seizures (grand-mal), complex partial seizures, and febrile convulsions. It is almost completely absorbed after oral or intramuscular administration. However, peak concentrations, similar in magnitude by both routes, are achieved in 12 to 18 h after oral and in 4 h after intramuscular doses. After intravenous administration, high concentrations occur rapidly in most tissues except the brain, where it may take as much as 1 h to reach equilibrium.

About 40 to 50% of phenobarbital is bound to serum proteins, but binding is considerably less in the normo-bilirubinemic neonate. In the hyperbilirubinemic neonate, binding is even further decreased and more than 70% may be free *(2)*. Concentrations in CSF approximate free concentrations in serum; salivary concentrations, however, are less than free drug concentrations because the pH of saliva is lower than the pH of serum *(1)*.

Metabolism of phenobarbital to the active metabolites *p*-hydroxy-phenobarbital and *N*-hydroxyphenobarbital occurs in the liver. These active metabolites subsequently are conjugated to glucuronide and excreted rapidly by the kidney. About 25% of phenobarbital is excreted unchanged in the urine. In infants and children the rate of excretion may be greater than in adults. Alkalinization of urine by intravenous administration of sodium bicarbonate may increase renal excretion as much as 10% by promoting ionization of the drug to a form resistant to reabsorption by the distal tubule. Although the inability of newborns to conjugate metabolites has been described, this appears to have little clinical significance *(3)*. Whether by competing for serum protein-binding sites or by inhibiting phenobarbital conversion, valproic acid increases phenobarbital concentrations *(4)*.

The half-life of phenobarbital is extremely variable, depending on the patient's age and the presence of other drugs. In newborns 24–48 h old, the half-life may be as long as 200 h, but by one week of age, the half-life is 115 h; by four weeks of age, the half-life approaches the adult value, about 67 h *(5)*. Children one to five years old have about the same phenobarbital half-life as adults, but the half-life is extremely variable. Some workers report that adults have longer phenobarbital half-lives than do children; these studies have been the basis for decreasing the dose needed to maintain therapeutic concentrations in children entering puberty. There is some suggestion that illness may be as important a determinant as age for concentration in serum; in some extremely ill newborns, metabolism of the drug is exceedingly prolonged *(3)*.

Phenobarbital apparently does not saturate the drug-metabolizing enzymes of the liver at therapeutic serum concentrations; even at concentrations as great as 100 μg/dL, saturation of this degradation pathway does not occur. By inducing the microsomal enzymes, phenobarbital may increase metabolic degradation of other drugs such as coumarin, cortisol, digitoxin, griseofulvin, valproic acid, and perhaps phenytoin.

Serum concentrations of at least 10 μg/mL are necessary to obtain a reasonable therapeutic effect, yet concentrations less than 15 μg/mL are frequently ineffective *(6)*. Serum concentrations of 10 to 30 μg/mL are generally therapeutic in older children and adults *(7)*; however, in some parts of Europe practitioners consider the range of 20 to 40 μg/mL to be therapeutic *(8)*. For febrile seizures in children, a minimum concentration of 15 μg/mL is needed *(9)* and, although some infants tolerate 40 μg/mL without sedation, this concentration is considered to be toxic. In adults, more than 30 μg/mL is associated with toxicity. The earliest clinical signs of toxicity are drowsiness, with or without ataxia, and may be seen with phenobarbital concentrations in the range of 35 to 80 μg/mL. Depressed reflexes occur in habitually intoxicated patients at serum concentrations of 65 to 117 μg/mL, and the absence of reflexes has been noted in concentrations exceeding 100 μg/mL. High phenobarbital values frequently are associated with a paradoxical increase in seizure frequency (2).

At the onset of phenobarbital therapy, drowsiness may occur even with quite low concentrations in blood, but subsides during continuous therapy. Malaise and a loss of concentration may or may not be dose-related. Initiation of phenobarbital therapy rarely is associated with idiosyncratic reactions, including rashes, agranulocytosis, aplastic anemia, jaundice, and hepatitis. Other toxic effects include paradoxical hyperactivity in about 15 to 20% of children, and osteomalacia.

Pregnancy appears to be associated with an increased requirement for phenobarbital to maintain serum concentrations at prepregnancy values *(10)*. After administration of the drug, barbiturates readily cross the placenta, and fetal blood concentrations approach those of the mother within a few minutes. With chronic oral administration, barbiturates are distributed throughout fetal tissues at concentrations slightly less than that of the mother. One of the most important side effects, although rare, is the occurrence of hemorrhages in newborns of mothers taking phenobarbital; this usually may be prevented by administering vitamin K to the mother. Barbiturates are excreted in the milk of nursing mothers, and nursing should be discontinued if infants of these mothers show signs of toxicity.

1. Schmidt, D., and Kupferberg, H. J., Diphenylhydantoin, phenobarbital, and primidone in saliva, plasma, and cerebrospinal fluid. *Epilepsia* **16**, 735–741 (1975).
2. Morselli, P. L., Pharmacokinetics of antiepileptic drugs during development. In *Antiepileptic Drug Monitoring,* C. Gardner-Thorpe, D. Janz, H. Meinardi, and C. E. Pippenger, Eds. Pitman Medical, Kent, England, 1977, pp 57–72.
3. Boreus, L. O., Jalling, B., and Kallberg, N., Phenobarbital metabolism in adults and in newborn infants. *Acta Paediatr. Scand.* **67**, 193–200 (1978).
4. Bruni, J., Wilder, B. J., Perchalaski, R. J., Hammond, E. J., and Villarreal, H. J., Valproic acid and plasma levels of phenobarbital. *Neurology* **30**, 94–97 (1980).
5. Heimann, G., and Gladtke, E., Pharmocokinetics of phenobarbital in childhood. *Eur. J. Clin. Pharmacol.* **12**, 305–310 (1977).
6. Kutt, H., and Penry, J. K., Usefulness of blood levels of antiepileptic drugs. *Arch. Neurol.* **31**, 283–288 (1974).
7. Buchthal, F., and Lennox-Buchthal, M. A., Phenobarbital. Relation of serum concentration to control of seizures. In *Antiepileptic Drugs,* D. M. Woodbury, J. K. Penry, and R. P. Schmidt, Eds. Raven Press, New York, NY, 1972, pp 335–344.
8. Van Dijk, A., and Uges, D. R. A., Analytical and pharmacokinetic aspects of phenobarbital, phenytoin, primidone and carbamazepine. *Excerpta Med.* **501**, 65–78 (1979).
9. Faerø, O., Kastrup, K. W., Lykkeggaard-Nielsen, E., Melchior, J. C., and Thorn, I., Successful prophylaxis of febrile convulsions with phenobarbital. *Epilepsia* **13**, 279–285 (1972).

10. Lander, C. M., Edwards, V. E., Eadie, M. J., and Tyrer, J. H., Plasma anticonvulsant concentrations during pregnancy. *Neurology* **27**, 128–131 (1977).

Phenylalanine

Specimen Tested:

P, S.

Laboratories Reporting:

3.

Reference (Normal) Values:

Age	mg/dL (mmol/L)	
	Lab. 1	Labs. 2, 3
1st wk	Up to 6 (0.36)	
Newborn		Up to 4 (0.242)
>1 wk	0.7–3.5 (0.042–0.212)	
Child		0.8–3.0 (0.048–0.182); 0.7–3.5 (0.042–0.212)

Sources of Reference (Normal) Values:

Institutional; Faulkner, W. R., Phenylalanine. *Stand. Methods Clin. Chem.* **5**, 199–209 (1965).

Specimen Volume, Collection, and Preservation:

50 to 100 μL. Heparin as anticoagulant. Presumably stable for 4 d at RT; increasing value on longer storage.

Analytical Method:

Lab. 1: Cation-exchange chromatography (see *Instrumentation*). **Labs. 2, 3:** Fluorometric; McCaman, M. W., and Robins, E., Fluorometric method for the determination of phenylalanine in serum. *J. Lab. Clin. Med.* **59**, 885–890 (1962); Faulkner, *op. cit.*

Instrumentation:

Lab. 1: Durrum (Dionex) 500 Amino Acid analyzer. **Labs. 2, 3:** Turner III, Aminco Bowman fluorometers; Micromedic diluter.

Commentary—Roger L. Boeckx

Classical phenylketonuria (PKU), first described by Fölling *(1)* in 1934, is only one of several inherited conditions manifested as hyperphenylalaninemia *(2)*. Classical PKU, the target of numerous newborn-screening programs, is caused by the absence of phenylalanine hydroxylase (EC 1.14.16.1), the enzyme that catalyzes the hydroxylation of phenylalanine to tyrosine. Incidence varies from country to country and region to region. The incidence in the United States is approximately 1 in 14 000 live births *(3)*. A diet low in phenylalanine, instituted as soon as possible after birth, is an effective form of treatment. Over 90% of untreated PKU patients will have an I.Q. of 50 or less *(4)*; in one study of three treated PKU children, the average I.Q. was 93 *(5)*.

Several other forms of hyperphenylalaninemia, related to a persistent or transient decrease in phenylalanine hydroxylase activity, have been described as benign *(2)*. Similarly, a deficiency of phenylalanine transaminase (EC 2.6.1.58) has been described as a benign condition in which the concentration of phenylalanine in plasma was increased *(6)*.

Recently, disorders related to deficiency or abnormal function of the dihydropteridine reductase (EC 1.6.99.7) system have been described. This enzyme catalyzes the reduction of biopterin, the coenzyme involved in the hydroxylation of phenylalanine to tyrosine *(7)*. Kaufman et al. *(8)* have also described another hyperphenylalaninemia variant due to biopterin deficiency. All of the dihydropteridine reductase- or biopterin-deficiency types of hyperphenylalaninemia are serious disorders presenting with ataxia and seizures; they are unresponsive to dietary treatment *(2)*. Some authors have reported promising results when dietary phenylalanine restriction is combined with the administration of the missing products of the enzymes affected by depressed biopterin concentrations, i.e., 3,4-dihydroxyphenylalanine and 5-hydroxytryptophan *(9)*. Early and accurate diagnosis of the various types of hyperphenylalaninemia is essential if these differing treatment regimens are to be correctly used.

Milstien et al. *(9)* have shown that the urinary excretion of tetrahydrobiopterin can serve to differentiate cases of classical PKU from cases of hyperphenylalaninemia related to dihydropteridine reductase deficiency. Kaufman *(10)* has reviewed other methods currently available for the differential diagnosis of the various forms of hyperphenylalaninemia.

In addition to these hereditary disorders, reportedly as many as 25% of all children born to mothers with PKU have congenital anomalies. Most infants born to PKU mothers have been retarded *(3)*. The effect on the fetus is related to the phenylalanine concentration in the mother, so that mothers with PKU should be on a low phenylalanine diet *(2)*.

1. Fölling, A., Uber Ausscheidung von Phenylbenztraubsäure in den Harn als Stoffwechselanomalie in Verbindung mit Imbezzillität. *Hoppe-Seyler's Z. Physiol. Chem.* **227,** 169–176 (1934).
2. Tourian, A. Y., and Sidbury, J. B., Phenylketonuria. In text ref. *11,* 4th ed., pp 240–255.
3. Scriver, C. R., and Rosenberg, L. E., *Amino Acid Metabolism and Its Disorders.* W. B. Saunders Co., Philadelphia, PA, 1973, pp 290–337.
4. Knox, W. E., Phenylketonuria. In text ref. *11,* 3rd ed., pp 266–295.

5. Dobson, J. C., Williamson, M. L., Azen, C., and Koch, R., Intellectual assessment of 3 four-year-old children with phenylketonuria. *Pediatrics* **60,** 822–827 (1977).
6. Auerbach, V. H., DiGeorge, A. M., Carpenter, G. G., and Wood, P., Phenylalaninemia. In *Amino Acid Metabolism and Genetic Variation,* W. L. Nyhan, Ed. McGraw-Hill, New York, NY, 1967, pp 11–68.
7. Kaufman, S., Holtzman, N. A., Milstien, S., Butler, I. J., and Kramholz, A., Phenylketonuria due to a deficiency of dihydropteridine reductase. *N. Engl. J. Med.* **293,** 785–790 (1975).
8. Kaufman, S., Berlow, S., Summer, G. K., Milstien, S., Schulman, J. D., Orloff, S., Spielberg, S., and Pueschel, S., Hyperphenylalaninemia due to a deficiency of biopterin. A variant form of phenylketonuria. *N. Engl. J. Med.* **299,** 673–679 (1978).
9. Milstien, S., Kaufman, S., and Summer, G. K., Hyperphenylalaninemia due to dihydropteridine reductase deficiency: Diagnosis by measurement of oxidized and reduced pterins in urine. *Pediatrics* **65,** 806–810 (1980).
10. Kaufman, S., Differential diagnosis of variant forms of hyperphenylalaninemia. *Pediatrics* **65,** 840–841 (1980).

Phenylalanine/Tyrosine Ratio

Specimen Tested:

P, S.

Laboratories Reporting:

2.

Reference (Normal) Values:

	Lab. 1	Lab. 2[a]
Controls:	0.62–1.18 (range)	<1.3
PKU heterozygote:	0.88–2.0 (range)	>0.9

[a] Individuals between 0.9 and 1.3 should be classified by considering phenylalanine concentration in addition to phenylalanine/tyrosine ratio.

Sources of Reference (Normal) Values:

Lab. 1: 18 controls, selected from amino acid reports. None were less than 13 years old, and none showed any amino acid abnormality. There were 18 obligate heterozygotes (mean ± 2SD = 1.46 ± 0.62). Also see Perry, T. L., Hansen, S., Tischler, B., and Bunting, R., Determination of heterozygosity for phenylketonuria on the amino acid analyzer. *Clin. Clim. Acta* **18,** 51–56 (1967). **Lab. 2:** Jackson, S. H., Hanley, W. B., Gero, T., and Gosse, G. D., Detection of phenylketonuric heterozygotes. *Clin. Chem.* **17,** 538–543 (1971).

Specimen Volume, Collection, and Preservation;
Patient Preparation:

0.1 to 1 mL. Heparin as anticoagulant. Deproteinize the P or S as soon as possible. Store in FR. Fast the patient according to age, 8 h for adults.

Analytical Method and Instrumentation:
Durrum (Dionex) 500 Amino Acid analyzer.

Commentary—Roger L. Boeckx

Several methods have been proposed for the detection of individuals heterozygous for phenylketonuria (PKU). The prevalence of PKU homozygotes is approximately 7:100 000 and, therefore, we should expect that the frequency of heterozygotes will be about 1:60. The identification of PKU heterozygotes can be of value in genetic counselling, case-finding, and confirmation of diagnoses.

Older approaches have made use of phenylalanine loading tests (1), in which the oral administration of phenylalanine (100 mg/kg of body weight) was followed by sequential analysis of serum samples for phenylalanine and tyrosine at 0, 1, 2, 3, and 4 h after the dose. Rampini et al. (1) developed a discriminant index, based on the phenylalanine/tyrosine (P/T) ratios obtained, that allowed them to identify heterozygotes with great accuracy.

Perry et al. (2) and Rosenblatt and Scriver (3) proposed a simpler procedure, with only one serum sample and no phenylalanine loading. Jackson et al. (4) later improved this procedure by plotting the P/T ratio vs phenylalanine concentration; by this approach the rate of misdiagnosis was less than 5%. A map of probabilities based on the aforementioned is shown in reference 5. Determining P/T or P^2/T ratios just before lunch but after a normal breakfast is now considered to be the best approach (6).

Test data from woman of fertile age should be interpreted cautiously. Both phenylalanine and P/T ratios are increased in pregnancy and in women taking oral contraceptives, which could lead to an erroneous classification of these individuals as being heterozygous.

1. Rampini, S., Anders, P. W., Curtius, H. C., and Marthaler, T., Detection of heterozygotes for phenylketonuria by column chromatography and discriminatory analysis. *Pediatr. Res.* **3**, 287–297 (1969).
2. Perry, T. L., Hansen, S., Tischler, B., and Bunting, R., Determination of heterozygosity for phenylketonuria on the amino acid analyzer. *Clin. Chim. Acta* **18**, 51–56 (1967).
3. Rosenblatt, D., and Scriver, C. R., Heterogeneity in genetic control of phenylalanine metabolism in man. *Nature* **218**, 677–678 (1968).
4. Jackson, S. H., Hanley, W. B., Gero, T., and Gosse, G. D., Detection of phenylketonuric heterozygotes. *Clin. Chem.* **17**, 538–543 (1971).
5. Scriver, C. R., and Rosenberg, L. E., *Amino Acid Metabolism and Its Disorders*. W. B. Saunders Co., Philadelphia, PA, 1973, p 320.
6. Griffin, R. F., and Elsas, L. T., Classic phenylketonuria: Diagnosis through heterozygote detection. *J. Pediatr.* **86**, 512–517 (1975).

Phenytoin (Dilantin, diphenylhydantoin)

Specimen Tested:

P, S.

Laboratories Reporting:

5.

Reference (Normal) Values:

Therapeutic range: 4 labs.: 10–20 mg/L (μg/mL); 1 lab.: 5–20
Toxic concentration: 25 mg/L

Note: mg/L × 3.964 = μmol/L

Sources of Data:

Institutional; see papers by Kutt and coworkers, under **Phenobarbital.**

Specimen Volume, Collection, Preservation; Analytical Method, and Instrumentation:

Same as for **Phenobarbital.**

Commentary—Peter J. and Joan H. Howanitz

Phenytoin, one of the oldest, most widely effective, and most extensively prescribed of the anticonvulsants, is used for major generalized seizures (grand mal), partial seizures with complex symptomatology (psychomotor), focal seizures, and temporal lobe epilepsy. The drug alone or in combination with phenobarbital remains the mainstay for the treatment of major motor seizures.

Peak phenytoin concentrations occur in 4 to 12 h, with the rate of absorption and amount absorbed depending on the pharmaceutical preparation. Absorption may be delayed by some antacids, tranquilizers, anticoagulants, and phenobarbital. Decreased absorption also has been described in pregnancy (1). Because neonates cannot absorb phenytoin for the first few months of life, other anticonvulsants are used in this age group (2). Intramuscular administration is unreliable because of erratic absorption from the injection site.

In blood, phenytoin is highly but reversibly bound to albumin, only about 10% of the drug remaining free (unbound). Salivary and cerebrospinal fluid concentrations have been found to approximate free drug concentrations in serum. Phenylbutazone, aspirin, and valproic acid can diminish binding by competing for carrier sites, while phenytoin itself displaces thyroxine from thyroxine-binding globulin. In addition, phenytoin binding is decreased in renal disease and in hepatic disease accompanied by hypoalbuminemia. Because most of the drug is protein bound, small alterations in protein binding will result in large changes in free phenytoin concentrations.

Phenytoin is widely distributed throughout the body and accumulates in most tissues in a greater concentration than in serum. About 60 to 70% of phenytoin is metabolized to an inactive, hydroxylated derivative (5-*p*-hydroxyphenyl-5-phenylhydantoin), which is conjugated and excreted in the urine. Phenytoin has several other metabolites, and only about 5% of the native drug appears in the urine unchanged. The half-life of phenytoin is about 24 h but varies from 10 to 45 h, depending on the patient's age and the concentration in serum.

Metabolism of phenytoin is inhibited by many commonly prescribed drugs, including isoniazid, bishydroxycoumarin, chloramphenicol, chlorpromazine, estrogens, benzodiazepines, and propoxyphene. At least one family has been reported in which the members have shown clinical toxicity from phenytoin accumulation because of a defect in hydroxylation (3). Increased clearance has been described during infectious mononucleosis (4). Newborns have a greatly diminished capacity to eliminate phenytoin (2), and pre-term infants have an even slower rate of drug elimination. Except in the newborn period, children younger than 10 years metabolize phenytoin at a more rapid rate than adults; however, this metabolism decreases markedly as children enter the early stages of puberty. By the time a child reaches adolescence, the rate of phenytoin metabolism is essentially identical to that in the adult population.

Poor correlation between concentrations in serum and doses is found not only among individuals, but also in the same individual under different circumstances. At low concentrations, the metabolism rate is proportional to the serum concentration, while in the therapeutic range (10–20 µg/mL), the biotransformation system becomes saturated and no further increase in elimination occurs.

It has been widely accepted that phenytoin concentrations of 10–20 µg/mL give maximum seizure control (5,6). Toxicity begins to occur at the higher end of the therapeutic range, with nystagmus appearing at approximately 20 µg/mL, ataxia at about 30 µg/mL, and disorientation and somnolence at concentrations exceeding 40 µg/mL. However, in children wider therapeutic ranges than in adults have been suggested, i.e., 5–20 µg/mL (7) and 12–25 µg/mL (8). Although a few children show side effects with subtherapeutic concentrations, side effects in children commonly are absent at 30–40 µg/mL; decreased levels of consciousness have been seen when concentrations exceed 50 µg/mL, and opisthotonos at concentrations >100 µg/mL (9). Paradoxical intoxication, a situation where seizure frequency increases as the concentration of the anticonvulsant in blood increases, has been described (10). Other toxic side effects not necessarily related to blood concentrations of the drug include skin eruptions, lymphadenopathy, hepatitis, blood dyscrasias, hypertrichosis, and gingival hyperplasia. In a patient with acute poisoning, hemodialysis was inefficient in removing phenytoin because most phenytoin is tissue-bound *(11)*.

To maintain therapeutic concentrations in serum, phenytoin requirements increase during pregnancy but decrease abruptly in the postpartum period. Concentrations in cord blood and the mother's blood are virtually identical at the time of delivery. In contrast to decreased elimination rates in most infants, newborns of epileptic mothers metabolize phenytoin as effectively as adults *(12)*. A group of findings termed the "fetal hydantoin syndrome," consisting of craniofacial anomalies, nail and digital hypoplasia, prenatal-onset growth deficiency, and mental retardation, has been described in infants born to women receiving phenytoin during pregnancy *(13)*. Because of the limited transport capacity of the mammary glands for phenytoin, phenytoin concentrations in breast milk are significantly less than in the mother's serum.

Therapeutic values of phenytoin for cardiac arrhythmias are similar to those found for seizure disorders: 75% of the responsive arrhythmias are abolished at serum concentrations of 10–18 μg/mL *(14)*.

1. Ramsay, R. E., Strauss, R. G., Wilder, B. J., and Willmore, L. J., Status epilepticus in pregnancy: Effect of phenytoin malabsorption on seizure control. *Neurology* **28**, 85–89 (1978).
2. Painter, M. J., Pippenger, C., MacDonald, H., and Pitlick, W., Phenobarbital and diphenylhydantoin levels in neonates with seizures. *J. Pediatr.* **92**, 315–319 (1978).
3. Vasko, M. R., Bell, R. D., Daly, D. D., and Pippenger, C. E., Inheritance of phenytoin hypometabolism: A kinetic study of one family. *Clin. Pharmacol. Ther.* **27**, 96–103 (1980).
4. Leppik, I. E., Ramani, V., Sawchuk, R. J., and Grumnit, R. J., Increased clearance of phenytoin during infectious mononucleosis. *N. Engl. J. Med.* **300**, 481–482 (1979).
5. Kutt, H., and Penry, J. K., Usefulness of blood levels of antiepileptic drugs. *Arch. Neurol.* **31**, 283–288 (1974).
6. Lund, L., Anticonvulsant effect of diphenylhydantoin relative to plasma levels. *Arch. Neurol.* **31**, 289–294 (1974).
7. Borofsky, B. G., Louis, S., Kutt, H., and Roginsky, M., Diphenylhydantoin: Efficacy, toxicity, and dose–serum level relationship in children. *Pediatr. Pharmacol. Ther.* **81**, 995–1002 (1972).
8. Norell, E., Lilienberg, G., and Gamstorp, I., Systemic determination of the serum phenytoin level as an aid in the management of children with epilepsy. *Eur. Neurol.* **13**, 232–244 (1975).
9. Morselli, P. L., Pharmacokinetics of antiepileptic drugs during development. In *Antiepileptic Drug Monitoring*, C. Gardner-Thorpe, D. Janz, H. Meinardi, and C. E. Pippenger, Eds. Pitman Medical, Kent, England, 1977, pp 57–72.
10. Troupin, A. S., and Ojemann, L. M., Paradoxical intoxication—a complication of anticonvulsant administration. *Epilepsia* **16**, 753–758 (1975).
11. Rubinger, D., Levy, M., Roll, D., and Czarzkes, J. W., Inefficiency of haemodialysis in acute phenytoin intoxication. *Br. J. Clin. Pharmacol.* **7**, 405–407 (1979).

12. Rane, A., Garle, M., Borga, O., and Sjoqvist, F., Plasma disappearance of transplacentally transferred diphenylhydantoin in the newborns studied by mass fragmentography. *Clin. Pharmacol. Ther.* **15,** 39–45 (1974).
13. Hanson, J. W., Myrianthopoulos, N. C., Harvey, M. A. S., and Smith, D. W., Risks to the offspring of women treated with hydantoin anticonvulsants, with emphasis on the fetal hydantoin syndrome. *J. Pediatr.* **89,** 662–668 (1976).
14. Bigger, J. T., Schmidt, D. H., and Kutt, H., Relationship between the plasma level of diphenylhydantoin sodium and its cardiac antiarrhythmic effects. *Circulation* **38,** 363–368 (1968).

Phosphogluconate Dehydrogenase
[EC 1.1.1.44; 6-phospho-D-gluconate:NADP+ 2-oxidoreductase (decarboxylating)]

Specimen Tested:

Erythrocytes.

Laboratories Reporting:

2.

Reference (Normal) Values:

Lab. 1: 6.8–12.0 U/g of hemoglobin (range)
Lab. 2: 1.9–2.5 U/mL of erythrocytes

Sources of Reference (Normal) Values:

Lab. 1: institutional study on 54 children; Nicholson, J. F., Bodourian, S. H., and Pesce, M. A., Measurement of glucose-6-phosphate dehydrogenase and 6-phosphogluconate dehydrogenase activities in erythrocytes by use of a centrifugal analyzer. *Clin. Chem.* **20,** 1349–1352 (1974). **Lab. 2:** institutional; in children <6 mo; this range is slightly higher than the adult range, possibly because of the increased reticulocyte values in younger patients.

Specimen Volume, Collection, and Preservation:

10 μL of hemolysate. Heparin and EDTA as anticoagulant. Although the enzyme is best analyzed immediately, blood may be stored at least 3 d in the RR, with claims for stability to 20 d in the RR (Beutler, E., *Red Cell Metabolism,* 2nd ed. Grune and Stratton, New York, NY, 1975, p 9).

Analytical Method:

Both labs use similar reactions but different conditions. **Lab. 1:** Nicholson et al., *op. cit.;* **Lab. 2:** Princeton Biomedix Erythrozyme kit.

Enzyme Data:

Lab. 1:

1. Enzyme unit definition: 1 IUB unit (U) will oxidize 1.0 μmol of 6-phospho-D-gluconate to D-ribulose 5-phosphate per minute.
2. Buffer, pH: triethanolamine, 7.6.
3. Substrate, pH: 6-phospho-D-gluconate, 7.4.
4. Reaction temperature: 37 °C.
5. Temperature reported: 37 °C.

Lab. 2:

1. Enzyme unit definition: same as Lab. 1.
2. Buffer, pH: glycylglycine, 8.0.
3. Substrate, pH: 6-phospho-D-gluconate, 8.0.
4. Reaction temperature: 30 °C.
5. Temperature reported: 30 °C.

Instrumentation:

Lab. 1: Union Carbide CentrifiChem Analyzer System 400. **Lab. 2:** Beckman Instruments, Inc., 35 spectrophotometer.

Commentary—Michael A. Pesce

The enzyme 6-phosphogluconate dehydrogenase (6-PGD) catalyzes the second reaction in the hexose monophosphate shunt and converts 6-phosphogluconate to ribulose 5-phosphate. Partial deficiency of 6-PGD in erythrocytes of certain subjects does not produce hemolytic anemia. The effects of severe 6-PGD deficiency are not well known.

6-PGD activity is determined in erythrocytes by conversion of 6-phosphogluconate to ribulose 5-phosphate with the concurrent reduction of $NADP^+$ to NADPH. The rate of increase in absorbance of NADPH is related to the activity of the enzyme *(1)*. 6-PGD is stable in heparinized blood stored at 4 °C for at least three days.

1. Nicholson, J. F., Bodourian, S. H., and Pesce, M. A., Measurement of glucose-6-phosphate dehydrogenase and 6-phosphogluconate dehydrogenase activities in erythrocytes by use of a centrifugal analyzer. *Clin. Chem.* **20**, 1349–1352 (1974).

Phospholipids

Specimen Tested:

S.

Laboratory Reporting:

1.

Reference (Normal) Values:

Cord blood: 0.48–1.60 g/L
2–13 yr: 1.66–2.47
3–20 yr: 1.93–3.38

Sources of Reference (Normal) Values:

Text ref. *1*.

Volume and Source of Specimen:

100 µL; capillary.

Analytical Method:

Text ref. *2*.

Instrumentation:

Beckman Model 25 spectrophotometer.

Phosphorus, Inorganic

Specimen Tested:

P, S.

Laboratories Reporting:

8.

Reference (Normal) Values:

Age	mg/dL (mmol/L)[a]	Age	mg/dL (mmol/L)[a]
Cord blood (1 lab.)	4.8–6.2 (1.55–2.00)	18 mo–3 yr	2.9–5.9 (0.94–1.90)
Premature		2–5 yr	3.5–6.8 (1.13–2.20)
Birth	5.6–8.0 (1.81–2.58)	3–15 yr	3.6–5.6 (1.16–1.81)
6–10 d	6.1–11.7 (1.97–3.78)	5–8 yr	3.1–6.3 (1.00–2.03)
20–25 d	6.6–9.4 (2.13–3.03)	Child	4.0–6.0 (1.29–1.94)
Full-term		10 yr	3.6–5.6 (1.16–1.81)
Birth	5.0–7.8 (1.65–2.52)	8–12 yr	3.0–6.0 (0.97–1.94)
3 d	5.8–9.0 (1.87–2.91)	12–16 yr	2.5–5.0 (0.81–1.61)
6–12 d	4.9–8.9 (1.58–2.87)	15–16 yr	2.4–5.4 (0.77–1.74)
Newborn	4.2–9.0 (1.36–2.91);	16 yr–adult	2.3–4.8 (0.74–1.55)
	4.2–8.2 (1.36–2.65)	Adult	3.0–4.5 (0.97–1.45)
0–2 yr	4.2–7.0 (1.36–2.26)		3.1–5.1 (1.00–1.65)
6 wk–18 mo	3.8–6.7 (1.23–2.16)		2.5–4.5 (0.81–1.45)
1 yr	3.8–6.2 (1.23–2.00)		

[a] Values based on measurements of phosphomolybdate (reduction or ultraviolet methods).

Sources of Reference (Normal) Values:

Text ref. *2*, p 253; Cheng, M. H., Lipsey, A. I., Blanco, V., Wong, H. T., and Spiro, S. H., Microchemical analysis for 13 constituents of plasma from healthy children. *Clin. Chem.* **25,** 692–698 (1979); institutional.

Specimen Volume, Collection, and Preservation:

Generally 10 to 20 μL. Heparin anticoagulant. Separate P or S as soon as possible after collection. Values increase after 1 d at RT or in RR. Separated P, in one report, may be stored in RR for 7 d.

Analytical Method:

Modification of Fiske, C. H., and Subbarow, Y., Colorimetric determination of phosphorus. *J. Biol. Chem.* **66**, 375–400 (1925); Taussky, H. H., and Schorr, E., A microcolorimetric method for the determination of inorganic phosphorus. *J. Biol. Chem.* **202**, 675 (1953); Harleco Phosphorus Reagent Set for use on Abbott ABA-100 Bichromatic Analyzer; Gindler, E. M., and Ishizaki, R. T., Rapid semimicro colorimetric determination of phosphorus in serum and nonionic surfactants. *Clin. Chem.* **15**, 807 (1969), abstract; Pierce Chemical Co. Manual Phosphorus Rapid Stat kit; Electro-Nucleonics Gemeni inorganic phosphorus kit; Hycel Inc. kit; Daly, J. A., and Ertingshausen, G., Direct method for determining inorganic phosphate in serum with the CentrifiChem. *Clin. Chem.* **18**, 263–265 (1972); Amador, E., and Urban, J., Simplified serum phosphorus analyses by continuous-flow spectrophotometry. *Clin. Chem.* **18**, 601–604 (1972); modification of Horwitt, B. J., Determination of inorganic serum phosphate by means of stannous chloride. *J. Biol. Chem.* **199**, 537 (1952); Shinowara, G. Y., Jones, L. M., and Reinhart, H. L., The estimation of serum inorganic phosphate and "acid" and "alkaline" phosphatase activity. *J. Biol. Chem.* **142**, 922–933 (1942); Kutner, T., and Cohen, H. R., Micro colorimetric studies. I. A molybdic acid, stannous chloride reagent. The micro estimation of phosphate and calcium in pus, plasma, and spinal fluid. *J. Biol. Chem.* **75**, 517–531 (1927).

Instrumentation:

Gilford Stasar II and III, Coleman Jr. II spectrophotometers; Abbott ABA-100 Bichromatic Analyzer; Electro-Nucleonics Gemeni centrifugal analyzer; Technicon SMA II and SMAC systems.

* * *

Laboratory Reporting:

1.

Reference (Normal) Values:

Age, yr	Sex	Percentile estimates, mg/dL (mmol/L)	
		5th	95th
4–8	F	3.9 (1.26)	5.4 (1.74)
4–9	M	3.8 (1.23)	5.4 (1.74)
9–13	F	3.5 (1.13)	5.1 (1.65)
10–15	M	3.4 (1.10)	5.3 (1.71)
14–20	F	2.8 (0.90)	4.3 (1.39)
16–20	M	2.5 (0.81)	4.4 (1.42)

Sources of Reference (Normal) Values:

Institutional study; Cherian, A. G., and Hill, J. G., Percentile esti-mates of reference values for fourteen chemical constituents in sera of children and adolescents. *Am. J. Clin. Pathol.* **69**, 24–31 (1978).

Analytical Method and Instrumentation:

Ammonium molybdate, ultraviolet method, modified from Greiner manual; Greiner Electronics Selective Analyzer II.

*   *   *

Laboratory Reporting:

1.

Reference (Normal) Values:

Newborn: 4.5–9.0 mg/dL (1.45–2.90 mmol/L)
Child: 4.0–6.5 (1.29–2.10)

Sources of Reference (Normal) Values:

Institutional.

Analytical Method and Instrumentation:

Enzymic; Pesce, M. A., Bodourian, S. H., and Nicholson, J. F., Enzy-matic method for determination of inorganic phosphate in serum and urine with a centrifugal analyzer. *Clin. Chem.* **20**, 332–336 (1974).

Note: See also Chapter 2 comments on inorganic phosphorus (p 9).

Phosphorus, Tubular Reabsorption of

Specimen Tested:

P, S, U.

Laboratory Reporting:

1.

Reference (Normal) Values:

78–97%

Sources of Reference (Normal) Values:

Text ref. *1*, p 992.

Analytical Method:

Text ref. *2*, p 252.

Porphyrins (Coproporphyrin, Porphobilinogen, Protoporphyrin, Uroporphyrin)

Specimen Tested:

Erythrocytes, feces, P, S, U.

Laboratories Reporting:

5.

Reference (Normal) Values:

	Copro-porphyrin	Protoporphyrin (free)	Uro-porphyrin	Por-phobilinogen
Erythrocyte	<0.03 μmol/L	upper limits reported to 60 μg/dL (<1.07 μmol/L of erythro-cytes); 1.0–5.0 μg/g of Hb	0.0	
Feces	0–0.06 μmol/g (dry wt.)	0–0.18 μmol/g (dry wt.)		
U				
Lab. 1			0–0.05 μmol/d	0–2 mg/d (0–8.8 μmol/d)
Child	<0.23 μmol/d			
Adult	<0.38 μmol/d			
Random U	0.46–0.61 μmol/d			
Lab. 2	0–160 μg/d		0–26 μg/d	

P, S total porphyrin (Lab. 2): <0.02 μmol/L

Note: See also δ-**Aminolaevulinate.**

Sources of Reference (Normal) Values:

Labs. 1, 4, 5: institutional. **Lab. 2:** Eales, L., Levey, M. J., and Swee-ney, M. B., The place of screening tests and quantitative investiga-tions in the diagnosis of the porphyrias, with particular reference to variegate and symptomatic porphyria. *South Afr. Med. J.* **40,** 63–71 (1966); Wranne, L., Free erythrocyte copro- and protoporphyrin: A methodological and clinical study. *Acta Paediatr.* **49,** Suppl., 119–124 (1960). **Lab. 3:** Preventing lead poisoning in young children. Cen-ter for Disease Control, USDHEW 00–2629, April, 1978.

Specimen Volume, Collection, and Preservation:

Protoporphyrin, free erythrocyte: 2 to 50 μL of B; **feces:** 1.5 g; **P, S:** 10 mL of B; **U:** aliquot of 24-h U or random sample. Store sample protected from light (covered with tinfoil) in FR. Urinary porphyrin is collected into a dark bottle containing Na₂CO₃ (alkalin-ized).

Note: Do not alkalinize for collecting porphobilinogen. *Acidify* to pH 1 (with HCl); stable for short time at RT, but best to freeze.

Analytical Method:

Lab. 1: Schwartz, S., Berg, M. H., Bossenmaier, I., and Dinsmore, H., Determination of porphyrins in biological materials. In *Methods of Biochemical Analysis*, **8,** D. Glick, Ed. Interscience, New York, NY, 1960, pp 221–293. **Lab. 2:** Eales et al. *op. cit.;* Wranne, *op. cit.;* Schwartz, et al., *op. cit.;* Martinez, C. A., and Mills, G. C., Spectrophotofluorometric determination of porphyrins in urine. *Clin. Chem.* **17,** 199–205 (1971); Assoc. Clin. Pathologists Broadsheet No. 70 (1971). **Lab. 3:** Caffo, A. L., and Lubin, A. H., Modified micromethod for erythrocyte protoporphyrin. *Clin. Chem.* **22,** 1412 (1976), letter. **Lab. 4:** Labbé, R. F., Finch, C. A., Smith, N. J., Doan, R. N., Sood, S. K., and Madan, N., Erythrocyte protoporphyrin/heme ratio in the assessment of iron status. *Clin. Chem.* **25,** 87–92 (1979). **Lab. 5:** Obernolte, R., and Sherwin, J. E., Ultramicro erythrocyte protoporphyrin determination using solvent extraction without sample transfer. *Clin. Chem.* **24,** 1058 (1978), abstract.

Instrumentation:

Zeiss, Varian Techtron spectrophotometers; Aminco-Bowman, Farrand, Turner 430 spectrofluorometers.

Commentary—Roger L. Boeckx

There are three conditions in which the concentration of erythrocyte protoporphyrin (EP) increases: lead poisoning, iron-deficiency anemia, and erythrocytic protoporphyria (EPP). Patients with EPP and lead poisoning both show EP concentrations as much as 100-fold normal, but patients with EPP are remarkably light-sensitive, whereas lead-poisoned individuals are not. Piomelli et al. *(1)* showed that the protoporphyrin that accumulates in EPP is bound as a free base to hemoglobin, but not at the heme-binding sites. On the other hand, the protoporphyrin that accumulates in lead poisoning and iron-deficiency anemia is present as a zinc chelate, firmly bound at the heme-binding sites *(2)*. Spectrophotometric data support these conclusions: erythrocytes from EPP patients emit fluorescence at 625 nm, whereas cells from patients with lead poisoning or iron-deficiency anemia fluoresce at 595 nm, suggesting that the porphyrins are present in different forms.

As erythrocytes age, the 625-nm fluorescence band associated with EPP disappears rapidly, but the 595-nm band observed in lead-poisoned erythrocytes remains constant throughout the life of the cell. Apparently, protoporphyrin accumulates in EPP erythrocytes in the later stages of maturation, and this more loosely bound protoporphyrin diffuses rapidly from the cell and reaches the skin, where it induces photosensitivity. In lead poisoning and iron-deficiency anemia, the last step in heme synthesis remains uncompleted and the protoporphyrin that accumulates is zinc protoporphyrin (ZPP). Because it is more tightly bound to hemoglobin, the ZPP remains in the erythrocyte throughout the life of the cell, and photosensitivity does not occur.

There are three common approaches to the measurement of ZPP: direct measurement in whole blood by direct fluorometry, extraction with ethanol or detergents, and extraction with acidic solvents. Unfortunately, many workers have referred to the measured compound as free erythrocyte porphyrin (FEP), when in fact the prophyrin is not "free" in the erythrocyte. Acid extraction, the first method developed to measure FEP, extracts the protoporphyrin from the erythrocyte, but the acid removes the chelated zinc and converts the ZPP to protoporphyrin IX. The Center for Disease Control has standardized the reporting of erythrocyte protoporphyrin results and uses the term erythrocyte protoporphyrin (EP) exclusively; this term is understood to refer to the protoporphyrin IX molecule extracted from the erythrocyte by means of an acidic solvent, as described by Piomelli (3), and is expressed as micrograms per 100 mL of whole blood.

As might be expected, ZPP, determined by the direct method (4) and expressed as micrograms of zinc protoprophyrin per 100 mL of whole blood, and EP, determined by the method recommended by the Center for Disease Control, correlate well. However, Joselow and Flores report that in lead poisoning ZPP concentration is 1.38-fold greater than EP (5), which they attribute to an incomplete extraction of EP. Peter et al. (6) reported that results obtained with a hematofluorometer were 9% lower than those obtained by the Piomelli extraction method; they noted that the extent to which blood was diluted and the composition of the extracting solvents could have pronounced effects on the completeness of extraction of EP from erythrocytes. Peter et al. (6) obtained better recoveries than did Joselow and Flores, which probably explains the differences in the EP/ZPP ratios observed by these two groups. Several groups have reported on comparisons of methods for EP determination. Hanna et al. (7) compared four extraction methods, and Joselow and Flores (5) and Peter et al. (6) compared direct measurements and extraction methods. Clearly, whatever method is used to determine EP, the procedure should be closely correlated with the Center for Disease Control reference method and results expressed as EP or EP equivalents, as recommended (8).

Increases of EP concentration may not appear until two weeks after exposure to lead, because the increase is due to events occurring during erythropoeisis. Measurement of EP concentration, therefore, is not a useful test in acute lead poisoning. In chronic lead poisoning, however, the increase of EP is the most reliable indicator of excessive lead exposure, next to the direct measurement of blood lead concentration. Also, EP concentrations may remain high for several weeks after chelation therapy, despite the fact that blood lead concentrations may have returned to normal during that period.

Numerous reports have shown good correlation between EP concentrations and blood lead burden. In a large study, Chisolm et al. determined the rate of false-negative results to be less than 2% *(9)*; however, a group of children containing more anemic individuals produced more false-positive results. This agrees with later reports that EP increases are common in iron-deficiency anemia. The mechanism of increasing EP is the same in lead poisoning and iron-deficiency anemia: in both cases, iron is not available to the erythrocyte.

The erythrocyte protoporphyrin/heme ratio has been shown to be a valuable test for the assessment of iron status. Labbé et al. *(10)* report that the molar ratio of protoporphyrin and heme in the erythrocyte correlates well with plasma iron, plasma ferritin, transferrin saturation, hemoglobin, and hematocrit. The FEP/hemoglobin ratio has also been proposed as a sensitive indicator of iron deficiency *(11)*.

In erythropoetic protoporphyria, there is marked increase in erythrocyte, plasma, and fecal protoporphyrin concentration. EP concentrations 100-fold normal have been reported. The metabolic defect appears to be a partial deficiency of ferrochelatase, which results in an overproduction of protoporphyrin IX. The disorder is relatively benign, being manifested primarily by acute solar urticaria and chronic solar eczema. Occasionally, gallstones and severe progressive liver disease are seen *(12)*.

1. Lamola, A., Piomelli, S., Poh-Fitzpatrick, M. B., Yamane, T., and Harber, L. C., Erythropoietic protoporphyria and lead intoxication: The molecular basis for difference in cutaneous photosensitivity. II. Different binding of erythrocyte protoporphyrin to hemoglobin. *J. Clin. Invest.* **56,** 1528–1535 (1975).
2. Lamola, A., and Yamane, T., Zinc protoporphyrin in the erythrocytes of patients with lead intoxication and iron deficiency anemia. *Science* **186,** 936–938 (1974).
3. Piomelli, S., A micromethod for free erythrocyte porphyrins: The FEP test. *J. Lab. Clin. Med.* **81,** 932–940 (1973).
4. Blumberg, W. E., Eisinger, J., Lamola, A., and Zuckerman, D. M., The Hematofluorometer. *Clin. Chem.* **23,** 270–274 (1977).
5. Joselow, M. M., and Flores, J., Comparison of zinc protoporphyrin and free erythrocyte protoporphyrin in whole blood. *Health Lab. Sci.* **14,** 126–128 (1977).
6. Peter, F., Growcock, G., and Strunc, G., Fluorometric determination of erythrocyte protoporphyrin in blood, a comparison between direct (hematofluorometric) and indirect (extraction) methods. *Clin. Chem.* **24,** 1515–1517 (1978).
7. Hanna, T. L., Dietzler, D. N., Smith, C. H., Gupta, S., and Zarkowsky, H. S., Erythrocyte porphyrin analysis in the detection of lead poisoning in children: Evaluation of four micromethods. *Clin. Chem.* **22,** 161–168 (1976).
8. *Preventing Lead Poisoning in Young Children.* Center for Disease Control, Atlanta, GA, 1978.
9. Chisolm, J. J., Mellits, E. D., Keil, J. E., and Barrett, M. B., A simple protoporphyrin assay—microhematocrit procedure as a screening tech-

nique for increased lead absorption in young children. *J. Pediatr.* **84,** 490–496 (1974).

10. Labbé, R. F., Finch, C. A., Smith, N. J., Doan, R. N., Sood, S. K., and Madan, N., Erythrocyte protoporphyrin/heme ratio in the assessment of iron status. *Clin. Chem.* **25,** 87–92 (1979).

11. Piomelli, S., Brickman, A., and Carlos, E., Rapid diagnosis of iron deficiency by measurement of free erythrocyte porphyrins and hemoglobin: The FEP/hemoglobin ratio. *Pediatrics* **57,** 136–141 (1976).

12. Meyer, U. A., and Schmid, R., The porphyrias. In text ref. *11,* 4th ed., pp 1196–1220.

Commentary—T. A. Blumenfeld

Erythrocyte Protoporphyrin

A final stage in the biosynthesis of hemoglobin involves the incorporation of iron into protoporphyrin IX to form heme. The unutilized protoporphyrin IX accumulates in circulating erythrocytes if iron is unavailable (in iron-deficiency states) or if there are disturbances at this stage of metabolism (as in lead poisoning). Because protoporphyrin IX is increased in latent iron deficiency and in subclinical lead poisoning, measurements of erythrocyte protoporphyrin are highly useful for the early detection of these conditions. Protoporphyrin extracted from erythrocytes has long been termed "free erythrocyte protoporphyrin." Of the porphyrin extractable from whole blood, 95% or more is protoporphyrin bound to erythrocytes *(1)*. The rest is composed of traces of protoporphyrin in plasma and coproporphyrin in erythrocytes and plasma. The "specificity" of simple microscale methods for protoporphyrin, which extract any porphyrin present, lies in the fact that, with rare exception, protoporphyrin from erythrocytes is the only porphyrin likely to be encountered in excess in human blood. For practical purposes, the terms "free erythrocyte protoporphyrin" and "free erythrocyte porphyrin" are the same and can be used interchangeably. In lead poisoning and iron deficiency, the predominant fraction of protoporphyrin in circulating erythrocytes is the metalloporphyrin, zinc protoprophyrin IX, whereas in the disease porphyria, protoporphyrin is present in the "free" state.

Metabolic disturbances in heme synthesis are the earliest well-recognized adverse effects attributable to lead. Increased erythrocyte protoporphyrin (EP) becomes evident in groups of children as the concentration of lead in whole blood increases to values of 30 to 50 μg/dL. Tests for EP permit detection and treatment of lead poisoning at the subclinical stage, before severe acute clinical lead poisoning appears, which in children may be followed by irreversible changes not amenable to chelation therapy.

Recently, a microtechnique requiring only 44.7 μL of heparinized capillary blood has been described for determining EP concentration *(2)*. The normal range was determined in 34 preschool children (mean age: two years, seven months). With hematocrits $\geqslant 36\%$ (36–42%) and blood lead values of <30 $\mu g/dL$, these children had EP values of 3.17 ± 1.36 $\mu g/dL$. In a second group of 118 children, 11 months to seven years old, from old housing areas in Charleston, SC, if the hematocrit was 30 to 35% and EP was $\geqslant 10.9$ $\mu g/dL$, the blood lead concentration was $\geqslant 50$ $\mu g/dL$; if the hematocrit was >35 and EP was $\geqslant 7.27$ $\mu g/dL$, the blood lead was $\geqslant 50$ $\mu g/dL$.

The tests for EP are more sensitive to an earlier sustained increase in lead absorption than are tests for δ-aminolaevulinate and coproporphyrin in random samples of children's urine. These urinary tests do not show comparable sensitivity until the blood lead concentration exceeds 80 $\mu g/dL$.

The clinical use of EP testing is as follows: If the test is positive, i.e., greater than the previously stated "cutoff" limits for corresponding hematocrits, blood should be obtained for lead measurement. If the EP value exceeds the normal by more than 10-fold, the patient should be referred promptly for diagnostic work-up. Studies of preliminary serial measurements of EP show that it reflects sustained assimilation of lead. The test provides a direct and sensitive metabolic index of increased lead absorption and serves as a metabolic signal of lead absorption.

Coproporphyrins

The coproporphyrins are tetrapyrroles. These compounds are formed after successive decarboxylation of the four acetic acid side-chains of the uroporphyrinogens. The colorless porphyrinogens can be oxidized to colored porphyrins that are not the same as the intermediates in heme biosynthesis. Coproporphyrin I excretion is increased when erythropoietic activity is increased, and also in infectious hepatitis and obstructive jaundice. Some increase in coproporphyrin III excretion is seen in infection, malignant disease, alcoholic cirrhosis, and after ingestion of certain chemicals. In lead poisoning, urinary excretion of coproporphyrin III is increased, the amount of which may be used to follow the course of the disease.

Uroporphyrins

Uroporphyrins are tetrapyrroles formed as by-products during heme synthesis. Uroporphyrin excretion is greatly increased in the acute porphyrias and may be increased in lead poisoning, cirrhosis of the liver, and hemochromatosis.

1. Chisolm, J. J., Jr., and Brown, D. H. (Schwartz, S., Mitchell, D. G., and Piomelli, S., evaluators), Micro-scale photofluorometric determination of "free erythrocyte porphyrin" (protoporphyrin IX). *Clin. Chem.* 21, 1669–1682 (1975). Proposed Selected Method.
2. Chisolm, J. J., Jr., Mellits, E. D., Keil, J. E., and Barrett, M. B., A simple protoporphyrin assay–microhematocrit procedure as a screening technique for increased lead absorption in young children. *J. Pediatr.* 84, 490–496 (1974).

Potassium and Sodium

Specimen Tested:

P, S, U.

Laboratories Reporting:

5.

Reference (Normal) Values:

Age	P, S (mmol/L)	
	K	**Na**
Cord	4.4–6.6	134–146
Premature		132–142
Newborn, full-term	5.0–7.5	132–142
2 d–3 mo	4.0–6.2	
Child–adolescent	3.8–5.0[a]	136–142[a]
Child–adult	3.5–5.5	135–145
	U (mmol/d)	
Infant		6–10[b]
		0.3–3.5
Child	25–120; 26–123	40–180
Adult		80–200; 27–287

[a] 5th-95th percentile.
[b] mmol/m² of body surface.

Sources of Reference (Normal) Values:

Institutional; Cherian, A. G., and Hill, J. G., Percentile estimates of reference values for fourteen chemical constituents in sera of children and adolescents. *Am. J. Clin. Pathol.* **69**, 24–31 (1978).

Specimen Volume, Collection, and Preservation:

10 to 50 μL. Heparin only as anticoagulant. When sterile, P, S, and U are stable for 2 wk at RT or in RR.

Analytical Method and Instrumentation:

Instrumentation Laboratory 343 flame photometer; Beckman Instruments Astra 8; Klina flame photometer; Technicon SMA II; Greiner Selective Analyzer II: Micromedic diluter.

Commentary—Garry M. Lum

Potassium

Serum. Potassium is the most abundant intracellular ion; serum potassium, therefore, reflects the status of body potassium and its apparent distribution. Despite a relatively low concentration outside the cells, such distribution plays a vital role in cell function. Maintaining serum concentrations of potassium within carefully regulated limits is essential for muscular function; conduction abnormalities of cardiac muscle, for example, arise with either high or low serum concentrations. Life-threatening cardiac arrhythmias can occur, therefore, with hypo- or hyperkalemia. The former may result from dietary restriction or use of diuretics, the latter from abundant administration, renal excretory deficiency, or rapid release by cells, as in hemolysis. Hemolysis during blood sampling may be the most common factor producing falsely high determinations.

Urine. The kidneys provide the primary route of excretion for potassium. Determination of urinary potassium may be useful in clinical conditions; for example, low urinary potassium may reflect severe total body deficit. Urinary potassium quantitation may be helpful when potassium excretion is suspected of being decreased or augmented as a result of deficient or exaggerated adrenal function. Overall, however, urinary potassium will reflect intake.

Sodium

Serum. Low serum sodium concentration (hyponatremia) primarily indicates that the amount of water in the serum (extracellular fluid) has increased relative to the amount of sodium. Thus, low serum sodium per se does not indicate whether the *total* body sodium is high, low, or normal. A low serum sodium value must therefore be viewed in light of the clinical situation. Factitious decreases of serum sodium can occur, most commonly in hyperlipemic states, for example, although three substances other than lipids—serum proteins, glucose, and urea—can cause a real or apparent alteration in serum sodium. This apparent alteration occurs, e.g., in the case of lipids because the concentration of serum sodium is expressed relative to serum volume, which includes water *plus* the volume occupied by lipids. Thus, actual concentration of sodium in the serum water will be underestimated if measured without taking into consideration the amount of water displaced by the lipids in the sample.

High serum sodium concentration (hypernatremia) usually suggests loss of total body water in excess of loss of sodium, but under some rarer circumstances might represent actual excess in total body sodium.

Urine. Urinary sodium will vary with intake, state of hydration or kidney perfusion, influences of drugs such as diuretics, or actual abnormalities of glomerular filtration or tubular function. Thus, determinations of urinary sodium can be extremely helpful if interpreted with knowledge of the clinical situation. Isolated values are of very little use except when extremely low (e.g., less than 20 mmol/L), suggesting renal avidity for sodium (as in dehydration) and likely normal renal function.

Pregnanetriol

Specimen Tested:

U.

Laboratories Reporting:

3.

Reference (Normal) Values:

Age (and Lab.)	mg/d (µmol/d)	Age (and Lab.)	mg/d (µmol/d)
Newborn–2 wk (1)	0–0.02 (0–0.06)	9–12 yr (1)	0–0.5 (0–1.5)
2 wk–1 yr (1)	0–0.05 (0–0.15)	12–16 yr (1),M	0.2–1.0 (0.6–3.0)
3 wk–6 yr (2)	<0.5 (<0.15)	F	0.2–1.0 (0.6–3.0)
Up to 6 yr (3)	(0–0.6)	16–20 yr (1),M	0.5–2.5 (1.5–7.4)
1–3 yr (1)	0–0.1 (0–0.3)	F	0.3–1.5 (0.9–4.5)
3–6 yr (1)	0–0.2 (0–0.6)	>16 yr (3)	(0.6–10.0)
6–9 yr (1)	0–0.3 (0–0.9)	Adult (1),M	0.5–2.0 (1.5–5.9)
6–16 yr (2)	<1.1 (<3.3)	F	0.3–2.0 (0.9–5.9)
7–16 yr (3)	(0.9–3.3)	(2)	<3.5 (<10.4)

Sources of Reference (Normal) Values:

Labs. 1, 2: institutional; Smith, E. K., A study of 119 healthy children, ages 3 to 17 yr, and 24 "normal" adults. **Lab. 3:** Bongiovanni, A. M., and Eberlein, W. R., Critical analysis of methods for measurement of pregnane-$3\alpha,17\alpha,20\alpha$-triol in human urine. *Anal. Chem.* **30,** 388–392 (1958).

Specimen Volume, Collection, and Preservation:

Aliquot (20 mL) of 24-h U. Collect U over 5 g of boric acid crystals.

Analytical Method:

Lab. 1: GLC, after chromatography on alumina; Kinoshita, K., Isurugi, K., Yoshiaki, K., and Hisao, T., Gas chromatographic estimation of urinary pregnanetriol, pregnanetriolone and pregnanetetrol in congenital adrenal hyperplasia. *J. Clin. Endocrinol. Metab.* **26,** 1219–1226 (1966). **Lab. 2:** Qazi, Q. H., Hill, J. G., and Thompson, M. W., Steroid studies on parents of patients with virilizing adrenal hyperplasia. *J. Clin. Endocrinol. Metab.* **33,** 23–26 (1971). **Lab. 3:** Phillipou, G., Seamark, R. F., and Cox, L. W., A procedure for comprehensive analysis of neutral urinary steroids in endocrine investigations. *Aust. N. Z. J. Med.* **8,** 63–68 (1978).

Instrumentation:

GLC; Hewlett-Packard 5711, FID detector; Perkin-Elmer F 30.

Commentary—Elizabeth K. Smith

Pregnanetriol is the urinary metabolite of 17-hydroxyprogesterone (17-OHP), a steroid intermediate in the biosynthesis of cortisol. Until the recent availability of reliable assay methods for plasma 17-OHP, the principal application of pregnanetriol determinations was in definitive diagnosis of congenital adrenal hyperplasia due to 21-hydroxylase deficiency, and in monitoring the adequacy of corticosteroid-replacement therapy. In the untreated patient with this disorder pregnanetriol excretion is markedly increased. In the older child with 21-hydroxylase deficiency, pregnanetriol excretion may exceed 50 mg/d, and roughly parallels the increases in 17-ketosteroids. With adequate corticosteroid therapy, values may be maintained near normal for age.

Normal infants excrete very small amounts of pregnanetriol, which usually are undetectable with sulfuric acid chromogen methods of analysis. With a specific and sensitive method such as GLC, concentrations in the range of 10–50 μg/d are measurable. Urine of newborns contains increased amounts of many unknown steroid metabolites that may interfere with the sulfuric acid chromogen method, especially in newborns with congenital adrenal hyperplasia. In these patients the typical GLC chromatogram often demonstrates increased amounts of pregnenetriol and 11-keto-pregnanetriol in quantities greater than pregnanetriol.

In the prepubertal child excretion values are low, but begin to increase at about eight years of age, reaching adult concentrations in puberty *(1)*. In adults very little sex difference is apparent, although values are slightly higher in men, and may be somewhat higher in the follicular phase of the menstrual cycle in women.

Pregnanetriol is excreted as its glucuronide conjugate, and must therefore be hydrolyzed with glucuronidase before extraction. Because the steroid is labile in the presence of strong acid, the collection bottle should contain a mild preservative such as boric acid.

1. Smith, E. K., and Tippit, D. F., Evaluation of steroid hormone metabolism. In text ref. 7, vol. **1**, p 325.

Primidone (Mysoline)[1]

Specimen Tested:

P, S.

Laboratories Reporting:

5.

---

[1] Phenobarbital, a major metabolite of primidone, should also be measured.

Reference (Normal) Values:

	mg/L (μg/mL)			
	2 labs.	1 lab.	1 lab.	1 lab.
Therapeutic range	5–12	6–12	4.4–10.9	4–10

Toxic value: 15 mg/L

Note: mg/L $\times$ 4.582 = μmol/L.

Sources of Data, Specimen Volume, etc., Analytical Method, Instrumentation:

Same as for **Phenobarbital.**

Commentary—Peter J. and Joan H. Howanitz

Primidone, a desoxybarbiturate, has been used since 1950 as an anticonvulsant for tonic-clonic seizures (grand mal) and for partial seizures with complex symptomatology (psychomotor). Primidone is absorbed rapidly from the gastrointestinal tract and converted mainly to two active metabolites, phenobarbital and phenylethylmalonamide (PEMA). After ingestion, peak serum primidone concentrations occur in about 3 h *(1)*, but there is wide variation among individuals. The mean half-life of primidone is about 10 to 12 h *(2)*, whereas the average half-life of its two active metabolites, phenobarbital and PEMA, are 96 and 24–48 h, respectively. However, some evidence indicates that, with chronic dosing, both the time to reach peak primidone concentration and the half-life may be prolonged. About two-thirds of serum primidone is bound to serum proteins. Salivary concentrations are close to those of serum, but CSF/serum ratios are quite variable and dependent on time of dosing *(3)*. About 20% of primidone is excreted in the urine unchanged. In children, the concentrations attained in serum are significantly less than in adults in response to comparable primidone dosage; for example, in children 1 mg of primidone per kilogram of body weight results in a value of about 0.5 μg/mL of serum, while in an adult this dose yields values up to 3 μg/mL *(4)*.

Investigations regarding the relationship between primidone concentrations and clinical efficacy or toxicity are relatively few. Primidone values exceeding 5 μg/mL usually are found in patients whose seizure control is improved *(5)*. Other investigators report that primidone values up to 12 μg/mL are associated with clinical improvement *(3)*. Maximum efficacy is achieved with serum primidone concentrations of 8–12 μg/mL *(6)*. The situation is complicated, however, by the active metabolites phenobarbital and PEMA, for which very little information is available.

When therapy with primidone is initiated, drowsiness, nystagmus, and unsteadiness of gait occur, but as the drug is continued, these manifestations soon disappear. If primidone values reach 15–20 μg/mL, however, those side effects may reappear *(3)*. It has been difficult to relate toxicity to the concentrations of primidone, phenobarbital, PEMA, or combinations of these. The ratio of phenobarbital to primidone is usually 2/1 or less in patients treated with primidone alone, but there is considerable interindividual variation. Concomitant phenytoin treatment results in a relatively higher concentration of phenobarbital from primidone *(7)*. In addition, isoniazid reportedly increases serum primidone concentration by inhibiting the metabolism of primidone to its active metabolites *(8)*. In a child with renal failure, who had primidone values in the therapeutic range, a 10-fold accumulation of PEMA was postulated as the cause of a syndrome of nystagmus, ataxia, emesis, lethargy, and weakness *(9)*. One distinguishing feature of acute primidone overdose is the occurrence of crystalluria, identified as primidone itself *(10,11)*.

Primidone has been shown to cross the placenta. In one case, a newborn whose mother was on chronic primidone therapy had a serum primidone concentration of 8 μg/mL. This newborn showed a neurologic syndrome that included tremulousness *(12)*.

1. Gallagher, B. B., and Baumel, I. P., Primidone. In *Antiepileptic Drugs,* D. M. Woodbury, J. K. Penry, and R. P. Schmidt, Eds. Raven Press, New York, NY, 1972, pp 357–366,
2. Booker, H. E., Hosokowa, K., Burdette, R. D., and Darcey, B., A clinical study of serum primidone levels. *Epilepsia* **11**, 395–402 (1970).
3. Schottelius, D. D., and Fincham, R. W., Clinical application of serum primidone levels. In *Antiepileptic Drugs: Quantitative Analysis and Interpretation,* C. E. Pippenger, J. Kiffin, J. K. Penry, and H. Kutt, Eds. Raven Press, New York, NY, 1978, pp 273–282.
4. Livingston, S., Pruce, I., and Pauli, L. L., Maintenance of drug therapy. *Pediatr. Ann.* **8**, 232–253 (1979).
5. Kutt, H., and Penry S. F., Usefulness of blood levels of antiepileptic drugs. *Arch. Neurol.* **31**, 283–288 (1974).
6. Penry, J. K., and Newmark, M. E., The use of antiepileptic drugs. *Ann. Intern. Med.* **90**, 207–218 (1979).
7. Reynolds, E. H., Fenton, G., Fenwick, P., Johnson, A. L., and Laundy, M., Interaction of phenytoin and primidone. *Br. Med. J.* **ii**, 594–595 (1975).
8. Sutton, G., and Kupferberg, H. J., Isoniazid as an inhibitor of primidone metabolism. *Neurology* **25**, 1179–1181 (1975).
9. Stern, E. L., Possible phenylethylmalondiamide (PEMA) intoxication. *Ann. Neurol.* **2**, 356–357 (1977).
10. Brillman, J., Gallagher, B. B., and Mattson, R. H., Acute primidone intoxication. *Arch. Neurol.* **30**, 255–258 (1974).
11. Cate, J. C., and Tenser, R., Acute primidone overdosage with massive crystalluria. *Clin. Toxicol.* **8**, 385–389 (1975).
12. Martinez, G., and Snyder R. D., Transplacental passage of primidone. *Neurology* **23**, 381–383 (1973).

Prolactin

Specimen Tested:

S.

Laboratories Reporting:

3.

Reference (Normal) Values:

Age	ng/mL		
	Lab. 1	**Lab. 2**	**Lab. 3**
Newborn			
Premature	169		
Full-term	280		
4 wk	75		
12 wk, full-term	adult range		
20 wk, premature	adult range		
Adult	0–30	0–20	M $<$ F
			F $<$ 25

Sources of Reference (Normal) Values:

Lab. 1: institutional; Perlman, M., Schenker, J., Glassman, M., and Ben-David, M., Prolonged hyperprolactinemia in preterm infants. *J. Clin. Endocrinol. Metab.* **47,** 894–897 (1978). **Lab. 2:** *Radioimmunoassay Manual,* 4th ed., Nichols Institute, San Pedro, CA, 1977, pp 307–309; Perlman et al., *op. cit.*

Specimen Volume, Collection, and Preservation:

50 μL. Collect B in chilled tubes. Transport in ice bath. Centrifuge B in refrigerated centrifuge and promptly remove S. Store in FR.

Analytical Method:

RIA, double antibody, ^{125}I-labeled prolactin; Nichols Institute; Precision Assays.

Instrumentation:

Gamma counter.

Commentary—Joan H. and Peter J. Howanitz

During the first trimester of pregnancy, when prolactin concentrations in the serum of the mother or fetus are 20 to 50 ng/mL, prolactin concentrations in amniotic fluid are as great as 10 000 ng/mL *(1)*.

Amniotic fluid prolactin steadily decreases between the 10th and 40th gestational weeks (2) and at term is usually in the range of 300 to 1500 ng/mL (1).

In the fetus, prolactin concentrations progressively increase from the 16th gestational week to term, reaching 300 to 500 ng/mL in late gestation (2,3). At delivery the mean cord prolactin concentration is about 165 ng/mL (3,4). During the first 30 min after birth, a significant prolactin surge occurs, peaking within the first 120 min of extrauterine life (4). In the full-term infant, prolactin values exceed those of premature infants the first day after birth (mean, 267 and 156 ng/mL, respectively), but are similar in both by the age of two to four weeks (mean for each, 69 ng/mL) (5). In full-term infants, prolactin concentrations decrease to a mean value of 24 ng/mL in four to 12 weeks, while in the premature infant, similar values are not reached until 12 to 20 weeks postnatally (5). Neonatal prolactin values show no sex-related differences (6,7).

After the newborn period, concentrations of prolactin during the remainder of the first year of life in both boys and girls have a mean value of about 10 ng/mL; by the age of two to 12 years, mean prolactin concentrations are about 5 ng/mL (7). Before puberty, there is no significant difference between prolactin concentrations in boys and girls (8); in men, however, prepubertal prolactin concentrations are maintained throughout life, while in normal women the higher prolactin concentrations reached during puberty are maintained until menopause (9).

Although prolactin deficiency is rare, it may occur in clinical situations such as pituitary necrosis or infarction (10). An undetectable prolactin concentration is not clinically significant in itself, occasionally occurring in normal persons. Low prolactin concentrations in cord blood may be important. It has been suggested that prolactin is involved in fetal lung maturation as well as surfactant formation (11). The incidence of respiratory distress syndrome is reportedly significantly greater in infants with low prolactin concentrations (11).

Prolactin increases occur in several circumstances, including in normal physiologic states, in patients treated with certain drugs, and in some pathologic conditions (Table 1). Sleep is an important physiologic factor affecting prolactin secretion. After the onset of sleep, prolactin increases progressively, reaching the highest concentrations in early morning (12). Altering the timing of the sleep period changes the prolactin secretory pattern, indicating that this is not an inherent neural rhythm. Prolactin concentrations also show random fluctuations of a brief episodic variety, and increase in response to stimuli such as hypoglycemia and stress (12).

Many drugs may cause hyperprolactinemia (Table 1), as may several pathologic conditions, including hypothyroidism and renal failure (12). Persistent hyperprolactinemia in the absence of obvious

Table 1. Some Causes of Increased Serum Prolactin Concentrations

Physiologic	Pharmacologic	Pathologic
Newborn	Estrogen	Prolactin-secreting
Stress (physical and	Haloperidol	pituitary tumors
mental)	Meprobamate	Hypothalamic disorders
Sleep	α-Methyldopa	Pituitary stalk section
Pregnancy	Monoamine oxidase in-	Acromegaly
Nursing	hibitors (clorgyline,	Nelson's syndrome
Luteal phase of	pargyline)	Hypothyroidism
menstrual cycle (?)	Phenothiazines	Renal failure
	Reserpine	Ectopic production by
	Thyrotropin-releasing	malignant tumors
	hormone (TRH; thyroliberin)	
	Tricyclic anti-depressants	

causes such as drug ingestion suggests a hypothalamic or pituitary lesion. Hyperprolactinemia occurs in a large percentage of patients with pituitary tumors. In a recently reported series, 79% of patients with pituitary tumors had increased prolactin concentrations *(13)*. Other studies indicate that patients with very high prolactin concentrations (greater than 300 ng/mL) have an extremely high incidence of pituitary tumors *(14)*.

To determine the etiology of hyperprolactinemia, investigators have studied the response of prolactin to various pharmacologic agents. Thyrotropin-releasing hormone (TRH; thyroliberin) and the phenothiazine drug chlorpromazine have been used to stimulate prolactin secretion, whereas drugs such as bromocriptine and L-dopa have been used to suppress its secretion. Several investigators suggest that prolactin response to stimulatory and inhibitory agents may be useful in determining the cause of hyperprolactinemia *(15,16)*.

1. Friesen, H., and Hwang, P., Human prolactin. *Ann. Rev. Med.* **24**, 251–270 (1973).
2. Winters, A. J., Colston, C., MacDonald, P. C., and Porter, J. C., Fetal plasma prolactin levels. *J. Clin. Endocrinol. Metab.* **41**, 626–629 (1975).
3. Aubert, M. L., Grumbach, M. M., and Kaplan, S. L., The ontogenesis of human fetal hormones. *J. Clin. Invest.* **56**, 155–164 (1975).
4. Sack, J., Fisher, D. A., and Wang, C. C., Serum thyrotropin prolactin and growth hormone levels during the early neonatal period in the human infant. *J. Pediatr.* **89**, 298–300 (1976).
5. Perlman, M., Schenker, J., Glassman, M., and Ben-David, M., Prolonged hyperprolactinemia in preterm infants. *J. Clin. Endocrinol. Metab.* **47**, 894–897 (1978).
6. Badawi, M., Van Exter, C., Delogne-Desnoeck, J., Van Meenen, F., and Robyn, C., Cord serum prolactin in relation to the time of day, the sex of the neonate and the birth weight. *Acta Endocrinol.* **87**, 241–247 (1978).
7. Guyda, H. J., and Friesen, H. G., Serum prolactin levels in humans from birth to adult life. *Pediatr. Res.* **7**, 534–540 (1973).

8. Thorner, M. O., Round, J., Jones, A., Fahmy, D., Groom, G. V., Butcher, S., and Thompson, K., Serum prolactin and oestradiol levels at different stages of puberty. *Clin. Endocrinol.* **7,** 463–468 (1977).
9. Prolactin update. *Br. Med. J.* **ii,** 846–848 (1977). Editorial.
10. Thorner, M. O., Prolactin. *Clin. Endocrinol. Metab.* **6,** 201–222 (1977).
11. Hauth, J. C., Parker, C. R., MacDonald, P. C., Porter, J. C., and Johnston, J. M., A role of fetal prolactin in lung maturation. *Obstet. Gynecol.* **51,** 81–88 (1978).
12. L'Hermite, M., Prolactin. In *Hormone Assays and Their Clinical Application,* J. A. Loraine and E. T. Bell, Eds. Churchill-Livingstone, Edinburgh, 1976, pp 293–332.
13. Antunes, J. L., Housepian, E. M., Frantz, A. G., Holub, D. A., Hui, R. M., Carmel, P. W., and Quest, D. O., Prolactin-secreting pituitary tumors. *Ann. Neurol.* **2,** 148–153 (1977).
14. Kleinberg, D. A., Noel, G. L., and Frantz, A. G., Galactorrhea: A study of 235 cases, including 48 with pituitary tumors. *N. Engl. J. Med.* **296,** 589–600 (1977).
15. Ayalon, D., Persitz, E., Ravid, R., Jedwab, G., Avidan, S., Cordova, T., and Harell, A., The diagnostic value of pharmacodynamic tests in the hyperprolactinaemic syndrome. *Clin. Endocrinol.* **11,** 201–215 (1979).
16. Cowden, E. A., Thomson, J. A., Doyle, D., Ratcliffe, J. G., MacPherson, P., and Teasdale, G. M., Tests of prolactin secretion in diagnosis of prolactinomas. *Lancet* **i,** 1155–1158 (1979).

Protein, Total, and Electrophoresis of

Total Protein in Cerebrospinal Fluid

Laboratories Reporting:

6.

Reference (Normal) Values:

	Total protein, mg/L	
Age	Labs. 1–4	Labs. 5, 6
Newborn	400–1200	400–1200
Up to 1 mo	200–800	
>1 mo	150–400	
Child–adult	150–450	150–450

Sources of Reference (Normal) Values:

Institutional; text ref. 2, p 287.

Specimen Volume, Collection, and Preservation:

Labs. 1–4: 50 μL to 1.00 mL; **Labs. 5, 6:** 50 μL. Proteins in CSF are presumed stable for 2 d at RT, 2 wk in RR, indefinitely in FR.

Analytical Method:

Labs. 1–4: nephelometry; Meulemans, O., Determination of total protein in spinal fluid with sulphosalicylic acid and trichloroacetic acid. *Clin. Chim. Acta* **5,** 757–761 (1960); text ref. *2,* p 287; Rice, E. W., and Arnold, L. H., Clinical nephelometry: 2. Accurate nephelometric ultramicro method for determination of total proteins in cerebrospinal fluid. *Clin. Biochem.* **7,** 91–93 (1944); *Gradwohl's Clinical Laboratory Methods and Diagnosis,* 6th ed., vol. **1,** S. Frankel and S. Reitman, Eds. C. V. Mosby Co., St. Louis, MO, 1963, pp 49–50. **Labs. 5, 6:** Pesce, M. A., and Strande, C. S., A new micromethod for the determination of protein in cerebrospinal fluid and urine. *Clin. Chem.* **19,** 1265–1267 (1973).

Instrumentation:

Gilford Stasar II, III, Beckman 25, Micromedic MS 2, Coleman Jr. II spectrophotometers; Hach Chemical Co. 2424 Clinical Nephelometer.

Electrophoresis of Proteins in Cerebrospinal Fluid

Laboratory Reporting:

1.

Reference (Normal) Values:

Fraction (adult)	% of total protein
Pre-albumin	4–6
Albumin	56–67
α_1-Globulin	3–6
α_2-Globulin	5–8.5
β-Globulin	10–17
γ-Globulin	6–10

Sources of Reference (Normal) Values:

Kaplan, A., and Savory, J., Cellulose acetate electrophoresis of proteins of serum, cerebrospinal fluid, and urine. *Stand. Methods Clin. Chem.* **6,** 13–30 (1970).

Specimen Volume:

5 μL. See preceding report for preservation information.

Analytical Method and Instrumentation:

Concentration of CSF by Amicon ultrafiltration to 4 g/dL; cellulose acetate electrophoresis, as with serum (see following report, p 382); Beckman R-101 Microzone electrophoresis equipment and R-110 densitometer.

Commentary—Leonard K. Dunikoski, Jr.

As for serum protein electrophoresis *(q.v.)*, cellulose acetate is the support medium most commonly used for CSF protein electrophoresis. Specimens may be concentrated by use of Amicon membrane (Amicon Corp.) or by ultrafiltration under reduced pressure (Schleicher & Schuell, Inc.). Cellulose acetate electrophoresis separates the CSF protein into six fractions, pre-albumin plus the five fractions seen in serum. Agarose gel yields increased resolution when used as a support medium (see Commentary on **Serum protein electrophoresis**). For cellulose acetate, about 75% of patients with multiple sclerosis have an increased CSF gamma-globulin. With agarose gel, however, more than 90% of patients with multiple sclerosis display two or more discrete IgG (oligoclonal IgG) in CSF; this oligoclonal pattern is not specific for the disease if similar bands are seen in serum, so agarose gel electrophoresis of serum should be performed at the same time *(1)*.

1. Johnson, K. P., Arrigo, S. C., and Nelson, B. J., Agarose electrophoresis of cerebrospinal fluid in multiple sclerosis. *Neurology* **27**, 273–277 (1977).

Commentary—Michael A. Pesce

CSF is a colorless liquid usually obtained by lumbar puncture. A yellow color is usually caused by bilirubin, methemoglobin, or oxyhemoglobin, whereas the presence of blood indicates either a traumatic puncture or a hemorrhage in the central nervous system. The normal range of CSF total protein varies with age, and in normal adults in less than 45 mg/dL. For full-term infants the range is from 40 to 120 mg/dL, and in normal premature infants CSF protein ranges between 50 and 200 mg/dL but may be as much as 400 mg/dL *(1)*. The values observed in the newborn rapidly decline and reach adult values at about five months. The nephelometric *(2)* and Ponceau S dye-binding methods *(3)* reported here require only 50 µL of CSF to measure protein concentrations. Bilirubin, up to 4 mg/dL, and the drugs sulfisoxazole, salicylate, and sulfadiazine do not interfere with this dye-binding method. The ratio of albumin to gamma-globulin in the CSF does not significantly affect the protein results obtained by this dye-binding technique.

Above-normal concentrations of protein in CSF are due either to increased synthesis of one or several proteins within the central nervous system or to damage to the blood/CSF barrier, resulting in increased passage of serum proteins into CSF. Increased concentrations of CSF proteins are usually observed in meningitis.

1. Bauer, C. H., New, M. I., and Miller, J. M., Cerebrospinal fluid protein values of premature infants. *J. Pediatr.* **66**, 1017–1022 (1965).

2. Rice, E. W., and Arnold, L. H., Clinical nephelometry: 2. Accurate nephelo-metric ultramicro method for determination of total proteins in cerebro-spinal fluid. *Clin. Biochem.* **7**, 91–93 (1974).
3. Pesce, M. A., and Strande, C. S., A new micromethod for determination of protein in cerebrospinal fluid and urine. *Clin. Chem.* **19**, 1265–1267 (1973).

Total Protein in Serum and Urine

Specimen Tested:

S, U.

Laboratories Reporting:

7.

Reference (Normal) Values:

Age	Total serum proteins, g/L	
	Labs. 1–5	**Labs. 6, 7**
Cord	53–67	
"At birth"		46–70
Premature, 1 wk	44–76; 43–76	
Full-term, 1 wk	47–74	
"Newborn"	40–68	
6 wk–18 mo	50–71	
<2 mo	54–74	
2 mo–2 yr	62–83	
3 mo		45–65
3–4 mo	42–74	
1 yr, premature	58–71	
1 yr, full-term	56–72; 61–67	54–75
18 mo–3 yr	55–71	
2–8 yr	65–87	
2 yr–adult		53–80
3–16 yr	58–77	
Child		55–80
4 yr–adult	59–80; 62–81	
8–12 yr	67–92	
>12 yr		M: 65–84 F: 63–83
12–14 yr	62–87	
14–16 yr	64–90	
16 yr–adult	65–85	
Adult	64–78	

U (1 lab.): >1 yr: <100 mg/m^2 of body surface per day

Sources of Reference (Normal) Values:

Labs. 1, 3, 5, 6: institutional. **Lab. 2:** a retrospective study of 449 pediatric and 150 adult patient charts. Subjects included in the data are free of infectious or inflammatory disease, malignancy, and ane-mia. **Lab. 4:** Cheng, M. H., Lipsey, A. I., Blanco, V., Wong, H. T., and Spiro, S. H., Microchemical analysis for 13 constituents of plasma from healthy children. *Clin. Chem.* **25,** 692–698 (1979).

Specimen Volume, Collection, and Preservation:

5 to 30 µL, generally. There is a claim of long stability at RT (1 wk), and 1 mo in RR.

Analytical Method:

Lab. 1–5: biuret method; Weichselbaum, T. E., An accurate and rapid method for the determination of proteins in small amounts of blood serum and plasma. *Am. J. Clin. Pathol.* **10,** 40–49 (1946); Kingsley, G. R., Procedure for serum protein determination with triphosphate biuret reagent. *Stand. Methods Clin. Chem.* **7,** 199–207 (1972); Koch, T. R., Johnson, G. F., and Chilcote, M. E., Kinetic determination of total serum protein with a centrifugal analyzer. *Clin. Chem.* **20,** 392–394 (1974); Technicon methodology manual; Skeggs, L. T., Jr., and Hochstrasser, H., Multiple automatic sequential analyses. *Clin. Chem.* **10,** 918–936 (1964); Gornall, A. G., Bardawill, C. J., and David, M. M., Determination of serum proteins by means of the biuret reaction. *J. Biol. Chem.* **177,** 751–766 (1949). **Labs. 6, 7:** refractometry.

Instrumentation:

Labs. 1–5: Gilford Stasar II spectrophotometer; Abbott ABA-100 Bichromatic Analyzer; Electro-Nucleonics Inc. Gemeni centrifugal analyzer; Technicon SMA II and SMAC. **Labs. 6, 7:** American Optical Total Solids Meter.

Commentary—Gregory J. Buffone

Normal Physiological Variation

1. *Neonatal and childhood period.* Total protein concentration gradually increases during gestation. By 35 to 39 weeks the protein concentration is usually between 45 and 65 g/L *(1,2)*. Hypoproteinemia of the neonate, usually seen in premature infants, is characterized by a decrease in all major protein fractions and a lag in the rate of increase in protein concentration during the first year of life. In the healthy newborn the major protein fractions, except the immunoglobulins, reach a steady-state concentration by age of six months. The concentrations of the five major immunoglobulin classes can vary significantly up to the age of three to five years. Immunoglobulin G is unique, in that IgG from the mother crosses the placenta and for the first few months of life provides the infant with IgG concentration and specificity very similar to that of the mother. The nadir in IgG concentration is usually seen at about three months of age *(3)*.

2. *Adolescence.* Changes in the concentrations of various hormones during early adolescence can directly and indirectly affect the concen-

tration of transport and storage proteins. Among the most notable examples of the changes seen with increased estrogen production or therapeutic administration is the increase in the concentration of α_2-macroglobulin and fibrinogen, and the decrease in antithrombin III concentration *(4,5)*. Likewise, the onset of menstruation and the associated chronic blood loss can influence changes in transferrin and ferritin concentration.

Methods

Total and specific protein measurements can be done on serum samples collected by skin puncture, and can be handled at ambient temperature for most of the proteins of clinical interest. Total protein is commonly measured by use of the biuret reaction. Because this method is "standard" for laboratory use, reagent formulation has become fairly uniform among laboratories *(6)*.

1. Baum, J. D., Eisenberg, C., Franklin, F. A., Jr., Meschia, G., and Battaglia, F. C., Studies on colloid osmotic pressure in the fetus and newborn infant. *Biol. Neonate* **18,** 311–320 (1971).
2. Baum, J. D., and Harris, D., Colloid osmotic pressure in erythroblastosis fetalis. *Br. Med. J.* **i,** 601–603 (1972).
3. Ritzmann, S. E., Immunoglobulin abnormalities. In *Serum Protein Abnormalities*, S. E. Ritzmann and J. C. Daniels, Eds. Little, Brown, and Co., Boston, MA, 1975, pp 351–486.
4. Horne, C. H. W., Howie, P. W., Goudie, R. B., and Weir, R. J., Effects of combined estrogen–progestogen oral contraceptives on serum levels of α_2-macroglobulin, transferrin, albumin and IgG. *Lancet* **i,** 49–50 (1970).
5. Fagerhol, M. K., and Abilgaard, U., Immunological studies on human antithrombin III. Influence of age, sex, and use of oral contraceptives on serum concentration. *Scand. J. Haematol.* **7,** 7–10 (1970).
6. Kingsley, G. R., Procedure for serum protein determinations. *Stand. Methods Clin. Chem.* **7,** 199–207 (1972).

Electrophoresis of Proteins in Serum

Laboratories Reporting:

2.

Reference (Normal) Values:

			g/L			
Age	**Total protein**	**Albu- min**	**α_1-Globu- lin**	**α_2-Globu- lin**	**β-Globu- lin**	**γ-Globu- lin**
At birth	46–70	32–48	1–3	2–6	3–6	6–12
Newborn, 1 wk	44–76	29–55	0.9–25	3–4.6	1.6–6	3.5–13
3 mo	45–65	32–48	1–3	3–7	3–7	2–7
3–4 mo	42–74	28–50	0.7–3.9	3.1–8.3	3.1–8.3	1.1–7.5
1 yr	56–72	39–51	1–3.4	2.8–8.0	3.8–8.6	3.5–7.5
	54–75	37–57	1–3	5–11	4–10	2–9
2 yr–adult	53–80	33–58	1–3	4–10	3–12	4–14
>4 yr	59–80	38–54	1–3.4	3.5–8.0	5–10	3.5–13

Sources of Reference (Normal) Values:

Institutional.

Specimen Volume, Collection, and Preservation:

0.6 to 5 μL. See preceding report for details.

Analytical Method and Instrumentation:

Beckman Microzone R101 Electrophoresis apparatus; R 101 and R 115 Densitometer; cellulose acetate electrophoresis.

Commentary—Michael A. Pesce

On cellulose acetate membranes at alkaline pH, proteins in normal serum are separated by electrophoresis into five fractions: albumin, α_1-globulins, α_2-globulins, β-globulins, and γ-globulins. Serum protein electrophoresis is useful in detecting nephrosis, liver damage, hypogammaglobulinemia, bisalbuminemia, and disorders involving abnormal production of immunoglobulins. In nephrosis the albumin and α_1-globulin fractions are decreased, and the α_2-globulin fraction is increased. In liver disease the γ-globulin fraction is usually increased and diffuse, and the albumin fraction is decreased. Bisalbuminemia is an asymptomatic genetic disorder characterized by two albumin peaks of about equal intensity. Hypogammaglobulinemia can be congenital, physiological, or secondary to other disorders and is characterized by γ-globulin concentrations of less than 0.25 g/dL. In adults a large monoclonal band migrating in the globulin region of the electropherogram is usually indicative of a plasma cell dyscrasia.

Normal values for the protein fractions vary with age. In newborns albumin concentration is low and the γ-globulins are high. Albumin values increase with age and reach adult concentrations by about 10 years of age. The γ-globulins decrease to their lowest values at about four months of age, then gradually increase and reach adult values by about age 13 years. Concentrations of the α_2- and β-globulins are low at birth and usually reach adult values by 12 months. The α_1-globulin concentrations are not significantly affected by age. Serum is ordinarily used to fractionate the proteins because plasma contains fibrinogen, which migrates as a sixth distinct fraction between the β- and α-globulin region of the electropherogram and is easily mistaken for an abnormal immunoglobulin. Serum stored at 4 °C for one week does not show any change in the protein patterns.

Commentary—Leonard K. Dunikoski, Jr.

Because agarose gel allows increased resolution, its use as a support medium for protein electrophoresis has increased dramatically in the clinical laboratory. With use of commercially available reagents (Worthington Diagnostics) and alkaline buffer containing calcium ion, plasma may be separated into nine to 12 distinct fractions. Because 12 major proteins constitute more than 95% of the plasma protein mass, a considerable amount of information may be obtained by this technique. Several of the fractions are so well resolved that they generally represent a single specific protein: prealbumin, albumin, α_1-antitrypsin, transferrin, C3 complement, and fibrinogen are in this category. Visual inspection of these fractions after staining can yield excellent estimations of plasma concentrations at a much lower cost than individual immunochemical assays. Quantitative data for α_1-antitrypsin and transferrin have been obtained by densitometric scanning of the agarose gel (1), but critical visual inspection can often provide more clinically relevant information than scanning, especially when combined with supplementary specific analysis of a few selected proteins (2). Unlike protein electrophoresis in geriatric adult populations, where serum is the specimen of choice, use of plasma is preferred here because it permits the estimation of fibrinogen content. The use of EDTA anticoagulation to obtain plasma also activates fewer proteases during venipuncture, therefore providing greater stability for labile C3 and C4 components.

1. Dunikoski, L. K., and Kiefer, L., Electrophoretic quantitation of alpha-1-antitrypsin and transferrin. *Clin. Chem.* **22,** 1200 (1976). Abstract.
2. Laurell, C. B., Electrophoresis, specific protein assays, or both in measurement of plasma proteins? *Clin. Chem.* **19,** 99–102 (1973).

Pyruvate

Specimen Tested:

B.

Laboratories Reporting:

2.

Reference (Normal) Values:

	Lab. 1	Lab. 2
Adult (fasting, venous B)	34–102 μmol/L	40–70 μmol/L

Sources of Reference (Normal) Values:

Text ref. 5, 2nd ed., p 941; Bio-Dynamics/*bmc* kit insert.

Specimen Volume, Collection, and Preservation; Patient Preparation:

1 to 2 mL. Collect B without stasis. Place B into 10% (100 mg/L) trichloracetic acid solution (**Lab. 1**) or into ice-cold perchloric acid (**Lab. 2**). The protein-free supernate is relatively stable. Sample should be obtained from a resting individual, which may necessitate use of an indwelling catheter so that the child is not disturbed by a venipuncture.

Analytical Method:

Lab. 1: enzymic; Scholz, R., Schmitz, H., Bucher, T., and Lampen, J. O., Uber die Wirkung von Nystatin auf backer Hefe. *Biochem. Z.* **331,** 71 (1959). **Lab. 2:** Bio-Dynamics/*bmc* kit insert; Bergmeyer, H. U., Ed., *Methods of Enzymatic Analysis,* **3,** 2nd English ed. Academic Press, New York, NY, 1974, p. 1446.

Instrumentation:

Zeiss and Varian 635 spectrophotometers.

Note: See Commentary for **Lactate.**

Pyruvate Kinase (EC 2.7.1.40; ATP:pyruvate 2-*O*-phosphotransferase)

Specimen Tested:

Erythrocytes.

Laboratories Reporting:

2.

Reference (Normal) Values:

Lab. 1:   7.4–15.7 U/g of hemoglobin
Lab. 2:   1.8–2.3 U/mL of erythrocytes

Sources of Reference (Normal) Values:

Lab. 1: Powell, R. D., and DeGowin, R. L., Relationship between the activity of pyruvate kinase and age of the normal human erythrocyte. *Nature* **205,** 507 (1965). **Lab. 2:** institutional.

Specimen Volume, Collection, and Preservation:

Lab. 1: 100 µL; **Lab. 2:** 5 µL. Heparin or EDTA as anticoagulant. The separated cells are stable for at least 2 wk in RR. There are claims that this enzyme is stable in Alsever's solution for 3.5 wk, or in heparin at RT for 8 d. Do *not* freeze.

Analytical Method:

Lab. 1: Tanaka, K. R., Valentine, W. N., and Miwa, S., Pyruvate kinase (PK) deficiency and hereditary nonspherocytic hemolytic anemia. *Blood* **19,** 267–294 (1962); Bucher, T., and Pfleiderer, G., Pyruvate kinase from muscle. In *Methods in Enzymology,* **1B,** S. P. Colowick and N. O. Kaplan, Eds. Academic Press, New York, NY, 1955, p 435. **Lab. 2:** Oski, F. A., and Diamond, L. K., Erythrocyte pyruvate kinase deficiency resulting in congenital nonspherocytic hemolytic anemia. *N. Engl. J. Med.* **269,** 763–770 (1963); Princeton Biomedix kit.

Enzyme Data:

Lab. 1:
1. Enzyme unit definition: 1 IUB unit (U) = 1 μmol of substrate transformed per minute.
2. Buffer, pH: Tris, 7.5.
3. Substrate: phosphoenolpyruvate.
4. Reaction temperature: 37 °C.
5. Temperature reported: 37 °C.

Lab. 2:
1. Enzyme unit definition: 1 IUB unit (U) = 1 μmol of substrate transformed per minute.
2. Buffer, pH: glycylglycine, 7.5.
3. Substrate, pH: phosphoenolpyruvate, 7.5.
4. Reaction temperature: 30 °C.
5. Temperature reported: 30 °C.

Instrumentation:

Beckman 25, 35 spectrophotometers.

Renin Activity, Plasma

Specimen Tested:
P.

Laboratories Reporting:
2.

Reference (Normal) Values:

Lab. (or ref.[a])	Age	ng/mL per hour[b]
Kotchen et al.	Newborn, 3–6 d	11.6 ± 2.8 (SEM)
Lab. 2	<3 mo	wide range, with values as high as 48 (particularly high in premature)
Lab. 2	3 mo–1 yr	<15
Stalker et al.	4 mo–3 yr	4.6 ± 1.6 (SEM)
Lab. 2	1–4 yr	<10
Lab. 1	3–8 yr	<6
Lab. 1	9–12 yr	<3
Lab. 2	4–15 yr	<6
Lab. 1	13–15 yr	<2
Lab. 2	Adult	<2
Kotchen et al.	Adult	0.70 ± 0.10 (SEM)

[a] Kotchen, T. A., Strickland, A. L., Rice, T. W., and Walters, D. R., A study of the renin–angiotensin system in newborn infants. *J. Pediatr.* **80**, 938–946 (1972); Stalker, H. P., Holland, N. H., Kotchen, J. M., and Kotchen, T. A., Plasma renin activity in healthy children. *J. Pediatr.* **89**, 256–258 (1976).

[b] Values based on samples taken from subjects on "normal" salt intake, supine after 2-h rest, and between 0900 and 1100 hours.

Sources of Reference (Normal) Values:

Lab. 1: Smith, E. K., Mauseth, R., and Kenny, M. A., Plasma renin activity in healthy children (unpublished data). **Lab. 2:** institutional; Kotchen et al., *op. cit.;* Stalker et al., *op. cit.*

Specimen Volume, Collection, and Preservation:

0.5 to 1.5 mL. EDTA as anticoagulant. Collect B in tube on ice. Centrifuge immediately in refrigerated centrifuge (4 °C). Promptly remove P, and without delay freeze the P for assay.

Analytical Method:

RIA; Haber, E., Koerner, T., Page, L. B., Kliman, B., and Purnode, A., Application of a radioimmunoassay for angiotensin I to the physiologic measurements of plasma renin activity in normal human subjects. *J. Clin. Endocrinol. Metab.* **29**, 1349–1355 (1969).

Instrumentation:

Gamma counter.

Commentary—Elizabeth K. Smith

Renin, a proteolytic enzyme produced in the juxtaglomerular apparatus of the kidney, acts on circulating renin substrate (angiotensinogen) from the liver to form the decapeptide angiotensin I. Enzymes in the lung convert angiotensin I to the octapeptide angiotensin II, which has potent biologic actions as a vasopressor and as a releaser of aldosterone from the zona glomerulosa of the adrenal cortex.

Plasma renin activity is measured by RIA of angiotensin I and reported as the quantity produced per milliliter of plasma per hour at 37 °C. Careful blood collection is imperative: blood must be collected with EDTA in a prechilled tube placed in ice and centrifuged as soon as possible at 4 °C, and the plasma must be separated immediately and stored frozen until assayed.

Renin activities vary widely in normal individuals; they are specifically influenced by posture (higher in upright than in recumbent position) (1), time of day (highest early in the day), salt intake (increased with low-sodium diet), and medication. Reference intervals usually are stated in relation to position and sodium intake. Plasma renin activity is age-dependent, being very high and widely variable in newborns and young infants (2). Healthy premature infants have even higher values; Sylyok et al. reported a mean of 18.2 ± 4.1 ng/mL per hour, which remains high until six weeks of age (3). Values decrease gradually during childhood to adult values.

The effect of age and posture upon plasma renin activity in children was demonstrated in a study of 38 healthy children, ages three to 15 years, who had a normal salt intake. Blood was drawn at 0800 hours with the subject ambulatory, and again after resting, supine, for 2 h. Differences among the three age groups and between upright and supine posture were statistically significant at $p < 0.01$ (4).

Age (and no.) of subjects	ng/mL per 3 h at 37 °C[a]	
	Ambulatory, upright	Resting 2 h, supine
3–8 yr (15)	3.47 ± 2.27	2.33 ± 1.63
9–12 yr (13)	3.00 ± 1.70	1.20 ± 0.73
13–15 yr (10)	2.66 ± 1.63	0.80 ± 0.50

[a] Mean ± 1 SD.

Measurement of plasma renin activity is useful in evaluation of hypertension; values tend to be increased in patients with hypertension of renal origin. In children these values are a useful guide to adequacy of mineralocorticoid-replacement therapy in the salt-losing form of congenital adrenal hyperplasia. Children with this disorder, untreated, have markedly increased plasma renin activity, the degree of increase being related to the severity of the deficiency of 21-hydroxylase. With appropriate mineralocorticoid therapy, plasma renin activity will return to normal limits for age.

1. Haber, E., Koerner, T., Page, L. B., Kliman, B., and Purnode, A., Application of radioimmunoassay for angiotensin I to the physiologic measurements of plasma renin activity in normal human subjects. *J. Clin. Endocrinol. Metab.* **29,** 1349–1355 (1969).

2. Kotchen, T. A., Strickland, A. L., Rice, T. W., and Walters, D. R., A study of renin-angiotensin system in newborn infants. *J. Pediatr.* **80,** 938–946 (1972).
3. Sylyok, E., Neneth, M., Tenyi, I., Csaba, I., Gyorgy, E., Ertl, T., and Varga, F., Postnatal development of renin–angiotensin–aldosterone system, RAAS, in relation to electrolyte balance in premature infants. *Pediatr. Res.* **13,** 817–820 (1979).
4. Mauseth, R., Smith, E. K., and Kenny, M. A., Plasma renin activity (PRA) in children: Supine versus ambulatory. *Clin. Res.* **28,** 95A (1980). Abstract.

Salicylate

Specimen Tested:

P, S.

Laboratories Reporting:

6.

Reference (Normal) Values:

Four labs. report that the therapeutic level (maximum anti-inflammatory effect) is 10–20 mg/dL (0.72–1.45 mmol/L). Toxicity may appear in the range of 20–30 (1.45–2.17), although 1 lab. regards this range as therapeutic. At >30 (2.17) toxicity will definitely occur.

Sources of Reference (Normal) Values:

Institutional: Levy, G., and Tsuchiya, T., Salicylate accumulation kinetics in man. *N. Engl. J. Med.* **287,** 430–432 (1972); see also the nomogram in Done, A. K., Salicylate intoxication. Significance of measurements of salicylate in blood in cases of acute ingestion. *Pediatrics* **26,** 800–807 (1960).

Specimen Volume, Collection, and Preservation:

10 to 100 μL, generally. Heparin or EDTA as anticoagulant. Salicylate is stable in P stored in RR for 2 mo.

Analytical Method:

Five labs use ferric ion–phenol reaction: MacDonald, R. P., Salicylate. *Stand. Methods Clin. Chem.* **5,** 237–243 (1965); Annino, J. S., *Clinical Chemistry: Principles and Procedures,* 4th ed. Little, Brown and Co., Boston, MA, 1976, pp 355–357; Trinder, P., Rapid determination of salicylate in biological materials. *Biochem. J.* **57,** 301–303 (1954); Keller, W. J., Jr., A rapid method for the determination of salicylates in serum or plasma. *Am. J. Clin. Pathol.* **17,** 415–417 (1947); text ref. 3. One lab. uses a microfluorometric procedure: Jacobs, J. C., and Pesce, M. A., Micromeasurement of plasma salicylate in arthritic children. *Arthritis Rheum.* **21,** 129–132 (1978).

Instrumentation:

Labs. 1–5: spectrophotometers: Gilford 300 N, Stasar II, III, Hitachi 102, Coleman Jr. II. **Lab. 6:** Farrand Mark 1 spectrofluorometer.

Commentary—Michael A. Pesce

Salicylates are among the most widely used analgesic drugs. Because of their widespread use and availability, salicylate intoxication is a frequent cause of accidental poisoning in children. As a therapeutic drug, salicylates are the mainstay of treatment for children with rheumatoid arthritis. Frequent monitoring of plasma salicylate concentrations in these children may be expected to provide greater therapeutic efficacy with less incidence of aspirin toxicity.

Salicylate can be measured in plasma either colorimetrically by reaction with ferric ions, or by a microfluorometric procedure involving precipitating the proteins and mixing an aliquot of the supernate with sodium hydroxide *(1)*. The salicylate values obtained with the microfluorometric system are about 7% lower than those obtained by the colorimetric method of Trinder *(2)*. Samples containing the drugs prednisone, erythromycin, ampicillin, penicillin G, and indomethacin did not interfere with this fluorometric system. With the microfluorometric method, blood can be collected by skin puncture. This is a distinct advantage over methods involving venipuncture techniques, especially in the management of young children with juvenile rheumatoid arthritis, who require frequent monitoring of their salicylate concentrations.

There is no difference in salicylate values obtained from serum or plasma. Salicylate is stable for at least one week in serum stored at 4 °C.

1. Jacobs, J. C., and Pesce, M. A., Micromeasurement of plasma salicylate in arthritic children. *Arthritis Rheum.* **21,** 129–132 (1978).
2. Trinder, P., Rapid determination of salicylates in biological materials. *Biochem. J.* **57,** 301–303 (1954).

Sedimentation Rate, Erythrocyte

Specimen Tested:

B.

Laboratory Reporting:

1.

Reference (Normal) Values:

Up to 2 yr: 1–5 mm/h
2 yr–adult: 1–8 mm/h

Sources of Reference (Normal) Values:

Institutional.

Specimen Volume, Collection, and Preservation:

200 μL. Sodium citrate anticoagulant. Sample must be mixed properly with anticoagulant, and free of clots.

Analytical Method:

Landau, A., Microsedimentation (Linzenmeier–Raunert) method, its serviceability and significance in pediatrics; use of a modified apparatus with simplified technic; also serviceable in ambulant practice. *Am. J. Dis. Child.* **45,** 691–734 (1933).

Instrumentation:

Micro Landau-sedimentation pipette, Fisher Scientific Co.

Somatomedin-C

Specimen Tested:

P.

Laboratory Reporting:

1.

Reference (Normal) Values:

Cord:	0.5 int. units/mL (mean)
Up to 2 yr:	rapid increase to adult values
Adolescent:	> adult; F > M
Adult > 18 yr:	0.4–2.0 int. units/mL

Sources of Reference (Normal) Values:

Studies made as follows: Cord P and P from young children—University of North Carolina; P from normal adolescents—Dr. Michael Preece, Institute for Child Health, London, England; 220 adults > 18 yr—Nichols Institute, San Pedro, CA, and the University of North Carolina. The assay standard used is a commercial preparation of pooled and lyophilized serum, calibrated to reflect the mean concentration in adult P, obtained from Ortho Diagnostics.

Specimen Volume, Collection, and Preservation:

200 μL. EDTA anticoagulant. Collect 5 mL of B directly into a tube containing EDTA, and place on ice. Centrifuge without delay in refrigerated centrifuge, and store in FR.

Analytical Method:

RIA; Furlanetto, R. W., Underwood, L. E., Van Wyk, J. J., and D'Ercole, A. J., Estimation of somatomedin-C levels in normals and patients with pituitary disease by radioimmunoassay. *J. Clin. Invest.* **60**, 648–657 (1977).

Commentary—J. J. Van Wyk and L. E. Underwood

The somatomedins are a family of insulin-like peptide growth factors, the serum concentrations of which are governed to a large extent by growth hormone (somatotropin) secretion. These substances stimulate cartilage growth in vitro and the proliferation of certain types of cells derived from extraskeletal tissues. The growth-promoting actions of somatotropin on the skeleton and on other tissues possibly are mediated through this family of peptides.

Although somatomedin-C was isolated as a small peptide (M_r about 7500), no detectable "free" somatomedin is present in whole blood; instead, somatomedin-C circulates in the form of macromolecular complexes, the most important of which has a relative molecular mass slightly less than the IgG fraction of blood. The biological significance of the somatomedin-binding proteins is the subject of active investigation in many laboratories.

The present RIA technique measures only "available" somatomedin-C, additional immunoreactive somatomedin-C being liberated from the macromolecular complexes by the action of serum proteases. Because EDTA inhibits the action of these proteases, the present data were obtained from EDTA-treated plasma. Although techniques to measure "total" somatomedin-C in serum are under development, the present techniques adequately discriminate between normal and pathologic values.

In 220 normal adults more than 18 years old, 95% of somatomedin-C values were between 0.4 and 2.0 int. units/mL. The values in this group followed a log-normal distribution. There was a significant sex-related difference within this group, women having greater values than men. There was a modest decrease in mean values between the third and seventh decade. Exercise, meals, and acute stress (needle insertion) apparently do not influence somatomedin-C concentrations, but the values during sleep are about 30% less than during waking hours. In normal children, the least values are encountered in cord blood (mean, about 0.5 int. units/mL). There is a positive correlation with birth weight in full-term infants. During the first two years of life, somatomedin-C concentrations increase rapidly, nearly to adult concentrations. Values during later childhood are greater than in the adult population, with the values in girls exceeding those in boys *(1)*. Normative data for both sexes during the first two decades are incomplete.

Somatomedin-C values appear to be uniformly increased in acromegaly. In a study of 57 patients with active acromegaly (2), the mean concentration of somatomedin-C was 10-fold greater than in a control group of 48 normal individuals; there was no overlap between normals and acromegalics. Somatomedin-C values are likewise increased in plasma from pregnant women after the 18th week of gestation, decreasing to normal values within a few days after delivery.

Somatomedin-C concentrations are low in hypopituitary dwarfs (3). The mean value in 36 untreated hypopituitary children was 0.10 int. units/mL (range, 0.03 to 0.23 int. units/mL). Therefore, values exceeding 0.30 int. units/mL probably exclude the diagnosis of hypopituitarism. Abnormally low serum concentrations of somatomedin-C are not necessarily diagnostic of hypopituitarism, however, because equally low concentrations have been observed in undernourished children and in children with short stature from causes other than hypopituitarism.

1. Van Wyk, J. J., and Underwood, L. E., The somatomedins and their actions. In *Biochemical Actions of Hormones*, 5, G. Litwack, Ed. Academic Press, New York, NY, 1978, pp 101–147.
2. Clemmons, D. R., Van Wyck, J. J., Ridgway, E. C., Kliman, B., Kjellberg, R. N., and Underwood, L. E., Evaluation of acromegaly by radioimmunoassay of somatomedin-C. *N. Engl. J. Med.* **301,** 1138–1142 (1979).
3. Furlanetto, R. W., Underwood, L. E., Van Wyk, J. J., and D'Ercole, A. J., Estimation of somatomedin-C levels in normals and patients with pituitary disease by radioimmunoassay. *J. Clin. Invest.* **60,** 648–657 (1977).

Sulfobromophthalein (BSP)[1]

Specimen Tested:

P, S.

Laboratories Reporting:

3.

Reference (Normal) Values:

Newborn:	Up to 15% retention in 45 min for a dose of 5 mg/kg of body weight
Child:	Up to 10%
Adult:	Up to 5%

---

[1] Hynson, Westcott and Dunning, Inc., has ceased manufacture of BSP, and now recommends use of their new dye product, Cardio-Green® (CG®), a sterile indocyanine green, USP. The newer dye is apparently far less hazardous to use, but unfortunately the analytical method for its determination has not yet been developed to the quality of the BSP test.

Sources of Reference (Normal) Values:

Institutional; Oppé, T. E., and Gibbs, I. E., Sulphobromophthalein excretion in premature infants. *Arch. Dis. Child.* **24,** 125–130 (1959); Lindquist, B., and Paulsen, L., Studies on the elimination rate of bromsulphtalein in infants and children. *Acta Paediatr.* **48,** 233–239 (1959); Seligson, D., and Marino, J., Sulfobromophthalein (BSP) in serum. *Stand. Methods Clin. Chem.* **2,** 186–191 (1958).

Specimen Volume, Collection, and Preservation; Patient Preparation:

100 to 500 μL. If venipuncture is performed, draw sample from arm opposite to the one used for BSP injection. Ideally, the patient should be fasting.

Analytical Method:

Seligson and Marino, *op. cit.*

Instrumentation:

Gilford Stasar II, Beckman 25, Bausch and Lomb Spectronic 100 spectrophotometers.

Sweat Electrolytes (Cl, K, Na)

Specimen Tested:

Sweat.

Laboratories Reporting:

6.

Reference (Normal) Values:

	mmol/L		
Age	Na	Cl	K
<8 d	range 24–59 (mean 40)	range 23–61 (mean 40)	range 8–33
5 wk–11 mo	15–24		4–18
1–9 yr	3–36		4–15
"Child"	Up to 50	Up to 50; <60 (1 lab.)	
10–16 yr	6–52		4–13
<17 yr	range 7–53 (mean 24)	range 7–52 (mean 23)	range 6–26
17–21 yr	range 12–55 (mean 34)	range 8–53 (mean 27)	range 7–20
17–60 yr	4–90		3–14
>21 yr	range 12–86 (mean 40)	range 9–72 (mean 31)	range 6–25
Borderline cystic fibrosis		50–60	
Cystic fibrosis	range 72–175 (mean 108)	range 77–174 (mean 119)	range 10–37

Sources of Reference (Normal) Values:

A combination of institutional experience at the Cystic Fibrosis Foundation (6000 Executive Blvd., Suite 309, Rockville, MD 20852) and published and private communications from H. Shwachman; see also *Disorders of the Respiratory Tract*, E. L. Kendig, Jr., Ed. W. B. Saunders, Co., Philadelphia, PA, 1977, p 776, and references below.

Specimen Volume, Collection, and Preservation:

50 μL preferred. Five labs use pilocarpine iontophoresis to collect sweat; Lab. 6 uses urecholine. The method for sweat induction and collection is described in Gibson, L. E., diSant'Agnese, P. A., and Shwachman, H., Procedure for the quantitative iontophoretic sweat test for cystic fibrosis. Cystic Fibrosis Foundation (address cited above); Gibson, L. E., and Cooke, R. E., A test for concentration of electrolytes in cystic fibrosis of the pancreas utilizing pilocarpine iontophoresis. *Pediatrics* **23**, 545–549 (1959); Shwachman, H., and Mahmoodian, A., Pilocarpine iontophoresis sweat testing: Results of seven years experience. *Bibl. Paediatr.* **86**, 158–182 (1967); Ibbott, F. A., Chloride in sweat. *Stand. Methods Clin. Chem.* **5**, 101–111 (1965). The sweat can be stored in the RR for 1 wk, if the container is tightly sealed against evaporation. (See also *Notes* below.)

Analytical Method and Instrumentation:

Chloride: Beckman CO_2/Cl analyzer; Buchler Instruments Chloridometer; American Instruments Co. 4–4411 Chloride Titrator; Heat Technology, Inc., Cystic Fibrosis Analyzer (1 lab.); for screening, 1 lab. uses Orion 417 skin chloride electrode and rechecks any value >35 mmol/L by use of a chloride-titrating apparatus. For **Na, K,** see instrumentation section of **Potassium and Sodium.**

Notes:

1. The major problem in performing sweat electrolytes is obtaining an adequate sample. Infants younger than six weeks may not sweat sufficiently. To overcome this, the sweat may be collected in duplicate (see Gibson et al., *op. cit.*). The leg may provide a better site than the arm for sweat collection in these infants.

2. The Gibson–Cooke iontophoresis apparatus may be made locally, or purchased from Farrall Instrument Co. (battery or a.c. converter) or from Dr. Harry Shwachman, Children's Hospital Medical Center, 300 Longwood Ave., Boston, MA 02115 (a.c. converter).

Commentary—J. Gilbert Hill

The demonstration of an increased electrolyte content of sweat is probably the single most important criterion in the diagnosis of pancreatic cystic fibrosis. Confirmed values for sweat chloride exceeding 60 mmol/L, or sweat sodium exceeding 70 mmol/L, are generally considered diagnostic of cystic fibrosis. It is recognized, however, that normal values may vary with age (see below) and that abnormally high values may occasionally be found other than in cystic fibrosis (e.g., in glucose-6-phosphatase deficiency, glycogen storage disease, hypothyroidism, untreated adrenal insufficiency, and malnutrition).

Hardy et al. *(1)* studied sweat sodium in the newborn and found the mean value on day 1 to be 51 mmol/L, decreasing to 35 mmol/L on day 2. Of the 72 babies tested on day 1, six had values exceeding 70 mmol/L; however, in five of these rechecked later, the sweat sodium value had declined to normal, and no evidence of cystic fibrosis was found. They concluded that an appreciable number of infants will show increased values for sweat electrolytes in day 1, but that most will subsequently be found to be normal. On the other hand, abnormally high sweat-electrolyte values on day 2 are unlikely in the absence of cystic fibrosis. Later in life there is a very gradual increase in sweat electrolyte concentration with age, reaching an average of about 55 mmol of sodium per liter by age 70 years *(2)*.

Technical problems abound in sweat testing, and the recent introduction of devices to simplify the test has been accused of leading to an increase in false-positive and false-negative results. Consequently, the pilocarpine iontophoresis procedure (Gibson–Cooke method) to stimulate sweating, followed by quantitation of the amount of sweat produced and the coulometric–amperometic measurement of chloride, is strongly recommended *(3)*.

1. Hardy, J. D., Davison, S. H. H., Higgins, M. U., and Polycarpou, P. N., Sweat tests in the newborn period. *Arch. Dis. Child.* **48,** 316 (1973).
2. Jones, J. D., Steige, H., and Logan, G. B., Variations of sweat sodium values in children and adults with cystic fibrosis and other diseases. *Mayo Clin. Proc.* **45,** 768–773 (1970).
3. Problems in Sweat Testing. "GAP" Conference-Feb. 6–7, 1975, Hilton Head, SC. Cystic Fibrosis Foundation, 3379 Peachtree Road, N.E., Atlanta, GA 30326.

Commentary—Michael A. Pesce

The sweat test is the most crucial laboratory assay used to diagnose cystic fibrosis. I and others *(1)* have found that patients are misdiagnosed because of improper collection and handling of sweat. The principal source of error is from the inexperience of the technicians. Sweat should be collected by those who are well trained in this procedure and in laboratories where the assay is frequently requested.

The differences between the sodium and chloride concentrations in sweat should be small. A gap of more than 30 mmol/L between the sodium and chloride values indicates an error either in calculation or analysis, or from contamination, and the sweat test should be repeated. If above-normal sodium and chloride values are obtained, the sweat test should be repeated to confirm the diagnosis. Borderline sweat test results must also be repeated. The diagnosis of cystic fibrosis should not be based entirely on the results of the sweat test, but must also be correlated with the clinical condition of the patient.

1. Shwachman, H., and Mahmoodian, A., Quality of sweat test performance in the diagnosis of cystic fibrosis. *Clin. Chem.* **25,** 158–161 (1979).

Testosterone

Specimen Tested:

P, S.

Laboratories Reporting:

3.

Reference (Normal) Values:

Labs. 1, 2:

	ng/dL (nmol/L)	
Age	**M**	**F**
Birth–prepuberty		<30 (<1.0)
1–15 d	<190 (<6.6)	
1–3 mo	<350 (<13.1)	
3–5 mo	<200 (<6.9)	
Prepubertal child	<100 (<3.5)	<40 (<1.4)
5–7 mo	<60 (<2.1)	
7 mo–puberty[a]	<30 (<1.0)	
Adult	>300 (>10.4)	<70 (<2.4)
	350–1100 (13.1–38.1)	20–70 (0.7–2.4)[a]

[a] Testosterone concentration increases during puberty to adult values, and is related to prepubertal stage or bone age rather than chronological age. Women may have values up to 95 ng/dL when treated with estrogens or progesterone and, on the average, values are higher during the luteal phase of the cycle than in the follicular phase. During puberty, girls experiencing anovulatory cycles have higher values than those cycling normally, but values should remain within the ranges indicated.

Lab. 3:
Adult: M, 10–33 nmol/L; F, 1.0–3.8 nmol/L
Prepubertal and pubertal males, according to testicular size:

Mean testicular size, mL	Testosterone, nmol/L
2	<0.4–2.0
3	0.8–2.8
4	1.0–2.9
5	1.7–3.2
6	2.2–5.4
8	2.4–8.5
15	9.3–11.0
18–23	12.8–20.0
>24	>23

Sources of Reference (Normal) Values:

Lab. 1: *Radioimmunoassay Manual,* 4th ed., Nichols Institute, San Pedro, CA, 1977, pp 311–313. **Lab. 2:** institutional; Sizonenko, P. C., Endocrinology in preadolescents and adolescents. I. Hormonal changes during normal puberty. *Am. J. Dis. Child.* **132,** 704–712 (1978). **Lab. 3:** institutional; Wang, C., Youatt, G., O'Connor, S., Dulmanis, A., and Hudson, B., A simple radioimmunoassay for plasma testosterone plus 5-alpha-dihydrosterone. *J. Steroid Biochem.* **5,** 551–555 (1974).

Specimen Volume, Collection, and Preservation:

M, 0.25 mL; F, 1.0 mL. Store in FR.

Analytical Method:

RIA. **Lab. 1:** Kinouchi, T., Pages, L., and Horton, R. A., A specific radioimmunoassay for plasma testosterone. *J. Lab. Clin. Med.* **82,** 309–316 (1973). **Lab. 2:** Endocrine Sciences. **Lab. 3:** Wang et al., *op. cit.;* institutional study of Montalto, J., Davies, H. E., and Connelly, J. F., Serum testosterone plus 5α-dihydrotestosterone and its relation to testicular volume from childhood to maturity (to be published).

Instrumentation:

Liquid scintillation counter.

Commentary—Elizabeth K. Smith

Cord serum values for testosterone are not significantly different in male and female infants *(1).* In both sexes, concentrations during the first week of life are significantly lower (mean, approximately 25 ng/dL) than in cord serum. In male infants, serum testosterone increases sharply in the second week to a maximum (mean, 175 ng/dL) at about two months, which lasts until six months of age *(1,2).* These data demonstrate that the testes are active in early infancy, corresponding to the increase in gonadotropins, especially lutropin (luteinizing hormone, LH), seen at one to two months of age. Testosterone concentrations decrease in the first week in female infants and remain low throughout infancy and early childhood *(1,3).*

At puberty serum testosterone increases dramatically in boys, in concert with increases in gonadotropins. Many studies have documented correlations with skeletal age and Tanner stage of puberty. Testosterone concentrations increase with onset of genital and pubic hair growth and voice change, and continue until pubertal development is complete and adult serum values are attained *(5).* Values relate to pubertal stage or skeletal age better than to chronological age. Good correlation also has been found between serum testosterone concentrations and testicular size (volume) *(6).*

Testosterone concentrations in serum display a diurnal or circadian variation, with highest mean concentrations at 0800 hours and lowest ones at 1900–2000 hours (7) or 2400–0400 hours (8). However, the magnitude of the variation is about 20% of that of the variation for cortisol. Nevertheless, care should be taken in interpreting small deviations from "normal," making sure that, in serial studies, blood is collected at the same time of day.

Although regulated primarily by gonadotropins, plasma testosterone also responds to corticotropin (ACTH). Age- and sex-related differences in this response have been reported (9), with increases in testosterone values in females at all ages and in prepubertal boys, but with decreases in males at periods of active testicular secretion— early infancy, puberty, and adulthood.

Clinical applications of serum testosterone tests in pediatrics include detection of hypogonadism in adolescent boys whose values are below normal; stimulation with human choriogonadotropin (HCG) should double the testosterone concentrations in a patient with normal testes. In pituitary or hypothalamic disease, where both testosterone and gonadotropin concentrations are low, clomiphene injections will act on the hypothalamus to increase both gonadotropin and testosterone concentrations twofold in the normal male. Virilization in girls usually is associated with increases in serum testosterone to more than 60 ng/dL. Increased testosterone concentrations associated with adrenal hyperplasia are suppressible with dexamethasone, but increases due to a virilizing tumor of the adrenal or ovary are not.

Plasma testosterone is largely protein-bound. Current RIA methods measure both free and bound (i.e., total) testosterone. In the first two weeks of life, there is significantly more unbound testosterone in male than in female infants; however, no sex difference in binding capacity or unbound testosterone concentration was observed in prepubertal children (10). Horst et al. (11) reported high sex-hormone-binding globulin capacity and percent binding in boys 0.5 to 8.0 years old, with a steady decrease thereafter until 18 years of age, when adult values were reached.

1. Winter, J. S. D., Hughes, I. A., Reyes, F. I., and Faiman, C., Pituitary-gonadal relations in infancy: 2. Patterns of serum gonadal steroid concentrations in man from birth to two years of age. *J. Clin. Endocrinol. Metab.* **42,** 679–686 (1976).
2. Forest, M. G., Sizonenko, P. C., Cathiard, A. M., and Bertrand, J., Hypophyso-gonadal function in humans during the first year of life. I. Evidence for testicular activity in early infancy. *J. Clin. Invest.* **53,** 819–828 (1974).
3. Sizonenko, P. C., Endocrinology in preadolescents and adolescents. I. Hormonal changes during normal puberty. *Am. J. Dis. Child.* **132,** 704–712 (1978).
4. Sizonenko, P. C., and Paunier, L., Hormonal changes in puberty III. Correlation of plasma dehydroepiandrosterone, testosterone, FSH, and LH, with stages of puberty and bone age in normal boys and girls and

in patients with Addison's diseases or hypogonadism or with premature or late adrenarche. *J. Clin. Endocrinol. Metab.* **41,** 894–904 (1975).

5. Lee, P. A., and Migeon, C. J., Puberty in boys: Correlation of plasma levels of gonadotropins (LH, FSH), androgens (testosterone, androstenedione, dehydroepiandrosterone and its sulfate), estrogens (estrone and estradiol) and progestins (progesterone and 17-hydroxyprogesterone). *J. Clin. Endocrinol. Metab.* **41,** 556–562 (1975).

6. Montalto, J., Davies, H. E., and Connelly, J. F., Serum testosterone plus 5 α-dihydrotestosterone and its relation to testicular volume from childhood to maturity. To be published.

7. Faiman, C., and Winter, J. S. D., Diurnal cycles and plasma FSH, testosterone and cortisol and men. *J. Clin. Endocrinol. Metab.* **33,** 186–192 (1971).

8. deLacerda, L., Kowarski, A., Johanson, A. J., Athanasiou, R., and Migeon, C. J., Integrated concentration and circadian variation of plasma testosterone in normal men. *J. Clin. Endocrinol. Metab.* **37,** 366–371 (1973).

9. Forest, M. G., Age-related response of plasma testosterone, Δ^4-androstenedione and cortisol to adrenocorticotropin in infants, children and adults. *J. Clin. Endocrinol. Metab.* **47,** 931–937 (1978).

10. Forest, M. G., Cathiard, A. M., and Bertrand, J. A., Total and unbound testosterone levels in the newborn and in normal and hypogonadal children: Use of a sensitive radioimmunoassay for testosterone. *J. Clin. Endocrinol. Metab.* **36,** 1136–1142 (1973).

11. Horst, H. J., Bartsch, W., and Dirksen-Thedens, I., Plasma testosterone, sex hormone binding globulin binding capacity and per cent binding of testosterone and 5α-dihydrotestosterone in prepubertal, pubertal and adult males. *J. Clin. Endocrinol. Metab.* **45,** 522–527 (1977).

Theophylline (Aminophylline)

Specimen Tested:

P, S.

Laboratories Reporting:

6.

Reference (Normal) Values:

Therapeutic ranges (mg/L; µg/mL):
  Apnea of newborn: 2 labs., 6–11; 1 lab., 7–14
  Asthma, child: 5 labs., 10–20; 1 lab., 8–16
Toxic concentration: 25 mg/L

(*Note:* mg/L $\times$ 5.545 = µmol/L.)

Sources of Reference (Normal) Values:

Institutional; Mitenko, P. A., and Ogilvie, R. I., Rational intravenous doses of theophylline. *N. Engl. J. Med.* **289,** 600–603 (1973); Shannon, D. C., Gotay, F., Stein, I. M., Rogers, M. C., Todres, I. D., and Moylan, M. B., Prevention of apnea and bradycardia in low-birth-weight infants. *Pediatrics* **55,** 589–594 (1975); Jenne, J. W., Pharmacokinetics of theophylline. *Clin. Pharmacol. Ther.* **14,** 509–513 (1973).

Specimen Volume, Collection, and Preservation:

5 to 100 μL. Heparin, EDTA, or oxlate as anticoagulant. Specimen is stable in RR for 1 wk, but best kept in FR.

Analytical Method and Instrumentation:

2 labs.: Syva EMIT, with Gilford 3500, Abbott ABA-100 Bichromatic Analyzer. **2 labs.:** HPLC; Jusko, W. J., and Poliszczuk, A., High-pressure liquid chromatographic and spectrophotometric assays for theophylline in biological fluids. *Am. J. Hosp. Pharm.* **33,** 1193–1196 (1976); DuPont 848 Liquid Chromatograph with Zipax SCX column; strong cation-exchange packing (DuPont); Soldin, S. J., and Hill, J. G., A rapid micromethod for measuring theophylline in serum by reverse phase high performance liquid chromatography. *Clin. Biochem.* **10,** 74–77 (1977); Waters HPLC ALC/GPC-204/6000 A, with a 440 detector (254 nm); RIA, double antibody, based on method of C. E. Cook, Chemistry and Life Sciences Division, Research Triangle Inst., North Carolina; Packard Tri-Carb liquid scintillation spectrometer; IEC PR-I centrifuge; LKB 2075 diluter. **1 lab.:** GLC, modified from multiple sources; Beckman GC-4 gas chromatograph; HP 3380 Recording Integrator; Damon-IEC PR 6000 centrifuge; Applied Science Mini-Aktor tubes.

Notes:

1. Time of sample collection is influenced by pharmacokinetic parameters, including drug dosage form, mode of administration, concomitant drug therapy, and biological variations affecting metabolism of the drug.

2. Samples for trough values should be drawn just before next dose. Drawing times for peak serum concentrations after various oral theophylline preparations are as follows: 1 h post-liquid form (e.g., elixir); 2 h post-conventional tablet; and 3 to 4 h post-sustained-release form. After an intravenous bolus, draw B in 1 h.

3. The steady-state serum concentration should be reached in 1 d. Much longer equilibration periods (up to 1 wk) are required in patients with liver disease.

Commentary—J. Gilbert Hill

Theophylline has been used for many years to treat asthma, but frequent reports of toxicity (headache, gastrointestinal upsets, convulsions, and even death) have discouraged some potential users. It is now recognized that most of these problems simply reflected the wide interindividual variations in the rate at which the drug is metabolized, and consequently in the concentration in blood achieved in response to a given dose of the drug. With the development of suitable methods for monitoring these blood concentrations, the hazards associated with theophylline therapy can be greatly diminished, and the full potential of the drug can be realized.

In the newborn, where the drug is important in the prevention of apnea, a plasma value between 5 and 15 mg/L is usually sought. In treating asthma in older children and adults, the usual therapeutic range is 10 to 20 mg/L. Values exceeding these are frequently associated with toxic effects, and call for immediate assessment of the clinical situation.

The most widely used measurement technique at the present time is homogeneous immunoassay (EMIT), but "high-performance" liquid chromatography, GLC, and RIA can also provide the sensitivity required to analyze micro-samples.

In the neonate, theophylline is distributed equally between plasma and erythrocytes, producing a whole-blood plasma concentration ratio of approximately 1. As a consequence, theophylline values in this age group, may be monitored in hemolyzed specimens, as long as the measuring technique itself is not affected by hemolysis (1). Of the methods mentioned, EMIT is subject to interference from hemolysis, and should not be used under these circumstances.

In children and adults, the theophylline concentration in erythrocytes is approximately one-half of the corresponding plasma concentrations; hemolyzed specimens should therefore be avoided, irrespective of the analytical technique to be used.

1. Koup, J. R., and Hart, B. A., Relationship between plasma and whole blood theophylline concentration in neonates. *J. Pediatr.* **94,** 320–321 (1979).

Thyroid Antibodies (Anti-microsomal/ anti-thyroglobulin antibodies; anti-M/anti-Tg)

Specimen Tested:

S.

Laboratory Reporting:

1.

Reference (Normal) Values:

Anti-M antibodies: ≤25 units/mL
Anti-Tg antibodies: ≤10 units/mL

Sources of Reference (Normal) Values:

Kriss, J. P., Competitive binding radioassay of serum anti-thyroglobulin and anti-microsomal antibodies. In *Radioimmunoassay Manual*, 4th ed., Nichols Institute, San Pedro, CA, 1977, pp 189–193.

Specimen Volume, Collection, and Preservation:

0.5 mL. Store frozen.

Analytical Method and Instrumentation:

Competitive protein binding; Mori, T., and Kriss, J. P., Measurements by competitive binding radioassay of serum anti-microsomal and anti-thyroglobulin antibodies in Graves' disease and other thyroid disorders. *J. Clin. Endocrinol. Metab.* **33,** 688–698 (1971); Gamma counter.

Thyrotropin (Thyroid-stimulating hormone; TSH)

Specimen Tested:

P, S.

Laboratories Reporting:

4.

Reference (Normal) Values:

Age	TSH, micro-int. unit/mL			
	Lab. 1	**Lab. 2**	**Lab. 3**	**Lab. 4**
Cord	3–22	30[a]		
Newborn–48 h[a]	2–3 X normal			
1–3 d				<40
3–7 d				<25
7–14 d				<10
3–14 yr	1.6–4.1			
All ages after newborn	<6		1.6–10.9	
All ages after 4 d		<10		
All ages after 14 d				<5

[a] **Lab. 1:** TSH increases to two- to threefold normal in the first 48 h, and returns to normal (adult) values in about 10 d; **Lab. 2:** TSH increases shortly after birth to a peak value as high as 50. Because of these rapid changes, results can be interpreted only in cord blood or in children more than 4 d old.

Sources of Reference (Normal) Values:

Lab. 1: institutional; and personal communication for cord blood and newborn from Prof. P. G. Walfish (see list of **Contributors**). **Labs. 2, 3, 4:** institutional.

Specimen Volume, Collection, and Preservation:

50 to 400 μL. Store in FR.

Analytical Method:

RIA; Bonnyns, M., Vanhaelst, L., and Golstein-Golaire, J., Correlation between radioimmunological and biological human thyrotropin measurements. *Horm. Metab. Res.* **3**, 409–414 (1971); Beckman Instruments, Inc., HTSH Bulletin and kit; Corning Medical Immo Phase kit; institutional.

Instrumentation:

Packard Auto-Gamma 5110, LKB 80 000, Nuclear Chicago gamma counters.

Note: Normal values may be influenced by crossreactivity of the primary antiserum, the type of second-antibody system, and the amount and type of protein used for standards. Therefore, each laboratory should establish its own range of "normal." Regardless of the antigen–antibody system used, TSH potencies for RIA should be standardized with an accepted reference TSH standard, preferably Medical Research Council World Health Organization human pituitary TSH. Results are expressed as international units of human TSH per milliliter of serum.

Commentary—William H. Hoffman

Measurement of serum TSH by RIA is a major advance in evaluating thyroid function in childhood. Because of the very sensitive negative-feedback mechanism between serum thyroid hormone concentrations and pituitary secretion of TSH, even small decreases in thyroid hormones normally result in an increase in serum TSH. Most cases of hypothyroidism involve a defect of the thyroid gland (primary hypothyroidism); therefore, TSH is a useful method for *(a)* identifying patients with primary hypothyroidism; *(b)* evaluating patients with clinically euthyroid goiters who may have impending primary hypothyroidism, i.e., normal serum thyroxine (T_4) at the expense of an increase in TSH *(1); (c)* helping to distinguish between primary and secondary/tertiary hypothyroidism; *(d)* monitoring patients with Graves' disease who are receiving thionamides or who have undergone subtotal thyroidectomy; *(e)* clarifying suspicious T_4 results obtained in screening programs for congenital hypothyroidism, as suggested by a committee of the American Thyroid Association *(2–4)*.

Serum TSH values decrease between the 30th and 45th week of gestation *(5)*. In newborns, regardless of the route of delivery, hypersecretion of TSH is most accentuated at 30 min of life, and persists at a lesser rate during the first 48 to 72 h of life *(6)*. This pattern appears to be quantitatively modified in the normal pre-term infant *(7)*. TSH concentration returns to the normal range by 14 days, the values then remaining fairly constant for infancy, childhood, adolescence, and adulthood of both sexes *(8)*. Serum TSH is increased in persons older than 60 *(9)*. The circadian variations of TSH reported in young adults are minor compared with fluctuations of other anterior pituitary hormones *(10)*.

TSH has been reported both as increased *(11)* and suppressed *(7)* in pre-term infants with respiratory distress syndrome; unlike the response in adults, TSH has been demonstrated to increase in newborns exposed to a cooler ambient temperature *(6)*, as well as in infants undergoing surgical hypothermia *(12)*. Both chronic renal and liver disease *(9)* and protein-calorie malnutrition *(13)* have been reported to increase serum TSH.

Pharmacologic and physiologic challenges have minimum effects on TSH release; however, pharmacologic doses of glucocorticoid significantly decrease serum TSH *(14)*. Thyroliberin (thyrotropin-releasing hormone) is the primary challenge in evaluating TSH reserve and may help in differentiating pituitary (secondary) from hypothalamic (tertiary) deficiency *(15)*.

TSH may be utilized to monitor effectiveness of L-thyroxine replacement in primary hypothyroidism; however, several points must be kept in mind:

1. A decreased sensitivity of the negative-feedback system in congenital hypothyroidism makes normalization of T_4 rather than TSH important *(16)*.

2. Suppression of TSH to the normal range in acquired hypothyroidism may take two to three months *(17)*.

3. Complete TSH suppression may reflect either an adequate (euthyroid) or excessive (hyperthyroid) replacement; clarification can be obtained by measuring serum T_4, which should be midway in the normal range for the child's age.

4. Individuals with Graves' disease receiving ^{131}I may not have increased TSH with the development of hypothyroidism *(18)*.

1. Greenberg, A. H., Czernichow, P., Hung, W., Shelley, W., Winship, T., and Blizzard, R. M., Juvenile chronic lymphocytic thyroiditis: Clinical, laboratory and histologic correlations. *J. Clin. Endocrinol. Metab.* **30,** 293–301 (1970).
2. Fisher, D. A., Burrow, G. N., Dussault, J. H., Hollingsworth, D. R., Larsen, P. R., Man, E. B., and Walfish, P. G., Recommendations for screening programs for congenital hypothyroidism. *J. Pediatr.* **89,** 692–694 (1976).
3. Dussault, J. H., Parlow, A., Letarte, J., Guyda, H., and Laberge, C., TSH measurements from blood spots on filter paper: A confirmatory screening test for neonatal hypothyroidism. *J. Pediatr.* **89,** 550–552 (1976).
4. Morissette, J., and Dussault, J. H., Commentary: The cutoff point for

TSH measurement or recalls in a screening program for congenital hypothyroidism using primary T₄ screening. *J. Pediatr.* **95,** 404–406 (1979).

5. Oddie, T. H., Fisher, D. A., Bernard, B., and Lam, R. W., Thyroid function at birth in infants of 30 to 45 weeks' gestation. *J. Pediatr.* **90,** 803–806 (1977).
6. Fisher, D. A., and Odell, W. D., Acute release of thyrotropin in the newborn. *J. Clin. Invest.* **48,** 1670–1677 (1969).
7. Uhrmann, S., Marks, K. H., Maisels, M. J., Friedman, Z., Murray, R., Kulin, H. E., Kaplan, M., and Utiger, R., Thyroid function in the preterm infant: A longitudinal assessment. *J. Pediatr.* **92,** 968–973 (1978).
8. Fisher, D. A., Sack, J., Oddie, T. H., Pekary, A. E., Hershman, J. M., Lam, R. W., and Parslow, M. E., Serum T₄, TBG, T₃ uptake, T₃, reverse T₃, and TSH concentrations in children 1 to 15 years of age. *J. Clin. Endocrinol. Metab.* **45,** 191–198 (1977).
9. Cuttelod, S., Lemarchand-Beraud, T., Magnenat, P., Perret, C., Poli, S., and Vannotti, A., Effect of age and role of kidneys and liver on thyrotropin turnover in man. *Metabolism* **23,** 101–113 (1974).
10. Alford, F. P., Baker, H. W. G., Burger, H. G., de Krester, D. M., Hudson, B., Johns, M. W., Masterton, J. P., Patel, Y. C., and Rennie, G. C., Temporal patterns of integrated plasma hormone levels during sleep and wakefulness. I. Thyroid-stimulating hormone, growth hormone, and cortisol. *J. Clin. Endocrinol. Metab.* **37,** 841–847 (1973).
11. Cuestas, R. A., Lindall, A., and Engel, R. R., Low thyroid hormones and respiratory distress syndrome of the newborn. *N. Engl. J. Med.* **295,** 297–302 (1976).
12. Wilber, J. F., and Baum, D., Elevation of plasma TSH during surgical hypothermia. *J. Clin. Endocrinol. Metab.* **31,** 372–375 (1970).
13. Pimstone, B., Becker, D., and Hendricks, S., TSH response to synthetic thyrotropin-releasing hormone in human protein-calorie malnutrition. *J. Clin. Endocrinol. Metab.* **36,** 779–783 (1973).
14. Re, R. N., Kourides, I. A., Ridgway, E. C., Weintraub, B. D., and Maloof, F., The effect of glucocorticoid administration on human pituitary secretion of thyrotropin and prolactin. *J. Clin. Endocrinol. Metab.* **43,** 338–346 (1976).
15. Costom, B. H., Grumbach, M. M., and Kaplan, S. L., Effect of thyrotropin-releasing factor on serum thyroid-stimulating hormone. *J. Clin. Invest.* **50,** 2219–2225 (1971).
16. Guyda, H., Letarte, J., Dussault, J. H., and Berge, C., Serum levels of T₄, T₃, and TSH during therapy of neonatal hypothyroidism. *Pediatr. Res.* **11,** 426 (1977).
17. Sutter, S. N., Kaplan, S. L., Aubert, M. L., and Grumbach, M. M., Plasma prolactin and thyrotropin and the response to thyrotropin releasing factor in children with primary and hypothalamic hypothyroidism. *J. Clin. Endocrinol. Metab.* **47,** 1015–1020 (1978).
18. Toft, A. D., Hunter, W. M., Seth, J., and Irvine, W. J., Plasma thyrotropin and serum thyroxine in patients becoming hypothyroid in the early months after iodine-131. *Lancet* **i,** 704–705 (1974).

Commentary—D. A. Fisher

Dr. J. F. Connelly of Melbourne, Australia (see list of **Contributors**), reports normal serum TSH values as follows:

Age, d	Thyrotropin (by RIA), micro-int. units/mL
1–3	<40
3–7	<25
7–14	<10
>14	< 5

The normal mean TSH value in cord blood is about 10 micro-int. units/mL. The neonatal TSH surge occurs in response to exposure to the (cold) extrauterine environment. Peak values (mean, about 80 micro-int. units/mL in full-term infants) occur at 30 min after birth, after which TSH decreases gradually to baseline values. In the United States, mean serum TSH concentrations are reported to be <20 micro-int. units/mL by 72 h. As Dr. Connelly indicates, the TSH surge values may remain above normal beyond three days of age. Seasonal variation in peak TSH range values has been reported *(1)*, perhaps related to temperature variations. The neonatal TSH surge also is observed in premature infants *(2)*.

Beyond the newborn period, serum TSH values remain within the normal adult range *(3)*, the absolute values being related to the TSH antibody utilized. With Odell antiserum *(4)* assays, normal values are <10–12 micro-int. units/mL; Parslow antiserum assays yield normal values of <5–6 micro-int. units/mL *(3)*.

1. Rogowski, P., Siersbach-Nielson, K., and Molholm-Hansen, J., Seasonal variation in neonatal thyroid function. *J. Clin. Endocrinol. Metab.* **39,** 919–922 (1974).
2. Klein, A. H., Foley, B., Kenny, F. M., and Fisher, D. A., Thyroid hormone and thyrotropin responses to parturition in premature infants with and without the respiratory distress syndrome. *Pediatrics* **63,** 380–385 (1979).
3. Fisher, D. A., Sack, J., Oddie, T. H., Pekary, A. E., Hershman, J. M., Lam, R. W., and Parslow, M. E., Serum T4, TBG, T3 uptake, reverse T3 and TSH concentrations in children 1 to 15 years of age. *J. Clin. Endocrinol. Metab.* **45,** 191–198 (1977).
4. Odell, W. D., Wilber, J. F., and Paul, W. E., Radioimmunoassay of thyrotropin in human serum. *J. Clin. Endocrinol. Metab.* **25,** 1179–1188 (1965).

Note: See also Chapter 9, **Screening for Neonatal Hypothyroidism.**

Thyroxine (T₄; total T₄)

Specimen Tested:

P, S.

Laboratories Reporting:

5.

Reference (Normal) Values:

| | T$_4$ range (and mean), μg/dL | | | | |
Age	Lab. 1	Lab. 2	Lab. 3	Lab. 4	Lab. 5
Cord	6.6–17.5 (10.8)				
0–3 d		11–23	peaks at 24 h, then decreases to 9–22 at 3 d		
1–3 d	11.0–21.5 (16.5)				
1–7 d				6–23	
4 d–3 wk			8–19		
1–4 wk	8.2–16.6 (12.9)	9–18		8–20	
3 wk–2 mo			7–16		
1–3 mo				7–20	
1–4 mo		7.5–16.5			
1–12 mo	7.2–15.6 (11.2)				
2–12 mo			5–14		
3–12 mo				4–16	
4–12 mo		6.5–14.5			
>1 yr				4–13	
1–5 yr	7.3–15.0 (10.5)				
1–6 yr		6.0–13.5			
1–15 yr			5–13		
Child					4.7–11
5–10 yr	6.4–13.3 (9.3)				
6–10 yr		5.5–12.5			
10–15 yr	5.6–11.7 (8.1)				
10 yr–adult		4.5–12.0			
15 yr and over			4–12		
15–20 yr	4.2–11.8 (8.0)				

Sources of Reference (Normal) Values:

Lab. 1: Fisher, D. A., and Oddie, T. H., Thyroxine (T$_4$). In *Radioimmunoassay Manual*, 4th ed., Nichols Institute, San Pedro, CA, 1977, p 322. **Lab. 2:** institutional study and literature. **Lab. 3:** institutional; Cuppett, C. C., and Rock, J. A., Normal range for serum thyroxine in neonates. *Clin. Chem.* **23,** 2170–2171 (1977); Garcia-Bulnes, G., Cervantes, C., Cerbón, M. A., Tudon, H., Argote, R. M., and Parra, A., Serum thyrotrophin, triiodothyronine and thyroxine levels by radioimmunoassay during childhood and adolescence. *Acta Endocrinol.* **86,** 742–753 (1977); Jacobsen, B. B., Andersen, H. J., Peitersen, A. B., Dige-Petersen, H., and Hummer, L., Serum levels of thyrotropin, thyroxine and triiodothyronine in fullterm small-for-gestational age and preterm newborn babies. *Acta Paediatr. Scand.* **66,** 681–687 (1977). **Labs. 4, 5:** institutional.

Specimen Volume, Collection, and Preservation:

20 to 100 μL. Heparin anticoagulant. Store in FR. There is a claim of stability of several days at RT, and 2 wk in RR.

Analytical Method:

RIA. **Lab. 1:** *Radioimmunoassay Manual, op. cit.,* p 143. **Lab. 2:** Yang Solid Phase T_4 RIA technical bulletin. **Lab. 3:** Corning Medical Immo Phase kit. **Lab. 4:** institutional. **Lab. 5:** Marsden, D. S., Radioimmunoassay separation techniques. *Lab. Manage.* **15,** 31 (1977); Beckman Instruments, Inc., kit.

Instrumentation:

Gamma counters: Nuclear-Chicago, Packard 5110 Auto-Gamma.

Commentary—D. A. Fisher

Cord-blood T_4 values increase progressively with gestational age. Between 30 weeks and term, this increase is not due to increased concentrations of thyroxine-binding globulin. T_4 values measured in cord blood of 2683 infants after 30 to 45 weeks' gestation (wt 1460–5250 g) showed an increase in mean T_4 values from 9.4 μg/dL at 30 weeks to 11.7 μg/dL at 45 weeks. Values for thyroxine-binding globulin varied from 3.1 to 11.4 mg/dL, without correlation with gestational age *(1).* The neonatal increase in T_4 values also occurs in premature infants *(2);* however, standards for T_4 values in premature infants during the perinatal period are not available. Neonatal values less than 5 μg/dL and greater than 17 μg/dL should probably be considered abnormal between 30 and 37 weeks' gestation *(1).*

Cord blood and neonatal T_4 values also exhibit seasonal variations *(3,4),* being about 15% higher in winter than summer *(4).* Values from reference standards for T_4 decrease progressively with storage (frozen) at a rate of about 5% per year *(4).*

1. Oddie, T. H., Fisher, D. A., Bernard, B., and Lam, R. W., Thyroid function at birth in infants of 30 to 45 weeks gestation. *J. Pediatr.* **90,** 803–806 (1977).
2. Klein, A. H., Foley, B., Kenny, F. M., and Fisher, D. A., Thyroid hormone and thyrotropin responses to parturition in premature infants with and without the respiratory distress syndrome. *Pediatrics* **63,** 380–385 (1979).
3. Rogowski, P., Siersback-Nielson, K., and Molholm-Hansen, J., Seasonal variation in thyroid function. *J. Clin. Endocrinol. Metab.* **39,** 919–922 (1974).
4. Oddie, T. H., Klein, A. H., Foley, T. P., and Fisher, D. A., Variation in values for iodothyronine hormones, thyrotropin and thyroxine binding globulin in normal umbilical cord serum with season and duration of storage. *Clin. Chem.* **25,** 1251–1253 (1979).

Note: See also Chapter 9, **Screening for Neonatal Hypothyroidism.**

Thyroxine-Binding Globulin (TBG)

Specimen Tested:

P, S.

Laboratories Reporting:

2.

Reference (Normal) Values:

Age	mg/dL	
	Lab. 1	Lab. 2
Cord	1.4–9.4	1.9–3.9 (mean, 2.9)
1 d–1 wk		1.4–4.1 (mean, 2.7)
1–4 wk	1.0–9.0	1.5–3.9 (mean, 2.6)
1–12 mo	2.0–7.6	2.2–4.2 (mean, 3.2)
1–5 yr	2.9–5.4	1.5–3.6 (mean, 2.6)
5–10 yr	2.5–5.0	1.4–3.0 (mean, 2.2)
10–15 yr	2.1–4.6	
10 yr–adult		1.2–3.0 (mean, 2.1)
15–20 yr	2.2–4.6	
Adult	2.1–5.2	

Sources of Reference (Normal) Values:

Lab. 1: *Radioimmunoassay Manual,* 4th ed., Nichols Institute, San Pedro, CA, 1977, p 322. **Lab. 2:** institutional study (to be published); Christine, M. J., Mason, R. D., Oldstrchel, G., and Doran, M. A., Solid phase radioassay for thyroxine binding globulin. *Clin. Chem.* **24,** 1038 (1978), abstract 251; Erenberg, A., Phelps, D. L., Lam, R., and Fisher, D. A., Total and free thyroid hormone concentrations in the neonatal period. *Pediatrics* **53,** 211–216 (1974); Fisher, D. A., Sack, J., Oddie, T. H., Pekary, A. E., Hershman, J. M., Lam, R. W., and Parslow, M. E., Serum T_4, TBG, T_3 uptake, T_3, reverse T_3, and TSH concentrations in children 1 to 15 years of age. *J. Clin. Endocrinol. Metab.* **45,** 191–198 (1977); Gershengorn, M. C. Larsen, P. R., and Robbins, J., Radioimmunoassay for serum thyroxine-binding globulin: Results in normal subjects and in patients with hepatocellular carcinoma. *J. Clin. Endocrinol. Metab.* **42,** 907–911 (1976).

Analytical Method:

Lab. 1: RIA, double antibody, ^{125}I-labeled TBG; Levy, R. P., Marshall, J. S., and Velayo, N. L., Radioimmunoassay of human thyroxine-binding globulin. *J. Clin. Endocrinol. Metab.* **32,** 372–381 (1971). **Lab. 2:** solid-phase RIA; Corning Medical, TBG by RIA, Directions for use: Immo-Phase TBG [125]I Radioimmunoassay Test System.

Instrumentation:

Searle Model 1185 Automatic Gamma System; Sorvall RC-3 refrigerated centrifuge.

Commentary—D. A. Fisher

TBG values are relatively high in the newborn period. Initially, this state of affairs was believed to be related to the high circulating concentrations of estrogen to which the fetus was exposed in utero. This seems not to be the case, because serum TBG concentrations remains high throughout infancy, decreasing gradually to adult values in late adolescence.

It is still possible to assess TBG concentrations with labeled-T_4-saturation and electrophoresis, reporting values as maximum T_4-binding capacity (micrograms per 100 mL of serum). Other methods proposed include rocket immunoelectrophoresis and radial immunodiffusion. However, measuring TBG by radioimmunoassay is simpler and more reliable.

Mean values of TBG of 3.6 and 2.9 mg/dL have been reported (1,2), but the "true" value probably approximates 1.5 mg/dL (3). The variations are probably related to the purity of the antisera or of the TBG utilized as reference standard. Serum TBG concentrations are distributed log-normal, accounting for the log-normal distribution of serum T_4 concentration (3).

1. Levy, R. P., Marshall, J. S., and Velayo, N. L., Radioimmunoassay of human thyroxine-binding globulin TBG. *J. Clin. Endocrinol. Metab.* **32**, 372–381 (1972).
2. Chopra, I. J., Solomon, D. H., and Ho, R. S., Competitive ligand-binding assay for measurement of thyroxine-binding globulin (TBG). *J. Clin. Endocrinol. Metab.* **35**, 565–573 (1972).
3. Gershengorn, M. C., Larsen, P. R., and Robbins, J., Radioimmunoassay for serum thyroxine-binding globulin: Results in normal subjects and in patients with hepatocellular carcinoma. *J. Clin. Endocrinol. Metab.* **42**, 907–911 (1976).

Thyroxine, Free (FT$_4$)

Specimen Tested:

S.

Laboratory Reporting:

1.

Reference (Normal) Values:

Child–adult: 1.3–3.8 ng/dL
Infants <1 mo: values are higher

Sources of Reference (Normal) Values:

Radioimmunoassay Manual, 4th ed., Nichols Institute, San Pedro, CA, 1977, p 163.

Specimen Volume, Collection, and Preservation:

0.5 mL. Store in FR.

Analytical Method and Instrumentation:

Dialysis and radioassay, ^{125}I-labeled thyroxine; gamma counter.

Commentary—D. A. Fisher

Adequate normal values for free thyroxine concentrations in infants and small children are not available. At present, adult standards are used. In premature infants with low thyroxine and low thyrotropin values, concentrations of thyroxine-binding globulin may also be low. In these infants measurement of free thyroxine probably is the best approach to assess thyroid status.

Triglycerides (Triacylglycerols)

Specimen Tested:

P, S.

Laboratories Reporting:

6.

Reference (Normal) Values:

Lab. 1:

	mg/L			
	M		**F**	
Age, yr	**White**	**Black**	**White**	**Black**
6–7	180–820	190–790	10–1410	270–830
8–9	70–1070	200–760	140–1260	160–960
10–11	180–980	180–980	240–1200	0–1410
12–13	70–1230	170–1010	250–1210	130–1250
14–15	110–1270	180–1020	180–1260	240–960
16–17	0–1560	270–990	60–1380	240–100

Note: mg/L $\times$ 0.00113 = mmol/L, if relative molecular mass of 885 is used (triolein); mg/L $\times$ 0.00133 = mmol/L, if mean relative molecular mass for triglyceride is 875.

Sources of Reference (Normal) Values:

Morrison, J. A., deGroot, I., Edwards, B. K., Kelly, K. A., Mellies, M. J., Khoury, P., and Glueck, C. J., Lipids and lipoproteins in 927 school children, ages 6 to 17 years. *Pediatrics* **62,** 990–995 (1978).

*   *   *

Reference (Normal) Values:

Lab. 2:

Age, yr	mg/L
≤19	100–1300
20–29	100–1400
30–39	100–1500
40–49	100–1600
50–59	100–1900

Sources of Reference (Normal) Values:

Chase, H. P., O'Quin, R. J., and O'Brien, D., Screening for hyperlipidemia in childhood. *J. Am. Med. Assoc.* **230,** 1535–1537 (1974).

*　　*　　*

Reference (Normal) Values:

Lab. 3:

Age	No.	mg/dL
Newborn	24	0–1710
6 wk–16 yr	385	60–1340
Adult	150	300–2000

Sources of Reference (Normal) Values:

An institutional, retrospective study of patients' charts. Patients studied were free of active infection, inflammatory disease, malignancy, and anemia.

*　　*　　*

Reference (Normal) Values:

Lab. 4: >1 yr: <1200 mg/L
Lab. 5: Unspecified age: 360–1650 mg/L

Sources of Reference (Normal) Values:

Lab. 4: institutional. **Lab. 5:** package insert, Worthington Diagnostics Triglycerides Reagent Set; Donabedian, R. K., Free glycerol interference in triglyceride determinations: Warning of a possible problem. *Clin. Chem.* **20,** 632 (1974), letter; Garland, P. B., and Randle, P. J., A rapid enzymatic assay for glycerol. *Nature* **196,** 987–988 (1962); Soloni, F. G., Simplified manual micromethod for determination of serum triglycerides. *Clin. Chem.* **17,** 529–534 (1971).

*　　*　　*

Specimen Volume, Collection, and Preservation; Patient Preparation:

5 to 100 μL, in general. Heparin or EDTA·Na₂ anticoagulant. Separated P or S may be stored 1 wk in RR, or several months in FR. Patient must be fasted for 12 to 16 h before blood collection.

Analytical Method and Instrumentation:

Lab. 1: Kessler, G., and Lederer, H., Fluorometric measurement of triglycerides. In *Automation in Analytical Chemistry,* Technicon Symposium 1965, New York, NY, Mediad, Inc., New York, NY, 1966, p 341; *Manual of Laboratory Operations,* Lipid Research Clinics Program. I. Lipid and Lipoprotein Analysis, DHEW Publication No. (NIH) 75–628; Technicon Instruments Corp. AutoAnalyzer II; Micromedic automatic diluter. **Lab. 2:** Bucolo, G., and David, N., Quantitative determination of serum triglycerides by the use of enzymes. *Clin. Chem.* **19,** 476–482 (1973); Calbiochem-Behring Enzymatic Triglycerides kit; Electro-Nucleonics Inc. Gemeni. **Lab. 3:** Technicon Instruments Corp. SMAC; modified method of Bucolo and David, *op. cit.* **Lab. 4:** Bucolo and David, *op. cit.;* Eggstein, M., and Kreutz, F. H., Eine neue Bestimmung der Neutralfette in Blutserum und Gewebe. *Klin. Wochenschr.* **44,** 262–267 (1966); Bio-Dynamics/*bmc* Reagent Set kit; Abbott ABA-100 Bichromatic Analyzer. **Lab. 5:** Worthington Diagnostics Triglycerides (500 nm) Reagent Set; Gilford Stasar spectrophotometer. **Lab. 6:** Abbott A-Gent; ABA-100 Bichromatic Analyzer; Bucolo and David, *op. cit.*

Commentary—K. W. Schmitt

Triglyceride concentrations in the (overnight) fasting individual vary slightly with age and sex. Values in the first two decades are slightly lower than those in subsequent years. Females have values about 10 mg/dL lower than for males *(1)*.

1. Frederickson, D. S., Levy, R. I., and Lees, R. S., Fat transport in lipoprotein—an integrated approach to mechanism and disorders. *N. Engl. J. Med.* **276,** 148–152 (1967).

Commentary—John E. Sherwin

Enzymic analysis of triglycerides may exhibit significant positive interference from the glycerol contained in some Vacutainer Tube (Becton-Dickinson) stoppers. Beckman Decision quality-control material also contains material that causes positive interference in the enzymic analyses.

Triiodothyronine (T₃)

Specimen Tested:

P, S.

Laboratories Reporting:

4.

Reference (Normal) Values:

	T_3 range (and mean), ng/dL		
Age	**Lab. 1,2**	**Lab. 3**	**Lab. 4**
Cord	14–86 (50)		
0–3 d		T_3 increases at birth from values <70 to 50–350 at 3 d	
1–3 d	100–470 (260)		
6 d–1 yr		90–300	
1–13 wk	99–130 (176)		
1–12 mo	105–245 (175)		
1–5 yr	105–269 (168)		
1–15 yr		90–270	
5–10 yr	94–241 (150)		
10–15 yr	83–213 (133)		
<11 yr			65–247
>15 yr		90–220	
15–20 yr	80–210 (130)		
Adult	70–204		72–176

Note: ng/dL $\times$ 0.01538 = nmol/L.

Sources of Reference (Normal) Values:

Labs. 1, 2: Oddie, T. H., Bernard, B., Klein, A. H., and Fisher, D. A., Comparison of T_4, T_3, rT_3 and TSH concentrations in cord blood and serum of infants up to 3 months of age. *Early Hum. Devel.* **3,** 239-244 (1979); Fisher, D. A., Sack, J., Oddie, T. H., Pekary, A. E., Hershman, J. M., Lam, R. W., and Parslow, M. E., Serum T_4, TBG, T_3 uptake, T_3, reverse T_3, and TSH concentrations in children 1 to 15 years of age. *J. Clin. Endocrinol. Metab.* **45,** 191-198 (1977); *Radioimmunoassay Manual,* 4th ed., Nichols Institute, San Pedro, CA, 1977, p 322. **Labs. 3, 4:** institutional.

Specimen Volume, Collection, and Preservation:

100 to 250 µL. Heparin anticoagulant. Store in FR.

Analytical Method:

Labs. 1, 2: RIA, double antibody, ^{125}I-labeled T_3; Chopra, I. J., Ho, R. S., and Lam, R., An improved radioimmunoassay of triiodothyronine in serum: Its application to clinical and physiological studies. *J. Lab. Clin. Med.* **80,** 729-739 (1972). **Lab. 3:** Corning Medical kit. **Lab. 4:** institutional.

Instrumentation:

Gamma radiation counters.

Commentary—D. A. Fisher

The dramatic increase in serum T_3 values at birth is due both to an increased conversion rate of thyroxine (T_4) to T_3 and to the thyrotropin-induced increase in thyroid gland T_3 secretion; the early increase at 3–4 h after birth is largely due to T_4 and T_3 conversion. An increase in T_3, like the T_4 surge, is seen in the premature infant *(1)*. The decrease in serum T_3 with age in children is associated with a decreasing concentration of thyroxine-binding globulin, but T_3 resin-uptake values remain stable. Thus calculated free T_3 concentrations, as well as total T_3 values, decrease progressively with age *(2)*.

Most (70–85%) of the circulating T_3 is derived from peripheral conversion of T_4 to T_3. However, in patients with Graves' disease or in patients with decreased thyroid reserve (and excessive thyrotropin stimulation) such as Hashimoto's thyroiditis, there is an increased ratio of T_3/T_4 thyroid gland secretion.

1. Klein, A. H., Foley, B., Kenny, F. M., and Fisher, D. A., Thyroid hormone and thyrotropin responses to parturition in premature infants with and without the respiratory distress syndrome. *Pediatrics* **63**, 380–385 (1979).
2. Fisher, D. A., Sack, J., Oddie, T. H., Pekary, A. E., Hershman, J. M., Lam, R. W., and Parslow, M. E., Serum T_4, TBG, T_3 uptake, T_3, reverse T_3, and TSH concentrations in children 1 to 15 years of age. *J. Clin. Endocrinol. Metab.* **45**, 191–198 (1977).

Triiodothyronine (T₃) Resin Uptake

Specimen Tested:

P, S.

Laboratories Reporting:

4.

Reference (Normal) Values:

Age	% of normal pool			
	Lab. 1	**Lab. 2**	**Lab. 3**	**Lab. 4**
Newborn–3 d	22–34			
<6 mo				75–115
Child–adult	25–35	22–32	25–40	
>6 mo				78–121

Sources of Reference (Normal) Values:

Institutional; Yang Bulletin.

Specimen Volume, Collection, and Preservation:

40 to 300 μL. Heparin anticoagulant. Store in FR.

Analytical Methods:

Lab. 1: Sterling, K., and Tabachnik, M., Resin uptake of I-131 triiodothyronine as a test of thyroid function. *J. Clin. Endocrinol. Metab.* **21,** 456–464 (1961); Yang Lab. Triiodothyronine Uptake Test. **Lab. 2:** Amersham Thyopac 3. **Lab. 3:** Mitchell, M. L., Harden, A. B., and O'Rourke, M. E., The in vitro resin sponge uptake of triiodothyronine from serum in thyroid disease and in pregnancy. *J. Clin. Endocrinol. Metab.* **20,** 1474–1483 (1960). **Lab. 4:** institutional.

Instrumentation:

Gamma counters: Packard Auto-Gamma 5110, Nuclear Chicago, LKB 80000.

Commentary—D. A. Fisher

T_3 resin-uptake values are relatively low in cord blood because of the relatively high concentrations of thyroxine-binding globulin (TBG) in serum. The neonatal thyroxine (T_4) surge saturates TBG binding sites and the T_3 resin-uptake result increases.

Re-equilibration occurs, in my experience, by one to two months of age, and values thereafter remain essentially similar to adult values *(1)*. T_3 resin-uptake results should not be reported in percent binding, but as a fraction (or a percent) of the binding in a reference pool, the latter being analyzed concomitantly with the unknown samples. This value, the "T_3 index," can be used to correct T_4 results for variations in TBG. The corrected T_4 is referred to as the "free T_4 index." T_3 resin uptake does not provide a reliable T_4 correction if TBG values are very low or very high. Thus, infants with TBG deficiency have low corrected T_4 results. If TBG deficiency is suspected, a direct measurement of TBG, preferably by RIA, is indicated.

Finally, the T_3 resin-uptake result can be used to correct the total T_3 result for TBG variations *(1)*. The calculation is similar to that for the free T_4 index.

1. Sawin, C. T., Chopra, D., Albane, J., and Azizi, F., The free triiodothyronine (T_3) index. *Ann. Intern. Med.* **88,** 474–477 (1978).

Trypsin (EC 3.4.21.4)

In Duodenal Fluid

Laboratory Reporting:

1.

Reference (Normal) Values:

Diluted 12.5-fold or greater, the specimen still will digest gelatin (160–180 μg of activated trypsin/mL of duodenal fluid).

Sources of Reference (Normal) Values:

Text ref. *1*.

Specimen Volume:

0.2 mL.

Analytical Method:

Varley, H., *Practical Clinical Biochemistry*, 3rd ed. Interscience, New York, NY, 1962, p 329.

In Feces

Laboratory Reporting:

1.

Reference (Normal) Values:

<1 yr: diluted 100-fold or greater, the specimen will still digest gelatin.

Sources of Reference (Normal) Values:

Text ref. *1*.

Amount of Specimen:

1.0 g (wet weight) required for dilution.

Analytical Method:

Varley, *op. cit.*, p 329.

*　　　*　　　*

Laboratory Reporting:

1.

Reference (Normal) Values:

20–950 U/g

Sources of Reference (Normal) Values:

Institutional.

Amount of Specimen:

Aliquot of 5-d collection.

Analytical Method:

Dyck, W. P., Titrimetric measurements of fecal trypsin and chymotrypsin in cystic fibrosis with pancreatic exocrine insufficiency. *Am. J. Dig. Dis.* **12**, 310–317 (1967).

Enzyme Data:

1. Enzyme unit definition: 1 IUB unit (U) = that enzyme activity hydrolyzing 1 μmol of substrate in 1 min at 37 °C.
2. Substrate: *p*-tosyl-L-arginine methyl ester hydrochloride.
3. Reaction temperature: 37 °C.
4. Temperature reported: 37 °C.

Instrumentation:

Metrohm Models E 300 B pH meter, E 473 Impulsomat, Dosimat, and recorder.

Note: See also **Chymotrypsin** and Chapter 8, **Laboratory Tests in Pediatric Gastroenterology.**

Tryptophan

Specimen Tested:

P.

Laboratory Reporting:

1.

Reference (Normal) Values:

Unspecified pediatric age: 41–67 μmol/L

Sources of Reference (Normal) Values:

Institutional.

Specimen Volume, Collection, and Preservation; Patient Preparation:

40 μL. Heparin anticoagulant. Fast patient overnight. Undetermined stability. Store P in FR.

Analytical Method and Instrumentation:

Measurement of the fluorescence of norharman produced from the oxidation of the product of tryptophan–formaldehyde condensation; Denckla, W. D., and Dewey, H. K., The determination of tryptophan in plasma, liver, and urine. *J. Lab. Clin. Med.* **69**, 160–169 (1967); Farrand Mark 1 spectrofluorometer.

Commentary—Roger L. Boeckx

The fluorometric method of Denckla and Dewey *(1)* is the most commonly used method for the measurement of tryptophan concentration. However, some reports have cited problems with this method *(2,3)*. In particular, Bloxam and Warren *(2)* report difficulties with the calibration curve and with the day-to-day precision. Modifications of the original Denckla and Dewey method have been proposed by Bloxam and Warren *(2)* and by Eccleston *(3)*.

Much has been written lately regarding the ratio of free to total tryptophan in plasma. Ultrafiltration *(3,4)* or equilibrium dialysis *(5)* has been used to separate free tryptophan from the plasma protein-bound fraction. Because binding is sensitive to pH and temperature, the different approaches have been shown to give different results *(5)*.

The measurement of free and total tryptophan concentrations is of interest in psychiatry. Decreased values for free tryptophan in plasma have been reported during depression *(6)*. On the other hand, free plasma tryptophan is increased in migraine *(7)* and in hepatic coma *(8)*.

Wood and Coppen *(6)* reported a mean total tryptophan concentration of 64.4 ± 2.5 μmol/L (mean ± standard error) in a group of control subjects. The free tryptophan concentration in this group was 6.08 ± 0.74 μmol/L, i.e., 9.4% of the total. In a group of "depressed" patients, the authors reported total tryptophan as 59.8 ± 4.4 μmol/L, and the free tryptophan concentration as 3.90 ± 0.29 μmol/L, or 6.5% of total.

1. Denckla, W. D., and Dewey, H. K., The determination of tryptophan in plasma, liver, and urine. *J. Lab. Clin. Med.* **69**, 160–169 (1967).
2. Bloxam, D. L., and Warren, W. H., Error in the determination of tryptophan by the method of Denckla and Dewey. A revised procedure. *Anal. Biochem.* **60**, 621–625 (1974).
3. Eccleston, E. G., A method for the estimation of free and total acid-soluble plasma tryptophan using an ultrafiltration technique. *Clin. Chim. Acta* **48**, 269–272 (1973).
4. Knott, P. J., and Curzon, G., Free tryptophan in plasma and brain tryptophan metabolism. *Nature* **239**, 452–453 (1972).
5. Wood, K., Swade, C., Harwood, J., Eccleston, E., Bishop, M., and Coppen A., Comparison of methods for the determination of total and free tryptophan in plasma. *Clin. Chim. Acta* **80**, 299–303 (1977).
6. Wood, K., and Coppen, A., The effect of clofibrate on total and free plasma tryptophan in depressed patients. *Neuropharmacology* **17**, 428–430 (1978).
7. Salmon, S., Fanciullacci, M., Bonciani, M., and Sicuteri, F., Plasma tryptophan in migraine. *Headache* **17**, 238–241 (1978).
8. Hutson, D. G., Ono, J., Dombro, R. S., Levi, J. U., Livingstone, A., and Zeppa, R., A longitudinal study of tryptophan involvement in hepatic coma. *Am. J. Surg.* **137**, 235–239 (1979).

Tyrosine

Specimen Tested:

P, S.

Laboratories Reporting:

2.

Reference (Normal) Values:

Age	Lab. 1	Lab. 2
Premature newborn	3.0–30.2 mg/dL	
Full-term newborn	1.7–4.7	
1–12 yr	1.4–3.4	
Child		2.5–4.0 mg/dL[a]

[a] Higher values in premature infant and in the neonatal period.

Note: mg/dL × 0.0552 = mmol/L.

Sources of Reference (Normal) Values:

Lab. 1: Hsia, D. Y.-Y., Litwack, L., O'Flynn, M., and Jacovcic, S., Serum phenylalanine and tyrosine levels in the newborn infant. *N. Engl. J. Med.* **267,** 1067–1070 (1962); Hsia, D. Y.-Y., Berman, J. L., and Slatis, H. M., Screening newborn infants for phenylketonuria. *J. Am. Med. Assoc.* **188,** 203–206 (1964). **Lab. 2:** Wong, P. W. K., O'Flynn, M. E., and Inouye, T., Micro methods for measuring phenylalanine and tyrosine in serum. *Clin. Chem.* **10,** 1098–1104 (1964); institutional.

Specimen Volume, Collection, and Preservation:

100 μL. Store in FR. Claims exist for long stability (4 d) at RT, with addition of NaF, 3 mg/mL of serum, prolonging stability to 7 d. Dried spot on paper, in closed container, is possibly stable at RT for 1 mo.

Analytical Method and Instrumentation:

Lab. 1: Wong et al., *op. cit.;* Sigma Chemical Co. tyrosine kit; Aminco-Bowman fluorometer. **Lab. 2:** modified method from Wong et al., *op. cit.;* Udenfriend, S., and Cooper, J. R., The chemical estimation of tyrosine and tyramine. *J. Biol. Chem.* **196,** 227–233 (1952); Varian 635 (UV-VIS) spectrophotometer.

Commentary—Roger L. Boeckx

Several disorders of tyrosine metabolism have been described. The normal catabolic pathway is affected in at least five conditions of clinical interest. In all cases, plasma and urine tyrosine concentrations are increased.

The most common form of tyrosinemia is the so-called "transitory tyrosinemia of the newborn," first described by Levine et al. *(1)* in 1939. It is now known that this condition is the result of retarded development or inhibition of p-hydroxyphenylpyruvic acid oxidase (p-HPPA) *(2)*. Vitamin C has been shown to relieve this condition and, in some cases, p-HPPA is believed to be inhibited by its own substrate *(3)*. As many as 30% of premature infants and 10% of full-term infants show increased values for tyrosine *(4)*. It is commonly thought that this condition is harmless.

Another benign but rare form of tyrosinosis, described by Medes *(5)* in 1932, was originally thought to be due to p-HPPA deficiency, but is now thought to be caused by a renal-specific deficiency of tyrosine aminotransferase (EC 2.6.1.5) *(2)*. Only one patient has been described *(5)*.

A third but more serious type of tyrosinemia, usually referred to as the "Oregon type," is manifested by a persistent hypertyrosinemia due to a deficiency of cytosol tyrosine aminotransferase activity *(6)*. Six patients with this disorder have been described. All were mentally retarded, and congenital anomalies were reported in some *(7)*.

Over 100 cases of the hepatorenal type of tyrosinemia have been reported. This is a serious disorder manifested by failure to thrive, rickets, vomiting, diarrhea, edema, ascites, hepatosplenomegaly, and occasionally mental retardation *(7)*. Liver failure and generalized renal reabsorption defects with Fanconi's syndrome are acute symptoms. Although some evidence suggests that the primary defect is a deficiency of p-HPPA, other workers have proposed instead that the p-HPPA deficiency is a secondary manifestation of another, as yet unidentified, metabolic defect *(8)*.

Finally, it must be emphasized that hypertyrosinemia is a common feature of liver disease, and that tyrosine alone or as one component of a generalized aminoacidemia is increased in many liver diseases *(7)*. It is also important to remember that plasma tyrosine concentrations can be decreased in some types of hyperphenylalaninemia *(9)*.

1. Levine, S. Z., Marples, E., and Gordon, H. H., A defect in metabolism of aromatic amino acids in premature infants: The role of vitamin C. *Science* **90**, 620–621 (1939).
2. Scriver, C. R., and Rosenberg, L. E., *Amino Acid Metabolism and Its Disorders*. W. B. Saunders Co., Philadelphia, PA, 1973, pp 338–369.
3. Zannoni, V. G., and La Du, B. N., Studies on the defect in tyrosine metabolism in scorbutic guinea pigs. *J. Biol. Chem.* **235**, 165–168 (1960).
4. Avery, M. E., Clow, C. L., Menkes, J. H., Ramos, A., Scriver, C. R., Stern, L., and Wasserman, B. P., Transient tyrosinemia of the newborn: Dietary and clinical aspects. *Pediatrics* **39**, 378–384 (1967).
5. Medes, G., A new error of tyrosine metabolism: Tyrosinosis. The intermediary metabolism of tyrosine and phenylalanine. *Biochem. J.* **26**, 917–940 (1932).

6. Kennaway, N. G., and Buist, N. R. M., Metabolic studies in a patient with hepatic cytosol tyrosine aminotransferase deficiency. *Pediatr. Res.* **5,** 287–294 (1971).
7. La Du, B. N., and Gjessing, L. R., Tyrosinosis and tyrosinemia. In text ref. *11,* 4th ed., pp 256–267.
8. Gaull, G. E., Rassin, D. K., Solomon, G. E., Harris, R. C., and Sturman, J. A., Biochemical observations on so-called hereditary tyrosinemia. *Pediatr. Res.* **4,** 337–344 (1970).
9. Tourian, A. Y., and Sidbury, J. B., Phenylketonuria. In text ref. *11,* 4th ed., pp 240–255.

Urea Clearance

Specimen Tested:

P, S, U.

Laboratory Reporting:

1.

Reference (Normal) Values:

Premature: 3.5–17.3 mL/min per 1.73 m^2 of body surface
Newborn: 8.7–33
2–12 mo: 40–95
2 yr and over: 52

Sources of Normal Values:

Text ref. *1.*

Analytical Method:

Text ref. *2.*

Commentary—Garry M. Lum

Urea is filtered by the glomerulus but is variably reabsorbed by the renal tubules. The concentration of urea in plasma is influenced by factors other than renal function. Because of the tubular reabsorption of urea, clearance of urea can be directly influenced by rate and volume of urine flow. Thus the variability in plasma urea, such as occurs with protein intake, catabolism, liver function, etc., and the alterations in urine concentration that occur with urine flow make the interpretation of urea clearance difficult and thus not very useful in most clinical situations. It is consequently equally difficult to derive normal values except in the most general sense. However, serum urea values certainly serve to draw attention to a possible decrease in glomerular filtration rate and, when interpreted in light of the concomitant serum creatinine value, may suggest the cause;

e.g., urinary obstruction usually results in serum urea/creatinine ratios greater than 20.

1. Schwartz, G. J., Haycock, G. B., and Spitzer, A., Plasma creatinine and urea concentrations in children: Normal values for age and sex. *J. Pediatr.* **88,** 828–830 (1976).

Urea Nitrogen

Specimen Tested:

P, S.

Laboratories Reporting:

8.

Reference (Normal) Values:

Age	mg/dL (mmol/L)
Cord (1 lab.)	5–11 (1.8–3.9)
<2 mo	4–15 (1.4–5.4)
2 mo–adult	5–23 (1.8–8.2)
1–2 yr	5–15 (1.8–5.4)
Child–adult, 2 SD range	5–25 (1.8–9.0); 6–20 (2.1–7.1); (2.5–6.7)
5th-95th percentile	9–18 (3.2–6.6)

Sources of Reference (Normal) Values:

Institutional; text ref. 2, p 347; Kaplan, A., Urea nitrogen and urinary ammonia. *Stand. Methods Clin. Chem.* **5,** 245–256 (1965); Cheng, M. H., Lipsey, A. I., Blanco, V., Wong, H. T., and Spiro, S. H., Microchemical analysis for 13 constituents of plasma from healthy children. *Clin. Chem.* **25,** 692–698 (1979); Cherian, A. G., and Hill, J. G., Percentile estimates of reference values for fourteen chemical constituents in sera of children and adolescents. *Am. J. Clin. Pathol.* **69,** 24–31 (1978).

Specimen Volume, Collection, and Preservation:

5 to 50 µL. Heparin anticoagulant; others may interfere with enzymic procedures for urea. Claims for stability: 1 to 3 d at RT. Fluoride or fluoride/thymol preserves for 5 d at RT, but should not be used if it interferes. Best stored less than 1 d in RR, or for prolonged periods in FR.

Analytical Method and Instrumentation:

Lab. 1: Fisher Diagnostics reagents for diacetyl monoxine method on Technicon SMA II. **Labs. 2, 3, 4:** conductivity rate method; Chin, W. T., and Kroontje, W., Conductivity method for determination of urea. *Anal. Chem.* **33,** 1757–1760 (1961); McClean, M. H., and Hearn,

D., Simultaneous measurement of glucose and urea nitrogen using an automated rate electrochemical system. *Clin. Chem.* **20**, 856–857 (1974), abstract 9; Beckman Instruments, Inc., B.U.N. Analyzer, Astra-8, System I Glucose/BUN Analyzer. **Lab. 5:** diacetyl monoxime; Marsh, W. H., Fingerhut, B., and Miller, H., Automated and manual direct methods for the determination of blood urea. *Clin. Chem.* **11**, 624–627 (1965); Technicon Instruments Corp. 6/60 (micro). **Lab. 6:** Talke, H., and Schubert, G. E., Enzymatische Harnstoffbestimmung in Blut und Serum im optischen Test nach Warburg. *Klin. Wochenschr.* **43**, 174–175 (1965); Herrera, L., The precision of percentiles in establishing normal limits in medicine. *J. Lab. Clin. Med.* **52**, 34–42 (1958); Reed, A. H., Henry, R. J., and Mason, W. B., Influence of statistical method on the resulting estimate of normal range. *Clin. Chem.* **17**, 275–284 (1971); Electro-Nucleonics Inc. GEMSAEC. **Lab. 7:** Greiner Electronics Selective Analyzer II, with urease–Berthelot reaction; Abbott A-Gent reagents with ABA-100 Bichromatic Analyzer.

Commentary—Robert L. Murray

Urea, the major nonprotein nitrogen component of plasma, can be determined either by condensation with substituted diketones (most commonly diacetyl monoxime) or more specifically by urease-catalyzed hydrolysis. Because fluoride inhibits urease, either separate samples must be drawn for glucose and urea determinations, or an alternative noninterfering antiglycolytic agent such as iodoacetate must be used. Diacetyl methods are sensitive to increased ammonia concentration only if phenazone or thiosemicarbazide is used to increase the sensitivity of the reaction.

Urea is the major end product of protein catabolism, synthesized chiefly in the liver and excreted via the kidneys, this path being the chief means of excreting surplus nitrogen. Although measuring urea is the most popular laboratory tool for evaluating renal function, its value is limited by the fact that urea concentration is affected by protein intake and the rate of urine formation. Because urea is reabsorbed in the tubules, low tubular flow rates result in increased reabsorption and increased plasma urea values. Owing to the reserve capacity of the kidneys, increases in plasma urea caused by renal impairment may not be seen until kidney function is as little as 50% of normal.

Consideration of the amount of protein intake is essential in the evaluation of normal limits derived from breast-fed vs formula-fed infants. Dale et al. *(1)* and Davies and Saunders *(2)* both report mean plasma urea concentrations in formula-fed babies (with or without additional solid supplement) that are double the concentration in breast-fed babies. This can be explained by the significantly greater protein intake of the formula-fed babies, caused by the higher concentration of protein in cow's milk (3.3 g/dL) than in human milk (1.1 g/dL), and perhaps by potential error in reconstituting a dry powder formula. On the other hand, when a breast-fed baby receives insufficient calories, the resulting starvation and dehydration can produce urea nitrogen values as great as 78 mg/dL (3).

Schwartz et al. have reported normal values for plasma urea nitrogen in 1398 healthy infants and children (4); their data, presented by sex and by single-year interval through age 17 years, document plasma urea values about one-half the adult value. Cheng et al. have published a similar study on a smaller population, and find no sex difference before age eight years and consistently increasing values for plasma urea for both sexes throughout childhood (5).

1. Dale, G., Goldfinch, M. E., Sibert, J. R., and Webb, J. K. G., Plasma osmolality, sodium, and urea in healthy breast-fed and bottle-fed infants in Newcastle-upon-Tyne. *Arch. Dis. Child.* **50,** 731–734 (1975).
2. Davies, D. P., and Saunders, R., Blood urea: Normal values in early infancy related to feeding practices. *Arch. Dis. Child.* **48,** 563–565 (1973).
3. Gilmore, H. E., and Rowland, T. W., Critical malnutrition in breast-fed infants. *Am. J. Dis. Child.* **132,** 885–887 (1978).
4. Schwartz, G. J., Haycock, G. B., Chir, B., and Spitzer, A., Plasma creatinine and urea concentration in children: Normal values for age and sex. *J. Pediatr.* **88,** 828–830 (1976).
5. Cheng, M. H., Lipsey, A. I., Blanco, V., Wong, H. T., and Spiro, S. H., Microchemical analysis for 13 constituents of plasma from healthy children. *Clin. Chem.* **25,** 692–698 (1979).

Uric Acid (Urate)

Specimen Tested:

P, S.

Laboratories Reporting:

10.

Reference (Normal) Values:

Lab. 1: Cord blood: 4.4–7.4 mg/dL (0.26–0.44 mmol/L)
Labs. 2–4: Child, adult F: 2.0–6.0 (0.12–0.36)
adult M: 3.0–7.0 (0.18–0.42)
Labs. 5–7: Child: 2.0–5.5 (0.12–0.33)
Lab. 8:

Age, yr	mg/dL (mmol/L)
0–2	2.0–7.0 (0.12–0.42)
2–12	2.0–6.5 (0.12–0.39)
12–14	2.0–7.0 (0.12–0.42)
14–adult, M	3.0–8.0 (0.18–0.48)
F	2.0–7.0 (0.12–0.42)

Lab. 9:
Age (unspecified), M: 2.9–8.5 mg/dL (0.17–0.51 mmol/L)
F: 2.4–6.5 (0.14–0.39)

Lab. 10:

Age	No.	2 SD range, mg/dL (mmol/L)
Newborn	24	1.2–8.8 (0.071–0.52)
6 wk–3 yr	72	2.0–7.6 (0.12–0.45)
3–12 yr	204	· 2.3–6.1 (0.14–0.36)
12–16 yr	142	3.1–7.6 (0.18–0.45)
Adult	150	M: 3.9–9.0 (0.18–0.54)
		F: 2.5–7.1 (0.15–0.42)

Sources of Reference (Normal) Values:

Five labs: institutional; 1 lab.: text ref. *5.* **Lab. 8:** Cheng, M. H., Lipsey, A. I., Blanco, V., Wong, H. T., and Spiro, S. H., Microchemical analysis for 13 constituents of plasma from healthy children. *Clin. Chem.* **25,** 692–698 (1979). **Lab. 9:** Natelson, S., Uric Acid. *Stand. Methods Clin. Chem.* **1,** 123–135 (1953); Dubbs, C. A., Davis, F. W., and Adams, W. S., Simple microdetermination of uric acid. *J. Biol. Chem.* **218,** 497–504 (1956); Young, D. S., Pestaner, L. C., and Gibberman, V., Effects of drugs on clinical laboratory tests. *Clin. Chem.* **21,** 1D-432D (1975). **Lab. 10:** retrospective studies of patients' charts. Included were patients free of infection, inflammatory disease, malignancy, and anemia.

Specimen Volume, Collection, and Preservation; Patient Preparation:

Generally 10 to 100 μL. Heparin anticoagulant. Stable for 7 d in RR, as long as 6 mo in FR. Claims are cited that uric acid in S is stable for 3 d at RT. Fluoride or fluoride/thymol preserves the specimen longer. Patient should be fasting for blood collection.

Analytical Method and Instrumentation:

Uricase methods: **Lab. 3:** Pesce, M. A., Bodourian, S. H., and Nicholson, J. F., Automated enzymatic micromethod for determination of uric acid in serum and urine with a centrifugal analyzer. *Clin. Chem.* **20,** 1231–1233 (1974); reagent kit of Union Carbide; Union Carbide CentrifiChem 400. **Lab. 4:** Beckman Instruments reagents adapted for use with Glucose Analyzer; oxygen rate method. **Lab. 5:** Kageyama, N., A direct colorimetric determination of uric acid in serum and urine with uricase–catalase system. *Clin. Chim. Acta* **31,** 421–426 (1971); Electro-Nucleonics Inc. Gemeni; SMI pipette; Clay-Adams adjustable volume Selectapette dispenser. **Lab. 6:** Bio-Dynamics/*bmc* URICA-QUANT kit; Electro-Nucleonics Inc. GEMSAEC. **Lab. 8:** Kageyama, *op. cit.;* Bio-Dynamics/*bmc* URICA-QUANT kit; Abbott ABA-100 Bichromatic Analyzer. **Lab. 9:** Worthington Diagnostics kit; Gilford 3500 automated system.

Phosphotungstate reduction method: **Lab. 1:** Fisher Diagnostics reagents; Technicon Instruments Corp. SMA II. **Lab. 2:** Henry, R. J., Sobel, C., and Kim, J., A modified carbonate–phosphotungstate method for the determination of uric acid and comparison with the spectrophotometric uricase method. *Am. J. Clin. Pathol.* **28,** 152–164, 645 (1957); Gilford Stasar III spectrophotometer. **Lab. 7:** Caraway, W. T., Uric acid. *Stand. Methods Clin. Chem.* **4,** 239–247 (1963); LKB 7400 absorptiometer. **Lab. 10:** Technicon Instrument Corp. SMAC.

Commentary—Robert L. Murray

Urate in body fluids has in the past been measured most frequently by reduction of phosphotungstate in alkaline pH to tungsten blue. It can also be measured enzymically by its uricase(EC 1.7.3.3)-catalyzed oxidation to allantoin. Either method is amenable to microadaptation. However, reducing substances such as acetaminophen, aminophenol, ascorbic acid, bilirubin, and salicylate, as well as purines such as caffeine, theophylline, and mercaptopurine, will reduce phosphotungstate, with consequent overestimation of uric acid concentration. Instability of the chromogen further complicates this assay. These difficulties have caused many to adopt the enzymic method. The uricase-mediated analysis of urate is considerably more specific and sensitive, with only certain purines (allopurinol, mercaptopurine, and xanthines such as caffeine and theophylline) reported to cause minor interference.

Urate appears in the plasma as the end product of excess nucleoprotein-derived purine catabolism, and is eliminated via renal excretion. Most of the purine initially degraded, however, is recirculated through the hypoxanthine–guanine phosphoribosyltransferase (EC 2.4.2.8) pathway. Consequently, diseases that involve increased cell turnover, such as leukemia or polycythemia, or decreased renal function result in increased concentrations of plasma urate. The former type of diseases will increase urinary urate concentrations, whereas the latter will initially decrease urinary concentrations.

Although severe renal failure can lead to urate concentrations in plasma as great as 35 mg/dL, the increase is variable and is not a useful index of renal insufficiency. Erythrocyte urate concentration is approximately one-half that of plasma, so hemolysis does not significantly change plasma concentration. Some urate circulates in plasma bound to albumin; consequently, its renal clearance is affected (inversely) by albumin concentration. Organic acids and certain drugs decrease renal clearance by competition with the tubular secretory system.

In the normal neonate, plasma urate increases transiently from day 1 to day 3 of life *(1),* perhaps because of hyperlacticacidemia resulting from initial stress. After this early period, excess urate is rapidly excreted, so that the urate concentration decreases to the normal value in children (less than the adult normal), which is consistent with the not-infrequent finding of urate crystals in urine of normal neonates *(2)*.

The lower plasma urate concentrations seen in preadolescents is attributed to the higher renal clearance in children *(3)*. Although the total excretion of urate increases between the ages of two and seven years (corresponding to the rapid increase in body mass), the amount excreted per kilogram of body weight decreases *(4)*. This decrease may be related to the infant's greater relative weight of internal organs, higher DNA/protein ratio, and accelerated growth.

The Lesch–Nyhan syndrome involves an absence of hypoxanthine–guanine phosphoribosyltransferase. Without this recirculating pathway, huge amounts of urate are lost in the urine. The amount of circulating urate, although frequently high, is quite variable.

1. Ahmadian, Y., and Lewy, P., Possible urate nephropathy of the newborn infant as a cause of transient renal insufficiency. *J. Pediatr.* **91**, 96–100 (1977).
2. Stapleton, F. B., Linshaw, M. A., Hassanein, K. M., and Gruskin, A. B., Uric acid excretion in normal children. *J. Pediatr.* **92**, 911–914 (1978).
3. Harkness, R. A., and Nicol, A. D., Plasma uric acid levels in children. *Arch. Dis. Child.* **44**, 773–777 (1969).
4. Stapleton, F. B., Hassanein, K. M., and Linshaw, M. A., Renal uric acid clearance and excretion during childhood. *Pediatr. Res.* **11**, 558 (1977).

Commentary—Michael A. Pesce

Urate is the end product of purine metabolism in humans. Hyperuricemia is caused by an increased production of uric acid, a defect in renal elimination, or a combination of both. Increased concentrations of urate in serum are found in renal failure, in disorders involving increased cellular destruction such as leukemia, in metabolic disorders, and in gout. In treating leukemia, serum urate must be monitored because abrupt and massive destruction of malignant cells by cytotoxic agents produces large amounts of uric acid. In disorders such as glucose-6-phosphatase deficiency and diabetic ketosis, there is an increased production of the weak organic acids lactic acid and β-hydroxybutyric acid, which compete with uric acid for renal tubular secretion and are responsible for hyperuricemia. Primary gout is predominantly an adult disease.

Urate is measured by reaction with phosphotungstate, or by enzymic procedures in which urate is oxidized by the enzyme uricase to hydrogen peroxide and allantoin. Quantitation is usually by *(a)* measuring the decrease in absorbance of urate at 293 nm, or *(b)* coupling the hydrogen peroxide with other reactions to form reaction products that can be measured spectrophotometrically. These enzymic systems can be adapted to discrete analyzers such as the ABA-100 (Abbott Labs.) or to centrifugal analyzers; these are ideal for use in pediatrics because small sample sizes can be used. Urate in serum is stable for seven days if stored at 4 °C *(1)*.

The normal values for uric acid in serum vary with age and sex. In normal infants, urate in serum obtained from cord blood averaged 6.0 mg/dL *(2)*; 24 h later, urate values increased to a mean of 7.0 mg/dL, decreasing to normal values (6.0 mg/dL) by the fourth day. In one study *(3)* urate values were shown not to change significantly in either sex from one month to 12 years of age, and ranged between 2.0 and 7.0 mg/dL. In another study *(4)* urate concentrations from ages five to 12 years were higher in girls than in boys: 2.3–7.1 and 2.3–6.3 mg/dL, respectively. From ages 13 to 17 years, urate concentrations in boys increased and were higher than in girls. By age 17 urate concentrations in both sexes reached adult values.

1. Pesce, M. A., Bodourian, S. H., and Nicholson, J. F., Automated enzymatic micromethod for determination of uric acid in serum and urine with a centrifugal analyzer. *Clin. Chem.* **20**, 1231–1233 (1974).
2. Raivio, K. O., Neonatal hyperuricemia. *J. Pediatr.* **88**, 625–630 (1976).
3. Cheng, M. H., Lipsey, A. I., Blanco, V., Wong, H. T., and Spiro, S. H., Microchemical analysis for 13 constituents of plasma from healthy children. *Clin. Chem.* **25**, 692–698 (1979).
4. Munan, M., Kelly, A., and PetitClerc, C., Serum urate levels between ages 10 and 14: Changes in sex trends. *J. Lab. Clin. Med.* **90**, 990–996 (1977).

Uroporphyrinogen I Synthase, Erythrocyte
[Uro-S; EC 4.3.1.8; porpho-bilinogen ammonia-lyase (polymerizing)]

Specimen Tested:

B.

Laboratory Reporting:

1.

Reference (Normal) Values:

2–18 yr, M: 15–47 arbitrary units
          F: 16–53
0–2 yr: values tend to be higher

Sources of Reference (Normal) Values:

An institutional study made on 120 male and 82 female ambulatory patients with no known hematologic or porphyrin disease. Samples assayed within 24 h of collection.

Sample Volume, Collection, and Preservation:

250 µL. Heparin anticoagulant. Avoid clotting and hemolysis. Store in RR. Assay within 48 h.

Analytical Method:

Fluorometric; Peterson, L. R., Hamernyik, P., Bird, T. D., and Labbé, R. F., Erythrocyte uroporphyrinogen I synthase activity in diagnosis of acute intermittent porphyria. *Clin. Chem.* **22,** 1835–1840 (1976).

Enzyme Data:

1. Enzyme unit definition: 1 arbitrary unit = 1 nmol of porphyrin formed per hour per milliliter of erythrocytes.
2. Buffer, pH: citrate–phosphate, 7.5.
3. Substrate: δ-aminolaevulinic acid.
4. Reaction temperature: 37 °C.
5. Temperature reported: 37 °C.

Instrumentation:

Turner 100 fluorometer, with filters: primary 110–812 (405), and secondary 110–820 (25).

Note: Uro-S activity in acute intermittent porphyria, whether the disease is clinically apparent or latent, is decreased to an average of 50% of normal values, and generally ranges between 5 and 20 arbitrary units. Lead intoxication will also decrease the activity, but dithiothreitol or Zn can reactivate it.

Valproic Acid (Depakene)

Specimen Tested:

P, S.

Laboratory Reporting:

1.

Reference (Normal) Values:

Therapeutic range: 50–100 mg/L (µg/mL)
Toxic concentration: 150 mg/L

Sources of Reference (Normal) Values:

Institutional.

Specimen Collection, etc.:

Same as for **Phenobarbital.**

Analytical Method and Instrumentation:

GLC, modified method of Dukhuis and Vervolet, as cited under **Phenobarbital;** Hewlett-Packard gas chromatograph.

Commentary—Peter J. and Joan H. Howanitz

Valproic acid is a branched-chain carboxylic acid; its mode of action may be mediated through its effects on the function of brain gamma-aminobutyric acid (GABA). Valproic acid, or its salt sodium valproate, is useful in treating a wide variety of seizures. In the United States, it has been approved for use in treating simple and complex absence seizures (as the sole drug), as well as seizure types that occur in conjunction with absence seizures (approved for adjunctive therapy) *(1)*.

After an oral dose, valproic acid is rapidly and completely absorbed, with peak serum concentrations attained between 1 and 4 h *(2)*. Simultaneous intake of food will delay but not decrease absorption. Although kinetic studies in man are scanty, serum half-lives range from 8 to 15 h *(2–4)*, with the half-life in children generally at the lower end of this range. The relatively short half-life predisposes to fluctuations throughout the day in serum concentrations of the drug. Valproic acid is tightly bound to serum albumin, with only 8 to 23% free (unbound), depending on its concentration in serum. Free fatty acids displace valproic acid from its serum-binding sites, and it has been suggested that this interaction may be clinically significant *(5)*. Valproic acid is extensively metabolized in the liver and then excreted by the kidney, mainly as the glucuronide conjugate.

The drug may be given once or three times daily; however, gastrointestinal side effects occur less often on the three times daily schedule *(6)*. When a daily dose of valproic acid was compared with a fasting morning serum value, no consistent relationship was observed *(8)*. Fifty to 100 μg/mL is usually considered to be within the therapeutic range *(1,2,7)*, but the relationships among serum concentration, therapeutic range, and side effects are not well established. In one well-controlled study, serum concentrations of 50 to 59 μg/mL were associated with better clinical response than were lower serum concentrations of the drug *(9)*. Although some patients have required valproic acid concentrations of 110 to 150 μg/mL of blood for seizure control, the upper limit of the therapeutic range has not been well defined.

Valproic acid often is used in combination with other drugs. When added to the regimen of a patient taking phenobarbital, it delays metabolism, thereby causing an increase in serum phenobarbital concentrations of about 20 to 50%; in patients taking primidone, valproic acid causes an increase in both primidone and phenobarbital concentrations. Addition of valproic acid to the therapeutic regimen decreases the total phenytoin concentration in serum *(10)*.

Reported side effects of valproic acid include thrombocytopenia, pancreatitis, abnormal hepatic function tests, hepatic failure, and coma. These reports, however, have not been well documented, and the relationship to serum values is unclear. In four patients reported to have abnormal hepatic function tests or hepatic failure, three had serum concentrations within the usual therapeutic range, and the fourth had 166 μg/mL *(11–13)*. A syndrome of altered behavior, confusion, and deteriorating seizure control may occur if concentrations exceed 100 μg/mL, although this apparently occurs rarely *(14)*. Two patients who ingested about 35 g of valproic acid developed coma that was managed successfully with conservative therapy. Increases in valproic acid half-life of up to 30 h have been reported in individuals attempting suicide with the drug *(15)*.

In a few patients reported to have received valproic acid during pregnancy, no increased incidence of congenital abnormalities was noted in the newborns. In one case, valproic acid concentration in breast milk was about 5 to 10% that of serum. Although this mother breast-fed her infant, serum valproic acid values, which had been about the same in both individuals at the time of delivery, became undetectable in the infant by one month of age *(16)*.

1. Bruni, J., and Wilder, B. J., Valproic acid. *Arch. Neurol.* **36,** 393–398 (1979).
2. Loiseau, P., Brachet, A., and Henry, P., Concentration of dipropylacetate in plasma. *Epilepsia* **16,** 609–615 (1975).
3. Schobben, E., van der Kleijn, E., and Gabreëls, F. J. M., Pharmacokinetics of di-*n*-propylacetate in epileptic patients. *Eur. J. Clin. Pharmacol.* **8,** 97–105 (1975).
4. Simon, D., and Penry, J. K., Sodium di-*n*-propylacetate (DPA) in the treatment of epilepsy. *Epilepsia* **16,** 549–573 (1975).
5. Patel, I. H., and Levy, R. H., Valproic acid binding to human serum albumin; determination of free fraction in the presence of anticonvulsants and free fatty acids. *Epilepsia* **20,** 85–90 (1979).
6. Schmidt, D., Fluctuation of dipropyl acetate plasma levels with one and three daily doses. *Pharm. Weekb.* **112,** 285–287 (1977).
7. Vajda, F. J. E., Drummer, O. H., Morris, P. M., McNeil, J. J., and Bladin, P. F., Gas chromatographic measurement of plasma levels of sodium valproate: Tentative therapeutic range of a new anticonvulsant in the treatment of refractory epileptics. *Clin. Exp. Pharmacol. Physiol.* **5,** 67–73 (1978).
8. Johannessen, S. I., Serum levels of di-*n*-propyl acetate in epileptic patients. *Pharm. Weekb.* **112,** 289 (1977).
9. Gram, L., Flachs, H., Wurtz-Jorgensen, A., Parnas, J., and Anderson, B., Sodium valproate, serum level and clinical effect in epilepsy: A controlled study. *Epilepsia* **20,** 303–312 (1979).
10. Browne, T. R., Valproic acid. *N. Engl. J. Med.* **302,** 661–666 (1980).
11. Willmore, L. J., Wilder, B. J., Bruni, J., and Villarreal, H. J., Effect of valproic acid on hepatic function. *Neurology* **28,** 961–964 (1978).
12. Gerber, N., Dickinson, R. G., Harland, R. C., Lynn, R. K., Houghton, D., Antonias, J. I., and Schimschock, J. C., Reye-like syndrome associated with valproic acid therapy. *J. Pediatr.* **95,** 142–144 (1979).
13. Suchy, F. J., Balistreri, W. F., Buchino, J. J., Sondheimer, J. M., Bates, S. R., Kearns, G. L., Stuhl, J. D., and Bove, K. E., Acute hepatic failure associated with the use of sodium valproate. *N. Engl. J. Med.* **300,** 962–966 (1979).

14. Chadwick, D. W., Cumming, W. J. K., Livingston, I., and Cartlidge, N. E. F., Acute intoxication with sodium valproate. *Ann. Neurol.* **6,** 552–553 (1979).
15. Pinder, R. M., Brogden, R. N., Speight, T. M., and Avery, G. S., Sodium valproate: A review of its pharmacological properties and therapeutic efficacy in epilepsy. *Drugs* **13,** 81–123 (1977).
16. Alexander, F. W., Sodium valproate and pregnancy. *Arch. Dis. Child.* **54,** 240–245 (1979).

Vanillylmandelic Acid
(VMA; 4-hydroxy-3-methoxymandelic acid)

Specimen Tested:

U.

Laboratories Reporting:

7.

Reference (Normal) Values:

Age, yr	mg/d (μmol/d)	μg/mg of creatinine[a]	μg/kg of body wt per day
Labs. 1–5:			
0–1	<1.8 (<9)		
<1	<1 (<5.1)	6–15	
1–4	<3 (<15)		
1–5		4–11	
1–15	1–6 (5.1–30)		
Child		2–12	31–135
4–10	<4.4 (<22)		
6–15	1.5–4.0 (7.6–20)	2–7	
>10	<7.1 (<36)		
>15–adult	2–7 (10.1–35)	1.5–4.5	
Adult	1.8–7.1 (9–36)		
	1.0–7.0 (5.1–35)	1.5–7.0	

Possible neural crest tumor: 1.5 × upper limit of normal.

Lab 6:			
Up to 1 mo			Up to 180
1 mo–2 yr			Up to 230
>2 yr			Up to 150

Lab. 7:		
1–12 mo	to 34.8; mean, 15.0	
1–2 yr	to 30.2; mean, 13.6	
2–5 yr	to 15.5; mean, 7.1	
5–10 yr	to 13.9; mean, 6.7	
10–15 yr	to 10.4; mean, 4.8	

[a] If data are reported as μg/mg of creatinine, a 12-h U collection may be used for small children from whom collection of a 24-h U is very difficult. However, this is much less than ideal because of the age-related change in urinary creatinine output (see Applegarth's Commentary on **Creatinine Clearance**).

Sources of Reference (Normal) Values:

Lab. 1: institutional, modified from Clark, A. C. L., Moore, A. E., and Niall, M., Metabolites of catecholamines in the urine of children with tumours of neural crest origin. *Aust. Paediatr. J.* **1**, 42–55 (1965). **Lab. 2:** Hakulinen, A., Urinary excretion of vanilmandelic acid of children in normal and certain pathological conditions. *Acta Paediatr. Scand.*, Suppl. 212, 1–67 (1971); Pisano, J. J., Crout, J. R., and Abraham, D., Determination of 3-methoxy-4-hydroxymandelic acid in urine. *Clin. Chim. Acta* **7**, 285–291 (1962). **Lab. 3:** institutional; Voorhess, M. L., Urinary catecholamine excretion by healthy children. *Pediatrics* **39**, 252–257 (1967). **Lab. 4:** institutional. **Lab. 5:** Addanki, S., Hinnenkamp, E. R., and Sotos, J. F., Simultaneous quantitation of 4-hydroxy-3-methoxymandelic (vanilmandelic) and 4-hydroxy-3-methoxyphenylacetic (homovanillic) acids in human urine. *Clin. Chem.* **22**, 310–314 (1976). **Lab. 6:** Hakulinen, *op. cit.* **Lab 7:** Haymond, R. E., Knight, J. A., and Bills, A. C., Normal values for urinary 3-methoxy-4-hydroxymandelic acid (VMA) in children. *Clin. Chem.* **24**, 1853 (1978).

Specimen Volume, Collection, and Preservation; Patient Preparation:

Aliquot of 24-h volume. Collect 24-h urine into bottle containing 10 to 15 mL of 6 mol/L HCl. Use 30 mL of HCl solution for adults. Adjust to pH 2 with 0.6 mol/L HCl. Store in RR during and after collection. Stable for 3 d in RR. There is a claim that VMA is stable for 1 wk at RT or in RR. **Precaution:** Do not administer aspirin for 3 d before collection; other drugs may also interfere. Diet, however, has little effect: Weetman, R. M., Rider, P. S., Oei, T. O., Hempel, J. S., and Baehner, R. L., Effect of diet in urinary excretion of VMA, HVA, metanephrine and total free catecholamine in normal preschool children. *J. Pediatr.* **88**, 46–50 (1976); Rayfield, E. J., Cain, J. P., Casey, M. P., Williams, G. H., and Sullivan, J. M., Influence of diet on urinary VMA excretion. *J. Am. Med. Assoc.* **221**, 704–705 (1972).

Analytical Method and Instrumentation:

Lab. 1: Varian 635 UV-Vis spectrophotometer. **Lab. 2:** Micromedic MS 2 spectrophotometer. **Lab. 3:** Gilford 300 N spectrophotometer. **Lab. 4:** Zeiss spectrophotometer. **Lab. 5:** Addanki et al., *op. cit.;* Varian 1440 GLC, with 600-cm (20-ft.) glass coil column. **Lab. 6:** Wybenga, D., and Pileggi, V. J., Quantitative determination of 3-methoxy-4-hydroxymandelic acid (VMA) in urine. *Clin. Chim. Acta* **16**, 147–154 (1967). **Lab. 7:** Beckman DB spectrophotometer.

Commentary—J. A. Knight

Neural crest tumors usually, although not always, produce excessive quantities of catecholamines (dopamine, norepinephrine, epinephrine), which are metabolized to various products before being excreted in urine. One of the most common of these is vanillylmandelic acid (VMA), a metabolite of epinephrine and norepinephrine that is excreted in increased amounts in most cases of neural crest tumors, regardless of whether the tumors are seen primarily in adults (pheochromocytoma) or children (neuroblastoma). VMA excretion is reportedly increased in about 77% of neuroblastomas. Homovanillic acid (HVA, 4-hydroxy-3-methoxyphenylacetic acid) excretion is increased in approximately the same percentage of cases. When both are measured, the proportion of cases detected approaches 95% *(1,2)*. Another advantage of measuring both substances is that the prognosis in disseminated disease reportedly correlates directly with the urinary VMA/HVA ratio. Ratios less than 1.5 apparently indicate a poorer prognosis than those greater *(3)*.

The excretion of VMA varies greatly with age, particularly in the first two years of life. Several studies have reported reference intervals for normal infants and children *(4–7)*. However, none of these have been entirely adequate for several reasons: *(a)* insufficient subjects were examined in each group; *(b)* the methodology varied considerably, with two studies involving results of semiquantitative two-dimensional paper chromatography; and *(c)* three of the studies were based on 24-h urine collections, which are almost impossible to obtain in infants and young children. (Because of the difficulty in obtaining an accurate 24-h collection, many investigators utilize a partial collection and relate the VMA concentration to milligrams of urinary creatinine.) A recent report *(8)*, in which Pisano's spectrophotometric method *(9)* was used, gives reliable data on random urine specimens, as follows:

	Normal values for urinary VMA in children, [a] μg/mg of creatinine				
	1–12 mo	**1–2 yr**	**2–5 yr**	**5–10 yr**	**10–15 yr**
Range	0.4–36.8	1.9–37.3	0.7–18.9	0.4–17.5	0.2–12.5
Mean	15.0	13.6	7.1	6.7	4.8
SD	9.9	8.3	4.2	3.6	2.8
Normal range ($\pm$2 SD)	0–34.8	0–30.2	0–15.5	0–13.9	0–10.4

[a] n = 41 for each age group.

Dietary influences can be a problem, but depend on the method used. Most of the colorimetric methods are influenced by prior intake of bananas, vanillin, coffee, and tea. However, the spectrophotometric method referred to above is not affected by diet *(10)*, and neither are the methods based on GLC *(11)*. Certain drugs and other substances, however, may stimulate increased catecholamine production and subsequent increased VMA excretion *(12)*. These may create diagnostic problems for the clinician, but are not methodological errors. Regardless of method, urine should be preserved with acid during collection to ensure stability.

Screening ("spot tests") for VMA is controversial. In my experience, the test tube method with *p*-nitroaniline *(13)* is the most reliable: the color is the easiest to interpret, and the reaction is the most specific *(14)*. A negative result, however, does not rule out tumor. There is now little to recommend screening tests, and the quantitative measurement of both VMA and HVA is appropriate when the clinician is concerned about either the presence of a neuroblastoma or its possible recurrence in a previously treated case.

1. Williams, C. M., and Greer, M., Homovanillic acid and vanilmandelic acid in diagnosis of neuroblastoma. *J. Am. Med. Assoc.* **183**, 134–138 (1963).
2. Bell, M., Newer chemical diagnostic tests. *J. Am. Med. Assoc.* **205**, 105–106 (1968).
3. Laug, W. E., Siegel, S. E., Shaw, K. N. F., Landing, B., Baptista, J., and Gutenstein, M., Initial urinary catecholamine metabolite concentrations and prognosis in neuroblastoma. *Pediatrics* **62**, 77–83 (1978).
4. McKendrick, T., and Edwards, R. W. H., The excretion of 4-hydroxy-3-methoxymandelic acid by children. *Arch. Dis. Child.* **40**, 418–425 (1965).
5. Voorhess, M. L., Urinary catecholamine excretion by healthy children. I. Daily excretion of dopamine, norepinephrine, epinephrine, and 3-methoxy-4-hydroxymandelic acid. *Pediatrics* **39**, 252–257 (1967).
6. Gitlow, S. E., Mendlowitz, M., Wilk, E. K., Wilk, S., Wolf, R. L., and Bertani, L. M., Excretion of catecholamine catabolites by normal children. *J. Lab. Clin. Med.* **72**, 612–620 (1968).
7. Borrell, S., Vega, P., Rivas, C., Collado, F., and Torreblanca, J., Urinary excretion of adrenaline, noradrenaline, and 3-methoxy-4-hydroxymandelic acid by children from one month up to eight years of age. *Ann. Endocrinol. (Paris)* **35**, 121–126 (1974).
8. Haymond, R. E., Knight, J. A., and Bills, A. C., Normal values for urinary 3-methoxy-4-hydroxymandelic acid (VMA) in children. *Clin. Chem.* **24**, 1853–1854 (1978).
9. Pisano, J. J., Crout, J. R., and Abraham, D., Determination of 3-methoxy-4-hydroxymandelic acid in urine. *Clin. Chim. Acta* **7**, 285–291 (1962).
10. Rayfield, E. J., Cain, J. P., Casey, M. P., Williams, G. H., and Sullivan, J. M., Influence of diet in urinary VMA excretion. *J. Am. Med. Assoc.* **221**, 704–705 (1972).
11. Brewster, M. A., Berry, D. H., and Moriarty, M., Urinary 3-methoxy-4-hydroxyphenylacetic (homovanillic) and 3-methoxy-4-hydroxymandelic (vanillylmandelic) acids: Gas–liquid chromatographic methods and experience with 13 cases of neuroblastoma. *Clin. Chem.* **23**, 2247–2249 (1977).
12. von Euler, U. S., Pathophysiological aspects of catecholamine production. *Clin. Chem.* **18**, 1445–1448 (1972).
13. Gitlow, S. E., Bertani, L. M., Rausen, A., Gribetz, D., and Dziedzic, S. W., Diagnosis of neuroblastoma by qualitative and quantitative deter-

mination of catecholamine metabolites in urine. *Cancer* **25,** 1377–1383 (1970).

14. Knight, J. A., Fronk, S., and Haymond, R. E., Chemical basis and specificity of chemical screening tests for urinary vanilmandelic acid. *Clin. Chem.* **21,** 130–133 (1975).

Vitamin A (Retinol)

Specimen Tested:

P, S.

Laboratories Reporting:

5.

Reference (Normal) Values:

	μg/dL (μmol/L)			
Age	**Lab. 1**	**Lab. 2**	**Labs. 3, 4**	**Lab. 5**
0–6 mo		>20 (>0.70)		
0–1 yr	20–90 (0.70–3.14)			
0–2 yr[a] 6 mo–adult		30–80 (1.05–2.79)		
1–5 yr	30–100 (1.05–3.50)			
6–16 yr	60–100 (2.09–3.50)			
Child			20–40 (0.70–1.40)	77–143 (2.7–5.0)
Adult	20–80 (0.70–2.79)			
4 h after loading dose			120–750 (4.2–26.2)	

[a] Value increases from 40 μg/dL (1.40 μmol/L) at birth to 70 (2.44) at 1 yr, then decreases slowly to 40 (1.40) by 2 yr (Labs. 3, 4).

Sources of Reference (Normal) Values:

Lab. 1: institutional study of 110 subjects, and literature. **Labs. 2, 4, 5:** institutional. **Lab. 3:** institutional; Fyfe, W. H., Vitamin-A levels in idiopathic hypercalcaemia. *Lancet* **i,** 610–612 (1956).

Specimen Volume, Collection, and Preservation; Patient Preparation:

0.15 to 2 mL. Heparin anticoagulant. Collect blood into tube protected from light (aluminum foil). Store P, S in dark in FR for no longer than 4 d. For 24 h before the test, the patient must not be receiving vitamin supplements that contain vitamin A, or foods containing vitamin A and carotene. Unless a vitamin-tolerance test is being performed, fast the patient overnight, if possible.

Analytical Method:

Lab. 1: Hansen, L. G., and Warwick, W. J., A fluorometric micromethod for vitamins A and E. *Am. J. Clin. Pathol.* **51,** 538–541 (1969). **Lab. 2:** Neeld, J. B., and Pearson, W. N., Macro and micro methods for the determination of serum vitamin A using trifluoroacetic acid. *J. Nutr.* **79,** 454–462 (1963). **Labs. 3, 4:** Bessey, O. A., Lowry, O. H., Brock, M. J., and Lopez, J. A., The determination of vitamin A and carotene in small quantities of blood serum. *J. Biol. Chem.* **166,** 177–188 (1946). **Lab. 5:** Steveninck, J. V., and DeGoeij, A. F. P. M., Determination of vitamin A in blood plasma of patients with carotenemia. *Clin. Chim. Acta* **49,** 61–64 (1973); Drujan, B. D., Castillon, R., and Guerrero, E., Application of fluorometry in the determination of vitamin A. *Anal. Biochem.* **23,** 44–52 (1968); Clausen, S. W., and McCoord, A. B., The determination of carotene and xanthophyll by a single distribution between liquid phases. *J. Biol. Chem.* **113,** 89–104 (1936).

Instrumentation:

Labs. 1, 5: Aminco-Bowman spectrophotofluorometer. **Labs. 2–4:** Zeiss PMQ II, Beckman 25 spectrophotometers.

Commentary—J. Gilbert Hill

Vitamin A is one of the essential fat-soluble vitamins, with important roles in vision, the biosynthesis of mucopolysaccharides, and bone growth. It occurs in nature as a provitamin (in the form of plant carotenes) or in the preformed state (especially in fish oils, liver, eggs, and dairy products). In man, conversion of carotenes to vitamin A takes place in the intestinal mucosa and the liver; in normal circumstances this mechanism can provide enough vitamin A to satisfy nutritional requirements.

Indications for the measurement of vitamin A include clinical suspicion of deficiency or excess of the vitamin. Both of these conditions are extremely rare in developed countries, but may increase in frequency with increased utilization of total parenteral nutrition. As a means of assessing fat absorption, measuring plasma vitamin A or conducting an oral vitamin A-tolerance test has a hallowed history, but these procedures have now been largely replaced by more specific tests.

The consumption of large amounts of carotene-rich foods may produce a yellow skin pigmentation. When this can not be distinguished from hyperbilirubinemia, a determination of plasma carotene concentration may be indicated.

Specimens to be used for vitamin A or carotene measurements should be collected with care, to minimize hemolysis and exposure to light, and the analyses should be performed promptly. Storage for as long as three weeks is possible, if the temperature is maintained at -20 °C.

Vitamin B$_1$ (Thiamine)

Specimen Tested:

B.

Laboratory Reporting:

1.

Reference (Normal) Values:

Age unspecified: 5.3–7.9 μg/dL (0.157–0.234 μmol/L)

Sources of Reference (Normal) Values:

Institutional.

Specimen Volume, Collection, and Preservation:

0.5 mL. Heparin anticoagulant.

Analytical Method and Instrumentation:

Fluorometric; Burch, H. B., Bessey, O. A., Love, R. H., and Lowry, O. H., The determination of thiamine and thiamine phosphates in small quantities of blood and blood cells. *J. Biol. Chem.* **198,** 477–490 (1952); Aminco-Bowman fluorometer.

Vitamin B$_2$ (Riboflavin)

Specimen Tested:

B.

Laboratory Reporting:

1.

Reference (Normal) Values:

Age unspecified: 3.7–13.7 μg/dL (98–363 nmol/L)

Sources of Reference (Normal) Values:

Yagi, K., Chemical determination of flavins. *Methods Biochem. Anal.* **10,** 319–356 (1962).

Specimen Volume, Collection, and Preservation:
0.5 mL. Heparin anticoagulant.

Analytical Method and Instrumentation:
Yagi. *op. cit.;* Aminco Bowman fluorometer.

Vitamin B$_{12}$ (Cobalamin)

Specimen Tested:
S.

Laboratory Reporting:
1.

Reference (Normal) Values:
Age unspecified: 130–785 pg/mL (96–579 pmol/L)

Sources of Reference (Normal) Values:
Kolhouse, J. F., Kondo, H., Allen, N. C., Podell, E., and Allen, R. H., Cobalamin analogues are present in human plasma and can mask cobalamin deficiency because current radioisotope dilution assays are not specific for true cobalamin. *N. Engl. J. Med.* **299,** 785–792 (1978).

Specimen Volume, Collection, and Preservation:
200 μL. Centrifuge in refrigerated centrifuge. Store S in RR for 1 d. For longer periods, store in FR.

Analytical Method and Instrumentation:
Radioassay, ^{57}Co; RIA Products, Inc., "Coat 57" kit; Packard gamma scintillation counter; Sorvall R-C centrifuge.

Vitamin E (Alpha-Tocopherol)

Specimen Tested:
P, S.

Laboratory Reporting:
1.

Reference (Normal) Values:
Child: 3.0–15 μg/mL (0.7–3.5 μmol/L)
Adult: 5.0–20 (1.2–4.6)

Sources of Reference (Normal) Values:

Hansen, L. G., and Warwick, W. J., A fluorometric micro method for serum tocopherol. *Tech. Bull. Regist. Med. Technol.* **36,** 131–136 (1966).

Specimen Volume, Collection, and Preservation:

100 μL. Heparin anticoagulant. Specimen stable 1 wk in RR, indefinitely in FR.

Analytical Method and Instrumentation:

Hansen and Warwick, *op. cit.;* G. K. Turner 430 spectrofluorometer.

Xylose Absorption

Specimen Tested:

B, U.

Laboratories Reporting:

5.

Reference (Normal) Values:

Dose, 0.5 g/kg of body weight (oral) to fasting child:
1-h B: <6 mo (1 lab.): 15 mg/dL (1.00 mmol/L)
       >6 mo: 30–50 (2.00–3.33); >20 (>1.33)
5-h U: <6 mo: 11–30% of ingested dose.
       6–12 mo: 20–32%
       1–3 yr: 20–42%
       Child (3 labs.): 16–33%
       3–10 yr: 25–45%
       >10 yr: 25–50%

Sources of Reference (Normal) Values:

Institutional; text ref. *2,* pp 10, 361; Rolles, C. J., Nutter, S., Kendall, M. J., and Anderson, C. M., One hour blood xylose screening test for coeliac disease. *Lancet* **ii,** 1043–1045 (1973); Benson, J. A., Culver, P. J., Ragland, S., Jones, C. M., Drummey, G. D., and Bougas, E., The D-xylose test in malabsorption syndromes. *N. Engl. J. Med.* **256,** 335–339 (1957); Reiner, M., and Cheung, H. L., Xylose. *Stand. Methods Clin. Chem.* **5,** 257–268 (1965); Lanzkowsky, P., Madenlioglu, M., Wilson, J. F., and Lahey, M. E., Oral D-xylose test in healthy infants and children. *N. Engl. J. Med.* **268,** 1441–1444 (1965); Hawkins, K. I., Pediatric xylose absorption test: Measurements in blood preferable to measurements in urine. *Clin. Chem.* **16,** 751–752 (1970).

Specimen Volume, Collection, and Preservation; Patient Preparation:

B, U: 100 to 200 μL. Heparin anticoagulant. Stability unreported. Infants should be fasted 4 h; others, overnight. Obtain fasting, 1-h, and other samples of B, as desired. Collect *complete* 5-h U.

Analytical Method:

Four labs.: furfural-*p*-bromoaniline reaction; Roe, J. H., and Rice, E. W., A photometric method for the determination of free pentoses in animal tissues. *J. Biol. Chem.* **173**, 507–512 (1948). **1 lab.:** by difference, using the *o*-toluidine reaction; Harleco glucose reagent kit.

Instrumentation:

Gilford Stasar II, III, Beckman 25, Coleman Jr. II spectrophotometers.

Note: Several gastrointestinal disturbances produce B values of 12–20 mg/dL (0.80–1.33 mmol/L). In true malabsorption, values are <10–12 mg/dL (0.67–0.80 mmol/L).

Commentary—K. W. Schmitt

The percentage of urinary xylose normally recovered (i.e., accounted for) analytically varies with age as follows *(1):*

	Percentage recovered	
Age	**Mean**	**Range**
<6 mo	17	11–30
6–12 mo	25	21–32
1–3 yr	25	19–42
3–6 yr	35	25–44
6–10 yr	34	25–44
10–16 yr	39	28–51
Adult	36	32–48

The lower analytical recovery (i.e., the lower proportion of the dose analytically accounted for) in the younger age groups reflects lower xylose absorption as well as smaller urinary volume. Determining recovery from urine is not recommended for children younger than six years because of difficulties in collecting urine *(1)*. Data on serum concentrations at 0.5, 1, and 2 h after dose ingestion are preferred for this age group; normal values for patients younger than six months are 10, 15, and 15 mg/dL, respectively, and 15, 20, and 20 mg/dL for older patients.

1. Lanzkowsky, P., Madenlioglu, M., Wilson, J. F., and Lahey, M. E., Oral ᴅ-xylose test in healthy infants and children. *N. Engl. J. Med.* **268**, 1441–1444 (1963).

Commentary—John F. Connelly and G. L. Barnes

A 1-h blood xylose test has been recommended as a screening test for celiac disease (1), but a normal 1-h value does not exclude this condition and is no substitute for an intestinal biopsy (2).

A change in the 1-h blood xylose after challenge with gluten or cow's milk may help confirm celiac disease or milk protein hypersensitivity (3).

1. Rolles, C. J., Nutter, S., Kendall, M. J., and Anderson, C. M., One hour blood xylose screening test for coeliac disease. *Lancet* ii, 1043–1045 (1973).
2. Lamabadusuriya, S. P., Packer, S., and Harries, J. T., Limitations of xylose tolerance test as a screening procedure in childhood coeliac disease. *Arch. Dis. Child.* 50, 34–39 (1975).
3. Morin, C. L., Buts, J.-P., Weber, A., Roy, C. C., and Bronchu, P., One hour blood xylose test in diagnosis of cow's milk protein intolerance. *Lancet* i, 1102–1104 (1979).

Zinc

Specimen Tested:

P, S.

Laboratories Reporting:

2.

Reference (Normal) Values:

	μg/dL (μmol/L)	
	Lab. 1	Lab. 2[a]
Child (S)	66–144 (10.1–22.0)	
Adult (P), M		83.5–87.9 (12.8–13.5)
F		85.3–90.5 (13.1–13.9)

[a] Lab. 2 also reports: F, taking oral contraceptives: 86.3–92.7 μg/dL (13.2–15.0 μmol/L); F, at 16 weeks' gestation: 66.2–70.2 (10.1–11.0); F, at 38 weeks' gestation: 53.9–58.1 (8.3–8.9).

Sources of Reference (Normal) Values:

Lab. 1: institutional. **Lab. 2:** Hambidge, K. M., and Droegemueller, W., Changes in plasma and hair concentrations of zinc, copper, chromium and manganese during pregnancy. *Obstet. Gynecol.* 44, 666–672 (1974).

Specimen Volume, Collection, and Preservation:

Lab. 1: 50 μL; **Lab. 2:** 120 μL. Heparin anticoagulant for P. Separate P, S as soon as possible after collection, and store in FR.

Analytical Method and Instrumentation:

Lab. 1: S, atomic absorption, institutional modification (unpublished); Varian 1200 atomic absorption spectrophotometer. **Lab. 2:** P, emission spectrometry; Hambidge and Droegemueller, *op. cit.;* Jarrell Ash-Fisher emission spectrometer.

Commentary—Roger L. Boeckx

The most reliable methods for the measurement of zinc in serum or plasma are atomic absorption spectrophotometric methods in which samples are diluted with water and aspirated directly into the flame. A fivefold dilution is common, and aqueous standards can be used if the viscosity of the standard solutions is increased to compensate for the difference in aspiration rates between aqueous solutions and diluted serum or plasma. Smith et al. *(1)* recommend use of plasma diluted fivefold with de-ionized water; they use aqueous standards of zinc nitrate prepared in 5% (50 mL/L) glycerol. In my experience dilutions as great as 10-fold give acceptable results, thereby allowing the use of smaller samples.

Zinc is ubiquitous and extreme care must be taken to prevent contamination of the sample during collection, dilution, and analysis. Zinc-free syringes must be used for venipuncture, which thus requires syringes that do not have rubber components. Similar contamination by the rubber stoppers used in evacuated collection tubes has been observed. The problem of sample contamination can be a serious stumbling block in establishing methods for trace-metal analysis, especially on a micro scale. A recent symposium has dealt with this problem in some detail *(2)*.

Zinc concentrations in serum and plasma differ significantly. Several authors report that zinc concentrations may be as much as 15 mg/dL greater in serum than in plasma *(3,4)*. In a study comparing venous and capillary plasma and serum samples collected from neonates, I have confirmed that serum has significantly higher zinc values. The mean concentration in plasma was 84 (SD 17) $\mu g/dL$, but in serum was 95 (SD 18) $\mu g/dL$. No significant difference between venous and capillary samples was detected. Plasma was prepared as recommended by Smith et al. *(1);* 30% sodium citrate (300 g/L) was used as the anticoagulant, 20 μL per milliliter of whole blood.

The significance of plasma or serum zinc concentrations is a complex issue. In whole blood, 90% of the zinc is in the erythrocytes. Of the plasma zinc, 30–40% is bound tightly to a specific α_2-globulin, 60–70% is bound loosely to albumin, and a smaller fraction is chelated to amino acids *(5)*. Although values for circulating zinc may not provide all information necessary to assess zinc nutritional status, the concentration of zinc in plasma may represent the exchangeable zinc that is available to metabolically active tissues. A review dealing with the assessment of zinc and copper nutriture has recently been published (5).

The fact that most solutions currently used for total parenteral nutrition are deficient in zinc has led to several investigations, to determine whether zinc deficiency is a consequence of long-term parenteral nutrition (6, 7). It now appears that significant zinc deficiency is a common consequence in premature infants; therefore, routine monitoring of zinc and perhaps other trace metals will become a requirement in the management of the critically ill premature infant.

1. Smith, J. C., Jr., Butrimovitz, G. P., and Purdy, W. C., Direct measurement of zinc in plasma by atomic absorption spectrophotometry. *Clin. Chem.* **25**, 1487–1491 (1979).
2. Koirtyohann, S. R., Integrity and processing of samples for trace-element analysis. *Clin. Chem.* **25**, 1048 (1979). Abstract.
3. Halsted, J. A., and Smith, J. C., Jr., Plasma zinc in health and disease. *Lancet* **i**, 322–324 (1970).
4. Reinhold, J. G., Trace-elements—a selective survey. *Clin. Chem.* **21**, 476–500 (1975).
5. Solomons, N. W., On the assessment of zinc and copper nutriture in man. *Am. J. Clin. Nutr.* **32**, 856–871 (1979).
6. Arakawa, T., Tamura, T., Igarushi, Y., Suzubi, H., and Sandstead, H. H., Zinc deficiency in two infants during total parenteral alimentation for diarrhea. *Am. J. Clin. Nutr.* **29**, 197–204 (1976).
7. Michie, D. D., and Wirth, F. H., Plasma zinc levels in premature infants receiving parenteral nutrition. *J. Pediatr.* **92**, 798–800 (1978).

Chapter 6. Free Bilirubin

T. A. Blumenfeld, J. A. Knight, and H. S. Cheskin

Bilirubin encephalopathy (kernicterus) is a potential hazard for high-risk newborns even when the unconjugated bilirubin concentration in serum is maintained at 15–20 mg/dL or less by phototherapy or exchange transfusion. Some high-risk newborns may develop kernicterus when bilirubin is <15 mg/dL, and later, subtle central nervous system dysfunction may occur in infants who have peak bilirubin concentrations of 15–20 mg/dL. Therefore, unconjugated bilirubin values alone are inadequate to identify those infants at risk for developing kernicterus. To identify those infants at risk and to avoid overtreatment of those at little or no risk, we need an indicator other than serum bilirubin concentration.

In vitro, bilirubin is toxic to cells and to specific cellular components such as mitochondria. The basis for this toxicity is unknown. However, albumin prevents toxicity when its molar concentration exceeds that of bilirubin. In animals, bilirubin toxicity usually does not occur unless the molar concentration of bilirubin exceeds that of albumin. Based on this information, the theory has been proposed that bilirubin not bound to albumin (free bilirubin) binds to cells and is a toxic fraction of the total bilirubin pool, whereas albumin-bound bilirubin cannot enter cells and is harmless. Consequently, efforts have been made to create clinically useful measurements of the bilirubin-binding properties of serum albumin in individual patients.

The terms used in the various laboratory tests for bilirubin-binding are as follows:

Binding capacity—the number of sites on the albumin molecule capable of binding bilirubin. Human albumin has a single high-affinity (tight) binding site for bilirubin and one or more, probably two, weaker sites.

Reserve binding capacity—the number of additional tight-binding sites available in a serum already containing some bound bilirubin.

Saturation of albumin—(a) the proportion of theoretical or demonstrated available tight-binding sites already occupied by bilirubin at a certain bilirubin concentration, and (b) the condition in which all available tight-binding sites are occupied.

Free bilirubin—the concentration of unconjugated bilirubin in solution or suspension in plasma not bound to any circulating or fixed protein or membrane.

Binding affinity—the strength of the bilirubin–albumin bond, most appropriately expressed as the concentration of bound and free bilirubin at chemical equilibrium.

Sera of healthy newborn infants generally have binding capacities of 0.8 to 1 mol of bilirubin per mole of albumin at the high-affinity site. Sick infants may have decreases in binding capacity, in binding affinity, or in both.

Several in vitro methods have been proposed for measurement of unbound or free bilirubin, relative or absolute saturation of albumin-binding sites with bilirubin, and the affinity of albumin for bilirubin, including the following:

1. *Hydroxybenzeneazobenzoic acid (HBABA) dye.* The binding of HBABA [also called 2-(4'-hydroxyazobenzene)benzoic acid (HABA)] to albumin is nonspecifically competitive with bilirubin; progressive displacement of the dye is quasi-linear with the addition of bilirubin and other albumin-bound anions.

2. *Direct Yellow 7.* This dye appears to be bound specifically to the bilirubin sites on albumin and undergoes a fluorescence enhancement when bound to albumin.

3. *Salicylate saturation index.* The salicylate saturation index is measured in dilute sera by the displacement in vitro of bilirubin from its albumin-binding sites by an excess of sodium salicylate. It is determined by the percent decrease in absorbance at 460 nm, the wavelength of maximum absorbance for albumin-bound bilirubin.

4. *Sephadex G-25 gel filtration.* Sephadex G-25 gel filtration is used to separate loosely bound bilirubin from tightly bound bilirubin. Loosely bound bilirubin is absorbed by the gel column; tightly bound bilirubin, presumably bound to the high-affinity first site, remains attached to albumin as it passes through the column.

5. *Free bilirubin.* The concentration of free bilirubin can be measured indirectly by oxidation of bilirubin with horseradish peroxidase.

6. *Albumin fluorescence.* Albumin fluoresces when exposed to appropriate wavelengths of ultraviolet light. Because bilirubin quenches this fluorescence, the quenching effect may be used to estimate binding factors.

7. *Front-faced reflectance fluorometry.* The fluorescence of bilirubin itself when bound to albumin is measured. The endpoint of the assay is indicated by a flattening of the fluorescence curve when the high-affinity binding sites are saturated.

At present, binding tests are not performed in a uniform fashion in different institutions, and there are no uniform laboratory standards for them. Differences in temperature, pH, instrumentation, and handling of specimens may prohibit valid comparisons of test results from different institutions. Various methods have been correlated with each other, but in some of these studies only low orders of correlation were achieved, suggesting that each method may be measuring a somewhat different aspect of the binding relationship. Although the status of some infants may need to be followed with frequent binding determinations, some of the methods described require blood volumes that are too large, or working times that are too long, to make repetitive measurements practical.

Conjugated bilirubin ≥2–3 mg/dL may interfere with the interpretation of free bilirubin test results by mimicking the effects of loosely bound or free bilirubin.

The ideal test for bilirubin-binding in neonatal serum should require a very small sample; be rapid, reproducible, and readily interpreted; and reliably guide further therapy. At present, not one of the described tests has been shown to be clearly superior to another in these respects.

Safe limits of reserve or total bilirubin-binding capacity, binding affinity, and free bilirubin have not been determined clinically. However, it does not seem appropriate to delay or defer treatment of jaundice on the basis of binding-test results alone, if treatment is warranted on reasonable clinical grounds. Even with further improvements, bilirubin-binding tests will augment, but not replace, serial bilirubin determinations and other pertinent clinical tests and observations.

In two recent thought-provoking reviews of free bilirubin, current knowledge was summarized as follows *(1,2)*:

1. The free-bilirubin theory proposes that unbound bilirubin binds to and enters the cells. The theory is simple, reasonable, and attractive, but at present there is no evidence to support the free-bilirubin theory over other possible mechanisms of kernicterus.

2. The measurement of free bilirubin is now technically possible for mixtures of purified bilirubin and albumin. Measurement in serum is promising, but proved methods still elude current capabilities.

3. At present there is no justification for the use of free-bilirubin tests in the management of jaundice. This applies to all related tests such as reserve-binding capacity, bilirubin-binding capacity, albumin saturation, loosely bound bilirubin, gel-bound bilirubin, and binding affinity.

4. For small premature infants, the total bilirubin concentration at which the risk of kernicterus exceeds the risk of treatment is unknown. In these cases, there is no scientific basis to guide the clinician in deciding when to institute treatment of jaundice.

5. Hyperbilirubinemia can lead to kernicterus. Whether it causes other milder forms of neurologic damage is unknown. At present there is no basis for treating jaundice with the hope of preventing such damage.

The recent literature on this topic is extensive, but a large number of these references are in the two excellent reviews cited.

1. Cashore, W. J., Gartner, L. M., Oh, W., and Stern, L., Clinical application of neonatal bilirubin-binding determinations: Current status. *J. Pediatr.* **93,** 827–833 (1978).
2. Levine, R. L., Bilirubin: Worked out years ago? *Pediatrics* **64,** 380–384 (1979).

Chapter 7. Tests for Fetal Lung Maturity

T. A. Blumenfeld, H. S. Cheskin, and R. I. Stark

The Lecithin/Sphingomyelin Ratio and Lung Profile

Reports of using the amniotic fluid lecithin/sphingomyelin (L/S)[1] ratio to predict fetal lung maturity first appeared in 1971. The rationale for this test is that, during gestation, lung development can be assessed from surfactant phospholipids secreted by the fetal lung into the amniotic fluid. The L/S ratio has been particularly useful in the management of pregnancies requiring repeated cesarean sections, those with uncertain gestational dates, those occurring after cessation of anti-fertility medication, those in which there has been no antepartum care, those where there is abnormal fetal growth, and those associated with various high-risk conditions involving the mother, the fetus, and the placenta.

Our review of several reports showed that mature L/S ratios predicted the absence of respiratory distress syndrome (RDS) in newborns with about 98% accuracy. Of 2170 infants with safe L/S ratios before delivery, 42 (less than 2%) had RDS. Most of these were born to mothers with gestational or types A-C diabetes mellitus, or had severe birth asphyxia or severe Rh disease, although some were idiopathic. However, the accuracy of a low L/S ratio in predicting RDS may be as low as 54%. In some series almost half of low and intermediate L/S ratios may be noninformative: low L/S ratios may not necessarily predict RDS, and intermediate values may not indicate how soon the lung will be mature.

Because of the deficiencies of the L/S ratio, a lung profile has been developed, based on the L/S ratio and the percentages of disaturated (acetone-precipitated) lecithin, phosphatidylinositol (PI) and phosphatidylglycerol (PG) in amniotic fluid *(1)*. It is thought that this profile will enhance the accuracy of diagnosis of fetal lung maturity and extend information about lung development. In a study of amniotic fluid specimens from 57 pregnancies with low L/S ratios, 69% were correctly diagnosed by the L/S ratio alone, whereas the lung profile correctly diagnosed 93% of the cases.

The extraordinarily high predictive accuracy (about 98%) from mature L/S ratios has been documented, even though there are varia-

---

[1] Abbreviations used in this chapter: L/S, lecithin/sphingomyelin ratio; RDS, respiratory distress syndrome; PI, phosphatidylinositol; PG, phosphatidylglycerol; PS, phosphatidylserine; PE, phosphatidylethanolamine; FSI, foam-stability index; DPH, 1,6-diphenyl-1,3,5-hexatriene.

tions in technique from that originally described. Variations in the method that omit acetone-precipitation may introduce large errors and, according to the original investigators, are not acceptable modifications. Acetone precipitates the surface-active, highly disaturated lecithin upon which the L/S ratio measurement is based. Omitting this step results in higher L/S ratios than when the acetone-precipitation is included, and serious and unpredictable errors may be introduced. This is especially important before 32 weeks' gestation, when most of the lecithin in surfactant may be unsaturated. Total lecithin isolated from lung and acetone-soluble lecithin do not lower the surface tension into the biological range of less than 15 dyn/cm; the acetone-precipitated fraction lowers the surface tension to 0–4 dyn/cm.

Some investigators have omitted the acetone-precipitation step and increased the cutoff for maturity to a L/S ratio of 3.5. This has the advantage of not missing immature fetuses but adds the significant disadvantage of increasing the number of low L/S ratios that falsely indicate immaturity in infants who will not develop RDS.

Although the L/S ratio alone is sufficient to monitor most normal pregnancies, the lung profile gives a clearer picture of fetal lung development. The advantages of the lung profile over the L/S ratio are as follows:

1. The high accuracy of a positive (mature L/S ratio alone) is further enhanced. When there is a mature L/S ratio with PG present, neither diabetes mellitus (gestational, class A) nor birth asphyxia appears to have any effect on the lung.

2. Use of the lung profile eliminates most of the noninformative low or intermediate L/S ratios.

3. The lung profile allows detection and evaluation of an abnormal pregnancy by indicating alterations from the expected mature pattern.

4. PG may appear early in pregnancies that are significantly immature by gestational age and have immature L/S ratios, but these infants have no RDS once PG is present at 30 g/L or more. This represents accelerated fetal lung maturation. Both PG and PI are highly surface-active, and surfactant containing PG and PI has lower compressibility on the modified Wilhelmy balance than surfactant containing PI only, suggesting that alveoli may be more stable at low lung volumes with the former surfactant. Investigators have shown that premature infants recovering from RDS before 34–35 weeks' gestation may not have PG in their tracheal aspirates but have an associated large increase in PI and lecithin.

5. PG is present in surfactant but not in blood; therefore, use of the lung profile is desirable if the amniotic fluid contains blood.

Lung profiles performed during complicated pregnancies *(2)* showed that in cases of *pregnancy-induced (class A) diabetes mellitus,* there was a statistically significant delay in the appearance of PG, a delay in maturation not related to lecithin; and PI concentrations remained high longer than normal. Other types of diabetes did not differ from normal except for accelerated maturation in class F and class R diabetes, and in these PG appeared before L/S ratios were mature (greater than 2). In cases with *prolonged rupture of membranes,* there was a significant acceleration of maturation, affecting both the L/S ratio and PG. In *hypertension* in pregnancy, including cases involving mild terminal pre-eclampsia, lung profiles were normal. A few patients with severe pregnancy-induced hypertension (chronic toxemia) showed accelerated maturation, sometimes with L/S ratios less than 2 and early PG. The appearance of PG signals the late or final maturation of surfactant, and a diabetic pregnancy of any class can safely be delivered free of RDS after PG appears.

Note that determining the L/S ratio alone has a coefficient of variation of about 16% at best; it is time-consuming and laborious and the quality of the results is greatly technique-dependent *(3)*. Performing these tests requires many steps, and in attempts to shorten the procedure, many variations from the original (Gluck) technique have been described. For laboratories not using Gluck's original method, especially those that omit acetone-precipitation, the cutoff values for their tests should be based on their own clinical experience with the method. It has now been shown that the complete lung profile— the L/S ratio, percentage of disaturated lecithin, PG, and PI—gives much more information than the L/S ratio alone. However, obtaining the lung profile requires use of two-dimensional thin-layer chromatography, which is technically more difficult and time-consuming than single-dimension chromatography and thus has even greater chance for technique-related problems and errors.

Fluorescence Polarization Test for Fetal Lung Maturity (Microviscosity of Amniotic Fluid)

Fluorescence polarization can be used to measure the microviscosity of liposomes. The technique involves 1,6-diphenyl-1,3,5-hexatriene (DPH), a molecular probe that is localized and becomes fluorescent in the hydrocarbon region of lipids. The degree of polarization of its fluorescence (P-value) is a reflection of the freedom of rotation of the molecular probe and is dependent on the viscosity of its microenvironment (microviscosity) in the liposomes. Microviscosity and surface tension are interrelated physical parameters dependent on the molecular packing of lipids. In many circumstances, changes in microviscosity parallel changes in surface tension.

The relative quantities of lecithin and sphingomyelin greatly influence the microviscosity of liposomes and the surfactant properties of amniotic fluid. Phospholipids in amniotic fluid, including lecithin and sphingomyelin, exist as liposomes. Therefore, changes in amniotic fluid surface tension may be detected by determining microviscosity. This is the rationale for the use of fluorescence polarization in the determination of fetal lung maturity.

The microviscosity measurement is performed with a fluorescence polarimeter, which indicates the P-value directly. Microviscosity can be estimated from the P-value by the formula:

$$\text{microviscosity} = 2P/(0.46 - P)$$

The microviscosity scale has the advantage of being linear, whereas P-values are not. However, each microviscosity value has only one associated P-value, and for purposes of determining fetal lung maturity, the P-value scale is more convenient.

The amniotic fluid P-value can be measured in 45 min (including a 30-min incubation period) and has a low coefficient of variation (0.45%). The procedure is easy to perform, mixing 0.5 mL of amniotic fluid with 2 mL of a single chemical reagent containing the DPH probe (4,5).

In normal term-pregnancies the phospholipid in greatest concentration in amniotic fluid is lecithin. Sphingomyelin, PG, PI, phosphatidylserine (PS), and phosphatidylethanolamine (PE) are also present. The relationships of the concentrations of all of these phospholipids are important indicators of fetal lung maturity. Besides the L/S ratio, the relative quantities of PG and PI are also an index to normal function of the newborn's lung. PG markedly improves the function of lung surfactant in stabilizing alveoli, and its absence may indicate fetal lung immaturity.

The microviscosity of sphingomyelin greatly exceeds that of lecithin over the temperature range 20–40 °C; values for PG, PI, PS, and PE are lower (6). The P-value is an excellent indicator of the L/S ratio in liposomes. In dispersions with known concentrations of egg lecithin, synthetic dipalmitoyl lecithin, and bovine brain sphingomyelin, there is an inverse relationship of the P-values and L/S ratios from 1 to 2.5. PG, PI, and PS added individually to dispersions with L/S ratios corresponding either to fetal lung immaturity or maturity significantly decrease the microviscosity; PG causes the greatest decrease in both mature and immature lungs.

Liposomal dispersions corresponding to the physiologic concentrations of lecithin, sphingomyelin, PG, PI, PS, and PE at gestational ages of less than 32 weeks, 32 to 35 weeks, and more than 35 weeks showed the following (7):

1. The microviscosity of the dispersions progressively decreased for increasing gestational ages.

2. Microviscosity values were the highest for each gestational period in dispersions without PG. As PG increased incrementally, the microviscosity values decreased in a step-wise pattern indicative of increasing maturity. However, even when maximum PG was present

at gestational ages of less than 32 weeks, it did not cause the microviscosity to be characteristic of a later gestational period and falsely indicate pulmonary maturity.

3. Physiologic percentages of PI decreased the microviscosity of dispersions of amniotic fluid phospholipids. However, in dispersions with contents characteristic of less than 32 weeks' gestation, even with maximum PI the microviscosity was not lowered to values characteristic of the more mature gestational periods.

Although clinical data have not yet been obtained, one can expect that, on the basis of these findings, an amniotic fluid with no PG, a borderline mature L/S ratio, and mean physiologic amounts of other phospholipids will have a microviscosity much higher than when PG is present in normal quantities. For this reason, amniotic-fluid microviscosity measurements may be a reliable index of the risk of RDS in infants of diabetic mothers.

Contamination of amniotic fluid with blood can significantly change the P-values. This is primarily caused by the serum, not the hemoglobin; therefore, the effect of blood contamination remains after blood cells have been removed from the specimen. The change in P-value caused by blood contamination depends on the volume of serum, the P-value of the serum, and the volume of amniotic fluid. When an amniotic-fluid specimen contains blood, these variables are unknown and their effect on the P-value cannot be predicted.

Meconium may also increase or decrease the amniotic fluid P-value. The magnitude of the change depends on the original amniotic fluid P-value, the quantity of meconium, the lipid content of the meconium, and the volume of the amniotic fluid. When amniotic fluid contains meconium, these variables are unknown and their effect on the P-value cannot be determined.

The amniotic fluid P-value is not affected by bilirubin, surgical lubricant, or amniotic fluid dilution.

During gestation the pattern of change of amniotic fluid microviscosity parallels the expected development of the surfactant system. Microviscosity is high during early gestation and abruptly decreases between the 28th and 36th week of gestation (mean, 30.4 weeks) (8). These findings indicate that changes in the fluorescence polarization value of amniotic fluid reflect the process of fetal lung maturation.

In amniotic fluid the L/S ratio and P-value have a significant correlation for values indicating fetal lung maturity and immaturity. In 161 specimens an amniotic-fluid P-value of 0.336 or less had a high positive correlation with an L/S ratio >2; therefore, this P-value can be used to indicate fetal lung maturity. The test results disagreed in only eight specimens, all of which had an L/S ratio indicating lung immaturity and a P-value indicating lung maturity. This finding suggests that in some cases the P-value may indicate fetal lung maturity earlier than the L/S ratio does.

In a prospective study, 161 amniotic fluid samples (distinct from those studied above) were obtained within 48 h of birth and the P-values compared with fetal outcome *(9)*. None of the 149 infants with a P-value $\leq$ 0.336 developed RDS, whereas eight of 12 with a P-value $>$ 0.336 developed RDS, indicating a significant relation (*p* $<$ 0.05) between the P-value and the risk of developing RDS. In this series, the test had a 0% false-negative rate and a 2.6% false-positive rate. In the same study P-values of 37 pregnancies with infants weighing less than 2500 g at delivery were analyzed separately because of these infants' high risk of developing RDS (an estimated prevalence of 14%). Correlation between the P-values and the risk of RDS in this group was also significant. In this low-birth-weight group the P-value had a false-negative rate of 0% and a false-positive rate of 8.1%, indicating that this is an excellent laboratory test for predicting the risk of RDS.

The ability of both L/S ratios and P-values to predict RDS was also compared. The two tests had an excellent correlation, predicting the same outcome in 88 of 96 cases. However, in eight cases where the tests indicated a different fetal outcome, the P-value was correct more often than the L/S ratio. The P-value predicted fetal lung maturity correctly in all cases, and the L/S ratio predicted fetal lung maturity incorrectly in two cases. The P-value falsely predicted RDS in three of nine cases and the L/S ratio did so in five of nine cases. Thus, the P-value correctly predicted the outcome in 93 of 97 cases (97%), and the L/S ratio correctly predicted the outcome in 89 of 96 cases (92%). A similar study of the two tests found that fluorescence polarization had a predictive value of 100%, but the predictive value of the L/S ratio was only 14% *(10)*.

In summary, studies of fluorescence polarization of amniotic fluid show that these measurements parallel the development of the surfactant system during gestation, reflect the relative concentration of lecithin and other phospholipids important for fetal lung maturity, and correlate well with L/S ratios. The amniotic-fluid P-value is an excellent predictor of the risk of RDS with a specificity comparable with or better than that of the L/S ratio. However, P-value determinations are faster, easier to perform, and have a much lower coefficient of variation. Consequently, the determination of fluorescence polarization in amniotic fluid appears to have diagnostic as well as technical advantages over the L/S ratio, the most frequently performed test for fetal lung maturity.

Foam-Stability Test

In 1972, Clements et al. *(11)* described a rapid, simple test to determine the presence of pulmonary surfactant in amniotic fluid. The test is based on the ability of pulmonary surfactant phospholipids to form a relatively long-lasting foam. The formation of foam by other amniotic fluid substances such as proteins, bile salts, and free fatty acids is inhibited by the presence of ethanol.

In this procedure, 1.0, 0.75, 0.5, 0.25, and 0.2 mL of amniotic fluid are pipetted into glass test tubes and enough 9 g/L saline is added to make the final volume in each tube equal to 1.0 mL, forming dilutions of 1/1, 1/1.3, 1/2, 1/4, and 1/5. To each tube is added 1 mL of 95% (950 mL/L) ethanol, and the tubes are capped, vigorously shaken for 15 s, and left undisturbed in a vertical position. After 15 min the air–liquid interface is examined for the presence of small, stable bubbles. A positive result is recorded if a tube shows a complete ring of bubbles on its surface.

Clements et al. demonstrated an abrupt increase in the amount of amniotic fluid surfactant at 30–35 weeks' gestation, indicated by an increase in the titer required for a positive test result. Results of tests performed within 24 h of birth indicated that a clearly nega- tive test for an undiluted sample (no addition of ethanol) was associ- ated with a high risk of RDS, and a clearly positive test at a twofold (1/2) dilution was associated with a low risk. An intermediate result (positive at undiluted and negative at twofold dilution) was associated with some probability of respiratory difficulty.

In 1973, Edwards and Baillie *(12)* recommended a simplification of the foam-stability test. After 1 mL of amniotic fluid is pipetted into a glass tube, 1 mL of fresh absolute alcohol is added and the tube is capped, vigorously shaken for 30 s, and examined 15 to 30 s later. Positive results are graded from 1+ (the presence of a single ring of small bubbles at the air–liquid interface) to 4+ (the presence of small bubbles completely covering the air–liquid interface); results are negative if the bubbles do not form a complete ring. In specimens obtained within 24 h of birth, Edwards and Baillie demonstrated that a positive test result was highly predictive of the absence of RDS; however, a negative result predicted the presence of RDS with considerably less accuracy.

In 1978, Sher et al. *(13)* described another modification of the foam- stability test, the foam-stability index (FSI) test. In this test 0.5 mL of amniotic fluid is added to a test tube containing 0.51 mL of 95% ethanol; the tube is capped, vigorously shaken for 30 s, and examined 15 s later. A result is positive when an uninterrupted ring of foam is present at the air–liquid interface. If the result is positive, the test is repeated with a tube containing more ethanol; if negative, it is repeated with less ethanol. The FSI value is defined as the highest volume fraction of ethanol that gives a positive result. Statland and Freer demonstrated that FSI values $\geq$ 0.48 give assurance of lung maturity, FSI values $<$ 0.44 indicate a high risk of RDS, and interme- diate values represent a "transition" range.

Although the foam-stability test is simple and rapid to perform, meticulous care must be given to the technique. A number of precau- tions must be considered to obtain meaningful results:

1. Because the final concentration of ethanol is critical, pipetting must be accurate. In addition, because absolute alcohol can absorb water, the ethanol used must be fresh and stored in a tightly stoppered container.

2. Glassware must be clean, without residues of detergents or biological fluids. The diameter of the test tubes used may influence the results and should be in the range of 8–15 mm. The influence of plastic tubes is not stated in the literature.

3. Tubes must be tightly stoppered to prevent evaporation from the foam. This is especially important for the test of Clements et al., because the tubes are inspected 15 min after shaking.

4. Tubes must not be moved after the foam is produced.

5. When ethanol is added to amniotic fluid, occasionally a precipitate forms, which must be differentiated from foam.

6. Amniotic fluid containing blood or meconium must not be used.

The evaluation of the results from this test are somewhat subjective, especially for the modified test (12). Strict criteria for the presence or absence of foam should be defined in every laboratory. Limiting the number of laboratory personnel performing the test will help to decrease variability in results due to variation in technique and evaluation.

A foam-stability test result that is positive for foam formation is very important, being associated with a very low incidence of RDS. However, the test has been criticized for its high proportion of results that are negative for foam formation when the fetus has sufficient surfactant for normal respiratory function, particularly between the 32nd and 37th weeks of gestation, and for the ambiguity of an intermediate test result.

Freer et al. (14) have shown that at various ethanol-volume fractions phospholipids can form stable foams in the following order: bovine brain sphingomyelin > dipalmitoyl lecithin > egg sphingomyelin > egg lecithin > PG. The effect of PI was not stated. These results pertain not only to the FSI test, but also to the original test (11) and its modification (12), which involve ethanol volume fractions of 0.475 and 0.50, respectively.

Of the three methods outlined above, the procedures of Clements et al. (11) and Sher et al. (13) are somewhat more quantitative than that of Edwards and Baillie (12), and may give more information. In the first method the amount of amniotic fluid surfactant is varied, whereas in the FSI method the ethanol volume fraction is varied. The results of Freer et al. (14) indicate that either procedure would lead to the same decision. Clements et al. indicate that foam from unsaturated lecithin breaks down in "a few seconds," whereas foam from saturated lecithin remains stable for several hours; in their method the foam is examined 15 min after shaking. The influence of unsaturated lecithin on the foam observed after 15–30 s for the other methods (12,13) is not stated.

In summary, the foam-stability test is a rapid, relatively simple test for fetal lung maturity, although it is not so simple a test that it obviates the need for experienced and careful laboratory personnel. The formation of foam is generally a good indication of maturity; however, for conditions in which PG production is delayed, such as diabetes, the results should be interpreted cautiously. The foam-stability test may therefore be used as a screening test, where other rapid methods such as fluorescence polarization are not available. When there is a negative result with no foam formation, fluorescence polarization or thin-layer chromatography should be performed.

1. Kulovich, M. V., Hallman, M. B., and Gluck, L., The lung profile I. Normal pregnancy. *Am. J. Obstet. Gynecol.* **135,** 57–63 (1979).
2. Kulovich, M. V., and Gluck, L., The lung profile II. Complicated pregnancy. *Am. J. Obstet. Gynecol.* **135,** 64–70 (1979).
3. Blumenfeld, T. A., Clinical laboratory tests for fetal lung maturity. In *Pathology Annual 1975*, S. C. Sommers, Ed., Appleton-Century-Crofts, New York, NY 1975, pp 21–36.
4. Blumenfeld, T. A., Stark, R. I., George, J. D., James, L. S., Shinitzky, M., Dyrenfurth, I., and Freda, V. J., Fetal lung maturity determined by fluorescence polarization of amniotic fluid. *Am. J. Obstet. Gynecol.* **30,** 782–787 (1978).
5. Shinitzky, M., Goldfisher, A., Bruck, A., Goldman, B., Stern, E., Barkai, G., Mashiach, S., and Serr, D. M., A new method for assessment of fetal lung maturity. *Br. J. Obstet. Gynaecol.* **83,** 838 (1976).
6. Blumenfeld, T. A., Cheskin, H. S., and Shinitzky, M., Microviscosity of amniotic fluid phospholipids and the importance of these values in determining fetal lung maturity. *Clin. Chem.* **25,** 64–67 (1979).
7. Cheskin, H. S., Blumenfeld, T. A., Beers, P. C., and Buddega, V., Effect of gestational variation of phosphatidylglycerol and phosphatidylinositol on the microviscosity of amniotic fluid phospholipids. *Clin. Chem.* **26,** 301–304 (1980).
8. Stark, R. I., Blumenfeld, T. A., George, J. D., Freda, V. J., and James, L. S., The relationship of amniotic fluid microviscosity determined by fluorescence polarization to gestational age. *Pediatrics* **63,** 213–218 (1979).
9. Stark, R. I., Blumenfeld, T. A., Cheskin, H. S., Dyrenfurth, I., and James, L. S., Amniotic fluid fluorescence polarization value as a predictor of respiratory distress syndrome. *J. Pediatr.* **96,** 301–304 (1980).
10. Elrad, H., Beydoun, S. N., Hagen, J. H., Cabalum, M. T., and Aubry, R. H., Fetal pulmonary maturity as determined by fluorescent polarization of amniotic fluid. *Am. J. Obstet. Gynecol.* **132,** 681–685 (1978).
11. Clements, J. A., Platzker, A. C. G., Tierney, D. F., Hobel, C. J., Creasy, R. K., Margolis, A. J., Thibeault, D. W., Tooley, W. H., and Oh, W., Assessment of the risk of the respiratory distress syndrome by a rapid test for surfactant in amniotic fluid. *N. Engl. J. Med.* **286,** 1077–1081 (1972).
12. Edwards, J., and Baillie, P., A simple method of detecting pulmonary surfactant activity in amniotic fluid. *S. Afr. Med. J.* **47,** 2070–2073 (1973).
13. Sher, G., Statland, B. E., Freer, D. E., and Kraybill, E. N., Assessing fetal lung maturation by the foam stability index test. *Obstet. Gynecol.* **52,** 673–677 (1978).
14. Freer, D. E., Statland, B. E., and Sher, G., Rational basis for foam-stability assays of amniotic fluid surfactant. *Clin. Chem.* **24,** 1980–1984 (1978).

Chapter 8. Laboratory Tests in Pediatric Gastroenterology

Emanuel Lebenthal and Ping-Cheung Lee

Pancreozymin–Secretin Test

In this test the pancreas is stimulated directly. Biochemical analysis of properly collected duodenal fluid provides useful information on exocrine pancreatic function. The test is particularly useful for assessing children with suspected pancreatic insufficiency or with steatorrhea without injury to small intestinal mucosa.

Children to be tested are usually fasted for 4 to 6 h. Children younger than 10 years of age should be appropriately sedated. We routinely use a mixture of Demerol (meperidine)/Phenergan (promethazine HC1)/Thorazine (chlorpromazine), 12.5/25.0/12.5 mg/mL, at a dosage of 0.1 mL/kg of body weight (maximum dose 2.0 mL) in our clinic. One hour after sedation, thread a double-lumen Dreiling tube (either nasal/duodenal or oral/duodenal) into the duodenum. Use fluoroscopy to confirm its placement in the duodenum. Collect two 10-min basal duodenal-fluid specimens and then slowly infuse intravenously a solution of purified porcine pancreozymin (purchased from Kabi Diagnostica, Sweden) at a dosage of 2 Ivy dog units/kg of body weight; total infusion time is about 2 min. Obtain three 10-min collections. Purified secretin (Kabi Diagnostica) can then be infused in the same way as pancreozymin, also at 2 clinical units/kg of body weight. Perform three additional 10-min collections. Collect all fluid specimens over ice and freeze them immediately in solid carbon dioxide after each collection; store at $-20\,°C$ for subsequent determination.

Continuously monitor the pH of all samples during the entire test. An alkaline pH and a yellowish-green color of the collected fluid indicate correct tube placement in the duodenum. A turbid sample or one with a pH much lower than 7 usually is contaminated with gastric juice and should be discarded. Perform a prior skin test on each subject for hypersensitivity to both hormones.

Enzymes determined in the collected duodenal fluids include trypsin, chymotrypsin, lipase, and amylase. A significant reduction in the activities of all enzymes is usually sufficient indication for pancreatic insufficiency such as Shwachman–Diamond syndrome and the majority of cases of cystic fibrosis. Clinical manifestations (e.g., steatorrhea) of pancreatic insufficiency will be apparent only if the pancreatic enzyme output is less than 10% of normal. A low output of pancreatic enzyme has also been shown in cases of malnutrition such as marasmus and kwashiorkor (1,2). Isolated cases of diarrhea may sometimes be a result of starch intolerance related to a low concentration or absence of amylase. This is exemplified by early introduction of cereal in the diet of infants less than four months old. Lipase deficiency is rare and in some instances may represent an insufficient colipase production (3). With low or absent proteolytic activities but normal lipase and amylase activities, one should measure enterokinase activities, to rule out the rare incidence of enterokinase deficiency. Measurement of immunoglobulins in duodenal fluid is useful in the differential diagnosis of chronic diarrhea that might be caused by secretory immunoglobulin deficiency.

Enterokinase

Enterokinase (EK) has been considered a brush border enzyme, but is also present in duodenal fluid. Thus it is important to distinguish between the EK activities in the mucosa and in the intraluminal fluid. Newborns have only 20% of the EK activity in the small intestinal mucosa that children one year and older have (4). In children with cystic fibrosis, EK activity is high intraluminally and in the mucosa (5,6). In celiac disease (6,7) and Shwachman–Diamond syndrome (5), both intraluminal and mucosal EK are normal. In intractable diarrhea of infancy with small intestinal mucosal injury, mucosal and intraluminal EK activities are low (7). A rare congenital disorder of EK deficiency occurs, in which mucosal and intraluminal activities are very low (8).

The assay for EK activity usually involves two steps: activating trypsinogen to trypsin, and measuring the trypsin formed. Because the amount of trypsin formed depends on the amount of EK present, an estimation of the final trypsin activity is an indirect measurement of the EK activity (see commentary on *trypsin*, below).

There are some inherent uncertainties about this indirect assay method. A more reliable method involves use of a new substrate, Gly-(Asp)$_4$-Lys-2-naphthylamide (9). This synthetic peptide contains an amino acid sequence similar to the peptide segment in trypsinogen, upon which EK acts specifically. The reaction of EK with this synthetic peptide results in the liberation of 2-naphthylamide, which can be quantitated fluorometrically. Interference by trypsin is eliminated by the addition of soybean trypsin inhibitor, making this assay a simple and direct measurement of EK activity. Unfortunately, the synthetic peptide substrate is not yet available commercially.

EK is very stable. Samples can be stored at $-20\ °C$ for several months without appreciable loss of enzyme activity. For the determination of its activity in duodenal fluid, separate the EK from the trypsin by Sephadex gel filtration, to avoid interference by trypsin.

Trypsin

The pancreas secretes trypsinogen, which is activated by EK from the duodenal mucosa to yield trypsin; duodenal fluid therefore contains various proportions of trypsin and trypsinogen. For the determination of total tryptic activity (i.e., trypsin and trypsinogen), the sample should first be activated with EK. Measuring the difference in trypsin activity before and after EK activation estimates the amount of trypsinogen in fluid.

Neonatal duodenal fluid has about 50% of the trypsin activity found in children at the age of one year and older. In congenital EK deficiency, trypsin activity in the duodenal fluid is low or absent *(10)*; the clinical presentation may simulate that of primary pancreatic insufficiency because of the absence of tryptic activity that is required for the activation of other pancreatic proenzymes. Prolonged feeding with a high-protein diet may increase the trypsin content in the pancreas and in duodenal fluid *(11)*.

Trypsin activity can be measured via the hydrolysis of *p*-tosyl-L-arginine methylester by a change in the absorbance at 247 nm, or by a change in pH caused by the production of carboxylic acids. Probably the most convenient method is to use a chromogenic substrate, *p*-benzoyl-DL-arginine-*p*-nitroanilide HCl. Hydrolysis of this substrate liberates *p*-nitroanilide, the intense yellow color of which can be monitored at 410 nm.

Normal serum has negligible trypsin activity. Higher trypsin activity is mainly associated with pancreatitis or direct insult to the pancreas. Accurate determination of trypsin in serum is difficult because: *(a)* the assay method is not sufficiently sensitive, *(b)* the substrates are not totally specific, and *(c)* serum protease inhibitor is present. In an alternative RIA technique *(12)* immunoreactive forms of human pancreatic cationic trypsin are measured in serum. Although this is a more sensitive and accurate method for determining trypsin in serum, it requires elaborate set-ups and techniques and is therefore not suitable for routine use. (See also the next section.)

Chymotrypsin and Carboxypeptidase

Both chymotrypsin and carboxypeptidase are secreted by the pancreas as zymogens, then activiated by trypsin in the duodenal fluid. Duodenal fluid, therefore, contains mainly the active forms of chymotrypsin and carboxypeptidase. To ascertain that the absence of their activities is not the result of nonavailable or low trypsin (see above), incubate the sample fluid with purified trypsin at 4 °C and then assay for chymotrypsin and carboxypeptidase.

Carboxypeptidase activity is usually very low in young infants. Even at the age of one month, carboxypeptidase activity is still about 30% of that in children one year and older. For chymotrypsin, newborns show 60 to 70% of the activity in children one year and older. Chymotrypsin and trypsin content in the pancreas increases after a high-protein diet, which may affect the chymotrypsin and trypsin activities in duodenal fluid *(11)*. In general, the measurement of trypsin and chymotrypsin activities is a better indicator than carboxypeptidase for pancreatic exocrine function in children.

The measurement is best made after intravenous injection of pancreozymin and secretin. Because newer techniques and equipment are available for collecting duodenal fluid, the assay for pancreatic proteases (trypsin, chymotrypsin, and carboxypeptidase) in stools is unnecessary, except in cases when fluid collection is not possible. Even at best, however, the measurement of fecal pancreatic proteases is a semiquantitative assessment of pancreatic enzyme secretion.

Lipase

Serum lipase activity is usually very low. High serum lipase activity often, but not always, indicates an acute attack of pancreatitis or trauma affecting the pancreas. Lipase activity in duodenal fluid, however, is high, except in patients with pancreatic insufficiency or in rare cases of congenital lipase deficiency *(13)*. In infants less than six months old, the lipase content in duodenal fluid is only 10 to 30% of the adult value *(14)*, gradually increasing to that of adults in subsequent development. A different range of reference (normal) values should be used for infants and children older than six months. Also, because comparison of units between different assays is difficult, each laboratory should set its own reference range, based on institutional experience.

Adaptation of lipase activity to prolonged feeding with a high-fat diet has been suggested, but definitive proof is still lacking.

Two methods are available for determining lipase: the turbidometric method of Vogel and Zieve *(15)* and the titrimetric method of Tietz et al. *(16)*. The turbidometric method is relatively simple and easy to use, but is not very suitable for samples with high lipase activity, e.g., duodenal fluid. The titrimetric method is more complicated and time-consuming but also more reliable. The titrimetric method measures ionized free fatty acids liberated by the action of lipase. The release of free fatty acids can be measured either after a fixed time of incubation, or continuously with an automatic pH titrator *(17)*. The latter method monitors the kinetics of the enzyme activity with time, which gives a better estimate of the lipolytic activity, but requires elaborate equipment and extra skill.

The substrate commonly used in both methods is purified olive oil. To attain a homogenous substrate solution, the olive oil is usually emulsified with deoxycholate or gum acacia. Deoxycholate, however, may inhibit lipolytic activity because bile salts inhibit pancreatic lipase *(18)*.

Amylase

Newborns and infants less than four months old have very low amylase activities in their duodenal fluid (14,19). Because the major portion of the serum amylase is derived from the pancreas, infants up to four months old also have a very low serum amylase. Although prolonged feeding with a high-starch diet has been claimed to increase the pancreatic content of amylase and its secretion, dietary adaptation of pancreatic amylase is still a controversial issue (11). Amylase in the duodenal fluid of older children is usually high except in cases of cystic fibrosis.

Amylase in the serum and urine of adults is usually low except in certain diseases, particularly in acute pancreatitis, hyperamylasemia, and acute parotiditis (mumps). To distinguish between the different diseases, serum isoamylase profiles should be performed to identify the pancreatic and salivary forms (20–22).

The three methods mostly used for amylase assay are: (a) the iodometric or amyloclastic method, which measures the disappearance of starch; (b) the saccharogenic method, which measures the production of maltose from starch; and (c) the chromogenic method, which measures the liberation of dye from a dye–starch complex.

The iodometric method has relatively low sensitivity and is interfered with by albumin (22).

Amylase requires Ca^{2+} and a neutral pH for optimum activity; EDTA and citrate should not be used during the collection of blood samples. Because albumin stabilizes amylase activity, amylase in serum is relatively stable, but in urine and duodenal fluid is not. To preserve the activity of amylase in urine and duodenal fluid, collect samples at 4 °C and assay soon after collection. We do not recommend storage of urine and duodenal-fluid specimens, even when they are frozen.

The diversity of substrates and methods for measuring amylase activity makes the standardization of enzyme units very difficult. Each institute should establish its own standard as the norm for its own reference. Obviously, different values are used for adults and infants.

Alkaline Phosphatase

Different tissues synthesize different isoenzymes of alkaline phosphatase. Serum alkaline phosphatases mainly originate from liver, bone, and intestine. High serum alkaline phosphatase activity is associated with skeletal disease, hepatic disorder, intestinal diseases, tumors, thyrotoxicosis, ingestion of anticonvulsant drugs, and rheumatoid arthritis (23). The capacity to distinguish between serum isoenzymes of alkaline phosphatase is important in differential diagnosis. Some isoenzymes exhibit characteristic properties that can be utilized for their identification. Alkaline phosphatase from bone tissue is more sensitive to heat *(24)* and urea *(25)* than the liver enzyme. The intestinal alkaline phosphatase activity is inhibited about 20% by 5 mmol of L-phenylalanine per liter, whereas the bone and liver enzymes are only slightly inhibited *(26)*. Different isoenzymes of alkaline phosphatase have also been separated by electrophoresis with various supporting media *(23)*. Results are conflicting, at least in part because of the different methods of extracting and preparing samples. Using polyacrylamide gel seems to resolve the isoenzymes better *(27)* and may be especially useful for detecting variants of alkaline phosphatase isoenzymes in the sera of tumor patients.

The activity of alkaline phosphatase in serum depends on the growth rate. In children, during a period of rapid growth, serum alkaline phosphatase activity has a higher normal upper limit.

The presence of phosphate inhibits the activity of alkaline phosphatase. Be careful not to introduce phosphate into the reaction mixture.

Measurement of alkaline phosphatase, correlated with disaccharidase activities in small intestinal biopsies, can serve as a good index of the integrity of the brush border of the mature villus cell in the small intestine.

Note: See also the Commentary on serum **Alkaline phosphatase** by G. N. Bowers (pp 73–77).

IgG, IgM, and IgA in Duodenal Fluid

See the Commentary on **Immunoglobulins in duodenal fluid,** p. 283.

1. Thompson, M. D., and Trowell, H. C., Pancreatic enzyme activity in duodenal contents of children with a type of kwashiorkor. *Lancet* **i,** 1031–1035 (1952).
2. Barbezat, G. O., and Hansen, J. D. L., The exocrine pancreas and protein in caloric malnutrition. *Pediatrics* **42,** 77–92 (1968).
3. Gaskin, K. J., Durie, P. R., Hill, R. E., Lee, L., and Forstner, G. G., Colipase in pancreatic insufficiency. *Gastroenterology* **78,** 1170 (1980). Abstract.
4. Antonowicz, I., and Lebenthal, E., Developmental pattern of small intestional enterokinase and disaccharidase activities in the human fetus. *Gastroenterology* **72,** 1299–1303 (1977).
5. Lebenthal, E., Antonowicz, I., and Shwachman, H., Enterokinase and trypsin activities in pancreatic insufficiency and diseases of the small intestine. *Gastroenterology* **70,** 508–512 (1976).
6. Morin, C. L., VanCaillie, M., Roy, C. C., and Lasalle, R., Mucosal enterokinase activity in pancreatic insufficiency and celiac disease. *Pediatrics* **60,** 114–116 (1977).
7. Lebenthal, E., Antonowicz, I., and Shwachman, H., The interrelationship of enterokinase activities in intractable diarrhea of infancy, celiac disease, and intravenous alimentation. *Pediatrics* **56,** 585–591 (1975).

8. Hadorn, B., Tarlow, M. J., Lloyd, J. K., and Wolff, O. H., Intestinal enterokinase deficiency. *Lancet* **i**, 812–813 (1969).
9. Hesford, F., Hadorn, B., Blaser, K., and Schneider, C. H., A new substrate for enteropeptidase. *FEBS Lett.* **71**, 279–282 (1976).
10. Hadorn, B., Tarlow, M. J., Lloyd, J. K., and Wolff, O. H., Intestinal enterokinase deficiency. *Lancet* **i**, 812–813 (1969).
11. Lebenthal, E., Pancreatic function and disease in infancy and childhood. *Adv. Pediatr.* **25**, 223–261 (1978).
12. Geokas, M. C., Largman, C., Brodrick, J. W., and Johnson, J. H., Determination of human pancreatic cationic trypsinogen in serum by radio-immunoassay. *Am. J. Physiol.* **236**, E77-E83 (1979).
13. Figarella, C., Negri, G. A., and Sardes, H., Presence of colipase in a congenital pancreatic lipase deficiency. *Biochim. Biophys. Acta* **280**, 205–210 (1972).
14. Zoppi, G., Andreotti, G., Pajno-Ferrara, F., Njai, D. M., and Gaburro, D., Exocrine pancreatic function in premature and full term infants. *Pediatr. Res.* **6**, 880–886 (1972).
15. Vogel, W. C., and Zieve, L., A rapid and sensitive turbidometric method for serum lipase based upon differences between the lipases of normal and pancreatitis serum. *Clin. Chem.* **9**, 168–181 (1963).
16. Tietz, N. W., Border, T., and Stepleton, J. D., An improved method in the determination of lipase in serum. *Am. J. Clin. Pathol.* **31**, 148–154 (1959).
17. Smeriva, M., Dufour, C., and Desnuelle, P., On the possible involvement of a histidine residue in the active site of pancreatic lipase. *Biochemistry* **10**, 2143–2149 (1971).
18. Desnuelle, P., The lipase colipase system. In *Lipid Absorption, Biochemical and Chemical Aspects*, K. Rommel, H. Goebell, and R. Bohmer, Eds. University Park Press, Baltimore, MD, 1976.
19. Auricchio, S., Rubino, A., and Murset, G., Intestinal glucosidase activities in the human embryo, fetus and newborn. *Pediatrics* **35**, 944–954 (1955).
20. Lebenthal, E., and Shwachman, H., The pancreas development, adaptation and malfunction in infancy and childhood. *Clin. Gastroenterol.* **6**, 397–413 (1977).
21. Merritt, A. D., and Karn, R. C., The human amylase. *Adv. Hum. Genet.* **8**, 135–244 (1977).
22. Skude, G., On human amylase isoenzymes. *Scand. J. Gastroenterol.* **12**, Suppl. 44, 1–37 (1977).
23. Warnes, T. W., Progress report: Alkaline phosphatase. *Gut* **13**, 926–937 (1972).
24. Posen, S., Neale, F. C., and Clubb, J. S., Heat inactivation in the study of human alkaline phosphatases. *Ann. Int. Med.* **62**, 1234–1243 (1965).
25. Bahr, M., and Wilkinson, J. H., Urea as a selective inhibitor of human tissue alkaline phosphatases. *Clin. Chim. Acta* **17**, 367–370 (1967).
26. Fishman, W. H., Green, S., and Inglis, H. I., L-Phenylalanine: An organ-specific inhibitor of human intestinal alkaline phosphatase. *Nature* **198**, 685–686 (1963).
27. Kaplan, M. M., and Rogers, L., Separation of human serum-alkaline-phosphatase isoenzymes by polyacrylamide gel electrophoresis. *Lancet* **ii**, 1029–1031 (1969).

Chapter 9. Screening for Neonatal Hypothyroidism

Paul G. Walfish

Neonatal hypothyroidism is a known cause of mental retardation that may be prevented by thyroid-hormone therapy before three months of age. The difficulty in diagnosis by clinical features alone before six months of age has justified routine laboratory-screening programs for early detection and therapy of neonatal hypothyroidism before its clinical recognition. According to recent reports from North America (1) and Europe (2), the incidence of neonatal hypothyroidism is between 1:3000 and 1:5000 live births, a frequency three- to fourfold greater than phenylketonuria.

Various sampling and transport techniques for the detection of neonatal hypothyroidism have been assessed (1,2). Although serum has several methodological advantages, most large-scale regional screening programs, because they involve mail transport of samples to a centralized laboratory, have utilized the same heel skin-puncture blood specimens spotted on filter paper (Schleicher and Schuell: no. 903 in North America, no. 2992 in Europe) as are taken at three to five days after birth for phenylketonuria and other inborn-error screening programs. Alternatively, cord-blood screening is as effective as heel-blood sampling in detecting neonatal hypothyroidism (3–5) and, by permitting an earlier screening diagnosis from a safe, non-invasive sampling technique, may have a number of advantages for those countries not screening for other inborn errors.

The methods for measuring thyroid hormones from the small amounts of serum within dried filter-paper discs must be modified from routine serum analytical methods to provide the necessary sensitivity. Very high specific activity ^{125}I tracer [1000 Ci/g for thyroxine (T_4) and 150 Ci/g for human thyrotropin (thyroid-stimulating hormone; TSH)][1] and antisera with the greatest possible affinity constant and hormone specificity must be used. Initially, T_4 was assayed from 10- to 13-mm diameter dried-blood discs (4–6), representing approximately 14 to 16 μL of plasma. Most North American centers are now using ⅛ " (3.2-mm) diameter discs representing 1.5 μL of plasma (8,9). Current blood TSH methods usually involve two ⅛ " (3.2-mm)

---

[1] Abbreviations used in this chapter: T_4, thyroxine; TSH, thyrotropin (thyroid-stimulating hormone); T_3, triiodothyronine; rT_3, reverse triiodothyronine; TBG, thyroxine-binding globulin.

diameter blood discs, representing 3 μL of plasma *(10–12)*, or a single ¼ " (6.4-mm) diameter disc *(13)*, representing approximately 6 μL of plasma. TSH assay sensitivity can be enhanced by reducing the final incubation volume from 1 to 0.5 mL or less *(10,12)*. The serum double-antibody TSH assay time may be shortened from five to two days by increasing the incubation temperatures from 4 °C to 20 or 37 °C *(14)*, and the dried-blood TSH assay time decreased from five to two days by using a solid-phase radioimmunoassay *(12)*.

Assays performed from dried-blood filter-paper discs have been generally reliable as screening tests, except at the extremes of hematocrit variation *(7,8)*, but require proper collection and saturation of both surfaces of the filter paper to avoid methodological errors *(7,9)*. Exposure to high (50 °C) temperatures for three or more weeks results in a significant decrease in blood TSH immunoassay values and could lead to false-negative results *(12)*. Also, falsely low dried-blood T_4 values (due to poor extractability of the red colors from the spots) can occur with specimens exposed to high ambient temperatures, high humidity, or sunlight *(15)*.

Screening for neonatal hypothyroidism on the basis of T_4 values alone has low specificity and sensitivity, owing to the high incidence of false-positive low T_4 results secondary to prematurity, hypo-TBG-emia, and methodological problems *(4–7,16)*; this leads to an impractically high (2 to 3%) burden of recall. In addition, "normal" T_4 results may occur in approximately 30 to 50% of cases with ectopic (lingual) thyroid dysplasia or goitrous biosynthetic causes of congential primary hypothyroidism *(2,5)*; these abnormalities could be detected by an above-normal TSH value obtained by either initial (primary) testing of all infants or an increased secondary TSH testing of the specimens with the lowest 5 to 15% of the T_4 initial screening tests *(2,5)*.

Because serum reverse triiodothyronine (rT_3) values are normally higher in newborn infants than in adults, several studies have assessed the value of initial cord or neonatal heel blood rT_3 screening for the detection of congenital hypothyroidism from abnormally low rT_3 results *(17)*. However, false-negative (normal) values were measured in approximately 50% of infants documented to have primary neonatal hypothyroidism *(17,19)*, and false-positive (low) values in infants without hypothyroidism secondary to idiopathic low T_4 and hypo-TBG-emia *(18)*. Although some infants with prematurity or systemic illness may have high cord-serum rT_3 values *(18)* that interfere with the specificity of the rT_3 screening test for detecting neonatal hypothyroidism, such co-existing conditions may be identified by their increased ratios for rT_3/T_4 *(18)* and rT_3/T_3 *(20)*. Hence, as an initial screening test, rT_3, like T_4, lacks specificity for the diagnosis of neonatal hypothyroidism; it is also more expensive, is less readily available, and offers no special advantage over initial primary T_4 screening *(17)*.

Although initial T_4 and rT_3 screening tests may theoretically detect secondary/tertiary hypothyroidism, this abnormality appears to represent less than 6% of the total neonatal hypothyroidism population *(1,2)* and requires a high (1%) follow-up recall burden to distinguish it from other causes of a falsely low T_4 value (as delineated above). Because secondary/tertiary hypothyroidism may not be necessarily associated with mental retardation and can be diagnosed by the clinical and laboratory manifestations of other accompanying pituitary gland deficiencies, many centers have abandoned routine follow-up recall of infants who have low T_4's but normal TSH screening values. These centers have altered the objectives of their screening program to detect only infants with primary hypothyroidism (low T_4 and high TSH), thereby reducing their infant recall rate to less than 0.3% of the screened population *(1,5)*.

The most specific and sensitive test for detecting primary neonatal hypothyroidism is TSH, which has a much lower false-positive incidence than screening for T_4 alone *(2–5)*. Initial TSH screening permits the detection of those infants with low normal T_4's but high TSH values from goitrous (biosynthetic) abnormalities and (or) ectopic (lingual) thyroid dysplasis *(2–5)*, who may have been missed by initial T_4 screening. False-positive increases of TSH values may occur more frequently in premature infants, particularly when a heel-blood sample is taken before three days of age, or after exposure to dietary or drug goitrogens, or after excessive stress from parturition or systemic illness *(4,5)*. Owing to the methodological detection limitations in distinguishing low from normal values for serum *(14)* or blood *(10–13)* TSH screening, primary TSH screening or even high-cutoff complementary secondary TSH screening will not detect the 6% or fewer infants who have congenital hypothyroidism due to low TSH hypothalamic–pituitary (secondary/tertiary) hypothyroidism *(1,2)*. TSH screening in which the cord-serum cutoff value is greater than 50 micro-int. units/mL *(3–5,14)* or a dried cord-blood value greater than 25 micro-int. units/mL *(12)* will require less than a 0.3% recall burden to detect cases with primary neonatal hypothyroidism. Heel-blood TSH screening in which cutoff values are 25 and 50 micro-int. units/mL (representing approximately 50 and 100 micro-int. units/mL of serum when corrected for hematocrit) will have recall incidences of 0.3% *(12)* and 0.04% *(13)*, respectively. Hence, primary TSH screening from either heel or cord blood may ultimately be the preferred and cost-effective screening test for detecting primary neonatal hypothyroidism.

Pending the availability of more automatable and cost-effective TSH methods suitable for large-scale centralized screening of more than 50 000 infants annually, initial primary T_4 testing, followed by secondary TSH testing on the lowest 3 to 5% of T_4 values, continues to be the most common screening program performed in most North American centers *(1)*. However, special studies from our laboratory have demonstrated some methodological limitations in blood T_4 assay reproducibility when single 3.2-mm diameter discs (as received for neonatal screening) are analyzed *(9)*. From these observations, we have recommended that a complementary secondary TSH test be performed on at least the lowest 10th centile (approximately −1.28 SD from the daily mean) of daily blood T_4 assays *(9)*. In our experience, an absolute daily T_4 cutoff value (e.g., 5 μg/dL) should not be used, owing to the day-to-day and seasonal variations observed for the blood T_4 assay *(9)*. Using a higher cutoff value for secondary TSH testing of T_4 results enhances the detection frequency of infants with low-normal T_4 values secondary to ectopic (lingual) or goitrous abnormalities *(5)* to frequencies similar to those of European centers that use primary blood TSH screening *(2)*, but theoretically may still miss some affected infants.

Primary or secondary blood TSH values that exceed 25 micro-int. units/mL (representing approximately 50 micro-int. units/mL of serum when corrected for hematocrit) should be recalled for repeat venous serum assessment *(2,5)*. Infants with blood TSH-screening values exceeding 50 micro-int. units/mL (representing approximately 100 micro-int. units/mL of serum) require immediate hospitalization for follow-up: they have a greater than 90% risk of having persistent primary hypothyroidism *(5)*. Hence, depending upon the facilities available for automation and the regionalization of statewide programs to be performed in a centralized laboratory to optimize quality control, we recommend that dried blood obtained from cord or neonatal heel-sampling sites have an initial T_4 test followed by selective secondary TSH testing on at least the lowest 10th centile of T_4 results—*or alternatively,* that all infants have initial TSH testing—to maximize the detection of primary neonatal hypothyroidism.

Infants with screening-test abnormalities require follow-up clinical and laboratory evaluation as previously described *(5)*, including venous serum T_4, T_3-uptake, and TSH tests. T_4 and T_3-uptake values should be assessed relative to the known higher values expected in the neonatal period and first few months of life compared with adult ranges. Serum TSH exceeding 10 micro-int. units/mL for infants more than 10 days old should be considered abnormal and suspect for transient or persistent primary hypothyroidism. Further anatomical assessment of infants with persistent follow-up abnormalities is recommended. Technetium-99m scintiscan or, preferably, ^{125}I can be used to classify the types of persistent primary hypothyroidism detected as well as assist in long-term management *(5)*. The presence of athyrosis (nonvisualization) of the thyroid gland, ectopic (lingual) thyroid dysplasia, or goitrous (biosynthetic) abnormalities indicates the need for long-term thyroid-hormone replacement therapy. Because congenital goitrous biosynthetic abnormalities and ectopic (lingual) thyroid dysplasia defects may be inherited, genetic counselling regarding future pregnancies is indicated. The appearance of hypoplasia or a normal-sized thyroid gland upon scintiscanning indicates that thyroid hormone should be withdrawn from such infants at two to three years of age, to differentiate transient from true persistent primary hypothyroidism. Infants with suspected secondary hypothyroidism may undergo special thyrotropin-releasing hormone (TRH; thyroliberin) stimulation (at doses of 3 to 5 $\mu g/kg$ of body weight intravenously) to confirm whether there is an abnormality in the hypothalamo–pituitary–thyroid axis.

Current screening programs confirm the diagnosis and institute therapy before three to four weeks of life in the majority of affected infants. Frequent follow-up assessment every one to two months in the first year of life is necessary to evaluate the adequacy of thyroid-hormone (thyroxine) replacement therapy and avoid insufficient or excessive treatment. Serial venous serum T_4 and T_3-uptake tests should be obtained at regular intervals to confirm that T_4 replacement therapy has produced serum T_4 values in the upper normal range expected for early infancy and childhood.

1. Fisher, D. A., Dussault, J. H., Foley, T. P., Klein, A. H., LaFranchi, S., Larsen, P. R., Mitchell, M. L., Murphey, W. H., and Walfish, P. G., Screening for congenital hypothyroidism: Results of screening one million North American infants. *J. Pediatr.* **94,** 700–705 (1979).
2. Report of the Newborn Committee on the European Thyroid Association. Neonatal screening for congenital hypothyroidism in Europe. *Acta Endocrinol.* **90** (Suppl. 223), 5–29 (1979).
3. Klein, A. H., Agustin, A. V., and Foley, T. P., Successful screening for congenital hypothyroidism. *Lancet* **ii,** 77–79 (1974).
4. Walfish, P. G., Evaluation of three thyroid function screening tests for detecting neonatal hypothyroidism. *Lancet* **i,** 1208–1211 (1976).
5. Walfish, P. G., Ginsberg, J., Rosenberg, R. A., and Howard, N. J., Results of a regionalized cord blood screening program for detecting neonatal hypothyroidism. *Arch. Dis. Child.* **54,** 171–177 (1979).
6. Dussault, J. H., Coulombe, P., Laberge, C., Letarte, J., Guyda, H., and Khoury, P., Preliminary report on a mass screening program for neonatal hypothyroidism. *J. Pediatr.* **86,** 670–674 (1975).
7. Walfish, P. G., Screening for neonatal hypothyroidism using dried capillary blood thyroxine method. Observations on methodological factors, selection criteria and preliminary results. In *Perinatal Thyroid Physiology and Disease,* D. A. Fisher and G. N. Burrow, Eds. Raven Press, New York, NY, 1975, pp 239–247.
8. Larsen, P. R., and Broskin, K., Thyroxine immunoassay using filter paper blood samples for screening neonates for hypothyroidism. *Pediatr. Res.* **9,** 604–609 (1975).
9. Walfish, P. G., Gera, E., and Wood, M. M., Methodological limitations on the measurement of thyroxine from small dried blood discs: Comparison of a double antibody and solid phase radioimmunoassay. In *Neonatal Screening for Inborn Errors of Metabolism,* H. Bickel, R. Guthrie, and G. Hammersen, Eds. Springer-Verlag, New York, NY, 1980, pp 229–239.
10. Larsen, P. R., Merker, A., and Parlow, A. F., Immunoassay of human TSH using dried blood samples. *J. Clin. Endocrinol. Metab.* **42,** 987–990 (1976).

11. Foley, T. P., Klein, A. H., and Agustin, A. V., Adaptation of TSH filter paper method for a regionalized screening for congenital hypothyroidism. *J. Lab. Clin. Med.* **90**, 11–17 (1977).

12. Walfish, P. G., and Gera, E., Experience with the application of a dried blood thyrotropin method for neonatal hypothyroidism screening: Comparative studies between double antibody and solid phase radioimmunoassays. In *Neonatal Screening for Inborn Errors of Metabolism* (see ref. *9*), pp 219–228.

13. Illig, R., Torresani, T., and Sobradillo, B., Early detection of neonatal hypothyroidism by serial TSH determination in dried blood. *Helv. Paediatr. Acta* **32**, 289–297 (1977).

14. Rosenberg, R. A., Gera, E., and Walfish, P. G., A rapid double antibody non-equilibrium serum thyrotropin radioimmunoassay suitable for primary neonatal hypothyroidism screening. *Clin. Chim. Acta* **92**, 209–219 (1979).

15. Davis, G., and Poholek, R., Stability of dried blood spots, as used in screening neonates for hypothyroidism. *Clin. Chem.* **25**, 24–25 (1979).

16. Gorodzinsky, P., Howard, N. J., Ginsberg, J., and Walfish, P. G., Cord serum thyroxine and thyrotropin values between 20 and 30 weeks gestation. *J. Pediatr.* **94**, 971–973 (1979).

17. Walfish, P. G., Ginsberg, J., and Chopra, I. J., Reverse T_3 cord serum screening. *J. Endocrinol. Invest.* **1**, 386 (1978). Letter.

18. Ginsberg, J., Walfish, P. G., and Chopra, I. J., Cord blood reverse T_3 in normal premature, euthyroid-low T_4 hypothyroid newborns. *J. Endocrinol. Invest.* **1**, 73–77 (1978).

19. Klein, A. H., Foley, T. P., Bernard, B., Ho, R. S., and Fisher, D. A., Cord blood reverse T_3 and congenital hypothyroidism. *J. Clin. Endocrinol. Metab.* **46**, 336–338 (1978).

20. Isaac, R. M., Hayek, A., Standefer, J. C., and Eaton, R. P., Reverse triiodothyronine to triiodothyronine ratio and gestational age. *J. Pediatr.* **94**, 477–479 (1979).

Chapter 10. Specific Proteins in Pediatrics

Gregory J. Buffone

Normal Physiological Variation

Neonatal and childhood period. Total protein concentration gradually increases during gestation. By 35 to 39 weeks' gestation, protein concentration is usually between 45 and 65 g/L *(1,2)*. Hypoproteinemia of the neonate is usually seen in premature infants and is characterized by a decrease in all major protein fractions and a lag in the rate of increase in protein concentration during the first year of life. In the healthy newborn, the major protein fractions, except for immunoglobulins, reach a steady-state concentration by six months of age.

The concentration of the five major immunoglobulin classes can vary significantly up to the age of three to five years. Immunoglobulin G is unique in that it crosses the placenta and for the first few months of life provides the infant with almost as much IgG concentration and specificity as in the mother. The nadir in IgG concentration usually occurs at about three months of age *(3)*.

Adolescence. Changes in the concentrations of various hormones during early adolescence can directly and indirectly affect the concentration of transport and storage proteins. Among the most notable examples of the changes seen with increased estrogen production or therapeutic administration is the increase in the concentration of α_2-macroglobulin and fibrinogen, and the decrease in antithrombin III concentration *(4,5)*. Likewise, the onset of menstruation and the associated chronic blood loss can influence changes in transferrin and ferritin concentration. (Further alterations in specific protein concentrations are reported in association with aging and the onset of menopause.)

The daily variation in the concentrations of 10 specific proteins has been studied in adults and was less than either method or between-individual variation *(6)*. Assuming this finding can be extrapolated to children, the use of population reference limits will significantly reduce the sensitivity of these measurements for differentiating health and disease. Because individual reference limits are not a practical consideration, multiple samplings during the period of observation are recommended, to detect increasing or decreasing *trends* in the concentration of a specific protein.

Table 1. Choice of Sample for Specific Protein Measurement

Plasma	Serum
Factor VIII	IgG, IgA, IgM, IgE
Antithrombin III	C3, C4, factor B
Prothrombin	Alpha-fetoprotein
Fibrinogen	α_1-Antitrypsin
	Albumin
	Total protein
	α_2-Macroglobulin
	Haptoglobin
	Transferrin

Collection and Preservation of Samples

Total and specific proteins can be measured in serum samples collected by skin puncture; these samples can be handled at ambient temperature for most of the proteins of clinical interest (Table 1). Notable exceptions include coagulation and complement proteins that are heat labile and also sensitive to degradation by endogenous plasma proteases (Table 1). For coagulation studies samples should be collected by venipuncture with a minimum of stasis. The blood should be carefully expressed from the syringe into a tube containing anticoagulant (e.g., heparin or citrate), and all handling should be at 4 °C. If fibrino-peptides are to be measured, an inhibitor of plasmin activity should be included in the collection tube (e.g., soybean trypsin inhibitor).

Immunochemical measurement of C3 and C4 can be done by skin puncture or venipuncture collection methods. For measurement of complement activity, either individual components or total hemolytic complement, samples should be collected by venipuncture and handled at 4 °C. Serum immunoglobulins are stable indefinitely if stored at −20 °C. Samples to be assayed for more labile proteins such as coagulation or complement components should be rapidly frozen and stored at −70 to −90 °C. Good data are not available for the selection of optimum storage conditions for other proteins such as α_1-antitrypsin, α_2-macroglobulin, ceruloplasmin, etc. However, in general, storage at ultra-low temperatures (−70 °C) will retard proteolytic degradation.

Methods and Instrumentation

Total protein and albumin are commonly measured with the biuret reaction and with bromocresol green (BCG) dye-binding, respectively (7). These methods are recommended as standard methods for laboratory use, and reagent formulation has become fairly uniform be-

Table 2. Quantitative Immunochemical Techniques

Technique	Method of Detection	Reference
Radial immunodiffusion	Precipitation	*12*
Nephelometry	Light scattering	*13, 14*
Enzyme-linked immunoassay	Absorbance or fluorescence	*15*
Fluorescent immunoassay	Excitation, emission	*16*
Radioimmunoassay	Emission	*17, 18*
Luminescent immunoassay	Emission	*19*

tween laboratories *(8,9)*. Variation in the time of the absorbance reading for the BCG procedure can cause significant differences in the results for patients' samples in which the α_1 and α_2 fractions are increased in concentration and the albumin is decreased (e.g., nephrotic syndrome and acute inflammation) *(10)*. Specificity of BCG dye-binding can be improved by measuring the absorbance before the α_1 and α_2 fractions begin to react with the dye (<20 s)*(10,11)*.

Specific proteins are best measured by immunochemical methods. The prevalent techniques include gel diffusion, light-scattering, and RIA (Table 2). Other techniques similar to RIA, but relying on fluorescent, enzyme, or bioluminescent labels instead of radioactive isotopes, are under development and should play an important role in clinical testing (Table 2). Regardless of the approach, variations in results can be expected from not only the choice of technique but also the antibody specificity and the material used for standardization *(20,21)*. The potential introduction of monoclonal antibodies as reagents may reduce variability from antibody specificity as well as improve analytical performance of many immunochemical methods. In any case, comparison of reference limits between laboratories should include not only the method but also the specific reagents, i.e., antiserum and calibrators.

Clinical Applications

Many authors have advocated the use of specific-proteins profiling as an improvement in laboratory methods of diagnosis *(22–24)*. However, the information provided is often redundant and nonspecific. Preliminary testing should consist of electrophoretic fractionation (preferably in agarose containing Ca^{2+}) to separate transferrin and C3, and quantitative measurement of albumin and specific immunoglobulins. Further evaluation of specific proteins should be based on the clinical presentation and the information provided by the electrophoresis pattern.

Examples of clinical uses of several specific proteins are shown in Tables 3 and 4. This list is meant to point out applications relevant to pediatrics and is not comprehensive.

Table 3. Associated Alteration in C3 and C4 Concentrations in Disease

Normal C4	Decreased C4
Normal C3	
Congenital complement deficiency other than C3 and C4 [a]	Hypergammaglobulinemia
	Cryoglobulinemia [a]
Circulating conversion products of C3 and(or) C4	Congenital C4 deficiency [a]
	Hereditary angioneurotic edema
	Treated SLE
	Immune complex disease
Decreased C3	
Acute glomerulonephritis (AGN)	Active SLE
Membrane proliferation (GN)	Serum sickness
Congenital C3 deficiency [a]	Chronic active hepatitis
C3 nephritic factor [a]	Subacute bacterial endocarditis
C3b–INA deficiency [a]	Immune complex disease
Immune complex disease	

[a] Rare disease entity.
SLE, systemic lupus erythematosus; INA, inactivator.

Simple immunochemical methods are often not sufficient to provide complete information for diagnostic purposes. In the case of Factor VIII-associated antigen, both Factor VIII-associated antigen and Factor VIII-procoagulant activity must be compared, to differentiate hemophilia carriers from the normal population *(30,31)*. Other examples include complement-component assays for C3, C4, and factor B, where the documentation of complement activation often necessitates demonstrating that complement split-products are present in vivo *(29)*. To confirm the diagnosis of α_1-antitrypsin deficiency, evaluation by a technique known as Pi-typing is required, in addition to results of a quantitative measurement *(24,25)*. In general, many proteins may be normal by immunochemical measurement and will require further evaluation by more sophisticated techniques to demonstrate an abnormality.

For a discussion of IgG, IgA, and IgM, the interested reader should refer to a more specific text *(3,33)*.

The usefulness of specific-protein measurements will be limited by the accuracy of the reference limits, the molecular idiosyncrasy of the protein of interest, and judicious sampling by the clinician during the disease course.

1. Baum, J. D., Eisenberg, C., Franklin, F. A., Jr., Meschia, G., and Battaglia, F. C., Studies on colloid osmotic pressure in the fetus and newborn infant. *Biol. Neonate* **18,** 311–320 (1971).
2. Baum, J. D., and Harris, D., Colloid osmotic pressure in erythroblastosis fetalis. *Br. Med. J.* **i,** 601–603 (1972).

Table 4. Specific Proteins: Clinical Applications

Protein	Clinical application	Relative change in concn	Ref.
Albumin	Shock	−	25
	Protein-losing enteropathy	−	
	Nephrosis	−	
	Inflammation	−	
	Malnutrition	−	
α_1-Antitrypsin	Inflammation	+	26, 27
	Congenital deficiency	−	
Alpha-fetoprotein	Neural tube defects[a]	−	28, 30
	Hepatocellular carcinoma	+	
Total complement	Complement deficiency	−, no change	31
	Complement consumption	−	
C3, C4	Complement consumption	−	31
Factor VIII-associated antigen	Screening for carriers of hemophilia	−[b]	32, 33
Fibrinogen	Inflammation	+	34
	Disseminated intravascular coagulation	−	
	Congenital deficiency	−	
IgG, IgA, and IgM	Infection	+	3, 35
	Immune deficiency	−, no change	
	Autoimmune disease	−, +, no change	
IgE	Reaginic disease	+	36, 38
	Parasitic infection	+	
	Polyarteritis nodosa	+	
	Wiskott–Aldrich syndrome	−	
	Ataxia telangiectasia	−	

[a] Amniotic fluid.
[b] Ratio of procoagulant activity to Factor VIII-associated antigen.

3. Ritzmann, S. E., Immunoglobulin abnormalities. In *Serum Protein Abnormalities*, S. E. Ritzmann and J. C. Daniels, Eds. Little, Brown and Co., Boston, MA, 1975, pp 351–486.
4. Horne, C. H. W., Howie, P. W., Goudie, R. B., and Weir, R. J., Effects of combined estrogen–progestogen oral contraceptives on serum levels of α_2-macroglobulin, transferrin, albumin and IgG. *Lancet* i, 49–50 (1970).
5. Fagerhol, M. K., and Abilgaard, U., Immunological studies on human antithrombin III. Influence of age, sex, and use of oral contraceptives on serum concentration. *Scand. J. Haematol.* **7**, 7–10 (1970).
6. Statland, B. E., Winkel, P., and Killingsworth, L. M., Factors contributing to intra-individual variation of serum constituents: 6. Physiological day-to-day variation in concentrations of 10 specific proteins in sera of healthy subjects. *Clin. Chem.* **22**, 1635–1638 (1976).
7. Reinhold, J. G., Total protein albumin and globulin. *Stand. Methods Clin. Chem.* **1**, 88–97 (1953).

8. Kingsley, G. R., Procedure for serum protein determinations. *Stand. Methods Clin. Chem.* **7,** 199–207 (1972).
9. Doumas, B. T., and Biggs, H. G., Determination of serum albumin. *Stand. Methods Clin. Chem.* **7,** 175 (1972).
10. Webster, D., Study of the interaction of bromocresol green with isolated serum globulin fractions. *Clin. Chim. Acta* **53,** 109–115 (1974).
11. Webster, D., The immediate reaction between bromocresol green and serum as a measure of albumin content. *Clin. Chem.* **32,** 663–665 (1977).
12. Mancini, G., Carbonara, A. O., and Heremans, J. F., Immunochemical quantitation of antigens by single radial immunodiffusion. *Int. J. Immunochem.* **2,** 235–254 (1965).
13. Kusnetz, J., and Monsberg, H. P., Optical considerations: Nephelometry. In *Automated Immunoanalysis,* R. F. Ritchie, Ed. Marcel Dekker, New York, NY, 1978, pp 1–44.
14. Buffone, G. J., Savory, J., and Hermans, J., Evaluation of kinetic light scattering as an approach to the measurement of specific proteins with the centrifugal analyzer. II. Theoretical considerations. *Clin. Chem.* **21,** 1735–1746 (1975).
15. Wisdom, B. G., Enzyme immunoassay. *Clin. Chem.* **22,** 1243–1255 (1976).
16. Curry, R. E., Heitzman, H., Riege, D. H., Sweet, R. V., and Simonsen, M. G., A systems approach to fluorescent immunoassays: General principles and representative applications. *Clin. Chem.* **25,** 1591–1595 (1979).
17. Zettner, A., Principles of competitive binding assays (saturation analyses). I. Equilibrium techniques. *Clin. Chem.* **19,** 699–705 (1973).
18. Zettner, A., and Duly, P. E., Principles of competitive binding assays (saturation analyses) II. Sequential saturation. *Clin. Chem.* **20,** 5–14 (1974).
19. Whitehead, T. P., Kricka, L. J., Cater, T. J. N., and Thorpe, G. H. G., Analytical luminescence: Its potential in the clinical laboratory. *Clin. Chem.* **25,** 1531–1546 (1979).
20. Buffone, G. B., and Lewis, S. A., Effect of analytical factors on immunochemical reference limits for complement component C3 in serum of a pediatric reference population. *Clin. Chem.* **23,** 994–999 (1977).
21. Buffone, G. B., Brett, E. M., Lewis, S. A., Iosefsohn, M., and Hicks, J. M., Limitations of immunochemical measurement of ceruloplasmin. *Clin. Chem.* **25,** 749–751 (1979).
22. Killingsworth, L. M., A report format for serum proteins. *Clin. Chem.* **24,** 728–729 (1978).
23. Blom, M., and Hjørne, N., Profile analysis of blood proteins with a centrifugal analyzer. *Clin. Chem.* **22,** 657–662 (1976).
24. Ritchie, R. F., What abnormal serum proteins may indicate. *Patient Care* 67–73 (May 15, 1974).
25. Beathard, G. A., Albumin abnormalities. In *Serum Protein Abnormalities* (see ref. *3*), pp 173–211.
26. Morse, J. D., Alpha₁-antitrypsin deficiency I. *N. Engl. J. Med.* **299,** 1045–1048 (1978).
27. Morse, J. D., Alpha₁-antitrypsin deficiency II. *N. Engl. J. Med.* **299,** 1099–1105 (1978).
28. Ruoslahti, E., and Sappala, M., Normal and increased alpha-fetoprotein in neoplastic and non-neoplastic liver disease. *Lancet* **i,** 228–279 (1972).
29. Purves, L. R., Branch, W. A., and Boes, F. G. M., Alpha-fetoprotein as a diagnostic aid. *Lancet* **i,** 1007 (1973).
30. Allen, L. D., Ferguson-Smith, M. A., Donald, I., Sweet, E. M., and Gibson, A. A. M., Amniotic fluid alpha-fetoprotein in the antenatal diagnosis of spina bifida. *Lancet* **ii,** 522–525 (1973).

31. Whicher, J. T., The value of complement assays in clinical chemistry. *Clin. Chem.* **24,** 7–22 (1978).

32. Firsheim, S. I., Hoper, L. W., Lazarchick, J., Forget, B. G., Hobbins, J. C., Clyne, L. P., Pitlick, F. A., Muir, W. A., Merkatz, I. R., and Mahoney, M. J., Prenatal diagnosis of classic hemophilia. *N. Engl. J. Med.* **300,** 937–940 (1979).

33. Zimmerman, T. S., Ratnoff, O. D., and Littell, A. S., Detection of carriers of classic hemophilia using an immunologic assay for antihemophilic factor (Factor VIII). *J. Clin. Invest.* **50,** 255–258 (1971).

34. Owen, C. A., Bowie, E. J. W., and Thompson, J. H., *The Diagnosis of Bleeding Disorders.* Little Brown and Co., Boston, MA, 1975, pp 369–380.

35. Hobbs, J. R., Immunoglobulins in clinical chemistry. *Adv. Clin. Chem.* **14,** 220–317 (1971).

36. Kjellman, N.-I. M., Predictive value of high IgE levels in children. *Acta Paediatr. Scand.* **65,** 465–471 (1976).

37. Kraus, H. F., Clausen, C. R., and Ray, C. G., Elevated immunoglobulin E in infantile polyarteritis nodosa. *J. Pediatr.* **84,** 841–845 (1974).

38. Homburger, H. A., The diagnostic usefulness of specific IgE antibody measurements. *Mayo Clin. Proc.* **53,** 459–462 (1978).

Appendix 1. Blood Volume

Specimen Tested:

P, B.

Laboratory Reporting:

1.

Reference (Normal) Values:

Premature: 98 mL/kg of body weight
1 yr: 86 (69–112)
Older child: 70 (51–86)

Sources of Reference (Normal) Values:

Text ref. *1*, p 988; Campbell, T. J., Frohman, B., and Reeve, E. B., A simple rapid and accurate method of extracting T-1824 from plasma, adapted to the routine measurement of blood volume. *J. Lab. Clin. Med.* **52,** 768 (1958).

Specimen Volume and Collection:

1.0 mL; venous.

Analytical Method:

Text ref. *2*, p 73; Brown Co. column with Solka Floc SW-40A.

Instrumentation:

Gilford Model 300-N or Beckman Model 25 spectrophotometer.

Commentary—S. Meites

Blood volume is not generally determined in the laboratories reporting here. On a weight basis, the low-birth-weight infant has a relatively high blood volume, 108 mL/kg of body weight, compared with the full-term newborn, 85 mL/kg. The volume at birth is influenced by transfer of blood from the placenta to the infant during labor and delivery *(1–3)*. In the newborn period the total blood volume may be about 8.0% of body weight, decreasing to about 7.5% in infants and young children. The total blood volume of children younger than one year has a mean of 80 and a range of 55–116 mL/kg *(4)*. For references to analytical methods see text ref. *9*, pp 246–264, and text ref. *3*, pp 179–182.

1. Schulman, I., The blood and blood forming organs. In text ref. *12*, p 1157.
2. Sinclair, J. C., Low-birth-weight infant. In text ref. *12*, p 96.
3. Shock, N. W., Physiological growth. In text ref. *10*, pp 151–152.
4. Text ref. *8*, pp 594–595.

Appendix 2. Daily Excretion of Urine

Specimen Tested:
U.

Laboratory Reporting:
1.

Reference (Normal) Values:

Age	Volume, mL/d
Full-term newborn, 1–2 d	15–60
2 mo	250–450
6–8 mo	400–500
1–2 yr	500–600
2–4 yr	600–750
5–7 yr	650–1000
8–15 yr	700–1500
Adult	1000–1600

Sources of Reference (Normal) Values:

Ross Laboratories, *Children Are Different,* 1st ed., Columbus, OH, 1972, p 25.

Appendix 3. Most Frequently Prescribed Drugs in a Children's Hospital[1]

* Acetaminophen
Acetazolamide (Diamox)
Allopurinol
Aminophylline
* Ampicillin
Ascorbic acid
* Aspirin
Calcium gluconate
Carbamazepine (Tegretol)
Carbenicillin disodium
Cefazolin sodium
Cephalexin
Chlorthiazide
* Dexamethasone
Diazepam (Valium)
Digoxin
Dioctyl sodium sulfosuccinate
Ferrous sulfate
* Furosemide (Lasix)
* Gentamicin sulfate
Guaifenesin (Glyceryl guaiacolate)
Hydroxyzine HCl
I. V. fat (Intralipid, 10%)

Metaproterinol sulfate
Methanenamine mandelate
Nafcillin sodium
* Penicillin G
Penicillin V
* Phenobarbital
Phenytoin (Dilantin)
Potassium chloride
Prednisone
Promethazine
Propoxyphene (Darvon)
Propranolol HCl
Sulfadiazine
Sulfamethoxazole/trimethoprim (SMX–TMP)
Sulfisoxazole (Gantrisin)
* Theophylline
Theophylline/guaifenesin (Quibron)
Trimethobenzamide HCl (Tigan)
Triprolidine HCl/pseudoephedrine HCl (Actifed)
Valproic acid (Depakene)
Vitamin E

---

[1] From the computerized dispensing records for 1978, Pharmacy Department, Children's Hospital, Columbus, OH; Thomas F. Hipple, R. Ph., Director. The nine most frequently prescribed drugs are marked with an *.

Appendix 4. General Comments on Leukocyte Preparation

Derek A. Applegarth

There are two excellent articles on the assay of lysosomal enzymes in leukocytes *(1,2)*, the first discussing the use of the fluorometric 4-methylumbelliferyl substrates and the latter the use of radioactively labeled natural substrates. The articles contain much useful assay information and some comments on the isolation techniques for leukocytes. The isolation technique involves differential sedimentation of whole blood with a dextran (polyglucose) polymer. The leukocyte-enriched plasma is removed and centrifuged, and the leukocytes are isolated by exposure to hypotonic, then hypertonic, saline to lyse the residual erythrocytes. These techniques usually yield cell populations that are mixtures of granulocytes, lymphocytes, and residual erythrocytes. Because each technique may yield different populations of these cells, each laboratory embarking on the investigation of lysosomal enzymes in leukocytes must establish its own reference values.

Variability in assay results may arise from the technique by which enzymes are solubilized from the lysosome of the cell, e.g., by *(a)* the use of a detergent such as Triton X-100, *(b)* the use of several cycles of freezing and thawing, *(c)* the use of ultra-sound to fracture the cells, or *(d)* combinations of the above.

Most of the lysosomal enzymes so solubilized are present in the supernate of a centrifuged, lysed leukocyte preparation. However, some of the enzymes are membrane-bound, e.g., β-glucosidase (the enzyme involved in Gaucher's disease) and galactosylceramide β-galactosidase (the enzyme involved in Krabbe's disease), so each laboratory must determine whether it is to analyze enzymes by using the total lysate or only a supernate. The results quoted in the text are obtained on sonicated preparations from the supernatant fraction of the cell lysate, centrifuged at between 1000 and 1500 $\times$ g. The protein used as a basis for the specific activity is also determined on the supernate of the lysate.

Blood samples are not especially stable, and the values quoted have been obtained from blood kept in ice water for no longer than 2 h before leukocyte isolation. Individual enzyme values may change during storage, and variable results may be obtained from a leukocyte preparation obtained from blood that has been stored at 4 °C overnight, or at ambient temperature when a sample is mailed to the laboratory. Unlysed pellets of leukocytes, stored frozen, appear to be stable for several days at -20 or -70 °C. Each laboratory must establish storage conditions for the enzymes assayed.

Representative enzymes are quoted, but as many as 15 enzymes may be analyzed. Let me stress, however, that the diagnosis of lysosomal enzyme diseases should not be undertaken lightly; it should be attempted only after much experience has been gained with the enzyme chosen for analysis.

In my laboratory we prefer to check for the presence of a particular disease by first using a leukocyte lysosomal enzyme assay. Because the lysosomal enzyme assays are diagnostic tests, it is desirable to perform some clinical screening before specific enzyme assays are considered. In general, the diagnosis should be confirmed by measurement of the enzymes in cultured skin fibroblasts. The cost of lysosomal enzyme testing in fibroblasts is very high, which is the main reason that assays of leukocyte enzymes are preferred in the initial attempt to make a diagnosis.

With all lysosomal enzyme diseases, the detection of carriers through leukocyte enzyme assays is not certain. Clearly, before embarking on carrier studies of members of a family, one must be certain to assess the activities of the particular enzyme in the mother and father of the affected child. Apparently, carrier detection is possible in some families, but not in others *(3)*. Use of ratios of activity of a particular lysosomal enzyme to one of the other enzymes quoted may be of help in assessing carrier status.

Arylsulphatase A. This enzyme is measured to diagnose metachromatic leukodystrophy. There are at least two soluble arylsulphatases (aryl sulfate sulfohydrolases, EC 3.1.6.1) in mammalian tissues: arylsulphatase A and arylsulphatase B. Both arylsulphatases may be determined by using *p*-nitrocatechol sulfate; to measure arylsulphatase A by this method, arylsulphatase B is inhibited by chloride ions. Because the reaction product, *p*-nitrocatechol, is unstable, the timing of the absorbance reading is critical: stopwatch accuracy is necessary. Normal values (see p 115) do not vary with age.

α-Galactosidase. This enzyme is deficient in Fabry's disease, an X-linked disease. Variable results may be expected in mothers and affected members of the family in whom this disease is suspected, presumably because of variable lyonization, which makes carrier detection in this disease even more difficult. The normal values quoted (see p 206) are for adults (for use in carrier detection). Preliminary studies indicate that the normal range for children may be as much as twice as high as for adults.

β-Galactosidase. This enzyme is used to diagnose generalized (GM_1) gangliosidosis. Normal values (p 206) do not vary with age.

α-Mannosidase. This enzyme is used to diagnose the disease known as mannosidosis. Normal values (see p 320) do not vary with age.

1. Kolodny, E. H., and Mumford, R. A., Human leucocyte acid hydrolases: Characterization of 11 lysosomal enzymes and study of reaction conditions for their automated analysis. *Clin. Chim. Acta* **70**, 247–257 (1976).
2. Svennerholm, L., Hakansson, G., Mansson, J. E., and Vanier, M. T., The assay of sphingolipid hydrolases in white blood cells with labelled natural substrates. *Clin. Chim. Acta* **92,** 53–64 (1979).
3. Lott, I. T., Dulaney, J. T., Milunsky, A., Hoefnagel, D., and Moser, H. W., Apparent biochemical homozygosity in 2 obligatory heterozygotes for metachromatic leukodystrophy. *J. Pediatr.* **89,** 438–440 (1976).

Appendix 5. Directory of Manufacturers Cited

Abbott Laboratories, Suite 101, 4757 Irving Blvd., Dallas, TX 75247.

American Can Co. (Parafilm M), American Lane, Greenwich, CT 06830.

American Instrument Co. (Aminco), Div. of Travenol Labs., Inc., 8030 Georgia Ave., Silver Spring, MD 20910.

American Monitor Corp., 5425 W. 84th St., P.O. Box 68505, Indianapolis, IN 46268.

American Optical Corp., Eggert Rd., Buffalo, NY 14215.

Amersham Corp, 2636 S. Clearbrook Dr., Arlington Heights, IL 60005.

Ames Division, Miles Labs., Inc., P.O. Box 70, Elkhart, IN 46515.

Amicon Corp., 21 Hartwell Ave., Lexington, MA 02173.

Applied Science Labs, P.O. Box 440, State College, PA 16801.

Atlantic Antibodies, Anderson Rd., Westbrook, ME 04092.

Baltimore Biological Labs. (BBL), Div. of Becton, Dickinson and Co., P.O. Box 243, Cockeysville, MD 21030.

Bausch & Lomb, Analytic Systems, 820 Linden Ave., Rochester, NY 14625.

Beckman Instruments, Inc., Clinical Instruments Div., 2500 Harbor Blvd., Fullerton, CA 92634.

Becton-Dickinson, Rutherford, NJ 07070.

Bio-Dynamics/bmc, 9115 Hague Rd., Indianapolis, IN 46250.

Bio-Rad Laboratories, 2200 Wright Ave., Richmond, CA 94804.

Bio-Science Laboratories, Inc., 7600 Tyrone Ave., Van Nuys, CA 91405.

Brown Co., Boston, MA.

Buchler Instruments, Inc., 1327 16th St., Fort Lee, NJ 07024.

Burroughs-Wellcome Co., Wellcome Reagents Div., 3030 Cornwallis Rd., Research Triangle Park, NC 27709.

Calbiochem-Behring Corp., 10933 N. Torrey Pines Rd., LaJolla, CA 92037.

Cary spectrophotometer (*see* Varian Instruments).

Clinical Assays, 620 Memorial Dr., Cambridge, MA 02139.

Chattanooga Pharmacal Co., Chattanooga, TN.

Coleman Instruments, 2000 York Rd., Oak Brook, IL 60521.

Consolidated Biomedical Labs, P.O. Box 2289, Columbus, OH.

Corning Medical, Medfield, MA 02052.

Corning Glass Works, Science Products Division, Corning, NY 14830.

Coulter Electronics, Inc., 600 W. 20th St., Hialeah, FL 33010.

Dade, Division American Hospital Supply Corp., P.O. Box 520672, Miami, FL 33152.

Damon Diagnostics, IEC Div., 115 Fourth Ave., Needham Heights, MA 02194.

Dow Diagnostics, The Dow Chemical Co., P.O. Box 68511, Indianapolis, IN 46268.

DuPont Co., Clinical Systems, Wilmington, DE 19898.

Durrum Instrument Corp., 1228 Titan Way, Sunnyvale, CA 94086.

Dynamed Corp., Elmsford, NY 10523.

Eberbach Corp., P.O. Box 1024, Ann Arbor, MI 48106.

Electro-Nucleonics, Inc., 386 Passaic Ave., Fairfield, NJ 07006.

Electro-Nucleonics Laboratories, Inc., Virgo Reagents, 4809 Auburn Ave., Bethesda, MD 20014.

Endocrine Sciences, 18418 Oxnard St., Tarzana, CA 91356.

Environmental Science Associates, 45 Wiggins Ave., Bedford, MA 02170.

Eppendorf Division, Brinkmann Instruments Inc., Cantiague Rd., Westbury, NY 11590.

Farrall Instrument Co., P.O. Box 1037, Grand Island, NE 68801.

Farrand Optical Co., Inc., 117 Wall St., Valhalla, NY 10595.

Fisher Scientific Co., 711 Forbes Ave., Pittsburgh, PA 15219.

Fiske Associates, Science Park, 134 Wheeler Rd., Burlington, MA 01803.

Gelman Instrument Co., 600 S. Wagner Rd., Ann Arbor, MI 48106.

General Diagnostics, Division of Warner-Lambert Co., 201 Tabor Rd., Morris Plains, NJ 07950.

Gilford Instrument Laboratories, Inc., 132 Artino St., Oberlin, OH 44074.

Greiner, Gasswerkstrasse 33, CH-4900, Langenthal, Switzerland.

Hach Chemical Co., P.O. Box 907, Ames, IA 50010.

Harleco, 60th and Woodland Ave., Philadelphia, PA 19143.

Helena Laboratories, P.O. Box 852, Beaumont, TX 77704.

Hitachi Scientific Instruments, 2672 Bayshore Frontage Rd., Mountain View, CA 94040.

Holland-Rantos Co., Inc., Piscataway, NJ 08854.

Honeywell Clinical Instruments, P.O. Box 5227, Denver, CO 80217.

Hospital Supply Corp., Piscataway, NJ 08854.

Hycel, Inc., 7920 Westpark, Houston, TX 77042.

Hyland Diagnostics, Div. of Travenol Labs., Inc., Bannockburn Executive Plaza, 2275 Half Day Rd., Deerfield, IL 60015.

ICL Scientific, 18249 Euclid St., Fountain Valley, CA 92708.

International (IEC) Damon/IEC Div., Damon Corp, 300 2nd Ave., Needham Heights, MA 02194.

Instrumentation Laboratory, Inc., Analytical Instrument Div., Jonspin Rd., Wilmington, MA 02173.
Instrumentation Laboratory, Inc., Biomedical Div., 113 Hartwell Ave., Lexington, MA 02173.
Isolab Inc., Drawer 4350, Akron, OH 44321.

Jarrell-Ash Division, Fisher Scientific Co., 590 Lincoln St., Waltham, MA 02154.
Jena Instruments (Toronto), Ltd., 199 Ashtonbee Rd., Toronto, Ontario, M1L 2P1 Canada.
Johnson & Johnson, New Brunswick, NJ.

Kabi Diagnostica, Sweden.
Kallestad Laboratories, Inc., 1000 Lake Hazeltine Dr., Chaska, MN 55318.
Kay Laboratories, Inc., P.O. Box 81571, San Diego, CA 92138.
Kew Scientific, Inc., 3824 April Lane, Columbus, OH 43227.

LKB Instruments, Inc., 12221 Parklawn Dr., Rockville, MD 20852.
The London Co., Radiometer Instruments, 811 Sharon Dr., Cleveland, OH 44145.

Mallinckrodt, Inc., Diagnostic Products Div., P.O. Box 5840, St. Louis, MO 63134.
Marine Colloids Division, FMC, P.O. Box 308, Rockland, ME 04841.
MED PAC Corp., Charleston, WV.
Meloy Labs, Diagnostics Division, 6715 Electronic Dr., Springfield, VA 22151.
Micromedic System, 102 Witmer Rd., Horsham, PA 19044.
Milton Roy Co., 5000 Park St. N, P.O. Box 12169, St. Petersburg, FL 33733.

New England Nuclear, 549 Albany St., Boston, MA 02118.
Nichols Institute Diagnostics, 1300 S. Beacon St., San Pedro, CA 90731.
Nuclear Chicago (*see* Searle Analytic, Inc.).

Organon Diagnostics, West Orange, NJ 07052.
Orion Research, Inc., 380 Putnam Ave., Cambridge, MA 02139.
Ortho Diagnostics, Inc., Raritan, NJ 08869.
Oxford Laboratories, 1149 Chess Dr., Foster City, CA 94404.

Packard (Hewlett-Packard) Instrument Co., 2200 Warrenville Rd., Downers Grove, IL 60515.
Perkin-Elmer Corp., Main Ave., Norwalk, CT 06856.
Pharmacia Diagnostics, Division of Pharmacia Inc., 800 Centennial Ave., Piscataway, NJ 08854.
Pierce Chemical Co., P.O. Box 117, Rockford, IL 61105.
Precision Assays, Swindon, Wiltshire, England.

Precision Systems, Inc., 60 Union Ave., Sudbury, MA 01776.
Princeton Biomedix, P.O. Box 2241, Princeton, NJ 08540.

Radiometer (*see* The London Co).
Ross Laboratories, Division of Abbott Labs. (USA), 625 Cleveland Ave., Columbus, OH 43216.

Schleicher & Schuell, Inc., 543 Washington St., Keene, NH 03431.
Scientific Industries, Inc., 70 Orville Dr., Airport International Plaza, Bohemia, NY 11716.
Scientific Products, 1210 Waukegan Rd., McGaw Park, IL 60085.
Searle Analytic, Inc., 2000 Nuclear Dr., Des Plaines, IL 60018.
Serono Laboratories, Inc., 11 Brooks Dr., Braintree, MA 02184.
Shandon Southern Instruments, Inc., 515 Broad St., Sewickley, PA 15143.
Sherwood Medical Industries, Inc., 1831 Olive St., St. Louis, MO 63103.
Sigma Chemical Co., P.O. Box 14508, St. Louis, MO 63178.
SmithKline Instruments, Inc. (SKI), P.O. Box 1947, Sunnyvale, CA 94086.
Sorvall (DuPont Instruments-Sorvall Biomedical Div.) DuPont Co., Pecks Lane, Newton, CT 06470.
Spectra Physics, Autolab Division, 2905 Spender Way, Santa Clara, CA 95051.
Standard Scientific, 385 Conners Lane, Hebron, KY 41048.
Syva Co., 3181 Porter Dr., Palo Alto, CA 94304.

Technicon Instrument Corp., 511 Benedict Ave., Tarrytown, NY 10591.
Turner Associates, 2524 Pulgas Ave., Palo Alto, CA 94304.

Union Carbide Corp., Med. Products Div., Clinical Diagnostics, 401 Theodore Fremd Ave., Rye, NY 10580.

Varian Instruments, 611 Hansen Way, Palo Alto, CA 94304.

Wang Laboratories, Inc., One Industrial Ave., Lowell, MA 01851.
Waters Associates, Inc., 34 Maple St., Milford, MA 01757.
Wescor, Inc., 459 S. Main St., Logan, UT 84321.
West Chemical Products, Inc., New York, NY.
Whitehall Laboratories, Ltd., Toronto, Canada.
Worthington Diagnostics, Division of Millipore Corp., Halls Mill Rd., Freehold, NJ 97728

Yang Laboratory, 13240 Northrup Way, Bellevue, WA 98005.
Yellow Springs Instrument Co., Box 279, Yellow Springs, OH 45387.

Carl Zeiss, Inc., 444 Fifth Ave., New York, NY 10018.

Appendix 6. Text References

1. O'Brien, D., and Rodgerson, D. O., Interpretation of biochemical values. In text ref. *16*, pp 970–994.
2. O'Brien, D., Ibbott, F. A., and Rodgerson, D. O., *Laboratory Manual of Pediatric Micro-Biochemical Techniques*, 4th ed. Hoeber, Hagerstown, MD, 1968.
3. Natelson, S., *Techniques of Clinical Chemistry*, 3rd ed. Charles C Thomas, Springfield, IL, 1971.
4. Henry, R. J., Cannon, D. C., and Winkelman, J. W., *Clinical Chemistry, Principles and Technics*, 2nd ed., 1974; 1st ed., 1964; Harper and Row, Hagerstown, MD.
5. Tietz, N. W., *Fundamentals of Clinical Chemistry*. W. B. Saunders, Philadelphia, PA, 1970 (2nd ed., 1976).
6. *Endocrine and Genetic Diseases of Childhood*, L. I. Gardner, Ed. W. B. Saunders, Philadelphia, PA, 1969.
7. *Metabolic, Endocrine and Genetic Disorders of Children*, Vols. 1–3, V. C. Kelley, Ed. Hoeber, Hagerstown, MD, 1974.
8. Wolman, I. J., *Laboratory Applications in Clinical Pediatrics*. McGraw-Hill, New York, NY, 1957.
9. Behrendt, H., *Diagnostic Tests in Infants and Children*, 2nd ed. Lea and Febiger, Philadelphia, PA, 1962.
10. *Human Development*, F. Faulkner, Ed. W. B. Saunders, Philadelphia, PA, 1966.
11. *The Metabolic Basis of Inherited Disease*, J. B. Stanbury, J. B. Wyngaarden, and D. S. Frederickson, Eds., 3rd ed. McGraw-Hill, New York, NY, 1972 (4th ed., 1978).
12. *Pediatrics*, 15th ed., H. L. Barnett and A. H. Einhorn, Eds. Appleton-Century-Crofts, New York, NY, 1972.
13. Hsia, D. Y.-Y., *Inborn Errors of Metabolism*, Part 1, 2nd ed. Yearbook Medical Publishers, Chicago, IL, 1966.
14. Hsia, D. Y.-Y., *Inborn Errors of Metabolism*, Part 2. Yearbook Medical Publishers, Chicago, IL, 1966.
15. *Duncan's Diseases of Metabolism*, P. K. Bondy and L. E. Rosenberg, Eds. W. B. Saunders, Philadelphia, PA, 1974.
16. Kempe, C. H., Silver, H. K., and O'Brien, D., *Current Pediatric Diagnosis and Treatment*, 3rd ed. Lange Medical Publications, Los Altos, CA, 1974.
17. *Nelson—Textbook of Pediatrics*, 10th ed., V. C. Vaughan III, R. J. McKay, Jr., and W. E. Nelson, Eds. W. B. Saunders, Philadelphia, PA, 1975 (11th ed., 1979; with R. E. Behrman).
18. Davidsohn, I., and Henry, J. B., *Clinical Diagnosis by Laboratory Methods*, 15th ed. W. B. Saunders, Philadelphia, PA, 1974 (16th ed., 1979).

Appendix 7. Author Index

Faulkner, W. R., 23, 317, 337, 349
Fayle, S. A., 193
Feigl, P., 138
Feldman, H., 239
Felsher, B. F., 92
Felton, H., 120, 169, 170, 231, 305, 306
Fenner, A., 174
Fenton, G., 373
Fenton, L. J., 25
Fenwick, P., 373
Ferguson-Smith, M. A., 476
Fernandez, F. J., 308
Fernandez, L., 193
Fessard, C., 345
Ficke, M., 299
Field, J. B., 100, 234
Fiereck, E. A., 313
Fies, H. L., 23
Figarella, C., 464
Filer, L. J., Jr., 126
Finch, C. A., 362, 365
Fincham, R. W., 142, 372
Findley, T. P., 56
Finegold, S. M., 145
Fingerhut, B., 424
Fink, D. J., 245
Finklea, J. F., 123
Finklestein, J. W., 243
Finley, P. R., 326
Firsheim, S. I., 477
Fischer, D. S., 293
Fischer, E., 25
Fishberg, E. H., 300
Fisher, D. A., 101, 103, 104, 108, 375, 404, 405, 406, 407, 408, 409, 414, 415, 469, 470
Fisher, D. S., 108
Fisher, J., 233
Fishman, W. H., 72, 79, 464
Fiske, C. H., 11, 359
Flachs, H., 432
Fleisher, G. A., 77, 79, 230
Fleming, L. W., 317
Flegg, H. M., 149
Flor, R., 302
Flor, R. V., 70
Flores, J., 364
Flueck, J., 344
Flynn, D. M., 24
Fogg, B. A., 77
Foley, B., 406, 408, 415
Foley, T. P., 408, 469, 470

Folin, O., 98
Follenius, M., 165
Fölling, A., 11, 350
Fomon, S., 126
Forbes, A. E., 243
Forbes, G. B., 177
Ford, S. H., 25, 251
Foreman, J. A., 99
Forest, M. G., 102, 103, 104, 165, 179, 181, 273, 274, 275, 398, 399
Forfar, J. O., 12
Forget, B. G., 477
Forman, D. T., 11, 23, 95
Fornaini, G., 201
Forsling, M. L., 108
Forster, B., 129
Forster, G., 169
Forstner, G. G., 463
Førte, O. H., 265
Foster, L. B., 163
Foti, A. G., 55
Fowler, K., 244
Fracassini, F., 288
Frand, M., 189
Frankel, S., 377
Frankenfeld, J. K., 77
Franklin, F. A., Jr., 381, 474
Franks, R. C., 167
Frantz, A. G., 108, 243, 376
Fraser, R., 68
Frasier, S. D., 241, 243
Frasier, S. E., 240
Frazier, T. M., 123
Freda, V. J., 457
Frederick, E. W., 339
Frederickson, D. S., 11, 77, 316, 413, 489
Free, A. H., 46
Free, H. M., 46
Freeman, J. M., 139
Freer, D. E., 120, 169, 170, 231, 305, 306, 457
Frenkel, L. D., 42
Frerichs, R. R., 151
Friedewald, W. T., 316
Friedland, M., 267
Friedman, G., 299
Friedman, H., 161
Friedman, M., 319
Friedman, M. A., 135, 319
Friedman, R. B., 331
Friedman, S., 213, 258
Friedman, Z., 405
Friel, P., 138

Friesen, H., 375
Friesen, H. G., 179, 375
Frigerio, A., 138
Friis-Hansen, B., 50, 126
Frohman, B., 479
Fronk, S., 437
Fu, P. C., 148
Fuchs, C., 317
Fukanoga, K., 335, 336
Fukishima, K., 273
Fukuchi, M., 243
Fukushima, D. K., 182
Funkenstein, B., 129
Furlanetto, R. W., 391, 392
Furman, M., 122
Fyfe, W. H., 437

Gabbay, K. H., 234, 235, 237
Gabreëls, F. J. M., 432
Gabriel, M., 25
Gabrilove, J. L., 68
Gaburro, D., 158, 464
Gaines, J., 25
Gal, E. M., 153
Galambos, J. T., 328, 331
Galen, R. S., 303
Gall, E. P., 159
Gallagher, B. B., 372
Gallop, P. M., 234, 237
Gambino, S. R., 24, 25, 48, 122, 228, 230
Gamstorp, I., 355
Gandy, G., 24
Ganguly, A., 68
Gant, P. W., 299
Ganten, D., 68
Gantz, M., 332
Garby, L., 256
Garcia, J. C., 211
Garcia, R., 140
Garcia-Bulnes, G., 407
Gardner, L. I., 489
Gardner-Thorpe, C., 348, 355
Garfield-Davies, D., 211
Garg, A. K., 24
Garland, P. B., 412
Garle, M., 356
Garnier, P. E., 238
Garrod, A. E., 12
Garrow, E., 23
Garry, P. J., 152
Gartner, L., 122

Appendix 8. Subject Index